**FOURTH EDITION**

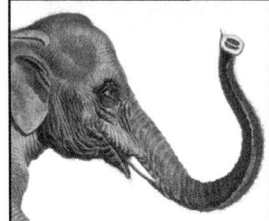

# APPLETON & LANGE
# OUTLINE REVIEW

# USMLE STEP 3

Joel S. Goldberg, DO
Assistant Professor of Medicine
Department of Medicine
Drexel University College of Medicine
Philadelphia, Pennsylvania

Appleton & Lange Reviews/McGraw-Hill
Medical Publishing Division

New York   Chicago   San Francisco   Lisbon   London   Madrid
Mexico City   Milan   New Delhi   San Juan   Seoul
Singapore   Sydney   Toronto

*The McGraw-Hill Companies*

**Appleton & Lange Outline Review for the USMLE Step 3, Fourth Edition**

Copyright © 2004 by The **McGraw-Hill** Companies, Inc. All rights reserved. Printed in the United States of America. Except as permitted under the United States Copyright Act of 1976, no part of this publication may be reproduced or distributed in any form or by any means, or stored in a data base or retrieval system, without the prior written permission of the publisher.

Previous editions copyright © 2001 by The McGraw-Hill Companies, Inc.; copyright © 1997, 1995 by Appleton & Lange

---

**Notice**

Medicine is an ever-changing science. As new research and clinical experience broaden our knowledge, changes in treatment and drug therapy are required. The authors and the publisher of this work have checked with sources believed to be reliable in their efforts to provide information that is complete and generally in accord with the standards accepted at the time of publication. However, in view of the possibility of human error or changes in medical sciences, neither the authors nor the publisher nor any other party who has been involved in the preparation or publication of this work warrants that the information contained herein is in every respect accurate or complete, and they disclaim all responsibility for any errors or omissions or for the results obtained from use of the information contained in this work. Readers are encouraged to confirm the information contained herein with other sources. For example and in particular, readers are advised to check the product information sheet included in the package of each drug they plan to administer to be certain that the information contained in this work is accurate and that changes have not been made in the recommended dose or in the contraindications for administration. This recommendation is of particular importance in connection with new or infrequently used drugs.

---

1 2 3 4 5 6 7 8 9 0 CUS/CUS 0 9 8 7 6 5 4 3

ISBN: 0-07-139019-7

The editor was Catherine A. Johnson.
The production supervisor was Richard Ruzycka.
Project Management was provided by Rainbow Graphics.
The index was prepared by Oneida Indexing.
Von Hoffmann Graphics was the printer and binder

This book is printed on acid-free paper.

**Library of Congress Cataloging-in-Publication Data**
    Appleton & Lange outline review for the USMLE step 3 / Joel S. Goldberg—4th ed.
      p. ; cm.
      Rev. ed. of: Appleton & Lange's outline review for the USMLE step 3. 3rd ed. © 2001.
      Includes bibliographical references and index.
      ISBN 0-07-139019-7 (alk. paper)
      1. Medicine—Examinations, questions, etc.  2. Medicine—Outlines, syllabi, etc.  I. Title: Appleton and Lange outline review for the USMLE step 3.  II. Title: Outline review for the USMLE step 3.  III. Goldberg, Joel S.  IV. Appleton & Lange's outline review for the USMLE step 3.  IV. Title.
      [DNLM: 1. Medicine—Examination Questions. 2. Medicine—Outlines. W 18.2 A6485 2003]
R834.5.115  2003
610'.76—dc21
                                                        2003044508

*For Mickey, Dan, and Kasey*

# Contents

*Contributors / vii*
*Preface / xi*
*Acknowledgments / xiii*
*How to Use This Book / xv*

1. CARDIOVASCULAR MEDICINE / 1
2. DERMATOLOGY / 45
3. ENDOCRINOLOGY / 87
4. DISEASES AND DISORDERS OF THE DIGESTIVE SYSTEM / 107
5. HEMATOLOGY AND ONCOLOGY / 167
6. IMMUNOLOGY AND ALLERGY / 197
7. INJURIES, WOUNDS, TOXICOLOGY, AND BURNS / 215
8. INFECTIOUS DISEASE / 247
9. MUSCULOSKELETAL AND CONNECTIVE TISSUE DISEASE / 269
10. NEUROLOGY / 301
11. MALE AND FEMALE REPRODUCTION / 339
12. OBSTETRICS / 363
13. OPHTHALMOLOGY / 391
14. PEDIATRICS / 419
15. PSYCHIATRY / 451
16. PULMONARY MEDICINE / 491
17. DISEASES OF THE RENAL AND UROLOGIC SYSTEMS / 527
18. SURGICAL PRINCIPLES / 561

19. ILL-DEFINED SYMPTOM COMPLEX / 621
20. OTOLARYNGOLOGY AND RESPIRATORY SYSTEM DISEASES / 645

*Index / 671*

# Contributors

**Monica Awsare, MD**
Resident
Department of Internal Medicine
Thomas Jefferson University Hospital
Philadelphia, Pennsylvania
*Chapter 19, "Ill-Defined Symptom Complex"*

**Siamak Barkhordarian, MD**
Vascular Fellow
Section of Vascular Surgery
Department of Surgery
Yale University School of Medicine
New Haven, Connecticut
*Chapter 18, "Surgical Principles"*

**Amy C. Brodkey, MD**
Clinical Associate Professor
Department of Psychiatry
University of Pennsylvania School of Medicine
Philadelphia, Pennsylvania
*Chapter 15, "Psychiatry"*

**Maria P. Childers, MD**
Instructor
Department of Pediatrics
Jefferson Medical College of Thomas Jefferson University
Philadelphia, Pennsylvania
*Chapter 14, "Pediatrics"*

**Christina M. Clay, MD**
Clinical Instructor
Department of Medicine
Jefferson Medical College of Thomas Jefferson University
Philadelphia, Pennsylvania
*Chapter 5, "Hematology"*
*Chapter 19, "Ill-Defined Symptom Complex"*

**Robert V. DeSilverio Jr., MD**
Resident
Department of Dermatology
Drexel University College of Medicine
Philadelphia, Pennsylvania
*Chapter 2, "Dermatology"*

**Thomas Fekete, MD**
Professor of Medicine
Section of Infectious Diseases
Departments of Internal Medicine and Microbiology
Temple University School of Medicine
Philadelphia, Pennsylvania
*Chapter 8, "Infectious Disease"*

**Jeffrey M. Finkelstein, MD, DMD, FACS**
Assistant Professor
Department of Otolaryngology and Bronchoesophagology
Temple University School of Medicine
Philadelphia, Pennsylvania
*Chapter 20, "Otolaryngology and Respiratory System Diseases"*

**Steven W. Fisher, MD**
Clinical Assistant Professor
Division of Surgery
Department of Otolaryngology
Temple University School of Medicine
Philadelphia, Pennsylvania
*Chapter 20, "Otolaryngology and Respiratory System Diseases"*

**Natali Franzblau, MD**
Assistant Professor
Department of Obstetrics and Gynecology
UMDNJ–Robert Wood Johnson School of Medicine
Camden, New Jersey
*Chapter 11, "Male and Female Reproduction"*
*Chapter 12, "Obstetrics"*

**Vivian Gahtan, MD**
Associate Professor
Section of Vascular Surgery
Department of Surgery
Yale University School of Medicine
New Haven, Connecticut
*Chapter 18, "Surgical Principles"*

**Jeffrey I. Greenstein, MD**
Chairman
Department of Neurology
Graduate Hospital
Philadelphia, Pennsylvania
*Chapter 10, "Neurology"*

**Victor A. Heresniak, DO**
Chairman
Department of Emergency Medicine
Crozer–Chester Medical Center
Upland, Pennsylvania
*Chapter 7, "Injuries"*

**Samuel L. Jacobs, MD**
Associate Professor and Clerkship Director
Division of Reproductive Endocrinology and Infertility
Department of Obstetrics and Gynecology
UMDNJ–Robert Wood Johnson School of Medicine
Camden, New Jersey
*Chapter 11, "Male and Female Reproduction"*
*Chapter 12, "Obstetrics"*

**Gary R. Kantor, MD**
Associate Professor of Medicine
Division of Dermatology
Department of Medicine
MCP–Hahnemann University School of Medicine
Philadelphia, Pennsylvania
*Chapter 2, "Dermatology"*

**Morris D. Kerstein, MD**
Professor and Vice Chairman
Division of General and Vascular Surgery
Department of Surgery
Mount Sinai Hospital and Medical Center
New York, New York
*Chapter 18, "Surgical Principles"*

**Margaret R. Khouri, MD, FACP**
Associate Professor of Medicine
Texas Tech University Health Science Center
Odessa, Texas
*Chapter 4, "Diseases and Disorders of the Digestive System"*

**Thomas Klein, MD**
Chief
Division of Allergy and Immunology
Delaware County Memorial Hospital
Drexel Hill, Pennsylvania
*Chapter 6, "Immunology and Allergy"*

**Joan A. Lit, MD**
Assistant Professor
Department of Family, Community and Preventative Medicine
Drexel University College of Medicine
Philadelphia, Pennsylvania
*Chapter 3, "Endocrinology"*

**S. Bruce Malkowicz, MD**
Associate Professor
Co-Director, Urology–Oncology Program
Division of Urology
University of Pennsylvania School of Medicine
Philadelphia, Pennsylvania
*Chapter 17, "Diseases of the Renal and Urologic Systems"*

**Joseph R. McClellan, MD, FACC, FACP**
Chairman
Department of Cardiovascular Medicine and Surgery
Executive Vice President and Director of Operations
Hamot Medical Center
Erie, Pennsylvania
*Chapter 1, "Cardiovascular Medicine"*

**Richard D. McDowell, MD**
Chairman
Department of Emergency Medicine
Crozer–Chester Medical Center
Upland, Pennsylvania
*Chapter 7, "Injuries, Wounds, Toxicology, and Burns"*

**Pekka A. Mooar, MD**
Associate Professor
Department of Orthopedic Surgery
Temple University School of Medicine
Philadelphia, Pennsylvania
*Chapter 9, "Musculoskeletal and Connective Tissue Disease"*

**Borislav Nikolov, MD**
Department of Neurology
Graduate Hospital
Philadelphia, Pennsylvania
*Chapter 10, "Neurology"*

**Charles A. Pohl, MD, FAAP**
Clinical Associate Professor and Associate Dean
Department of Pediatrics
Jefferson Medical College of Thomas Jefferson University
Philadelphia, Pennsylvania
*Chapter 14, "Pediatrics"*

**Ernane D. Reis, MD**
Assistant Professor
Department of Surgery
Mount Sinai School of Medicine
New York, New York
*Chapter 18, "Surgical Principles"*

**Daniel L. Ridout III, MD**
Clinical Assistant Professor
Division of Gastroenterology
Department of Medicine
Temple University School of Medicine
Philadelphia, Pennsylvania
*Chapter 4, "Diseases and Disorders of the Digestive System"*

**Andrea M. Saxon, MD**
Assistant Professor
Division of Ophthalmology
Drexel University College of Medicine
Philadelphia, Pennsylvania
*Chapter 13, "Ophthalmology"*

**Edward S. Schulman, MD**
Professor
Division of Pulmonary and Critical Care Medicine
Drexel University College of Medicine
Philadelphia, Pennsylvania
*Chapter 16, "Pulmonary Medicine"*

**Michael Sherman, MD**
Associate Professor
Division of Pulmonary and Critical Care Medicine
Drexel University College of Medicine
Philadelphia, Pennsylvania
*Chapter 16, "Pulmonary Medicine"*

**Richard L. Spielvogel, MD**
Professor and Chair
Department of Medicine
Director
Division of Dermatology
Allegheny University of the Health Sciences
Philadelphia, Pennsylvania
*Chapter 2, "Dermatology"*

**Christopher A. Williams, MD**
Chief
Department of Ophthalmology
Crozer–Chester Medical Center
Upland, Pennsylvania
*Chapter 13, "Ophthalmology"*

# Preface

The typical review book is written in a question-and-answer–type format. It has long existed as the sole product for student examinations, until now. In 1992, I formulated my concept of a rapid-reading review manual, conceived out of the tremendous need for a succinct, yet complete review text. The key component was the extensive coverage of the USMLE "high-impact" disease list, with the inclusion and incorporation of all pertinent test material. In addition, it was necessary to present this material in a concise, easily assimilated format, to allow for a swift and highly effective review.

This text, *Appleton & Lange Outline Review for USMLE Step 3,* Fourth Edition exists as a result of the tremendous popularity and widespread use of the Step 2 text, called *The Instant Exam Review for USMLE Step 2*. After the Step 2 text received extraordinary acceptance and acclaim by students and educators across the United States and abroad, I was asked by Appleton & Lange to create a new study book for the Step 3 exam. Thus, *Appleton & Lange Outline Review for USMLE Step 3!*

In this review manual, my original concept and ideals remain unchanged. Once again, the material in this book encompasses the key test facts, diseases, and disorders listed by the National Board of Medical Examiners for the new Step 3 examination. Our categories in this revised edition have changed to reflect the new examination content, with each chapter encompassing the Board's new list of diseases and disorders.

Finally, I have enlisted as contributors an exceptional group of physicians, widely renowned for their clinical and educational proficiency. These authors have completely revised this book.

Please note that this book was not designed to teach general medicine, nor was it to be a substitute for accepted methods of medical education. Like its predecessor, it was designed as a unique study tool to assist you, the student, in passing the Step 3 examination.

*Joel S. Goldberg*
*Philadelphia, Pennsylvania*

# Acknowledgments

I would like to extend my sincere appreciation to Ms. Catherine Johnson and the staff at McGraw-Hill for their assistance with this project. They were always available for counsel and support during the task of manuscript preparation, copyediting, review of page proofs, and production of bound books.

I wish to thank my coauthors for their willingness to participate in this complex endeavor and investing extensive time and effort in the construction of their chapters, despite their busy professional and personal schedules. They are a group of physicians dedicated to medicine, and their commitment to education is clear.

Finally, I would like to express my gratitude to the staff and faculty of Drexel University College of Medicine for their assistance and unselfish dedication to both the clinical practice of medicine and the education of young physicians in training.

# How to Use This Book

This book is an innovative and practical study guide designed to be used in both the initial phase of USMLE Step 3 examination preparation as a comprehensive study outline and in the final few days and hours before the exam as a quick review manual.

## USING THE BOOK AS A STUDY OUTLINE

When you begin to study, turn to the Contents to obtain an overview of this text. Review the material supplied by your school and the National Board of Medical Examiners, including the "Step 3 General Instructions, Content Description, and Sample Items." It is important to have a full understanding of the design of the exam and the type of questions that will be asked.

Once you begin to study, *do not* omit any chapters in this text, but instead start at the beginning and read the book in its entirety. Notice that the outline format is streamlined to allow the rapid assimilation of facts in a minimal amount of reading time. Because extraneous and time-consuming information and phrasing have been omitted, working with *Appleton & Lange Outline Review for the USMLE Step 3* for 1 hour will provide a database equivalent to that procured from several hours' study of any other review text. Because the text is concise, it is vital that you be well rested and in a proper frame of mind for study and concentration. A quiet, comfortable, bright study area without glare is vital (with plenty of snacks nearby, of course!).

## USING THE BOOK AS A QUICK REVIEW

In the final several weeks and days prior to your examination, *Appleton & Lange Outline Review for the USMLE Step 3* will serve as a rapid review tool. As in the Step 2 text, this revolutionary new format, which completely covers the "high-impact" fact list, will allow the handbook to be read quickly, with successful, easy assimilation of the core facts necessary for exam success.

# Cardiovascular Medicine | 1

I. **ISCHEMIC HEART DISEASE** / 3
   A. Acute / 3
   B. Chronic / 6

II. **HEART FAILURE (HF)** / 8
   A. Left-Sided / 8
   B. Right-Sided / 9

III. **HYPOTENSION AND ACUTE CIRCULATORY COLLAPSE (SHOCK)** / 10
   A. Cardiogenic Shock / 10
   B. Hypovolemic Shock / 11
   C. Obstructive Shock / 12
   D. Distributive Shock / 12

IV. **MYOCARDIAL DISEASES** / 13
   A. Dilated Cardiomyopathy / 13
   B. Hypertrophic Cardiomyopathy / 14
   C. Restrictive Cardiomyopathy / 15

V. **CARDIAC ARRHYTHMIAS** / 16
   A. Supraventricular Arrhythmias / 16
   B. Ventricular Arrhythmias / 18

VI. **PERICARDIAL DISEASES** / 20
   A. Acute Pericarditis / 20
   B. Pericardial Effusion / 20
   C. Cardiac Tamponade / 21
   D. Constrictive Pericarditis / 22

VII. **VALVULAR DISEASES** / 22
   A. Acute / 22
   B. Chronic / 24

VIII. CARDIAC TRANSPLANTATION / 25

IX. CONGENITAL HEART DISEASE / 25
    A. Ventricular Septal Defect / 25
    B. Atrial Septal Defect / 26
    C. Tetralogy of Fallot / 27
    D. Coarctation of the Aorta / 27

X. CARDIAC LIFE SUPPORT / 28

XI. HYPERTENSION / 29
    A. Essential Hypertension / 29
    B. Secondary Hypertension / 30
    C. Malignant Hypertension / 31

XII. LIPOPROTEINS AND ATHEROSCLEROSIS / 32
    A. Hyperlipoproteinemia / 32
    B. Atherosclerosis / 34

XIII. PERIPHERAL ARTERIAL VASCULAR DISEASE / 34
    A. Chronic Atherosclerotic Occlusion / 34
    B. Acute Arterial Occlusion / 35
    C. Vasculitis Syndromes / 36

XIV. PERIPHERAL VENOUS VASCULAR DISEASES AND PULMONARY EMBOLISM / 37
    A. Venous Thrombosis / 37
    B. Pulmonary Embolism / 38

XV. DISEASES OF THE AORTA / 39
    A. Aneurysms / 39
    B. Aortic Dissection / 40
    C. Aortic Occlusion / 41
    D. Aortitis / 42

**BIBLIOGRAPHY / 44**

# I. ISCHEMIC HEART DISEASE

## A. Acute

### 1. Unstable Angina

▶ **H&P Keys**

Chest pain with accelerating pattern including new onset or rest symptoms. Often a midsternal squeezing or heaviness that may radiate to the left shoulder or arm, jaw, neck, etc. Symptoms may be similar to those present previously; however, usual alleviating factors (eg, nitroglycerin [NTG], rest) may no longer be effective. Associated symptoms, eg, diaphoresis, nausea, dyspnea, are common. Reduction in left ventricular (LV) compliance may allow auscultation of an $S_4$ gallop. With coexisting LV dysfunction an $S_3$ may be heard. In the presence of global ischemia or LV dysfunction, a dyskinetic cardiac impulse may be palpated. Ischemia-induced papillary muscle dysfunction may cause the murmur of mitral regurgitation (MR). Ischemia-induced elevations in cardiac filling pressures often cause pulmonary congestion, allowing auscultation of rales.

▶ **Diagnosis**

Electrocardiogram (ECG): ST depression or elevation or T wave inversion. Exercise stress testing (ETT; not performed in patients with unstable angina). ETT or pharmacologic stress testing is combined with an imaging agent, such as thallium, that permits the visualization of myocardial perfusion, coronary angiography. Invasive evaluation and treatment is indicated for patients with high risk clinical features.

▶ **Disease Severity**

High risk clinical features are advanced age, ST segment depression, signs of heart failure and elevation of biomarkers of cell damage (troponins). Response to therapy and duration of symptoms dictate evaluation. Patients easily stabilized on medical therapy can often be closely followed clinically. Patients not medically stabilized or whose symptoms reemerge on therapy and those with prominent ischemic ECG findings usually undergo coronary angiography. Location and severity of stenoses (eg, left main, three-vessel) dictate management.

▶ **Concept and Application**

The vast majority of patients with unstable angina have underlying coronary atherosclerosis (CAD). Conversion from stable to unstable symptoms is usually caused by plaque rupture with superimposed thrombosis. Platelet aggregation at site of plaque rupture with release of vasoconstricting mediators plays an important role.

▶ **Treatment Steps**
1. Continuous ECG monitoring.
2. Bed rest, mild sedation, and treatment of extracardiac precipitants of increased oxygen demand (eg, hypoxia, sepsis, anemia, uncontrolled hypo- or hypertension, etc).

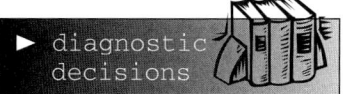

### ▶ diagnostic decisions

**ISCHEMIC HEART DISEASE**

**Acute myocardial infarction**
Sudden onset of typical squeezing or crushing substernal chest pain; ECG with S-T segment elevation in 2 or more leads; increased CPK-MB isoenzymes and troponins.

**Angina pectoris**
Chest pain lasting 1–15 minutes precipitated by exertion relieved by rest; associated ECG changes with S-T segment depression. Abnormal exercise stress test or abnormal perfusion on nuclear scan.

**Unstable angina**
Angina that increases in frequency or severity, is of new onset or occurs at rest. Coronary angiography defines the extent and severity of disease and need for intervention; exercise testing with perfusion imaging useful for risk stratification and treatment decisions.

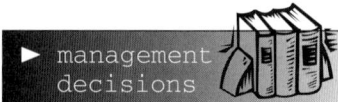

## management decisions

### ISCHEMIC HEART DISEASE

**Acute myocardial infarction**
Open the occluded artery to restore cardiac blood flow with thrombolytic therapy or angioplasty; monitor and treat serious dysrhythmias, aspirin to decrease clot formation, beta-blockers to decrease myocardial oxygen needs, oxygen and pain relief.

**Angina pectoris**
Drug therapy with nitrates, β-blockers, aspirin to prevent acute MI; calcium antagonists are second-line therapy. Intervention with bypass surgery or coronary intervention for patients with refractory symptoms or severe coronary disease.

**Unstable angina**
Drug therapy for stabilization with intravenous nitroglycerin, aspirin, heparin, clopidogrel, glycoprotein IIB/IIIA inhibitors, and β-blockers. Coronary interventions and coronary bypass surgery for severe coronary disease.

3. Intravenous nitrates, heparin, thienopyridines, and aspirin (acetylsalicylic acid [ASA]) and IIB/IIIA inhibitors are of proven efficacy. Thienopyridines, especially clopidogrel, reduces adverse events including death, MI, and stroke. Agents that block the platelet glycoprotien IIB/IIIA receptor substantially reduces mortality and the occurrence of acute MI primarily in patients who undergo coronary intervention. Intravenous NTG often is successful when other routes fail. β-blockers are useful and also reduce the incidence of acute MI.
4. Calcium channel blockers can provide symptomatic relief but do not decrease event rates.
5. Intra-aortic balloon counterpulsation (IABP) is often used as a bridge to percutaneous transluminal coronary angioplasty (PTCA) or coronary artery bypass graft (CABG) and is effective in stabilizing medically refractory patients.
6. Lipid-lowering therapy with HMG-CoA reductase inhibitors should be started for patients with LDLs greater than 100 mg/dL.

## 2. Myocardial Infarction

### ▶ H&P Keys
Chest pain, often midsternal squeezing or crushing. The pain may radiate to the neck, jaw, shoulders, arms, etc. Diaphoresis is frequent. Approximately 20% of episodes occur in the absence of pain (silent). Displaced and even dyskinetic cardiac impulse can be palpated. Ischemia-induced papillary muscle dysfunction may allow auscultation of a MR murmur. In the presence of associated right ventricular (RV) infarction, jugular venous distention (JVD) can be seen. Elevations in cardiac filling pressures often cause pulmonary congestion, allowing auscultation of pulmonary rales.

### ▶ Diagnosis
ECG: transmural or Q wave myocardial infarction. (MI): ST segment elevation and T wave inversions with subsequent evolution of Q waves. Nontransmural or non-Q MI: ST depression and T wave inversions are seen. Elevations in cardiac enzymes: creatine kinase (CK), specifically CK-MB and isoforms, peaks at 24 hours; troponins I and T, and myoglobin can detect cell injury early in the course of MI. L-lactate dehydrogenase (LDH) peaks at 3 to 5 days after MI. A ratio of $LDH_1:LDH_2$ greater than 1:0 suggests that MI has occurred. If a question of diagnosis of MI exists, 2D echocardiography and technetium nuclear scans can be valuable in detecting abnormalities in heart function and blood flow.

### ▶ Disease Severity
Mortality increases with the number of ECG leads showing ST segment elevation. Cardiac imaging with echocardiography (echo) or radionuclide ventriculography (RVG) can help assess the extent and prognosis of infarction by measuring LV systolic function and ejection fraction. Echo aids in diagnosis of MI complications, eg, LV thrombus or aneurysm, pericardial effusion, free wall and septal rupture, and mitral regurgitation (MR).

▶ Concept and Application

MI results from the abrupt cessation of myocardial blood flow and oxygen delivery. The vast majority of cases of MI are due to CAD. Plaque rupture leads to thrombosis and coronary occlusion. Platelet aggregation and release of mediators further hinder flow and contribute to spasm. Elevation of myocardial oxygen demand (eg, tachycardia) can increase myocardial cell damage. Irreversible cell death occurs, usually within 6 hours, if therapy is not given to restore blood flow or if spontaneous improvement does not occur. Nonatherosclerotic causes of MI, such as embolism, trauma, vasculitis, or hypercoagulable states, are less common.

▶ Treatment Steps

1. Supplemental oxygen, establishing intravenous access, and continuous monitoring to detect potentially lethal dysrhythmias in the cardiac care unit (CCU) are important first steps.
2. Analgesia should be administered as necessary.
3. Thrombolysis (streptokinase, tissue plasminogen activator [TPA], acylated streptokinase–plasminogen complex [APSAC]), especially early administration, reduces mortality. PTCA is effective, especially if thrombolysis is contraindicated.
4. Aspirin should be given on day 1 of AMI to all patients without a contraindication.
5. Heparin and ASA are useful in conjunction with thrombolysis.
6. Intravenous nitroglycerin is helpful in decreasing oxygen demand and increasing supply.
7. β-Blocker therapy should be administered to all patients without a contraindication within 12 hours of the onset of the MI.
8. Coronary angiography and revascularization wih PTCA or CABG is recommended if the patient is in shock, has a large infarct, or is unresponsive to medical therapy. Catheterization may also be required for the diagnosis and treatment of complications.

3. Spasm (Prinzmetal's or Variant Angina)

▶ H&P Keys

Anginal-type chest pain, typically occurring at rest. High percentage of patients with isolated coronary spasm are cigarette smokers or cocaine abusers. Patients tend to be younger than those with exertional angina. When the patient is asymptomatic, the cardiac exam is usually normal.

▶ Diagnosis

ECG: typically shows ST elevation during symptomatic periods. Coronary spasm in response to the vasoconstrictor ergonovine, usually during coronary angiography, is the gold standard diagnostic test.

▶ Disease Severity

Severity judged by symptom frequency and response to ergonovine.

▶ Concept and Application

Most patients have CAD, and spasm occurs in close proximity to a diseased segment, although approximately one third have angiographically normal coronaries. Diseased coronary vasculature loses the ability to manifest endothelial-dependent vasodilation and may react paradoxically to what are normally vasorelaxant stimuli.

▶ Treatment Steps

1. Cigarette smoking and cocaine use are to be avoided.
2. Nitrates and calcium channel blockers are usually effective; the effect of β-blockers is unpredictable; in some they can precipitate spasm.
3. Alpha-adrenergic β-blockers (eg, prazosin) can be helpful.

## B. Chronic

### 1. Stable Angina Pectoris

▶ H&P Keys

Episodic chest discomfort, often described as heaviness or squeezing lasting 1–15 minutes. Pain may radiate to the jaw, neck, shoulder, or the left arm. Symptoms typically are precipitated by exertion, cold weather, or emotional upset, and relieved by rest. Family history of premature CAD, diabetes, hyperlipidemia, hypertension, cigarette smoking. Exam may be normal, but if the patient is examined during an ischemic episode, reduction in LV compliance may allow auscultation of an $S_4$. An $S_3$ may be heard if coexisting LV dysfunction is present. In the presence of global ischemia or LV dysfunction, a dyskinetic cardiac impulse may be palpated. Ischemia-induced papillary muscle dysfunction may give rise to MR murmur. Ischemia-induced elevations in filling pressures often lead to pulmonary congestion with auscultation of rales.

▶ Diagnosis

ECG may be normal if patient is asymptomatic, but evidence of prior MI may be seen. If patient is symptomatic, ischemic ST and T wave changes may be noted. ETT, pharmacologic stress testing, or exercise echo are useful.

▶ Disease Severity

Global ECG changes suggest multivessel CAD. Quantitation of ischemic burden can be accomplished with perfusion imaging. Coronary arteriography documents presence, extent, and severity of CAD and suitability for revascularization.

▶ Concept and Application

Angina results from myocardial oxygen supply-demand imbalance. Obstructive coronary lesions limit the blood flood to myocardial segments. Dilatation of myocardial arteriolar resistance vessels mitigates ischemia, but this mechanism eventually is inadequate as stenosis severity increases. Angina can be precipitated in the absence of CAD in patients with augmented myocardial oxygen demand, eg, thyrotoxicosis, hypertrophy or aortic stenosis.

▶ Treatment Steps
1. Reduction of ischemic precipitants and treatment of coexisting illnesses (eg, hyperthyroidism) that increase oxygen demand.
2. Sublingual nitroglycerin (NTG) is valuable for prompt relief of anginal symptoms.
3. Aspirin reduces the risk of future adverse events by 33%.
4. Lipid-lowering therapy with HMG CoA reductase inhibitors also substantially reduce the risk of future fatal and non-fatal MI.
5. β-Blockers stimultaneously improve angina and ischemia while also preventing MI and death.
6. Calcium channel blocking drugs also relieve ischemic symptoms.
7. PTCA and CABG relieve symptoms and improve outcomes in appropriate patients.

2. **Silent Ischemia**

▶ H&P Keys
Patients are most frequently asymptomatic, and the physical exam in the absence of ischemia is usually normal.

▶ Diagnosis
Holter monitoring can uncover ambulatory ST segment changes indicative of ischemia, as can ETT.

▶ Disease Severity
Degree of ST segment depression and number of leads involved can suggest disease extent; nocturnal ST segment depression often means multivessel CAD.

▶ Concept and Application
Two populations exist, those with entirely asymptomatic ischemia and those with both symptomatic and asymptomatic episodes. In patients with symptomatic CAD, most episodes are asymptomatic. Whether an abnormal pain mechanism or a heightened pain threshold is responsible for silent ischemia is unknown; however, it appears to occur with higher frequency in diabetic patients.

▶ Treatment Steps
1. Medical therapy, as outlined for angina pectoris, is often used; however, specific therapy depends on extent of disease, patient's age, occupation, etc.
2. Most patients develop symptomatic angina before additional adverse events occur.

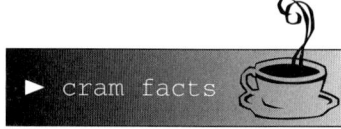

## cram facts

### TREATMENT DECISIONS

**Heart Failure**

**Left-sided heart failure**
Find and treat or correct any precipitating or underlying cause, eg, valvular heart disease. Medical treatment with angiotensin-converting enzyme inhibitors, diuretics, digoxin, and β-blockers. Anticoagulation with severe dysfunction. Severe decompensation may require sympathomimetic agents, a left ventricular assist device or cardiac transplantation.

**High-output heart failure**
Find and treat the underlying cause, eg, thyrotoxicosis and/or arteriovenous fistula; diuretics.

**Right-sided heart failure**
Correct underlying problems that resulted in pulmonary obstruction or hypertension; diuretics and treatment similar to left-sided failure.

## II. HEART FAILURE (HF)

### A. Left-Sided

1. **Low Output**

   ▶ **H&P Keys**
   History may elicit cause, eg, CAD, prior MI, hypertension, or valvular disease. Symptoms: fatigue, weakness, reduced exercise tolerance, exertional or rest dyspnea, paroxysmal nocturnal dyspnea (PND), orthopnea, nocturia. Physical findings: displaced cardiac impulse; $S_3$ murmurs, especially MR; rales; rarely Cheyne–Stokes respiration.

   ▶ **Diagnosis**
   Most often made by history and exam. Confirmation can be made by chest roentgenogram, echo, or radionuclear angiogram (RNA). In patients with a prior MI, Q waves may be seen on ECG. Pulmonary artery catheterization documents the hemodynamic derangements.

   ▶ **Disease Severity**
   Determined by degree of symptomatic incapacity and of LV impairment (systolic dysfunction), degree of hemodynamic impairment, indicated by elevated filling pressures (systolic and diastolic dysfunction) and impaired cardiac output.

   ▶ **Concept and Application**
   In systolic dysfunction, the heart delivers inadequate oxygen to meet metabolic needs; in diastolic dysfunction ventricular filling is compromised. Systolic and diastolic dysfunction commonly coexist. In predominantly systolic dysfunction, activation of sympathetic nervous system, renin–angiotensin–aldosterone axis, and hormonal (antidiuretic hormone [ADH]) elaboration occurs.

   ▶ **Treatment Steps**
   1. Search for precipitating causes of decompensation (infection, MI, uncontrolled hypertension, dietary indiscretion, etc.). Correct underlying diseases, eg, valvular disease, ischemia, arrhythmia. Salt restriction.
   2. Pharmacologic therapy is tailored to the stage of the disease (A, high risk to develop CHF; B, structural disease without symptoms; C, prior or current symptoms; D, refractory symptoms requiring special intervention).
   3. Most symptomatic patients should be managed with a combination of four drugs: diuretics, ACE inhibitors, β-blockers, and digitalis.
   4. Diuretics decrease symptoms related to volume overload in patients with evidence of fluid retention.
   5. ACE inhibitors are used to reduce afterload, increase cardiac output, and decrease mortality (Stages B–D).
   6. Digoxin augments contractility and reduces symptoms but does not improve prognosis (Stage C and D)

7. β-blockers help modulate neurohumoral activation, blunt excess sympathetic tone and are used in all stable, symptomatic patients (Stage C and D)
8. With severe decompensation sympathomimetic amines (dobutamine) or phosphodiesterase inhibitors (milrinone) are used.
9. B-naturetic hormone therapy is also valuable to rapidly relieve symptoms and improve hemodynamics.
10. Stage D patients may require cardiac transplantation or a left ventricular assist device.

2. **High Output**

▶ H&P Keys

Signs of hyperdynamic circulation, eg, brisk pulses. Dyspnea, orthopnea often present. Angina in patients with CAD.

▶ Disease Severity

Assessed primarily on degree of disability.

▶ Concept and Application

Patients often have an underlying syndrome causing elevation in metabolic demands and/or cardiac output, eg, arteriovenous fistulas, Paget's disease, hyperthyroidism, anemia.

▶ Treatment Steps

Treatment of underlying cause, medical therapy: often diuresis.

B. **Right-Sided**

▶ H&P Keys

Seen with history of LV failure, RV infarction, lung disease, pulmonic stenosis, pulmonary emboli, myocarditis, etc. Clinical findings: fatigue, RV heave and gallops, JVD, hepatomegaly, ascites, edema, atrial arrhythmias.

▶ Diagnosis

Signs and symptoms of RV or biventricular failure in setting of predisposing condition. ECG may show RV or right atrial (RA) hypertrophy. Echo may show RV dilatation and hypokinesis.

▶ Disease Severity

Often suggested by degree of edema and JVD on exam. Ascites suggests more severe decompensation. Echo and RVG can quantitate the degree of functional impairment and dilatation. Right heart catheterization quantitates the degree of hemodynamic impairment and response to therapy. Arterial blood gases (ABG) and pulmonary function tests (PFTs) document the degree of pulmonary disability, if any.

▶ Concept and Application

RV outflow obstruction (eg, pulmonic stenosis), pulmonary hypertension resulting from chronic LV failure, obstructive lung disease, chronic pulmonary emboli (cor pulmonale), etc, lead to chronic overload of the RV. LV cardiac output is also reduced. Elevated pressures in systemic vasculature lead to accumulation of fluid in the extravascular space. See Figure 1–2.

▶ Treatment Steps
1. Treatment of underlying condition.
2. Diuretics lead to symptomatic improvement.
3. Oxygen supplementation.
4. ACE inhibitors.
5. Antiarrhythmics, anti-ischemics, anticoagulation as needed.

## III. HYPOTENSION AND ACUTE CIRCULATORY COLLAPSE (SHOCK)

Occurs in a wide array of conditions that ultimately lead to inadequate oxygen delivery to the organs, tissues, and cells. Impairment in oxygen transport results from increases in demand or inability to maintain normal oxygen supply. Shock is classified according to the primary hemodynamic derangement as cardiogenic, hypovolemic, obstructive, and distributive. In all forms, physical examination reveals hypotension defined as mean pressure less than 60 mm Hg with evidence of peripheral hypoperfusion, including vasoconstriction, with cool and mottled extremities and other evidence of poor organ perfusion, including abnormal mentation and decreased urine output.

### A. Cardiogenic Shock

Inadequate cardiac output as a result of an abnormality in intrinsic cardiac function or an anatomic derangement in cardiac structure, for example, acute valvular heart disease.

▶ H&P Keys
During an MI, patients will have acute chest pain, dyspnea, diaphoresis, evidence of peripheral hypoperfusion, $S_3$ gallop, elevated venous pressure, or a murmur of MR or ventricular septal defect. Other entities, eg, acute valvular endocarditis, will produce a characteristic clinical picture and new cardiac murmurs.

▶ Diagnosis
ECG to confirm MI, echo to evaluate global LV function, regional abnormalities, and structural abnormalities, eg, ventricular septal defect or acute MR. Hemodynamic monitoring with Swan–Ganz catheter often required for characterization.

▶ Disease Severity
Level of blood pressure, organ perfusion including urine output, metabolic acidosis, or elevated serum lactate.

▶ Concept and Application
With fatal cardiogenic shock, 40% of the functioning myocardium is lost. Reduction in coronary perfusion pressure leads to a downward spiral, with progressive loss of contractility. Mechanical derangements, including rupture of the ventricular sep-

---

▶ diagnostic decisions

**HYPOTENSION AND ACUTE CIRCULATORY COLLAPSE**

Cardiogenic shock
Diagnosis of acute MI or severe acute valvular heart disease with ECG and echocardiogram also useful to define severity of cardiac dysfunction and extent of valvular disease. Hemodynamic monitoring with balloon flotation catheter to define therapy, immediate surgery may be necessary.

Hypovolemic shock
Hypotension or postural hypotension with tachycardia; blood loss evidenced by a low hemoglobin; illness resulting in fluid loss, eg, severe diarrhea.

Obstructive shock
Echocardiogram to diagnose pericardial effusion and cardiac tamponade; ventilation-perfusion lung scan or pulmonary angiogram for suspected pulmonary embolus.

Distributive shock
Source of acute infection, blood cultures, WBC count, or source of anaphylaxis. Hemodynamic monitoring to characterize cardiac output.

tum or mitral valve apparatus at any level, eg, papillary muscle or chordae, result in elevation of venous pressure, pulmonary congestion, reduced cardiac output, and organ hypoperfusion.

▶ Treatment Steps
1. The most effective therapy for MI is acute restoration of blood flow with thrombolysis or coronary angioplasty.
2. Hemodynamic management is guided by placement of a balloon flotation catheter with determinations of pulmonary capillary wedge pressure and cardiac output.
3. If pulmonary capillary wedge pressure is low, volume is administered.
4. If pulmonary capillary wedge pressure is high and cardiac output is low, treatment is needed to augment cardiac output and improve organ perfusion at reduced filling pressures.
5. Intraaortic balloon pump augments coronary perfusion and produces systolic unloading of the ventricle.
6. Dopamine or dobutamine may be helpful to produce augmentation of cardiac output and maintenance of peripheral perfusion. Oxygenation must be maintained. Mortality remains high, in spite of modern management techniques, unless effective myocardial blood flow can be restored or a mechanical complication is repaired.

## B. Hypovolemic Shock

Inadequate circulatory volume caused by hemorrhage or dehydration. Common with trauma, surgery, vomiting, diarrhea, and some skin disorders.

▶ H&P Keys

Weakness, postural light-headedness in setting of blood loss or fluid loss, eg, history of hemorrhage, melena. Postural hypotension and tachycardia, low jugular venous pressure.

▶ Diagnosis

Measurement of postural blood pressure and heart rate changes, nasogastric aspiration, hemoglobin, blood urea and nitrogen (BUN):creatinine ratio.

▶ Disease Severity

Level of blood pressure, severity of impaired organ perfusion, mentation, hourly urine output.

▶ Concept and Application

Cardiac output is dependent on preload or venous return. An initial reduction in volume is compensated by an increase in heart rate and arterial and venous vasoconstriction. As volume reduction progresses, compensatory mechanisms are unable to compensate, and the blood pressure falls.

▶ Treatment Steps
1. Acute, rapid volume restoration with blood, crystalloid, or colloid solutions.
2. Temporary maintenance of peripheral perfusion pressure with vasoconstrictors.

3. Next, identification of cause or source of blood loss or fluid loss and control of site of bleeding, eg, with endoscopy, arterial cauterization, surgery.

## C. Obstructive Shock

Impairment of venous return to the right ventricle or left ventricle occurs secondary to obstruction in the venous system, pulmonary artery, or pericardium. Observed with acute pulmonary embolus, or tamponade with a pericardial effusion. Effusion is caused by trauma, infections, malignancy, connective tissue disease, and renal failure.

▶ H&P Keys

Dyspnea, orthopnea, elevated venous pressure, chest pain, hemoptysis, pulsus paradoxus, faint and distant heart sounds, or pulmonary hypertension.

▶ Diagnosis

Echo for effusion or tamponade, ECG with electrical alternans, analysis of pericardial fluid for etiology. Analysis for source of embolus, venous Doppler probe, ventilation-perfusion lung scan.

▶ Concept and Application

During pericardial tamponade, elevation of the intrapericardial pressure raises pressure in the cardiac chambers, leading to a reduction in venous return to the right and left heart and reduced cardiac output. Venous obstruction or pulmonary artery embolus also prevents adequate flow and venous return to the left heart with reduction in cardiac output.

▶ Disease Severity

Level of blood pressure, mentation, peripheral perfusion.

▶ Treatment Steps
1. Acute volume administration.
2. Administration of beta-agonist to increase heart rate and stroke volume.
3. Definitive therapy requires drainage by pericardiocentesis, guided by hemodynamic monitoring or two-dimensional echo, or subxiphoid or anterior pericardiectomy. Pulmonary embolus with shock has a high mortality. Thrombolytic therapy with streptokinase infusion over 24 hours is favored over acute embolectomy.

## D. Distributive Shock

Characteristic of sepsis, also anaphylaxis and neurogenic, toxic, or endocrinologic shock.

▶ H&P Keys

Fever, chills, rigor, respiratory alkalosis, bee sting or toxic ingestion, hypotension, peripheral vasodilation with warm extremities.

▶ Disease Severity

Level of blood pressure, evidence of poor organ perfusion.

▶ Diagnosis

Blood cultures, white blood count, ABG, pH, lactate, toxin screen, hemodynamic monitoring to determine venous pressure and cardiac output.

▶ Concept and Application

Diffuse arterial and venous dilatation in response to endotoxins, exotoxins, and cytokines. Other mediators include kinins, histamine, and prostaglandins. Cardiac output is increased and peripheral oxygen demand also markedly increased. Inadequate tissue oxygen delivery and failure of microcirculation, with inappropriate vasodilatation and vasoconstriction. Later, sepsis leads to depression in myocardial function.

▶ Treatment Steps

1. Antibiotic coverage, including two bacteriocidal agents for likely organisms.
2. Initial rapid volume infusion with crystalloid and colloid solutions and blood to maintain hemoglobin- and oxygen-carrying capacity.
3. Vasoactive drugs including dopamine to maintain perfusion pressure of 60 mm Hg.
4. Initial characterization of the site of infection and appropriate treatment, eg, drainage of an abscess.

## IV. MYOCARDIAL DISEASES

### A. Dilated Cardiomyopathy

▶ H&P Keys

Symptoms suggest low cardiac output and congestion of systemic and pulmonary vasculature: dyspnea, fatigue, orthopnea, PND, edema. Exam often reveals hypotension, tachycardia, cool extremities, pulmonary rales, displaced cardiac impulse often of diminished intensity, and $S_3$, mitral, or tricuspid murmur. Signs of RV failure (edema, ascites, elevated JVD) often present.

▶ Diagnosis

Chest roentgenogram often shows cardiomegaly, often with signs of congestion, possibly with pleural effusions. ECG often shows signs of ventricular or atrial enlargement, atrial fibrillation; premature ventricular complexes (PVCs) are often seen. Echo and RNA often show ventricular or four chamber enlargement with diffuse hypocontractility and reduced cardiac output.

▶ Disease Severity

Symptoms may correlate poorly with degree of ventricular impairment. Echo and RNA document degree of ventricular dilatation and dysfunction. Echo documents associated valvular abnormalities. Cardiac catheterization documents degree of hemodynamic abnormality and presence of CAD. In absence of CAD, catheterization rarely alters therapy.

▶ Concept and Application

Various etiologies, most common being idiopathic. Other etiologies include ischemic (postinfarction), viral (eg, coxsackie), peripartum, toxic (eg, alcohol, doxorubicin). Myocyte injury occurs, causing reduction in contractility, leading to ventricular dilation, with compensation by activation of sympathetic nervous system and renin–angiotensin–aldosterone axis.

▶ Treatment Steps

1. Removal of inciting cause (eg, discontinue alcohol) if one can be found.
2. Diuresis improves symptoms and relieves pulmonary and systemic congestion.
3. ACE inhibition.
4. β-Blockers have been shown to improve survival and quality of life.
5. Enhancement of myocardial contractility with digoxin.
6. Anticoagulation in patients with atrial fibrillation or cardiac embolism.
7. Salt restriction.
8. Implantable cardioverter-defibrillator in select patients with severe ventricular arrhythmias.
9. Cardiac transplantation may ultimately be required.

## B. Hypertrophic Cardiomyopathy

▶ H&P Keys

Often patients are younger; history of sudden death of a relative during exertion may be obtained. Symptoms: exertional dyspnea, chest pain, syncope, light-headedness, sudden death, especially during exertion. Exam may reveal $S_4$, double or triple apical impulse, a crescendo–decrescendo systolic murmur that is increased by the Valsalva maneuver and by rising from recumbency, decreased by squatting.

▶ Diagnosis

ECG may show left ventricular hypertrophy (LVH) and possibly large Q waves in inferior and lateral leads; giant negative T waves are occasionally seen in the midprecordium. Characteristic echo findings are: (1) asymmetric septal thickening or hypertrophy (ASH), (2) systolic anterior motion of the anterior mitral leaflet, and (3) MR. Holter monitoring may document atrial fibrillation, which is poorly tolerated, or ventricular arrhythmias, which may precede sudden death.

▶ Disease Severity

Echocardiography can quantitate the degree of hypertrophy especially with ASH, the most common form. Doppler studies can quantify the amount of outflow obstruction. The presence and magnitude of a pressure gradient can also be documented in the cardiac catheterization lab.

▶ Concept and Application

A massively hypertrophied LV wall results in a noncompliant, stiffened chamber with impaired filling. Increased myocardial mass leads to increased myocardial oxygen demand and frequently angina. Patients with ASH often have dynamic LV obstruction and frequently MR. Hypertrophic cardiomyopathy (HCM) can be both spontaneous, inherited, or the result of long-standing hypertension.

▶ Treatment Steps
1. Beta- and calcium channel blockers are effective in decreasing the intraventricular gradient, myocardial oxygen demand, and ventricular stiffness.
2. Competitive sports are generally prohibited because of the risk of sudden death.
3. Dual-chamber pacing has been shown to be effective in decreasing the amount of outflow obstruction in these patients.
4. Surgery (septal myectomy) is effective in patients with obstructive HCM.
5. Implanting a cardiac defibrillator may help to prevent sudden cardiac death.

## C. Restrictive Cardiomyopathy

▶ H&P Keys
Patient may have an underlying disease (eg, hemachromatosis, sarcoid, amyloid, or cancer). Symptoms: fatigue, weakness, dyspnea. Physical findings: elevated jugular venous pressure; Kussmaul's sign; edema; ascites; enlarged, tender liver; distant heart sounds; $S_3$ and $S_4$ are common.

▶ Diagnosis
ECG often shows low voltage, with echo showing thickened LV walls, often with a "speckled" appearance in patients with amyloidosis.

▶ Disease Severity
Echo shows LV thickening and systolic impairment (if any). Doppler and cardiac catheterization can show augmented early diastolic filling. Catheterization demonstrates lowered cardiac output and abnormal RV filling with a typical "dip and plateau" morphology in the right ventricular diastolic pressure tracing. RV biopsy can identify a specific cause.

▶ Concept and Application
Restrictive cardiomyopathy is the least common of the cardiomyopathies. Systemic disorders (eg, hemachromatosis, sarcoid, amyloid, metastatic cancer), patients with thoracic radiation or with other disorders (eg, endomyocardial fibrosis) caused by myocardial infiltration, fibrosis, etc, have elevated filling pressures, which lead to signs and symptoms of right and left heart congestion. Reduced cavity size causes decreased cardiac output.

▶ Treatment Steps
1. Identify and treat the underlying illness if possible (eg, steroids in sarcoid or chelation therapy in hemachromatosis).

2. Symptomatic treatment includes diuretics and salt restriction. Digitalis is often not helpful and may be harmful in these disorders.
3. The prognosis depends on the severity of the underlying condition.

## V. CARDIAC ARRHYTHMIAS

### A. Supraventricular Arrhythmias

Rhythm disturbances involving sinus node, atria, and atrioventricular (AV) node.

1. Bradyarrhythmias

   a. Sinus Node Dysfunction (Sick Sinus Syndrome)—Heart rates less than 60 beats per minute (bpm) or inappropriate rise in rate for level of activity (chronotropic incompetence). Includes sinus arrest, sinus exit block, bradycardia–tachycardia syndrome (rapid atrial fibrillation or flutter with long pauses).

   ▶ H&P Keys
   Fatigue, dizziness, weakness, syncope, low rhythm, and pulse.

   ▶ Diagnosis
   ECG, cardiac rhythm monitoring, electrophysiologic studies.

   ▶ Disease Severity
   Depressed mental status, fatigue, limitation of activity, shortness of breath.

   ▶ Concept and Application
   Disruption of normal structures and conduction pathways resulting from collagen deposition, hypertension, ischemia, atrial stretch, idiopathic causes, autonomic nervous system.

   ▶ Treatment Steps
   1. Acute symptomatic: temporary intravenous pacemaker or external pacing device.
   2. Chronic symptomatic: permanent pacemaker, withdrawal of offending drugs.

   b. AV Node

   *First-degree AV Block*—PR interval > 0.20 seconds. May or may not be associated with bradyarrhythmia.

   *Second-degree AV Block*—Intermittent failure of atrial activity to reach ventricles:
   - Mobitz Type I (Wenckebach). Usually at level of AV node, progressive PR prolongation prior to blocked QRS. Does not include blocked premature atrial contraction.
   - Mobitz Type II Block. Usually distal to AV node (bundle of His). High risk for complete AV block. Often associated with wide QRS.

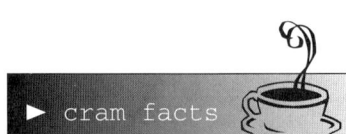

### TREATMENT DECISIONS

**Cardiac Arrhythmias**

**Bradyarrhythmias**
Withdrawal of medications that produce bradycardia; temporary intravenous or external pacemaker for acute management; permanent pacemaker for definitive treatment.

**Atrial fibrillation**
β-Blockers, calcium channel blockers for rate control; anticoagulation with coumadin if underlying structural heart disease; DC cardioversion or antiarrhythmic drugs such as amiodarone or sotalol to restore sinus rhythm. Catheter-based radiofrequency ablation techniques are also useful in restoring and maintaining sinus rhythm.

**Ventricular tachycardia**
Immediate DC cardioversion if patient is hemodynamically unstable; drugs including lidocaine, procainamide, amiodarone, or pronestyl. Implantable defibrillator to treat high risk patients.

**Ventricular fibrillation**
Immediate DC cardioversion.

*Complete (Third-degree) AV Block*—May be at level of AV node, bundle of His, or bundle branches. Atrial and ventricular activity are independent and atrial rate faster than ventricular escape rate. QRS usually wide. Often associated with symptoms.

▶ H&P Keys

Fatigue, shortness of breath, congestive heart failure, dizziness, syncope. Slow or irregular pulse.

▶ Diagnosis

ECG, intermittent cannon A waves and complete heart block, cardiac rhythm monitoring, electrophysiologic studies.

▶ Disease Severity

Heart rate, blood pressure, mentation, level of activity.

▶ Concept and Application

Influence of autonomic nervous system, medications, hypertension, associate valve diseases (calcific), ischemic heart disease, Lev's and Lenegre's degenerative diseases of the conduction system, electrolyte disturbances (potassium).

▶ Treatment Steps

1. Temporary pacemaker in unstable patients.
2. Withdrawal of offending medications.
3. Permanent pacemakers for patients with symptomatic bradycardia or asymptomatic Mobitz II or third-degree heart block.

2. Tachyarrhythmias

   a. Premature Atrial Complex (PAC)—Found in over 60% of normal adults. Usually benign and asymptomatic. May be associated with the initiation of atrial fibrillation, flutter, or atrial tachycardias.

   b. Premature Junctional Complex (PJC)—Early beat originating in AV node. Narrow QRS.

   c. Sinus Tachycardia—Rate > 100 bpm. Normal or abnormal response to metabolic demand.

   d. Atrial Fibrillation—Relatively common disorder characterized by irregularly irregular rhythm and absence of identifiable P waves. Sometimes seen in normal patients, often associated with various cardiac abnormalities and thyroid disease.

   e. Atrial Flutter—Usually associated with atrial fibrillation. Organized atrial activity with rates 250 to 300 bpm. Sawtooth atrial activity on ECG. Variable conduction to ventricles (2:1, 3:1, 4:1).

   f. Atrial Tachycardia—Rates > 100 bpm inappropriate for activity level. Originate from within left or right atrium.

   g. AV Reentry (AVRT; Wolff–Parkinson–White Syndrome) and AV Nodal Reentrant Tachycardias (AVNRT)—Reentrant arrhythmias dependent on the AV node. Classic models for reentry.

▶ **H&P Keys**

Palpitations: rapid heart rate is irregularly irregular for atrial fibrillation and often regular for other forms of sustained supraventricular tachycardia. Fatigue, shortness of breath, dizziness, syncope.

▶ **Diagnosis**

Long-term ECG recording, electrophysiologic studies.

▶ **Disease Severity**

Frequency of symptoms, including fatigue, lethargy, dizziness, chest pain, shortness of breath, syncope. Stroke is associated with atrial fibrillation.

▶ **Concept and Application**

Automatic mechanism for PACs, PJCs, and some atrial tachycardia. Reentry is a predominant mechanism for most supraventricular tachycardia. May be congenital (Wolff–Parkinson–White) or associated with other forms of structural heart disease, eg, hypertension, ischemic heart disease, congenital heart disease (atrial septal defect). May be seen in normal patients.

▶ **Treatment Steps**

1. Direct-current cardioversion if unstable, radiofrequency ablation to maintain or convert to sinus rhythm.
2. Digoxin, calcium channel blockers, and β-blockers for rate control.
3. Antiarrhythmic drugs, eg, amiodarone and sotalol.
4. Maintenance of sinus rhythm or control of ventricular rate.

### B. Ventricular Arrhythmias

Disorders of rhythm isolated to ventricles.

#### 1. Bradyarrhythmias

Conduction disturbances within the His–Purkinje system and bundle branches. Often symptomatic. Usually caused by second- and third-degree heart block.

▶ **H&P Keys**

Light-headedness, fatigue, syncope, intermittent cannon A waves in jugular venous pulse exam (third-degree heart block), slow pulse (intermittent or chronic).

▶ **Diagnosis**

ECG, auscultation (dissociation of atrial [$S_4$] and ventricular [$S_1$ and $S_2$] activity), electrophysiologic studies.

▶ **Disease Severity**

Frequency of symptoms including dizziness, light-headedness, fatigue, shortness of breath, chest pain, syncope. Trifascicular block may be asymptomatic but predictive of complete heart block.

▶ **Concept and Application**

Lenegre's disease (sclerodegenerative disease of the conduction system), myocardial infarction, cardiomyopathies, drugs, infections (myocardial abscess).

▶ Treatment Steps
1. Temporary pacemaker for stabilization of symptomatic patients.
2. Withdrawal of offending medications.
3. Permanent pacemaker for patients at high risk of developing third-degree heart block, patients with trifascicular block, or symptomatic bradycardia.

2. **Tachyarrhythmias**

PVCs may be seen in normal patients. Often associated with ischemic heart disease, congestive heart failure, electrolyte abnormalities, and cardioactive drugs.

a. **Ventricular Tachycardia (VT)**—May be nonsustained, eg, 3 beats ≤ 30 seconds, or sustained, eg, > 30 seconds. May be uniform (regular); or polymorphic (irregular). Rate > 100 bpm and usually < 250 bpm.

b. **Ventricular Fibrillation**—Chaotic ventricular tachycardia with rate > 250 bpm. Most common cause of cardiac arrest.

▶ H&P Keys

Palpitations, sudden-onset weakness, dizziness, syncope, and cardiac arrest. Often associated with ischemia, congestive heart failure, cardiomyopathy. Cardiac arrest victim is pulseless and without respirations.

▶ Diagnosis

ECG, signal-averaged ECG, invasive electrophysiologic studies.

▶ Disease Severity

Cardiac arrest has a high recurrence rate if untreated. Prognosis related to LV function, CAD. Two-dimensional echo, cardiac catheterization to assess severity of LV dysfunction.

▶ Concept and Application

Most ventricular arrhythmias are due to reentry and are associated with acute or chronic ischemic heart disease or congestive heart failure (CHF). Rarely seen in structurally normal heart. Other forms (automatic, triggered activity) are associated with medications or electrolyte abnormalities (torsade de pointes) or are idiopathic.

▶ Treatment Steps

*Sustained Ventricular Tachycardia*
1. Low-energy cardioversion (50 to 200 J); or
2. Antiarrhythmic drugs, including lidocaine, amiodarone, bretylium, and procainamide.

*Ventricular Fibrillation*
1. Rapid defibrillation with 200 to 360 J.

*Chronic Management*
1. Stabilization of underlying disease.
2. Correction of electrolyte imbalances.
3. Antiarrhythmic drugs, especially amiodarone.
4. Implantable cardioverter defibrillator in patients at risk for sudden death.

## VI. PERICARDIAL DISEASES

### A. Acute Pericarditis

Most common pericardial disorder, consisting of acute inflammation of the pericardium from a wide variety of causes.

▶ H&P Keys

Retrosternal and left precordial sharp chest pain, often radiating to the back and left trapezius, with strong pleuritic component. Dyspnea is common. Symptoms often are worse in supine position, alleviated by sitting forward. Friction rub (three-component) best heard in left precordium while patient sitting forward during held exhalation.

▶ Diagnosis

ECG can show evolutionary changes consisting of widespread ST elevations with upward concavity and depressed PR interval, reduction of T wave amplitude or T wave inversion; with large associated pericardial effusions, reduction and respiratory variation in R wave amplitude (electrical alternans). Tests for etiology, eg, antinuclear antibodies (ANA), purified protein derivative (PPD).

▶ Disease Severity

The underlying disease is an important determination of outcome. Echo used to assess for presence and degree of associated pericardial effusion.

▶ Concept and Application

Pericardial inflammation caused by a variety of factors. Most common cause is idiopathic, although serologic studies have suggested these cases may be due to viral infection. Tuberculous pericarditis now reemerging, especially in AIDS patients. Purulent (bacterial) pericarditis is a fulminant disease with a poor prognosis. Other causes are post-MI injury (Dressler's syndrome), malignant neoplasia, radiation, uremia, and collagen vascular diseases.

▶ Treatment Steps
1. In idiopathic or viral cases, anti-inflammatory agents are used.
2. Rarely, steroids are used in recalcitrant cases.
3. Large effusions producing hemodynamic compromise require drainage.
4. Purulent pericarditis requires complete drainage and antibiotics.
5. Other treatment depends on the specific etiology.

### B. Pericardial Effusion

Fluid accumulation in the pericardial space. The amount of fluid and the rapidity of accumulation of the effusion determines the observed signs and symptoms.

▶ H&P Keys

Symptoms of pericarditis, or patient may be asymptomatic. Previously present friction rub may diminish in intensity. In large effusion, heart sounds may be muffled.

▶ **Diagnosis**

Chest roentgenogram shows cardiomegaly with "water bottle" shape. ECG, especially in large effusions, shows reduced QRS amplitude; electrical alternans may be seen. Echo for direct visualization of size and presence of effusion.

▶ **Disease Severity**

Determined by rapidity of accumulation and size of effusion. Echo documents size of effusion and extent of the hemodynamic impairment; hemodynamic effects can be also documented by cardiac catheterization.

▶ **Concept and Application**

Any cause of pericarditis can lead to the formation of a pericardial effusion. Pericardial effusion can also occur with a variety of systemic disorders such as hypothyroidism.

▶ **Treatment Steps**

1. Pericardiocentesis for diagnosis and treatment.
2. Treatment of underlying cause.
3. Removal of the pericardium may be required to prevent recurrent tamponade.

**C. Cardiac Tamponade**

An accumulation of pericardial fluid under high pressure, which limits the ability of the heart to fill.

▶ **H&P Keys**

May have antecedent history of pericarditis or chest trauma. Symptoms: dyspnea, fatigue. Physical findings: JVD, hypotension, shock, distant heart sounds, tachycardia, pulsus paradoxus.

▶ **Diagnosis**

Echo documents effusion, often with diastolic collapse of RA and RV. Cardiac catheterization documents elevated pericardial pressure and equivalence of this pressure to the diastolic pressures in all four chambers. RA pressure tracing typically shows amputation of the Y descent (compromised early ventricular filling).

▶ **Disease Severity**

Can be assessed by degree of symptomatic or hemodynamic impairment.

▶ **Concept and Application**

Pericardial fluid under high pressure compresses the heart, impairing its ability to fill. This leads to signs and symptoms of pulmonary and systemic venous congestion and ultimately obstructive shock.

▶ **Treatment Steps**

1. Immediate pericardiocentesis or surgical drainage with removal of the fluid, usually during echocardiographic and hemodynamic monitoring.
2. In recurrent cases, pericardiectomy may be necessary.

### D. Constrictive Pericarditis

Obliteration of pericardial space or scarring of pericardial tissue, causing cardiac enclosure, resulting in compromised cardiac filling.

▶ H&P Keys

Symptoms: fatigue, hypotension, weakness. Physical signs: ascites, edema, JVD, often with Kussmaul's sign (elevation of venous pressure during inspiration), pericardial knock in diastole, reduced amplitude of apical impulse.

▶ Diagnosis

ECG may show a low voltage QRS complex with diffuse T wave changes. Chest roentgenogram may show pericardial calcification, present in approximately 50% of patients. Echo and Doppler demonstrate normal cavity size with enhanced early diastolic filling. Pericardial thickening can be suggested by echo; however, computed tomography (CT) and magnetic resonance imaging (MRI) are more accurate in diagnosis.

▶ Disease Severity

Degree of thickening can be judged noninvasively, but confirmation of constrictive physiology is by catheterization. Hemodynamic features seen during catheterization include elevation and equalization of all diastolic pressures; LV and RV pressure tracings are equal in diastole and have a dip and plateau configuration (square root sign); RA pressure tracing shows an M configuration with prominence of the Y descent.

▶ Concept and Application

Historically, tuberculosis was the most common cause; current common causes are idiopathic and radiation. The scarred encasing pericardium restricts cardiac filling, leading to signs of reduced cardiac output and systemic venous congestion.

▶ Treatment Steps
1. Pericardial resection is the definitive therapy.
2. Diuretics can afford symptomatic improvement. Risks of the operation and prognosis postoperatively depends on the degree of involvement of the epicardium in the scarring, calcific process.

## VII. VALVULAR DISEASES

### A. Acute

#### 1. Rheumatic Fever

Delayed sequel to pharyngeal infections with group A streptococci. Pathology involves the heart, joints, central nervous system (CNS), skin, and subcutaneous tissues.

2. **Endocarditis**
Native valve endocarditis usually with prior valve pathology; endocarditis in prior drug users; and prosthetic valve endocarditis are the most common forms. May be acute or subacute. Acute endocarditis is often caused by *Staphylococcus aureus* and is rapidly destructive, and often fatal (if untreated) in less than 6 weeks. Subacute endocarditis has a longer, smoldering course and is frequently caused by viridans streptococci. Without effective treatment, death usually occurs in 2 to 6 months.

3. **Ischemic**
Acute valvular decompensation resulting from ischemic heart disease, eg, acute ischemia or myocardial infarction: may lead to cardiac decompensation and death. Usually acute MR caused by posterior papillary muscle ischemia or infarct.

▶ **H&P Keys**

*Acute Rheumatic Fever*—Arthritis, heart murmurs, congestive heart failure, fever, arrhythmias, CNS disorders, subcutaneous nodules, and skin rash.

*Endocarditis*—Fever, malaise, weakness, congestive heart failure, cardiac murmurs, splinter hemorrhages under fingernails, skin manifestations (Osler's nodes, Janeway lesions), embolic episodes, and petechiae.

*Ischemic-related Acute Valvular Decompensation*—Acute-onset CHF, hypotension, and shock; new cardiac murmur may not be heard.

▶ **Diagnosis**
Blood cultures, elevated white blood cell count, erythrocyte sedimentation rate (ESR), liver and muscle enzyme levels. Streptococcal antibody titer for rheumatic fever. Echocardiography, cardiac catheterization.

▶ **Disease Severity**
Depends on the chronicity, extent, and severity of valvular damage. Frequently involves multiple valves. Organism causing the endocarditis often key to severity. Degree of involvement of subvalvular apparatus (papillary muscle) determines severity of CHF in patients with ischemia-related MR.

▶ **Concept and Application**
Destruction of valvular and subvalvular apparatus, and the production of inflammatory myocarditis. Systemic embolization, as well as involvement of other organ systems, with both the infecting agent and inflammatory response responsible for other disease manifestations. Acute volume overload results from acute mitral or aortic valve rupture.

▶ **Treatment Steps**
1. Penicillin to prevent recurrent rheumatic fever.
2. Prolonged course of appropriate antibiotics for endocarditis.
3. Hemodynamic stabilization in the acutely ill patient.
4. Surgical valve replacement in patients with progressive valvular heart disease.

## B. Chronic

Degeneration of cardiac valvular structures over a prolonged time. Progressive dilation of the LV or RV. Chronic degenerative disorders including mitral valve prolapse (myxomatous degeneration) and calcific valvular disease in the elderly. Mitral and aortic valves are most commonly involved in endocarditis and degenerative valvular disorders including mitral regurgitation (MR), aortic regurgitation (AR), aortic stenosis (AS). Acquired mitral stenosis (MS) occurs almost exclusively from rheumatic fever. Pulmonary and tricuspid valves less often involved. Bicuspid aortic valve is a common congenital abnormality predominantly in men, and is associated with AS later in life.

### ▶ H&P Keys

CHF, shortness of breath, fatigue, pedal edema, cardiac murmurs consistent with severe stenotic or regurgitant lesions, elevated JVP, pulse alterations, eg, delayed upstroke with aortic stenosis, bounding pulse with aortic insufficiency.

### ▶ Diagnosis

Chest roentgenogram, echo, cardiac catheterization.

### ▶ Disease Severity

Heart rate, respiratory rate, ascultatory findings peripheral edema, pulmonary rales, blood pressure, oxygen saturation, level of consciousness.

### ▶ Concept and Application

*AS*—Obstruction of LV ejection producing pressure overload, LV hypertrophy, and ultimately reduced cardiac output.

*MS*—Obstruction of blood flow resulting in elevated LA and pulmonary pressures, plumonary edema, and impaired cardiac output.

*AR*—Dilated aorta, hypertension; large volume of blood in reverse direction from aorta to left ventricle resulting in LV dilation and reduced forward flow.

*MR*—Mitral valve prolapse; large volume of blood in reverse direction from left ventricle to left atrium and pulmonary veins resulting in pulmonary congestion, pulmonary edema and reduced cardiac output.

### ▶ Treatment Steps

*Acute MR and AR*
1. Diuretics.
2. Afterload reduction.
3. IABP for MR but contraindicated in AR.
4. Valve replacement surgery.

*Chronic MR and AR*—In less severe cases,
1. Diuretics.
2. Afterload reduction.

*Symptomatic AS and MS*
1. Treated surgically with valve replacement.
2. MS can also be treated with catheter-based balloon dilation of the stenotic valve.

## VIII. CARDIAC TRANSPLANTATION

Reserved for patients who are severely compromised by CHF despite maximal medical therapy. Approximately 2,500 heart transplants are performed worldwide yearly; limitation to wider application of transplantation is primarily due to an undersupply of donor hearts. Major contraindications to cardiac transplantation include factors that increase short- and intermediate-term morbidity or mortality, eg, associated diseases such as diabetes with end-organ complications or lung disease with pulmonary hypertension. A compliant patient able to adhere to the rigorous post-transplant rejection surveillance program and a strong social support system are important factors in selecting potential candidates for this therapy.

Immunosuppression is critical in preventing rejection in the post-transplant period, and cyclosporin has been a major advancement since its introduction in 1980. Sequential endomyocardial biopsies are performed to assess transplant rejection; based on biopsy results, doses of cyclosporin, prednisone, and azathioprine are adjusted. Severe rejection is often treated with short courses of T-cell suppression. One- and 5-year survival rates continue to improve and are now over 90% and 70%, respectively.

Complications associated with cardiac transplantation include rejection, infection, accelerated atherosclerosis, and hypertension.

## IX. CONGENITAL HEART DISEASE

Result of aberrant embryonic development of a normal structure or failure of such structure to develop beyond early stage of embryonic or fetal development. Malformations are complex and multifactorial and include genetic (chromosomal), environmental (eg, maternal rubella infection), and toxic (eg, anticoagulants) factors.

### A. Ventricular Septal Defect

One or more openings in the membranous or muscular septum (VSD). Most common congenital heart disease in adults.

▶ H&P Keys

Harsh systolic murmur at left sternal border radiating to right percordium, palpable thrill over percordium. Large left to right shunt associated with CHF. Pulmonary hypertension causes reversal of flow (right to left shunt), resulting in the Eisenmenger syndrome characterized by cyanosis, pedal edema, syncope, and CHF.

▶ Diagnosis

Physical exam, chest roentgenogram, oxygen saturation of blood in the ventricles, two-dimensional echo, cardiac catheterization, and angiography.

▶ Disease Severity

Mentation, heart rate, cyanosis, growth retardation. In children, 30% to 50% spontaneous closure. May be asymptomatic if shunt is small.

▶ Concept and Application

The size of the defect and the amount of blood shunted between the chambers determines the physiologic consequences.

*Left-to-right Shunt*—Large volume of blood from LV to RV causes volume overload of pulmonary circulation and decreased LV output.

*Right-to-left Shunt*—Large volume of unsaturated blood from RV to LV and systemic circulation, causing cyanosis, fatigue, right heart failure, embolic phenomenon.

▶ Treatment Steps
1. Small shunts do not require treatment.
2. Large shunts should undergo surgical repair.
3. Because bacterial endocarditis may be associated with VSD, endocarditis prophylaxis is warranted.

**B. Atrial Septal Defect**

Persistent opening in septum (ASD).

1. **Secundum ASD**

    In region of fossa ovalis.

2. **Primum ASD**

    Involves lower atrial septum.

3. **Sinus Venosus ASD**

    In region of sinus node.

    ▶ H&P Keys

    Often asymptomatic. Murmur heard at upper left sternal border. Associated with fixed and widely split $S_2$. May be associated with trisomy 21. Dyspnea, fatigue, atrial arrhythmias, right heart failure. May be associated with severe pulmonary hypertension and Eisenmenger's syndrome. Primum ASD may be associated with mitral and tricuspid valve disorders.

    ▶ Diagnosis

    Physical exam, chest roentgenogram, ECG (RV hypertrophy), two-dimensional echo, cardiac catheterization.

    ▶ Disease Severity

    CHF, pedal edema, elevated jugular venous pulse, fatigue, palpitations, dizziness, paradoxic emboli.

▶ Concept and Application

Shunting of blood at level of atria. Again, the size of the defect and amount of blood shunted between the chambers determines the consequences. Usually a left-to-right shunt develops, but reversal of flow may develop if pulmonary artery and right ventricular pressure increases. Disease severity correlates with size of shunt and symptoms.

▶ Treatment Steps
1. Observation of small shunts in asymptomatic patients but systemic emboli are a risk.
2. Closure for larger, symptomatic shunts.
3. Current catheter-based techniques allow less traumatic closure for many defects.

## C. Tetralogy of Fallot

Most common congenital heart lesion over the age of 1 year characterized by the following four signs:

1. VSD
2. RV outflow narrowing
3. Overriding aorta
4. RV hypertrophy

▶ H&P Keys

Growth retardation, cardiac murmurs, cardiac arrhythmias, polycythemia and cyanosis, exercise limitation with squatting maneuver to restore normal breathing, clubbing, thrill at left sternal border.

▶ Diagnosis

Physical exam, chest roentgenogram, ECG (RV hypertrophy), two-dimensional echo, cardiac catheterization.

▶ Disease Severity

Activity level, growth, ABG, mentation, heart rate, cyanosis and pedal edema, heart size, CHF, syncope.

▶ Concept and Application

Caused by the combination and severity of characteristic abnormalities; the degree of obstruction at the right ventricular outflow tract (RVOT), shunting at the level of the VSD, amount of blood from RV and LV to the aorta.

▶ Treatment Steps
1. Total surgical correction.
2. Bacterial endocarditis prophylaxis.

## D. Coarctation of the Aorta

Narrowing of aortic lumen, usually at level just below left subclavian artery (ligamentum arteriosum).

▶ H&P Keys

More common in males. Differential development of upper and lower body, differential pulses in upper and lower extremities, a cause of secondary hypertension.

▶ Diagnosis

Brachial and femoral artery pulses, blood pressure in upper versus lower extremities, chest roentgenogram (rib notching), two-dimensional echo in children, aortography, CT scan.

▶ Disease Severity

Depends on extent of luminal narrowing. Severe hypertension may result, producing headache, CHF, CNS hemorrhage. Lower extremity claudication, aortic rupture possible. May be associated with bicuspid aortic valve (AS or AR).

▶ Concept and Application

Congenital. Narrowing of aorta at the level of the ligamentum arteriosum.

▶ Treatment Steps

1. Surgical correction optimally at age 4 to 8.
2. Bacterial endocarditis prophylaxis.

## X. CARDIAC LIFE SUPPORT

Cardiopulmonary arrest is the cessation of effective cardiac function resulting in hemodynamic collapse. In children, a pulmonary etiology is most common, whereas in adults a cardiac etiology (eg, ventricular tachycardia or ventricular fibrillation) is the most common.

▶ H&P Keys

Dizziness, dyspnea, palpitations, chest pain may precede cardiac arrest and loss of consciousness that is not spontaneously terminated. Examination: cyanotic, pulseless, unconscious, or unarousable patient with absent or agonal respirations. Children often are cyanotic.

▶ Diagnosis

Most cardiopulmonary arrests occur outside the hospital and are fatal. Only 25% of cardiopulmonary arrest victims survive to hospital admission. Cardiopulmonary arrest victims are identified as unresponsive and pulseless patients. ECG, electrolytes, myocardial enzymes, and cyanosis.

▶ Disease Severity

Duration of cardiopulmonary arrest time, ie, time to resuscitation.

▶ Concept and Application

*Children*—Sudden infant death syndrome (SIDS) may be multifactorial; pulmonary failure may be secondary to obstruction of airways.

*Adult*—VT or ventricular fibrillation (VF) secondary to acute and chronic CAD. Often associated with depressed LV function resulting from acute or prior MI.

▶ Management

*Basic Life Support (BLS)—ABC*
1. Airway: Check for patency and obstruction.
2. Breathing: Ventilate.
3. Circulation: Reestablish with external compression.
4. Repetitive cycles of ventilation and external compression, punctuated by assessing for spontaneous ventilation and pulse, continued until Advanced Cardiac Life Support team available.

*Advanced Cardiac Life Support (ACLS)*
1. Arrhythmia recognition ("quick look" with defibrillator paddles or ECG) and appropriate treatment with electrical cardioversion (VT: 50 to 200 J), or defibrillation (VF: 200 to 360 J).
2. Continued BLS.
3. Use of adjunctive equipment including performing endotracheal intubation for improved ventilation and placement of intravenous lines.
4. Initiation of pharmacologic therapy, including IV fluids (normal saline) epinephrine (1:10,000), lidocaine, procainamide, amiodarone, dopamine, norepinephrine.

## XI. HYPERTENSION

Hypertension is defined as a diastolic pressure greater than 90 and a systolic pressure greater than 140. Severe hypertension includes a diastolic blood pressure greater than 115. Hypertension is an important public health problem and a major cause of CHF. Uncontrolled hypertension is associated with a marked reduction in life expectancy.

### A. Essential Hypertension

The etiology is unknown in 95% of patients with essential hypertension. There is a strong family occurrence.

▶ H&P Keys

The vast majority of patients are asymptomatic. Symptoms of occipital headache are seen with severe hypertension. Other associated symptoms reflect end-organ damage, eg, hematuria, blurring of vision, CHF. Exam is tailored to detect evidence of end-organ damage, eg, retinal hemorrhages, $S_4$, $S_3$.

▶ Diagnosis

All patients with hypertension should have urinalysis for protein, blood, potassium, creatinine, BUN, and an ECG for evidence of LV hypertrophy. Other testing is performed to exclude a suspected secondary cause.

▶ Disease Severity

Evidence of end-organ damage including CNS, renal, and cardiac dysfunction.

*CNS*—Lacunar infarcts and stroke.

*Renal*—Elevated creatinine, BUN.

*Cardiac*—LV hypertrophy, cardiomegaly. CHF, MI, aortic enlargement, and aortic dissection. Natural history depends on the level of blood pressure and the extent and severity of organ involvement.

### ▶ Concept and Application

The cause of essential hypertension remains unknown. Possible mechanisms include complex multifactorial genetic factors as well as abnormal responsiveness to sodium and calcium. Associated with diabetes and obesity.

### ▶ Treatment Steps

Both isolated systolic and diastolic hypertension should be treated.

1. In general, weight reduction in the obese patient and some restriction in salt are often very valuable in control. Step therapy has been evaluated over a 25-year period, with evidence of improved life expectancy.
2. Diuretics and β-blockers improve outcomes and are recommended as the initial drug choices.
3. Other agents including ACE inhibitors and calcium antagonists are useful as secondary agents.
4. As severity increases, anti-adrenergic drugs such as clonidine and vasodilators (eg, minoxidil) may be valuable.

## B. Secondary Hypertension

A host of disease entities produce hypertension, including endocrine abnormalities, such as adrenal cortical hyperfunction (Cushing's disease), primary hyperaldosteronism, and pheochromocytoma; neurogenic, renal vascular, and parenchymal diseases; and entities associated with increasing stroke volume, eg, hyperthyroidism and aortic insufficiency.

### ▶ H&P Keys

Wide-ranging disease process may be detected such as Cushingoid features, episodic marked elevation in blood pressure in pheochromocytoma, polyuria, polydipsia, and muscle weakness secondary to hypokalemia.

### ▶ Diagnosis

BUN, creatinine level, thyroid-stimulating hormone (TSH) level, renal artery Doppler flow studies or angiography, urine and plasma catecholamine levels, plasma renin activity, serum and urine catecholamine levels.

### ▶ Disease Severity

Depends on specific etiology and its natural history as well as response of the blood pressure to therapy.

### ▶ Concept and Application

Elevations of catecholamine levels, activation of the renin–angiotensin system with vasoconstriction, excessive sodium retention in primary and secondary aldosteronism, and excessive glucocorticoid production.

### ▶ Treatment Steps
1. Renal artery stenosis may respond to angioplasty or surgery, especially in patients with high renin from the affected kidney and suppression of renin production in the uninvolved kidney.
2. Other secondary forms, eg, pheochromocytoma and Cushing's disease, can be cured with surgical removal of the tumor.
3. ACE Inhibitors may worsen renal functions in patients with bilateral renal artery stenosis, and renal function must be followed in everyone who receives these agents.

## C. Malignant Hypertension
Sudden and severe elevation of blood pressure with evidence of acute end-organ damage. Includes hypertensive encephalopathy, rapidly deteriorating renal function, and acute CHF.

### ▶ H&P Keys
Visual disturbances, severe headache, confusion, coma, seizures, edema, dyspnea, blood pressure greater than 200/115, papilledema, hemorrhage, and spasm on ophthalmoscopic exam, $S_3$ gallop, oliguria.

### ▶ Diagnosis
BUN, creatinine levels, peripheral smear for microangiopathic hemolytic anemia, chest roentgenographic evidence of CHF.

### ▶ Disease Severity
Depends on the extent and severity of end-organ damage and may include stroke, refractory pulmonary edema, and progressive oliguric renal failure.

### ▶ Concept and Application
The trigger for malignant hypertension is unknown. There is widespread fibrinoid necrosis of the arterial walls. Cerebral autoregulation is impaired and cerebral blood flow is increased, which contributes to the encephalopathy.

### ▶ Treatment Steps
*Acute*
1. Nitroprusside infusion in doses of 0.5 to 8 mg/kg/min can produce rapid, graded control of blood pressure and is recommended initial therapy.
2. Also, continuous labetolol infusion in doses in the range of 2 mg/min have been effective.

*Long-Term*—Other agents for long-term control are needed.
1. Diuresis is useful to contract volume and decrease blood pressure and also to assist with CHF and encephalopathy.
2. β-Blockers, ACE inhibitors, and calcium antagonists are all effective. Renal function may deteriorate in the early phase of treatment, but persistent blood pressure control is needed to resolve the arterial lesions.

## XII. LIPOPROTEINS AND ATHEROSCLEROSIS

### A. Hyperlipoproteinemia

A wide array of disorders resulting from abnormalities in metabolism of the lipoproteins, that transport exogenously and endogenously produced cholesterol and triglycerides. The major lipoproteins are chylomicrons and very-low-density lipoproteins (VLDL), which transport triglycerides (TG), and intermediate-, low-, and high-density lipoproteins (IDL, LDL, HDL), which primarily transport cholesterol. Hyperlipoproteinemias occur as a result of a genetic defect in synthesis or degradation or secondary to diabetes, hyperthyroidism, and excessive alcohol ingestion. Classification is based on the recognized abnormality in lipoproteins and the type of lipid that accumulates in the serum (see Table 1–1).

Most important are accumulations in LDL, which are associated with premature atherosclerosis.

▶ H&P Keys

Cutaneous, tendinous, tuberous, and eruptive xanthomas, premature atherosclerosis, lipemia retinalis, and pancreatitis.

▶ Diagnosis

Examination of serum for creamy, chylomicron layer, measurement of serum lipids, eg, cholesterol, TG, HDL, and LDL. High LDL is associated with an increased risk of atherosclerosis and MI. Occasionally, lipoprotein electrophoresis is required for definitive characterization.

▶ Disease Severity

The extent of atherosclerosis and its complications include MI, stroke, peripheral vascular disease. Patients with high level of TG frequently develop recurrent pancreatitis.

▶ Concept and Application

In familial hypercholesterolemia, premature, accelerated atherosclerosis and MI occurs in the third or fourth decade. The hyperlipoproteinemias are genetically transmitted as a result of single or multiple gene disorders.

### 1-1 LIPOPROTEIN ABNORMALITY TYPES

| Type | Lipoprotein Abnormality | Lipid Accumulation |
| --- | --- | --- |
| I | Chylomicrons | TG |
| IIA | LDL | Cholesterol |
| IIB | LDL and VLDL | Cholesterol and TG |
| III | Chylomicrons and IDL | TG and cholesterol |
| IV | VLDL | TG |
| V | VLDL and chylomicrons | TG and cholesterol |

▶ Treatment Steps

*General*
1. Dietary restriction of fats and weight reduction.
2. Control of secondary factors, eg, cessation of alcohol, optimum control of diabetes.
3. Elimination of other risk factors for CAD.

*Drug Therapy*—Dependent on lipid abnormality, severity, other coronary risk factors, and associated disease. In patients with known atherosclerosis or significant, multiple risk factors, lipid therapy should be considered when the LDL > 100 mg/dL. HMG Co A reductase inhibitors are the most effective agents and have been demonstrated to substantially reduce atherosclerotic event rates and are widely used for both primary and secondary prevention. Available agents include:

1. Cholestyramine. Not absorbed. Binds bile acids in the gut, stimulating conversion of cholesterol to bile.
2. Nicotinic acid. Reduces production of VLDL by liver and lowers LDL, HDL, and TGs.
3. 3-Hydroxy-3-methylglutaryl coenzyme A (HMG CoA)-reductase-inhibitors. Lower LDL by blocking endogenous cholesterol biosynthesis.
4. Fibric acid derivatives gemfibrozil and clofibrate. Increase breakdown of VLDL and IDL, hence lower TGs and increase HDL cholesterol.

## B. Atherosclerosis

Results as a response to injury of vascular endothelium with thrombus formation. Initially, isolated macrophages or foam cells infiltrate endothelium. Later, lipid-rich lesions with smooth muscle and fibrous collagen cap form mature atheromatous plaque. Acute coronary syndromes (unstable angina and MI) occur when there is acute plaque rupture and thrombus formation.

▶ H&P Keys

Anginal chest pain, stroke syndromes with neurologic deficits, including motor or sensory abnormalities, intermittent claudication, reduction in peripheral pulses and pressure.

▶ Diagnosis

ECG, stress testing, and myocardial perfusion imaging, noninvasive vascular assessment, including carotids, arterial Doppler, cardiac catheterization, and angiography (Fig. 1–1).

▶ Disease Severity

Extent of motor and sensory deficit after stroke, impairment in cardiac function after MI, exercise limitation, claudication.

▶ Concept and Application

The development of atherosclerosis is multifactorial and related to injury of the endothelium as well as the factors that enhance thrombosis. Endothelial cells produce a variety of substances that cause vasoconstriction and smooth-muscle proliferation. Acute plaque disruption occurs as a result of alterations of stress at the

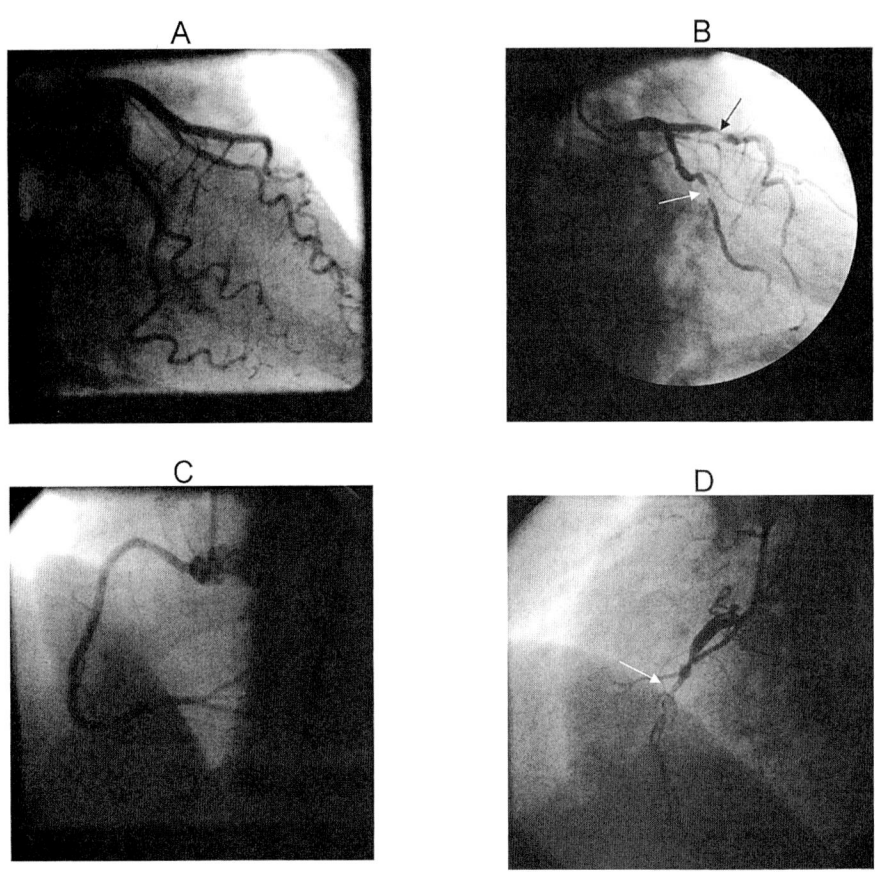

Figure 1–1. Normal coronary angiogram of left coronary (A) and right coronary (C). Figure B and D arrows point to atherosclerotic narrowing in abnormal left and right coronary arteries.

plaque surface. Exposure of damaged vessel wall leads to the adherence of platelets, development of thrombus, and ultimately, occlusion of the vessel.

▶ Treatment Steps
1. Prevention of atherosclerosis and plaque rupture with thrombosis is complex and requires multiple interventions. Major risk factors include cigarette smoking, hypertension, diabetes, and elevated cholesterol. Management is directed at eliminating these risk factors. Thrombosis is enhanced by catecholamines (stress), cigarette smoking, and familial predisposition.
2. Aspirin therapy is effective in both primary and secondary prevention.

## XIII. PERIPHERAL ARTERIAL VASCULAR DISEASE

### A. Chronic Atherosclerotic Occlusion

Associated with generalized atherosclerosis and frequently coexists with CAD as well as cerebral vascular disease.

▶ H&P Keys

Intermittent claudication (exertional calf, thigh, and buttocks discomfort), rest pain with more severe reduction in blood flow, subclavian steal syndrome, reduction in blood pressure in affected limb (or limbs), decreased or absent pulses, vascular bruits over subclavian aorta or femoral arteries. Elevational pallor, dependent rubor, and prolonged venous filling time of the legs. Ulcers and gangrene.

▶ Diagnosis

Doppler pressure measurements before and after exercise and calculation of ankle-brachial index, pulse volume recordings (PVR), peripheral angiography, computed tomography, and magnetic resonance angiography.

▶ Disease Severity

Severe if ankle-brachial index less than 0.4. Resting ischemia, ulcerations, and gangrene. Recurrent neurologic symptoms with subclavian steal syndrome.

▶ Concept and Application

Progressive atherosclerotic lesions produce reduction in blood flow to the affected limbs. Associated with generalized atherosclerosis. Steal syndrome (exercise induced neurologic symptoms, eg, presyncope) results from a lesion in left subclavian before the vertebral artery and exercise results in "steal" of blood from the cerebral circulation to the arm.

▶ Treatment Steps

*Medical*
1. Control of atherosclerotic risk factors.
2. Smoking cessation most important.
3. Exercise may stimulate collateral blood flow. Vasodilators are generally ineffective.
4. Pentoxifylline improves exercise ability in approximately one third of patients.

*Surgical*
1. Revascularization with bypass procedure or angioplasty for limiting symptoms or for limb salvage.
2. Sympathectomy for pain relief.
3. Amputation for serverely damaged ischemic limbs.

## B. Acute Arterial Occlusion

Sudden cessation of blood flow as a result of an embolus, acute thrombosis, or vasospasm.

▶ H&P Keys

Appropriate setting with sudden onset of pain, then loss of sensation, paralysis and cool, cyanotic, mottled limb.

▶ Diagnosis

Doppler studies, angiography, two-dimensional echo to evaluate thrombolytic source.

▶ **Disease Severity**
Occlusion of an artery to an extremity leads to paralysis, cyanosis, and loss of viability with tissue necrosis, ulceration, and gangrene.

▶ **Concept and Application**
Majority of emboli are from cardiac sources. Intracardiac thrombosis occurs in MI and atrial fibrillation; also in valvular disease, especially MS and prosthetic valves. Acute and chronic bacterial endocarditis and vegetations may embolize. A "paradoxical" embolus may occur with an ASD. Large-vessel occlusion occurs with bulky vegetations, especially in fungal endocarditis. Acute thrombosis occurs in some infectious diseases, especially rickettsial, eg, Rocky Mountain spotted fever, connective tissue disease, and hypercoagulable states.

▶ **Treatment Steps**
1. Heparin administration.
2. Prompt evaluation with arteriography and embolectomy.
3. After reperfusion, especially in the leg muscle compartments, fasciotomy may be necessary to relieve compressive symptoms.
4. Additional therapy may be required after the source of embolus is identified, eg, valve replacement for mitral stenosis or acute endocarditis.

## C. Vasculitis Syndromes

Encompasses a wide variety of conditions, characterized by inflammation of the blood vessel wall. The syndromes include:

1. Necrotizing vasculitis: polyarteritis nodosa.
2. Hypersensitivity angitis.
3. Giant cell arteritis: Takayasu's, temporal arteritis.
4. Other: thromboangiitis obliterans; mucocutaneous lymph node syndrome.

▶ **H&P Keys**
Wide-ranging because arterial thrombosis can affect any organ system. Systemic signs and symptoms include: fever, weight loss, arthritis, organ dysfunction from occlusion of cerebral vessel limb or digital arteries, absent or decreased pulses, differential blood pressures, vascular bruits. Also, elevated sedimentation rate, leukocytosis.

▶ **Diagnosis**
Arterial biopsy, eg, in temporal arteritis to confirm vessel inflammation. Arterial Doppler studies, PVR, and aortography.

▶ **Disease Severity**
Dependent on extent and severity of organ dysfunction or compromising blood flow to the limbs. Patients may develop stroke, gangrenous bowel, MI, ischemia to limbs and digits.

▶ **Concept and Application**
In general, vasculitis occurs because of immune injury. There is a deposition of immune complexes in the arterial wall, which initiates an acute inflammatory response that leads to thrombosis. There also may be cell-mediated vascular injury.

▶ Treatment Steps
1. Many of these entities respond partially to treatment with systemic glucocorticoids, eg, temporal arteritis and Takayasu's disease.
2. Occasionally, responses are seen from other cytotoxic agents.
3. Cessation of smoking in thromboangiitis.
4. Sympathectomy is of value to relieve pain.

## XIV. PERIPHERAL VENOUS VASCULAR DISEASES AND PULMONARY EMBOLISM

### A. Venous Thrombosis

Occurs in a wide variety of settings. Predisposing factors include trauma or surgery, especially orthopedic, prolonged bed rest for any reason, pregnancy, and a variety of neoplasms. The disease commonly affects the lower extremities, although upper extremities can be involved.

▶ H&P Keys

Recognition of the appropriate setting and predisposing factors. Clinical signs, calf swelling, tenderness, and warmth, are nonspecific and frequently missed.

*Superficial Venous Thrombosis*—Hot, red, swollen visible vein.

*Chronic*—Leg swelling and superficial varicosities.

▶ Disease Severity

*Acute*—Pulmonary embolus is the primary risk; however recurrent deep venous thrombosis (DVT) can lead to a chronic state.

*Chronic*—Refractory edema, stasis ulceration with superimposed chronic cellulitis.

▶ Diagnosis

Impedance plethysmography, Doppler ultrasonography, ventilation perfusion lung scan, spiral CT, and pulmonary angiography.

▶ Concepts and Application

Virchow described the triad of venous thrombosis: (1) abnormality of the vascular wall; (2) stasis of blood flow; and (3) hypercoagulable state. Thrombosis may occur because of deficiency of antithrombin III or fibrinolytic proteins C and S, a circulating lupus anticoagulant, and homocystinuria.

▶ Treatment Steps

*Acute*
1. Heparin in continuous infusion for 7 to 10 days, adjusted so partial thromboplastin time (PTT) is approximately two times control value.

*Chronic*
1. Anticoagulation for 6 to 12 months with warfarin, longer (indefinite) if DVT recurs.
2. Elevation of legs when possible.
3. Full waist-length, graduated compression stockings.
4. Meticulous skin care.

*Prophylaxis*
1. With 5,000 U heparin every 8 to 12 hours in high-risk clinical situations needs to be initiated prior to surgical procedure.
2. Below-the-knee thrombosis can be followed if no proximal venous disease is detected; anticoagulation may not be required.

## B. Pulmonary Embolism

A common event in hospitalized patients, frequently unrecognized, with high morbidity and mortality.

### ► H&P Keys
Sudden dyspnea, pleuritic chest pain, hemoptysis, syncope, unexplained tachycardia, supraventricular dysrhythmias, pulmonary hypertension with a right ventricular lift, wide, persistent splitting and loud pulmonic component of the second heart sound.

### ► Diagnosis

*ECG*—Nonspecific ST-T wave changes, right axis deviation.

*Chest Roentgenogram*—Dilatation of pulmonary artery, abrupt cutoff. Ventilation perfusion lung scan, pulmonary angiogram, detection of DVT.

### ► Disease Severity
The size of the embolus and the resultant extent and severity of obstruction of the pulmonary arteries. Hemodynamic deterioration can occur with shock and peripheral hypoperfusion and is more severe with preexisting heart or lung disease. Impairment of gas exchange and arterial hypoxemia.

### ► Concept and Application
The majority of pulmonary embolisms occur in the setting of DVT. Embolization of clot from below the knee is unusual. The best approach to the disease is prophylaxis, prevention, early detection, and treatment of DVT.

### ► Treatment Steps
1. Heparin, with initial dose of 5,000 U and continuous infusion to maintain PTT approximately two times control.
2. Intermittent regimens can be employed.
3. With recurrent embolization or contraindication to anticoagulant therapy, venal caval filter or plication is effective in prevention of further emboli.
4. If severe hemodynamic compromise occurs, thrombolytic therapy with streptokinase (initial bolus of 250,000 U and 24-hour infusion) is favored over acute embolectomy.

## XV. DISEASES OF THE AORTA

### A. Aneurysms

Pathologic dilatation of a segment of a blood vessel. A true aneurysm involves all three layers of the vessel wall and is distinguished from a pseudoaneurysm, which involves only the intima and media. Classified by their location and gross appearance: thoracic versus abdominal, and fusiform versus saccular.

▶ **H&P Keys**

Most aneurysms are asymptomatic. Symptoms of pain may be produced by expanding aneurysms; often a harbinger of rupture and an acute medical emergency. Acute rupture may occur without warning and is always life threatening. Compression of contiguous blood vessels may result in other symptoms, including stroke from compression of carotid vessels in thoracic aortic aneurysms and impairment of lower-extremity blood flow in expanding abdominal aortic aneurysms.

*Abdominal Aortic Aneurysms*—Presence of palpable, pulsatile, and tender abdominal mass with abdominal bruit.

*Thoracic Aortic Aneurysms*—Tracheal deviation, hoarseness, and CHF because of aortic dilatation and resulting aortic regurgi-

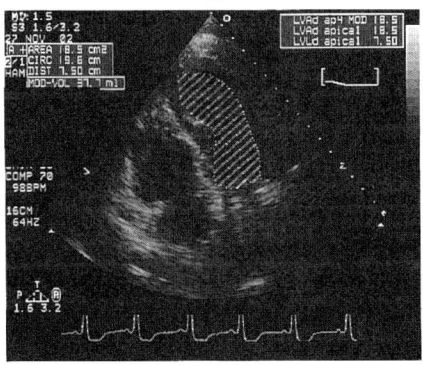 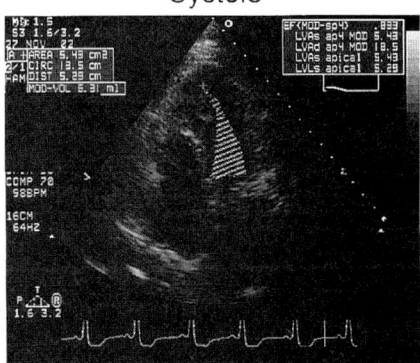
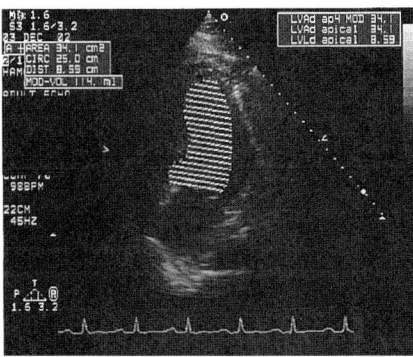 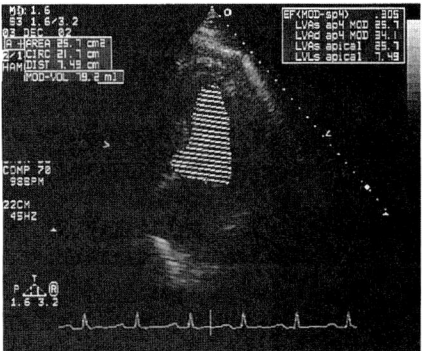

Figure 1–2. Echocardiograms recorded in end-diastolic and end-systolic in a normal ventricle (upper panel) with uniform systolic contraction and a normal ejection fraction and an abnormal ventricle with reduced contraction during systole. The cross-hatched areas outline the left ventricular cavities.

tation. Patients with abdominal aneurysms may also have distal arterial embolization and lower-extremity claudication. Most abdominal aneurysms occur distal to the renal arteries.

### ▶ Diagnosis

Radiography including chest roentgenogram and abdominal films may demonstrate the enlarged aorta sometimes outlined by calcium. More definitive studies include thoracic and abdominal ultrasonography, CT scan, and MRI scan. Thoracic and abdominal aortography are often performed prior to surgery to outline the extent of aneurysm.

### ▶ Disease Severity

Determined by location, size of aneurysm, and rate of dilatation. For abdominal aneurysms exceeding 6 cm in diameter, the 2-year mortality related to rupture is approximately 50%, and for those 4 to 6 cm in diameter, 25%.

### ▶ Concept and Application

Atherosclerosis is the most common cause of aortic aneurysm. Abdominal aortic aneurysms are almost always due to atherosclerosis, whereas those of the ascending thoracic aorta may be caused by cystic medial necrosis, atherosclerosis, syphilis, bacterial infections, or rheumatic aortitis. Aneurysms of the descending thoracic aorta that are contiguous with infradiaphragmatic aneurysms are usually due to atherosclerosis.

### ▶ Treatment Steps

1. Location and extent of the aneurysm using radiographic imaging techniques (CT scan, MRI, aortography).
2. Followed by operative excision of the aneurysm and replacement with graft.
3. Reimplantation of branch vessels is often necessary.

## B. Aortic Dissection

Caused by a transverse or circumferential tear of the aortic intima in areas with high shear forces (left subclavian artery and right lateral ascending aortic wall).

- Type 1. Dissection in proximal aorta, may extend into the arch.
- Type 2. Dissection limited to aortic arch.
- Type 3. Dissection begins distal to left subclavian artery and extends for variable distance inferiorly.

### ▶ H&P Keys

Acute dissection is characterized by a sudden onset of severe and tearing pain associated with diaphoresis. Pain usually from front of chest to interscapular area. May be associated with syncope, dyspnea, or weakness. Blood pressure may be high or low. Other signs include differential pulses, pulmonary edema, neurologic symptoms (stroke or spinal cord compression), aortic regurgitation producing CHF. Abdominal aortic dissection may be accompanied by bowel ischemia and hematuria, whereas thoracic dissection may be accompanied by superior vena caval syndrome, hoarseness, airway compromise, dysphagia, inferior MI with hemopericardium and cardiac tamponade.

▶ Diagnosis
Chest roentgenogram, ECG, CT scan, MRI, and aortography.

▶ Disease Severity
Physical examination for involvement of brain, peripheral arteries, kidneys, spinal cord, heart. Continued pain or symptoms of compromise to major arterial branches indicate active propagation of dissection. Hypotension or shock, oliguria, mentation.

▶ Concept and Application
Disruption of aortic intima, possibly related to medial hemorrhage at areas with high shear forces. Pulsatile flow dissects along elastic laminar plates of aorta, creating false lumen. Underlying condition may be related to cystic medial necrosis of aortic wall or collagen dysfunction (Marfan syndrome).

▶ Treatment Steps
1. Emergency operation is indicated for patients with symptoms indicating propagating dissection. Emergency operation carries a high mortality, but active propagation is often fatal if not stabilized.
2. Stabilization with medical therapy, including β-blockers and afterload-reducing agents (nitroprusside), is preferred for ≥ 14 days if possible before surgical correction.
3. For patients with stable and uncomplicated distal aortic dissection, medical therapy is preferred and includes long-term use of β-blockers and orally administered afterload-reducing agents.

## C. Aortic Occlusion
Chronic occlusive disease that generally involves the distal abdominal aorta below the renal arteries.

▶ H&P Keys
Claudication, impotence in males (Leriche's syndrome). Symptoms vary depending on presence and adequacy of collateral blood flow. Physical findings include absent or depressed femoral and distal pulses and presence of bruits over abdominal aorta and femoral arteries. Lower-extremity skin loss, atrophic skin changes, cool extremities, peripheral skin ulcerations.

▶ Diagnosis
Physical examination, noninvasive Doppler evaluation of arterial blood flow, ankle-brachial index (ABI) (sphygmomanometry). Abdominal aortography to define anatomy prior to revascularization.

▶ Disease Severity
Dependent on collateral blood flow.

▶ Concept and Application
Atherosclerotic; nonatheromatous disease may be associated with smoking (Buerger's disease or thromboangiitis obliterans) or homocystinuria, especially in young adults.

▶ Treatment Steps
1. Preoperative assessment by aortography and surgical revascularization.
2. Cessation of smoking and modification of diet are important in stabilizing this progressive disease.

### D. Aortitis
Syphilitic, rheumatic, Takayasu's disease, giant cell aortitis.

#### 1. Syphilitic Aortitis
Usually affecting the proximal aorta, resulting in aortic root dilatation and aneurysm formation.

▶ H&P Keys
Often asymptomatic. As it progresses, may cause compression and erosion into adjacent structures; rupture may occur.

▶ Diagnosis
Chest roentgenogram, two-dimensional echo, cardiac catheterization, immunologic screening, rapid plasma reagin (RPR), Venereal Disease Research Laboratory (VDRL).

▶ Disease Severity
Long latency period: 15 to 30 years after initial infection. Symptoms may occur from aortic regurgitation or narrowing of coronary ostia or from compression to adjacent structures (esophagus), or rupture. Serologic tests confirm diagnosis. Evaluation includes chest roentgenogram, ultrasonography, CT scan, MRI, and aortography.

▶ Concept and Application
Destruction of collagen elastic tissue, leading to dilatation of aorta with scar formation and calcification, is due to obliterative endarteritis of the vasa vasorum in the adventitia. This is an inflammatory response to invasion of the adventitia by spirochetes.

▶ Treatment Steps
1. Antibiotic treatment (penicillin).
2. Surgical excision and repair.

#### 2. Rheumatic Aortitis
Includes rheumatoid arthritis, ankylosing spondylitis, psoriatic arthritis, Reiter's syndrome, Behçet's syndrome, relapsing polychondritis, and inflammatory bowel disorders.

#### 3. Takayasu's Aortitis
An inflammatory disease of the aortic arch resulting in obstruction of the aorta and its major branches. Also termed pulseless disease, a panarteritis with marked intimal hyperplasia. Usually found in young females of Asian descent and associated with fever, malaise, weight loss, and other systemic symptoms. ESR is elevated. Symptoms chronically include upper-extremity claudication, syncope, cerebral ischemia. No definitive therapy; the disease is progressive. Surgical bypass of stenotic arteries may be necessary, and anticoagulation to prevent thrombosis may be advisable.

4. Giant Cell Aortitis

An inflammatory disorder infecting large and medium-sized arteries and resulting in focal granulomatous lesions. It may be associated with polymyalgia rheumatica. Obstruction of medium-sized arteries, including the temporal and ophthalmic arteries, may occur.

▶ H&P Keys

Fever, malaise, myalgias, headache, jaw pain, scalp tenderness, visual changes.

▶ Diagnosis

Elevated ESR, anemia. Biopsy of arterial wall.

▶ Disease Severity

Symptoms related to involvement of branch vessels.

▶ Concept and Application

Inflammation, poorly understood.

▶ Treatment Steps

1. Long-term corticosteroids.

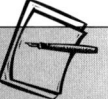

▶ on rounds

## CARDIOLOGY AT A GLANCE

### Myocardial Infarction
- Chest pain, diaphoresis, 20% without pain
- Transmural or Q wave has ST segment elevation and T wave inversions
- Non-transmural has ST segment elevation and T wave inversions.
- CK-MB peaks at 24 hours
- AST or SGOT peaks at 48–72 hours
- LHD peaks at 3–5 days

### Prinzmetal's or Variant Angina
- Angina at rest
- Younger patients
- ECG positive for ST elevation during symptoms
- Gold standard diagnostic test: Spasm on angiography
- Treatment: Nitrates, calcium channel blockers, stop smoking, avoid cocaine

### Signs of Heart Failure
#### Left Side, Low Output
- Fatigue, dyspnea, PND, orthopnea
- $S_3$ or $S_4$, displaced cardiac impulse, CXR, echo

#### Left Side, High Output
- Brisk pulse, dyspnea, orthopnea, hyperdynamic circulation

#### Right Side
- Fatigue, RV heave, JVD, hepatomegaly, atrial arrhythmias
- ECG may show RV or RA hypertrophy
- Echo may show RV dilation and hypokinesis

# BIBLIOGRAPHY

ACC/AHA Guidelines
1. Guidelines for the early management of patients with acute myocardial infarction. *Circulation* 1999;100:1016.
2. Guideline update for the management of patients with unstable angina and non-ST segment elevation myocardial infarction. *J Am Coll Card* 2002;40:1366.
3. Guidelines for the evaluation and management of chronic heart failure in the adult. *Circulation* 2001;104:2996.

Braunwald E. *Heart Disease: A Textbook of Cardiovascular Medicine*. 6th ed. Philadelphia: Saunders; 2001.

Fuster V et al (eds.) *Hurst's The Heart*. 10th ed. New York: McGraw-Hill Information Services Co; 2000.

Loh E, McClellan JR. Congestive heart failure. In: Conn et al (eds.) *Current Diagnosis*. Orlando, FL: Saunders; 2003.

McClellan JR: Clinical approach to the patient in shock. In Chizner M (ed) Cedar Grove, NJ: Laennec Publishing; 1996.

# Dermatology 2

I. **ACUTE EXANTHEMS / 46**
   A. Varicella (Chickenpox) / 46
   B. Varicella Zoster (Shingles) / 46

II. **OTHER SKIN INFECTIONS / 47**
   A. Mycoses / 47
   B. Bacterial Infections / 49
   C. Viral Infections / 51
   D. Secondary Syphilis / 52

III. **SKIN ERUPTIONS / 53**
   A. Inflammatory Conditions of Skin / 53
   B. Blistering Diseases / 58
   C. Other Diseases of the Skin and Subcutaneous Tissues / 61
   D. Symptoms Involving the Skin / 62
   E. Insect Bites (Nonvenomous) and Ectoparasites / 63

IV. **NAILS AND HAIR / 66**
   A. Ingrowing Nails / 66
   B. Other Diseases of Hair and the Hair Follicle / 67

V. **TUMORS OF THE SKIN / 69**
   A. Premalignant and Malignant Neoplasms of Skin / 69
   B. Benign Neoplasms / 72
   C. Follicular Cyst (Epidermal, Pilar, Sebaceous Cyst) / 75

VI. **OTHER CONDITIONS / 76**
   A. Acquired Keratoderma (Tylosis) / 76
   B. Decubitus Ulcer / 77
   C. Ulcers of the Lower Limbs / 77
   D. Cutaneous Manifestations of Systemic Disease / 79
   E. Cutaneous Signs of Internal Malignant Neoplasms / 83
   F. Nail Signs and Disease / 84
   G. Diseases and Disorders of Newborns / 85

**BIBLIOGRAPHY / 86**

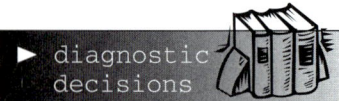

## diagnostic decisions

### VESICULAR ERUPTIONS

**Varicella**
Constitutional symptoms, recent exposure, nonclustered teardrop vesicles on pink base, older lesions crusted, generally heal without scar, favor head and trunk, multinucleated giant cells on Tzanck smear, culture shows VZV. Direct fluorescent antibody test is rapid and specific.

**Zoster**
Prodrome of pain and paresthesia at site, prior Varicella infection, grouped vesicles on pink base distributed linearly within a single dermatome, unilateral, heals with crusts and often scars. Trigeminal zoster associated with conjunctivitis and keratitis. Sacral involvement can lead to urine retention, post-herpetic neuralgia common, multinucleated giant cells on Tzanck smear, culture shows VZV. Direct fluorescent antibody test is rapid and specific.

**Herpes simplex**
Primary infection in childhood asymptomatic, secondary infection commonly manifests as recurrent cold sores on the lip (herpes labialis), many triggers including systemic illness and sunlight, small clustered vesicles preceded by pruritus and discomfort in the involved area, heals with erosions and crusts, multinucleated giant cells on Tzanck smear, culture shows HSV. Direct fluorescent antibody test is rapid and specific.

## I. ACUTE EXANTHEMS

### A. Varicella (Chickenpox)

▶ **H&P Keys**
Rash begins on face and scalp and rapidly spreads to trunk, with relative sparing of extremities. Typical lesions are vesicles with a pink base, but presence of lesions at all stages of development (macules, papules, vesicles, pustules, crusted lesions) is characteristic. Fever, chills, malaise, and headache may accompany. Mucous membranes may be affected.

▶ **Diagnosis**
History and physical exam. Confirm if necessary with Tzanck smear demonstrating multinucleated giant cells, viral culture, direct fluorescent antibody test.

▶ **Disease Severity**
Mildest cases in infants and most severe cases in adults. Fever correlates with disease severity. Prolonged fever may be associated with complications such as pneumonia. Scarring is more likely in adults.

▶ **Concept and Application**
Viral entry through mucosa of upper respiratory tract and oropharynx, primary (incubation) and secondary (infection) viremia. Humoral and cellular immune response terminates viremia; immunity is complex and antibody alone does not guarantee total immunity. A live attenuated vaccine is available.

▶ **Treatment Steps**
1. Symptomatic: cool compresses, topical anti-pruritic lotion, antihistamines, analgesics (acetaminophen in children).
2. Antibiotics if secondary infection develops. Acyclovir or derivative for infections in adult or immunocompromised. Varicella-zoster immune globulin can be used in immunocompromised patients up to 3 days after exposure.

### B. Varicella Zoster (Shingles)

▶ **H&P Keys**
Prodrome of pain and paresthesia in involved dermatome (may simulate pleurisy, myocardial infarction, peptic ulcer, renal colic); typical rash is localized, unilateral, does not cross midline, grouped vesicles on a pink base that evolve into pustules and crusts (Fig. 2–1).

▶ **Diagnosis**
Same as varicella.

▶ **Disease Severity**
Pain is more severe in elderly patients; disease is more severe in immunocompromised (skin necrosis and scarring, postherpetic neuralgia, dissemination).

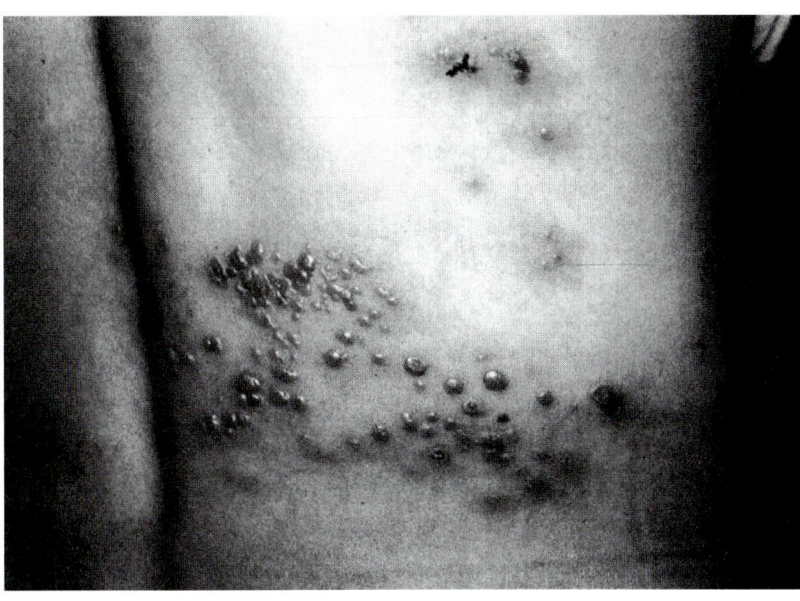

Figure 2–1. Varicella-zoster. Some lesions in this example are hemorrhagic.

▶ Concept and Application
Infection is a recrudescence of latent infection with varicella-zoster virus, passed to the skin and mucosa by sensory nerves from dorsal ganglia; cellular immunity is more important in host resistance (increased incidence of infection in patients with HIV or defects in cellular immunity).

▶ Treatment Steps
1. Acyclovir or derivative for 7 days, analgesics, topicals as in varicella.
2. Post-herpetic neuralgia: capsaicin cream, tricyclic antidepressants, gabapentin. For severe pain, consider nerve blocks.

## II. OTHER SKIN INFECTIONS

### A. Mycoses

#### 1. Dermatophytosis

▶ H&P Keys
Contact with infected person or animals, typical annular reddish scaly plaques with central clearing, hair loss with scalp involvement (tinea capitis); fissures, scales, or blisters with foot involvement (tinea pedis).

▶ Diagnosis
Potassium hydroxide (KOH) preparation, fungal culture, Wood's light (some cases of tinea capitis).

▶ Disease Severity
Toenails involved (onychomycosis) usually with tinea pedis; hand infection usually accompanied by tinea pedis; extensive or

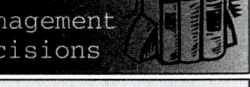
▶ management decisions

**FUNGAL INFECTIONS**

**Tinea capitis**
Topicals ineffective. Treat with systemic agents for 4–8 weeks or until cultures are negative. Griseofulvin is the gold standard, but other oral agents, itraconazole, terbinafine, and fluconazole are alternatives. Addition of shampoo such as selenium sulfide improves outcome.

**Tinea corporis, tinea pedis, tinea manuum**
Mild, localized cases respond to treatment with topical imidazole or allylamine. More extensive disease requires systemic treatment.

**Onychomycosis**
Topical therapies not effective. Itraconazole pulse dosed (first week of the month for 3 months) or terbinafine daily for 6 weeks (fingernails) or 12 weeks (toenails).

**Tinea versicolor**
Mild or localized cases often respond to topical treatment with ketoconazole and/or selenium sulfide, zinc pyrithione or sulfur shampoos. For more extensive disease, oral ketoconazole or itraconazole.

chronic involvement in immunodeficiency states and endocrine disorders (Cushing's diabetes).

▶ **Concept and Application**
Infection dependent on climatic conditions (tinea pedis more common where occlusive footwear is used; tinea corporis more common in hot, humid climates under occlusive garments), host factors (men are more susceptible), virulence of organisms.

▶ **Treatment Steps**
1. Topical antifungals for most limited infections, oral agents (eg, griseofulvin) for extensive disease and tinea capitis. Onycomycosis can be treated with itraconazole or terbinafine.
2. Recurrence or treatment failure: add or switch oral agent, check culture.

2. **Candidiasis, Oral (Thrush)**

   ▶ **H&P Keys**
   Asymptomatic, white patches resembling milk curds or cottage cheese on tongue or oral mucosa; fissuring and redness at corners of mouth (perlèche).

   ▶ **Diagnosis**
   KOH preparation, culture.

   ▶ **Disease Severity**
   Associated with use of broad-spectrum antibiotics, diabetes, malignant neoplasms, and HIV infection.

   ▶ **Concept and Application**
   *Candida albicans* is a saprophyte that colonizes the oropharynx, gastrointestinal tract, and vagina in most individuals. Susceptability to infection related to diminished host defenses.

   ▶ **Treatment Steps**
   1. Nystatin suspension or clotrimazole troches; eliminate predisposing factors.
   2. Fluconazole or itraconazole, but long-term use in immunocompromised might be associated with drug resistance.

3. **Candidiasis, Cutaneous**

   ▶ **H&P Keys**
   *Acute*—Inflammatory plaques with satellite pustules in moist, macerated folds of skin (eg, axillae, submammary).

   *Chronic*—Same as acute, but also can develop heavily crusted lesions on skin and thickened nail plate.

   ▶ **Diagnosis**
   KOH preparation, culture, pathologic studies.

   ▶ **Disease Severity**
   *Acute*—Increased predisposition in obesity, diabetes, and certain occupations (wet work: waitresses, dishwashers, housecleaners).

*Chronic*—Associated with endocrinopathies (hypoparathyroidism, hypoadrenalism, hypothyroidism), circulating autoantibodies, chronic active hepatitis, thymoma.

▶ Concept and Application
See candidiasis, oral (above). In chronic types, cell-mediated immune defect selective for *Candida*.

▶ Treatment Steps
1. Nystatin powder, topical imidazole (clotrimazole, econazole).
2. Fluconazole or itraconazole.

*Canistan*

## B. Bacterial Infections

### 1. Cellulitis, Abscess of Finger or Toe (Paronychia)

▶ H&P Keys
Redness, swelling, and/or local pus collection in nail fold.

▶ Diagnosis
Gram stain of pus, bacterial and fungal culture.

▶ Disease Severity
May cause nail-plate deformity.

▶ Concept and Application
Barrier function of nail fold (cuticle) altered by trauma and moisture. *Staph, Strep*, or *Candida* usually causative.

▶ Treatment Steps
1. Antiseptic soaks (Burow's solution), topical imidazole.
2. β-Lactamase-resistant penicillins, fluconazole.

### 2. Cellulitis, Abscess, or Other Local Infections

▶ H&P Keys

*Cellulitis*—Local area of redness, tenderness, warmth, and edema; may be accompanied by constitutional symptoms.

*Abscess*—Local pus collection with tenderness and fluctuation.

▶ Diagnosis
Culture, Gram's stain.

▶ Disease Severity
Systemic toxicity suggests bacteremia.

▶ Concept and Application

*Cellulitis*—Breaks in skin allow entry of organism; β-hemolytic *Strep* or *Staph* common in adults (erysipelas); *Haemophilus influenzae* seen in children under 2.

*Abscess*—Most often arises from an infected hair follicle (furuncle); *Staph* most common organism.

▶ Treatment Steps
1. Beta-lactamase resistant penicillin intravenously. Add gram-negative coverage in the case of underlying disease such as diabetes mellitus. Incision and drainage for abscess.
2. Adjust oral antibiotic according to culture results.

3. Impetigo

▶ H&P Keys

Golden-yellow, crusted lesions on face, nose, or around mouth (β-hemolytic *Strep, Staph*); bullous variant (*Staph*) (Fig. 2–2).

▶ Diagnosis

Bacterial culture, Gram stain.

▶ Disease Severity

Spread by close contacts. Secondary infection of preexisting skin lesions (insect bites, abrasions, herpes simplex, eczematous dermatitis) is common.

▶ Concept and Application

Highly communicable infection in which the organism induces a superficial skin blister that rapidly ruptures, forming a crust. Crowding, poor hygiene, neglected wounds, and minor trauma contribute to spread. Bullous variant caused by phage group II type 71 *Staphylococcus*.

▶ Treatment Steps
1. Topical antibiotic ointments, including mupirocin. β-Lactamase-resistant antibiotics for bullous type.

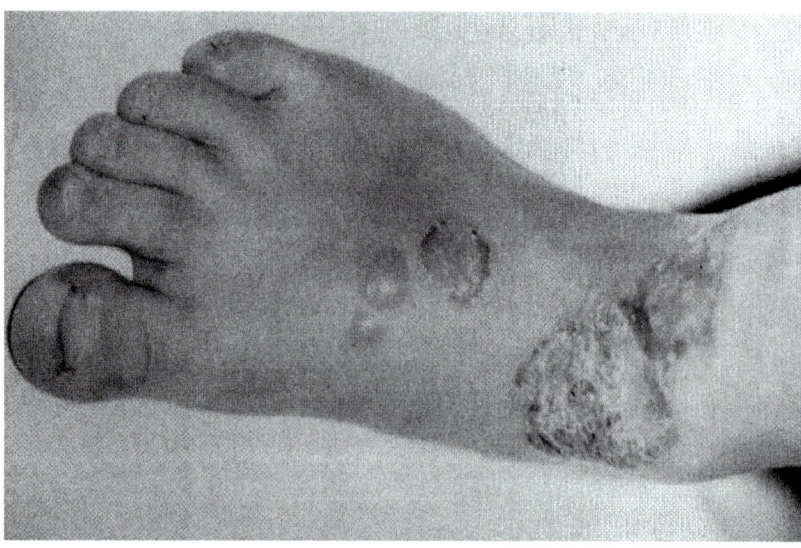

Figure 2–2. Bullous impetigo.

## C. Viral Infections

### 1. Verrucae (warts)

▶ **H&P Keys**
Common wart (verruca vulgaris), palmoplantar wart (verruca palmaris/plantaris), flat wart (verruca plana), genital wart (condyloma acuminatum); spread by trauma.

▶ **Diagnosis**
History and physical exam; biopsy confirmatory.

▶ **Disease Severity**
Disseminated lesions associated with immunodeficiency; certain viral types (16, 18, 31, 33) associated with squamous cell carcinoma.

▶ **Concept and Application**
Human papillomavirus (HPV) infection. Most treatment modalities involve destruction of involved tissue. Imiquimod induces a specific immune response locally.

▶ **Treatment Steps**
1. Topical acids (eg, salicylic acid) daily. Imiquimod for genital warts.
2. Liquid nitrogen (multiple treatments may be necessary), paring, topical acids.
3. Excision, laser.

### 2. Molluscum Contagiosum

▶ **H&P Keys**
Discrete umbilicated pearly papules in children and adults; may be transmitted sexually.

▶ **Diagnosis**
History and physical exam, biopsy confirmatory.

▶ **Disease Severity**
Numerous, large, and disfiguring in AIDS patients.

▶ **Concept and Application**
DNA poxvirus infection.

▶ **Treatment Steps**
Same as for warts.

### 3. Herpes Simplex

▶ **H&P Keys**
Grouped vesicles on base of erythema. Occurs anywhere on the skin, but mostly perioral or genital. Local discomfort and possible prodrome or systemic symptoms (Fig. 2–3).

▶ **Diagnosis**
History and physical exam. Vesicle for culture or direct fluorescent antibody assay, PCR. Tissue biopsy.

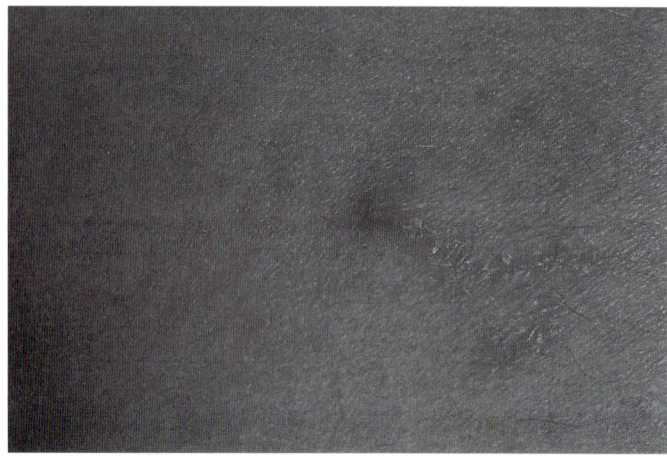

Figure 2-3. Herpes simplex.

▶ Disease Severity
Primary infection can be accompanied by fever, malaise, and lymphadenopathy. Herpetic keratoconjunctivitis can lead to blindness. EM minor usually related to outbreak of orolabial herpes. Dissemination to CNS seen mostly in immunosuppressed.

▶ Concept and Application
HSV is a DNA virus spread by physical contact. HSV-1 causes most orolabial disease and almost all adults are seropositive. HSV-2 associated with genital herpes with 20% seropositive. After initial infection, virus is harbored in sensory nerves and shed both during outbreaks and in asymptomatic periods.

▶ Treatment Steps
1. Acyclovir or derivative PO at first sign of outbreak. Local care.
2. Suppressive therapy with daily acyclovir if more than 6 episodes per year.

### D. Secondary Syphilis

▶ H&P Keys
Lesions appear 6 to 12 weeks after onset of chancre (primary stage). Associated lymphadenopathy. Great imitator—many cutaneous expressions: Macules, brownish-red papules, variable scale. Palms and soles often involved (Fig. 2-4).

▶ Diagnosis
History and physical exam, darkfield microscopy, serology, biopsy.

▶ Disease Severity
Associated findings: mucous patches, condylomalta, pharyngitis, iritis, periostitis, arthralgias, hepatosplenomegaly.

▶ Concept and Application
Sexually transmitted disease caused by the spirochete, *Treponema pallidum*. Untreated, it may progress to tertiary phase (granulomas, gummas).

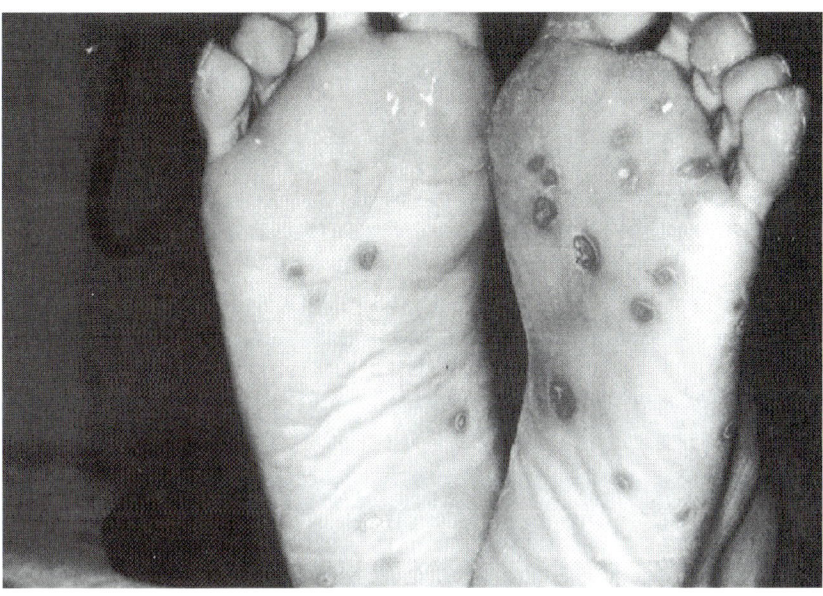

Figure 2–4. Secondary syphilis.

▶ Treatment Steps
1. Benzathine penicillin (tetracycline or doxycycline in penicillin allergic). Beware of Jarisch–Herxheimer rection (acute exacerbation of disease with treatment).
2. Sexual partners should be screened.
3. HIV test recommended for all patients with syphilis.

## III. SKIN ERUPTIONS

### A. Inflammatory Conditions of Skin

1. Psoriasis

   ▶ H&P Keys
   Well-demarcated reddish plaques with adherent silvery scale (Fig. 2–5). Typically chronic, symmetric, and familial. Variable itching, shows Koebner's phenomenon (lesions occur after trauma). Sites: elbows, knees, scalp, buttocks, nails. Variants: pustular, erythrodermic, guttate, palmoplantar.

   ▶ Diagnosis
   History and physical exam, biopsy to confirm.

   ▶ Disease Severity
   Arthritis may be associated. Pustular and erythrodermic variants associated with systemic toxicity. Guttate psoriasis triggered by *Strep* pharyngitis. Some drugs (β-blockers, lithium, withdrawal of systemic steroids) cause flare.

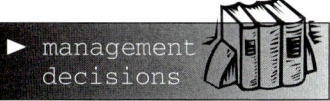

### PSORIASIS

Topical halogenated corticosteroids are a principle mode of therapy, however prolonged use is associated with skin atrophy. Topical retinoids, keratolytics, calcipotriene (vitamin D derivative), and tars are useful alone or in combination with a steroid. Resistant psoriasis usually responds to the addition of UVB or PUVA. If still no significant response, consider systemic treatment with acitretin, methotrexate or cyclosporine. Etanercept indicated for psoriatic arthritis.

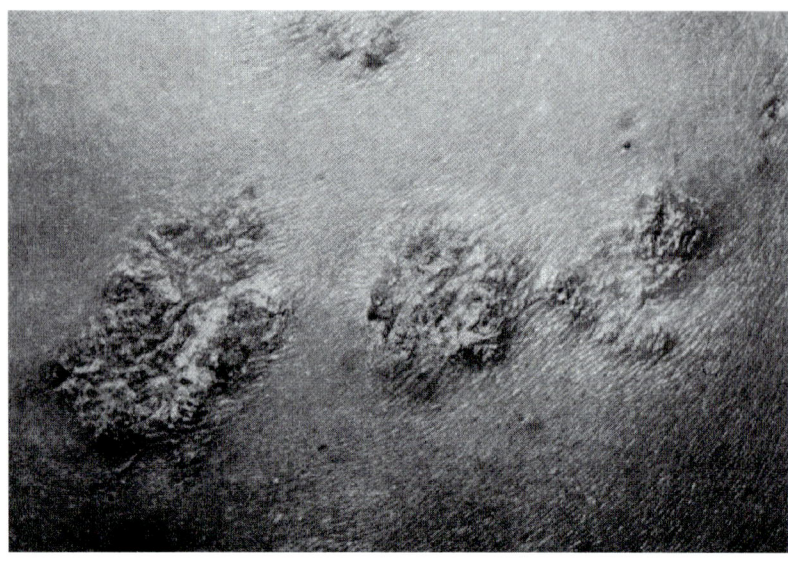

Figure 2–5. Plaques of psoriasis.

▶ Concept and Application

Hyperproliferation of epidermis. Multiple mediators involved, including cyclic nucleotides, polyamines, proteases, and leukotrienes. Recent research indicates a strong role for cell-mediated immunity. Topical corticosteroids modulate hyperproliferation. New systemic agent etanercept targets immune aspect of pathogenesis.

▶ Treatment Steps

*Topical*—Tars, corticosteroids, anthralin, calcipotriene ointment, topical retinoids, keratolytics, emollients.

*Phototherapy*—UVB, psoralen plus UVA (PUVA).

*Systemic*—Acitretin, methotrexate, cyclosporine. Etanercept for psoriatic arthritis.

1. Start with topicals. If guttate, add course of antibiotic that covers Strep. If pustular, start acitretin.
2. Add phototherapy. If pustular disease unresponsive to acitretin, consider other systemic agent.
3. Start systemic agent.

2. Seborrheic Dermatitis

▶ H&P Keys

The mildest form is flaking of scalp (dandruff). Scale is yellowish and greasy. Variable erythema. Also affects external ear canal, eyebrows, nasal crease. Occasionally involves presternal area, axillae, umbilicus, and groin. In infant, referred to as cradle cap.

▶ Diagnosis

History and physical exam. Biopsy excludes other disorders.

▶ Disease Severity
May be severe and treatment resistant in HIV patients. More frequent and severe in neurologic disorders (eg, Parkinson's disease).

▶ Concept and Application
Oily skin is a predisposing factor, but the disorder is not a disease of sebaceous glands. Worse in fall and winter. The yeast *Pityrosporum ovale* is abundant in lesions and may be a trigger.

▶ Treatment Steps
1. Ketoconazole 2% cream and shampoo and/or shampoo containing selenium sulfide or zinc pyrithione. Low-potency steroid.
2. Tars, salicylic acid, sulfur compounds.

3. Contact Dermatitis

▶ H&P Keys
Linear, pruritic, erythematous plaques with or without blisters. Rhus plants (poison ivy, oak, sumac) most common cause. Nickel (costume jewelry) (Fig. 2–6), neomycin (Neosporin), and fragrances (perfumes) are frequent causes. Twenty-four- to 48-hour delay from contact to development of rash.

▶ Diagnosis
History and physical exam, biopsy, patch tests.

▶ Disease Severity
May be generalized. Pruritus can be severe. Can become chronic if precipitating cause not eliminated. Frequent cause for work disability.

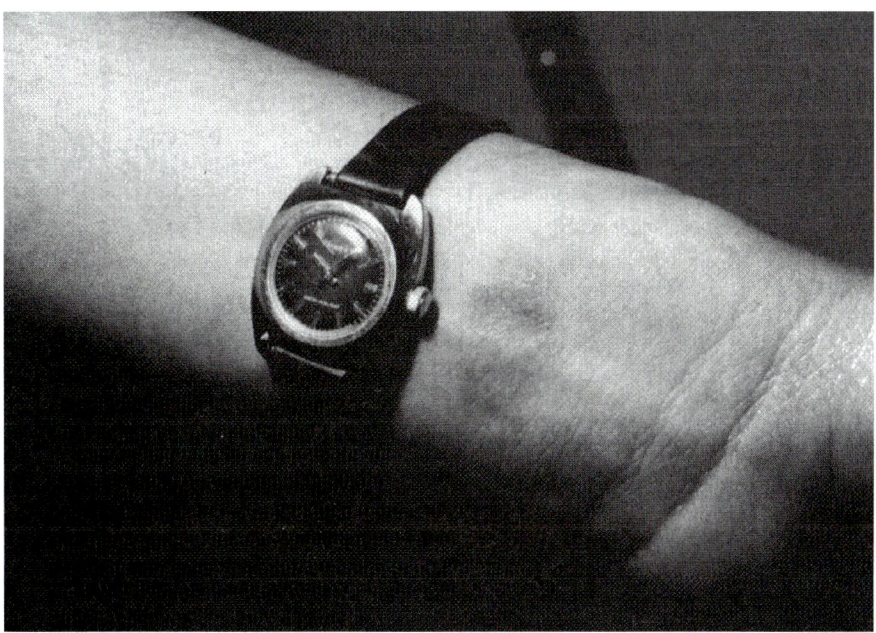

Figure 2–6. Allergic contact dermatitis from nickel.

▶ Concept and Application
Type IV delayed hypersensitivity. Occasionally type I hypersensitivity (contact urticaria to foods, latex).

▶ Treatment Steps
1. Topical steroids for acute flare, systemic for severe cases; avoidance of precipitating antigen; antihistamines.
2. Consider patch testing.

4. Atopic Dermatitis

▶ H&P Keys
Personal or family history of atopy. Marked pruritus. May begin in infancy. Excoriations and erythematous plaques in antecubital and popliteal fossae, posterior neck. Redundant eyelid fold, hyperlinear palmar creases, dry skin, and cataracts are associated findings.

▶ Diagnosis
History and physical exam, biopsy, blood eosinophilia, IgE levels.

▶ Disease Severity
May generalize (erythroderma). *Staphylococcus aureus* is a frequent colonizer and may trigger flares. Increased susceptibility to herpes infection (Kaposi's varicelliform eruption) and fungal infection.

▶ Concept and Application
Unknown cause. In some patients, allergens (eg, foods) may provoke itching, dermatitis, and bronchospasm.

▶ Treatment Steps
1. Moisturizers, topical corticosteroids, sedating antihistamines, avoidance of irritants. Antibiotics if secondary infection present or if staphylococcal related flare suspected.
2. Tar preparations, higher potency topical steroids. Topical tacrolimus and pimecrolimus.
3. UVB, PUVA, systemic steroids only rarely.

5. Eczematous Dermatitis (Eczema)

▶ H&P Keys
Many different etiologies. Contact dermatitis and atopic dermatitis are subtypes. Lesions are erythematous plaques with variable minute blisters, scale, excoriation, and crust. Round configuration resembling ringworm (nummular dermatitis) (Fig. 2–7). When present on legs with venous stasis and varicosities (stasis dermatitis), associated with hyperpigmentation and ulcers. Type related to severe dry skin (asteatotic dermatitis, eczema craquele).

▶ Diagnosis
History and physical exam, biopsy.

▶ Disease Severity
May generalize (autoeczematization). Itching may be severe and interfere with daily living and sleep.

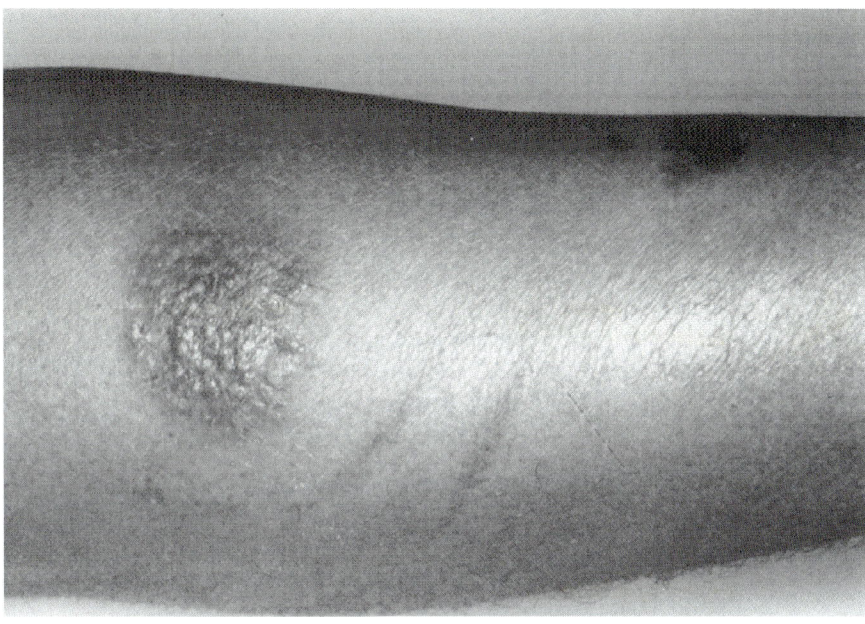

Figure 2-7. Nummular dermatitis.

▶ Concept and Application
Unknown. Dry skin exacerbates all forms of eczema.

▶ Treatment Steps
1. Moisturizers (ointments better than creams), oral antihistamines, topical steroids, treatment of infection if present. If stasis dermatitis, leg elevation and compression stockings.
2. Tars, systemic steroids, intralesional steroids for localized process (eg, nummular dermatitis), UVB. Consider patch testing.

6. Urticaria (Hives)

▶ H&P Keys
Acute or chronic (> 6 weeks). Lesions are fleeting (usually hours) in duration. Pruritic, pink, edematous papules (wheals). Precipitating cause may be known to patient.

▶ Diagnosis
History and physical. Biopsy in chronic cases to rule out vasculitis. Differentiate from dermographism (hives occurring after scratching).

▶ Disease Severity
May be associated with laryngeal spasm or bronchospasm. Angioedema (deep swelling in skin) may be associated (if prominent feature, rule out hereditary angioedema associated with C1 esterase inhibitor deficiency).

▶ Concept and Application
Numerous causes. Both type I and II hypersensitivity implicated. Mast cell degranulation leads to edema and vascular permeability.

▶ Treatment Steps
1. Elimination of cause if known (drugs, foods, insect bites most common), oral antihistamines, avoid systemic corticosteroids.
2. Switch antihistamine to $H_1/H_2$ blocker (doxepin) or add $H_2$-blocking antihistamine, consider patch testing.

7. **Drug Reactions**

   ▶ H&P Keys
   Variable presentation. Disseminated pruritic pink macules and papules (morbilliform) are typical (eg, mononucleosis patient given amoxicillin). Time course of rash usually corresponds to offending medication. Other presentations: urticaria, erythema multiforme (targetoid lesions), photosensitivity, vasculitis, fixed (lesions recur in same spot with rechallenge).

   ▶ Diagnosis
   History and physical exam. Biopsy. Some drugs are more frequent offenders (trimethoprim–sulfamethoxazole, phenytoin, thiazides, penicillins).

   ▶ Disease Severity
   May generalize (erythroderma). Itching may be severe. Erythema multiforme (Stevens–Johnson syndrome, toxic epidermal necrolysis) may be life threatening. Systemic vasculitis may be associated with cutaneous lesions (palpable purpura).

   ▶ Concept and Application
   Immunologic (types I to IV) and nonimmunologic mechanisms.

   ▶ Treatment Steps
   1. Cessation of offending medication.
   2. Antihistamines, soothing topical emollient lotions (Sarna), topical steroids. Systemic corticosteroids should be used with caution.

B. **Blistering Diseases**

1. **Bullous Pemphigoid**

   ▶ H&P Keys
   Elderly patients; pruritus; large, tense blisters and urticarial plaques; negative Nikolsky's sign (cannot induce blister with blunt pressure).

   ▶ Diagnosis
   Biopsy for routine studies and direct immunofluorescence, serum for indirect immunofluorescence (to detect circulating autoantibody).

   ▶ Disease Severity
   Blisters can be large and leave large eroded areas; mucosal lesions are painful; pruritus can be severe.

► Concept and Application
Autoimmune mechanisms with IgG and complement infiltrating skin; immunosuppressives used for treatment. Rarely, may be caused by drugs (furosemide).

► Treatment Steps
1. Local skin care; superpotent topical corticosteroids for limited disease.
2. Systemic steroids, tetracyclines, or other immunosuppressives for generalized disease.
3. Taper as tolerated.

2. Herpes Gestationis

► H&P Keys
Clinical presentation identical to bullous pemphigoid except occurs in second or third trimester of pregnancy.

► Diagnosis
History and physical exam, skin biopsy and immunofluorescence (differentiate from pruritic urticarial papules and plaques of pregnancy [PUPPP], which begins on abdomen [usually striae] and occurs late in pregnancy).

► Disease Severity
May increase fetal mortality or premature delivery; fetus may be born with skin lesions.

► Concept and Application
Autoimmune mechanism. Not related to herpes virus. Oral contraceptives may exacerbate disease in patients with documented disease.

► Treatment Steps
Some cases of mild disease can be managed with antihistamines and topical steroids. Most patients require systemic steroids.

3. Pemphigus

► H&P Keys
Two types: superficial (foliaceus) and common (vulgaris). Vulgaris type shows fragile blisters and Nikolsky's sign. Oral lesions are common and often presenting feature. Lesions usually tender or painful, not pruritic. Increased frequency in people of Jewish or Mediterranean origin (Fig. 2–8).

► Diagnosis
History and physical exam, skin biopsy for histology and direct immunofluorescence, serum for indirect immunofluorescence.

► Disease Severity
Oral lesions may interfere with intake of solid foods; large eroded raw surfaces may develop; can be fatal if diagnosis and treatment are not established.

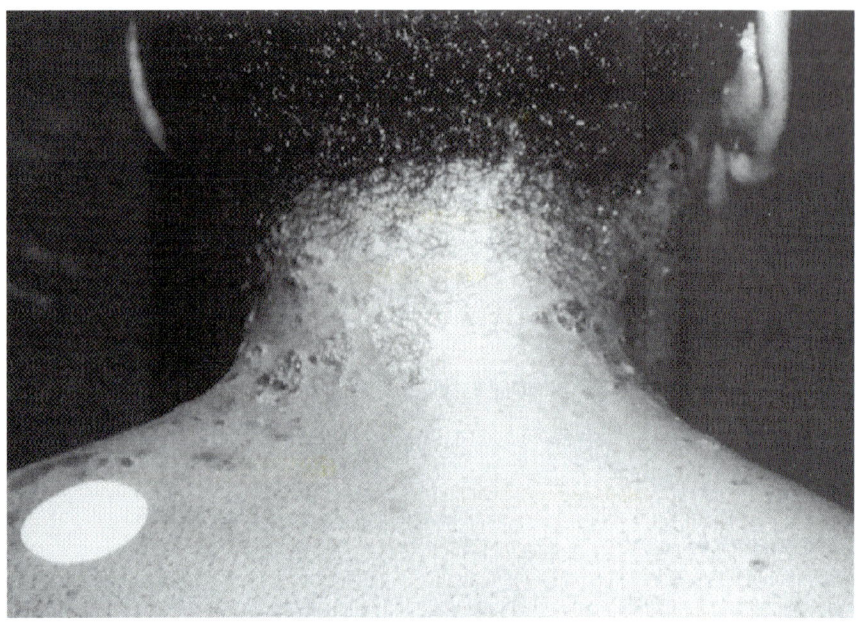

Figure 2–8. Fragile blisters and erosions in pemphigus vulgaris.

▶ Concept and Application

Autoimmune mechanism with antibodies to intercellular substrate of epithelium (skin and mucosae). Immunosuppressives mainstay of treatment. Pemphigus associated with malignant neoplasms (paraneoplastic pemphigus) can resemble erythema multiforme.

▶ Treatment Steps
1. High-dose systemic steroids, local skin care, antibiotics for secondary infection.
2. Add "steroid-sparing" agent such as azathioprine, dapsone.
3. Taper steroid as tolerated.

4. Dermatitis Herpetiformis

▶ H&P Keys

Markedly pruritic dermatosis characterized by symmetric grouped blisters (often excoriated) on extensor surfaces of skin (elbows, knees, scalp, back). Associated with gluten-sensitive enteropathy (usually subclinical).

▶ Diagnosis

History and physical exam; skin biopsy for histology and immunofluorescence.

▶ Disease Severity

Itching usually severe. Associated steatorrhea, anemia.

▶ Concept and Application

Strong HLA predisposition identical to that seen in celiac disease. IgA in skin probably has gut origin.

▶ Treatment Steps
1. Dapsone. Gluten-free diet is beneficial and may reduce need for dapsone.
2. Taper dapsone as tolerated.

## C. Other Diseases of the Skin and Subcutaneous Tissues

### 1. Erythema Multiforme

▶ H&P Keys
Target lesions (irislike) are typical. Lesions usually on palms and soles but can involve remainder of skin. May show central blister. Two forms: minor and major (Stevens–Johnson syndrome). Major form involves two or more mucosal surfaces and systemic symptoms (Fig. 2–9).

▶ Diagnosis
Physical examination, skin biopsy.

▶ Disease Severity
Major form causes significant morbidity. Toxic epidermal necrolysis (which resembles major form in early stages) produces widespread denudation resembling a burn, and it is associated with mortality from fluid loss and infection.

▶ Concept and Application
Minor form usually associated with oro-labial herpes simplex infection (immune complexes found in skin). Major form associated with drugs and *Mycoplasma* infection.

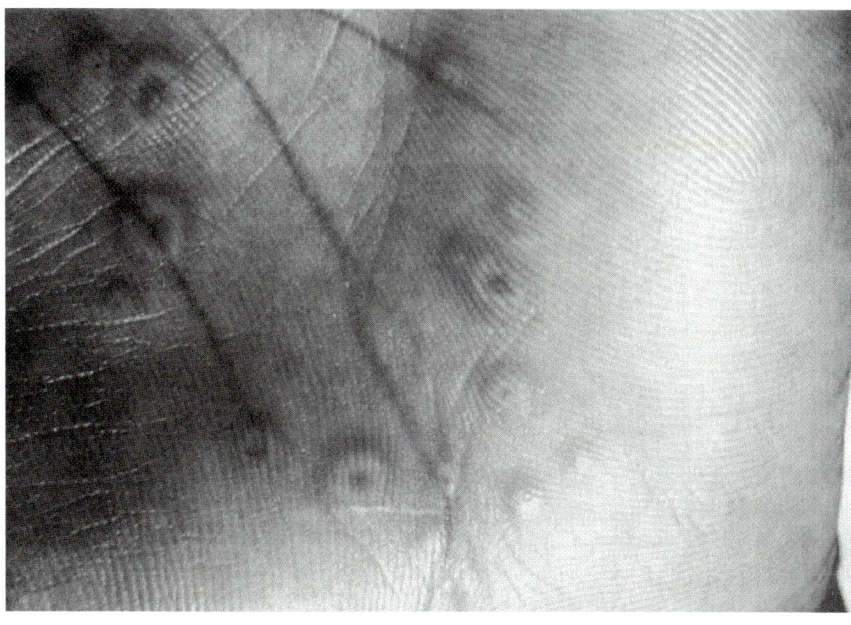

Figure 2–9. Targetoid lesions of erythema multiforme.

▶ Treatment Steps
1. Local skin care, antihistamines, chronic, suppressive dose of acyclovir or derivative if associated with herpes simplex infection.
2. Admit patients with major form or TEN to burn center.
3. Use of systemic steroids controversial.

2. Erythema Nodosum

▶ H&P Keys
Tender, red, warm nodules on legs; may show bruising; nonulcerating; heal without scarring.

▶ Diagnosis
Incisional biopsy for confirmation in atypical cases. To search for underlying cause: antistreptolysin-O (ASO) titer, throat culture (*Strep*), chest roentgenogram (sarcoidosis), purified protein derivative (PPD) (tuberculosis).

▶ Disease Severity
Extratibial sites occasionally involved. Associated fever, chills, malaise, arthralgias.

▶ Concept and Application
Immunologic.

▶ Treatment Steps
1. Bed rest, nonsteroidal anti-inflammatory drugs (NSAIDs), potassium iodide, systemic steroids if etiology not infectious.

D. Symptoms Involving the Skin

1. Pruritus (Itching), Generalized

▶ H&P Keys
Excoriations (no primary lesions) in accessible areas. No rash in nonreachable areas (eg, mid-back "butterfly sign"). Examine for lymphadenopathy and signs for systemic cause.

▶ Diagnosis
History most helpful in determining cause. When unaccompanied by rash, drugs or systemic causes are possible. If systemic cause considered, rule out uremia, hepatobiliary obstruction, polycythemia vera, hyperthyroidism, and Hodgkin's disease.

▶ Disease Severity
Severe pruritus interferes with quality of life and sleep. Secondary psychiatric disease (eg, depression) may be present.

▶ Concept and Application
Cause undetermined in many cases.

▶ Treatment Steps
1. Treatment of underlying condition, if known. For unknown causes, antihistamines (hydroxyzine, doxepin), soothing emollient lotions (Sarna).
2. UV light is helpful in refractory cases.

2. Pruritus Ani

   ▶ H&P Keys
   Itching around rectum with excoriations.

   ▶ Diagnosis
   History and physical exam. Cellophane tape applied to area may show pinworms.

   ▶ Disease Severity
   Bleeding and fissures.

   ▶ Concept and Application
   Irritation from stool (possibly related to diet) on skin and mucosae.

   ▶ Treatment Steps
   Avoidance of external irritants (soaps, medication), meticulous anal hygiene, soothing lotions (Balneol).

3. Pruritus, Localized

   ▶ H&P Keys

   *Acute*—Excoriations.

   *Chronic*—Nodules (prurigo nodularis) or scaly plaques (lichen simplex chronicus).

   ▶ Diagnosis
   History and physical exam, biopsy will confirm.

   ▶ Disease Severity
   Disfiguring scars. In factitial dermatitis (self-inflicted), bizarre configuration of lesion is characteristic.

   ▶ Concept and Application
   In some cases, an inciting event (insect bite, rash) leads to self-perpetuating itch–scratch cycle.

   ▶ Treatment Steps
   1. Break the itch–scratch cycle, corticosteroids (triamcinolone acetonide) injected into nodules. Superpotent topical corticosteroids for lichen simplex chronicus.
   2. Reinject as necessary. Psychologic counseling in severe cases.

## E. Insect Bites (Nonvenomous) and Ectoparasites

1. Scabies

   ▶ H&P Keys
   Marked pruritus (especially in the evening); papules, vesicles, and burrows in typical sites (interdigital web spaces, volar wrists, axillae, areolae, umbilicus, genitals, knees, ankles) (Fig. 2–10).

   ▶ Diagnosis
   Skin scraping with a drop of mineral oil on slide will demonstrate mites or their products.

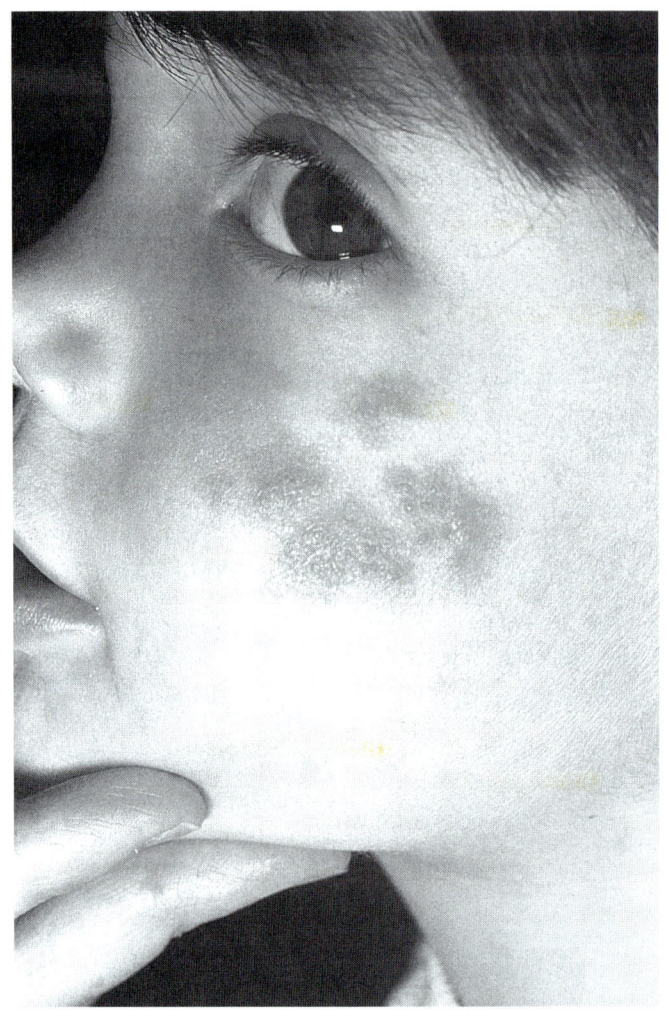

Figure 2–10. Burrow typical of scabies.

▶ Disease Severity
Itching may interfere with sleep and daily activities and can persist for several weeks after successful treatment. Variant (Norwegian scabies) produces crusted, scaly lesions and is found in elderly, mentally retarded, or immunocompromised patients.

▶ Concept and Application
May be sexually transmitted.

▶ Treatment Steps
1. Permethrin 5% cream or Lindane 1% (associated with neurotoxicity in kids) lotion. Antihistamines and topical steroids for itching. Treat contacts. Consider HIV testing if sexually transmitted.
2. Repeat course if necessary or ivermectin PO.

2. Pediculosis

   ▶ H&P Keys

   Pruritus, excoriation, and secondary infection of affected sites. Head lice (*Pediculosis capitis*), pubic lice (*Pediculosis pubis*) (Fig. 2–11), body lice (*Pediculosis corporis*). Nits on hair. Adult lice can be seen with hand lens.

   ▶ Diagnosis

   Presence of nits or adult lice on physical examination.

   ▶ Disease Severity

   Lice can transmit some rickettsial diseases.

   ▶ Concept and Application

   Transmitted by casual or sexual contact. Often epidemic in schools (head lice).

   ▶ Treatment Steps
   1. Elimite 5% or 1%, nit removal, 1% malathion powder to clothing for body lice, treat contacts.
   2. Lindane 1% if above treatment ineffective.

3. Mosquitoes and Flies

   ▶ H&P Keys

   Pruritic papules on exposed areas.

   ▶ Diagnosis

   History and physical exam, skin biopsy for atypical lesions.

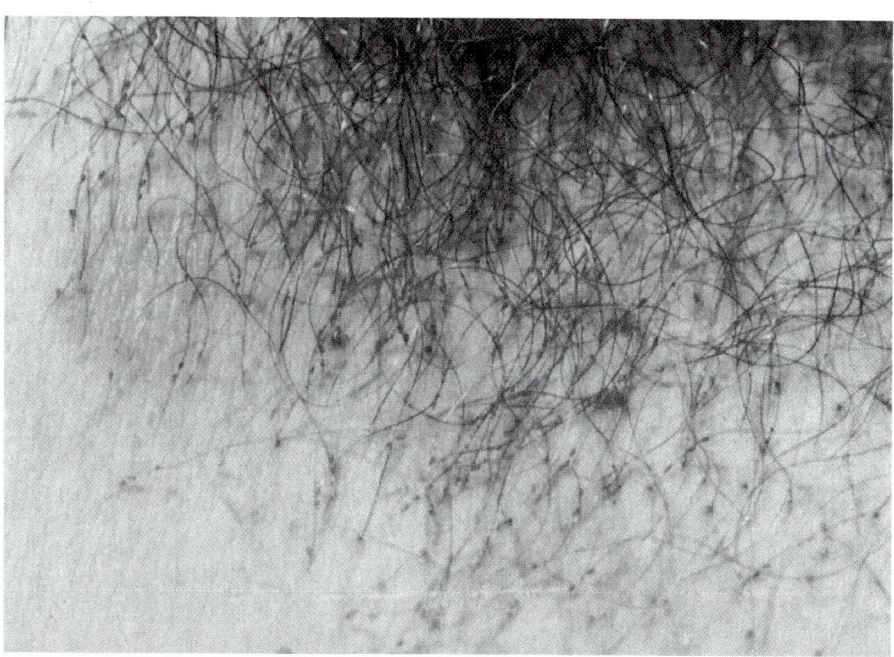

Figure 2–11. *Pediculosis pubis* with nits and lice.

▶ Disease Severity
Spectrum of cutaneous findings dependent on host sensitivity. Organisms largely responsible for transmission of disease (malaria, yellow fever, encephalitis, dengue, West Nile virus).

▶ Concept and Application
Female inserts blood tube through skin and injects anticoagulant. Mosquitoes attracted to scents and bright colors. Diethyltoluamide (DEET) is an effective repellent.

▶ Treatment Steps
1. Local care, antihistamines, topical steroids.

4. Fleas

▶ H&P Keys
Pets (cats, dogs, birds) in household. Characteristic pattern of lesions grouped in threes ("breakfast, lunch, dinner"). Blisters in severely allergic individuals.

▶ Diagnosis
History and physical exam.

▶ Disease Severity
Can see generalized reaction in some individuals (papular urticaria).

▶ Concept and Application
Survival of adult fleas for months in the absence of an animal host makes fleaborne epidemics difficult to eradicate.

▶ Treatment Steps
1. Veterinary care of pet, good housecleaning, symptomatic treatment with antihistamines, and topical steroids.

## IV. NAILS AND HAIR

### A. Ingrowing Nails

▶ H&P Keys
Great toe most common; painful inflammatory soft-tissue swellings; ill-fitting footwear and improper nail care.

▶ Diagnosis
History and physical exam.

▶ Disease Severity
Interferes with ambulation; secondary cellulitis.

▶ Concept and Application
Overcurvature or developmental abnormality of nail plate with trauma and improper nail care causes nail plate to embed into soft tissue. This provokes an inflammatory response and predisposes to secondary infection.

▶ Treatment Steps
1. Antiseptic soaks, analgesics, rest, antibiotics, elevating of nail plate corner with cotton.
2. Surgical treatment.

## B. Other Diseases of Hair and the Hair Follicle

### 1. Acne Vulgaris

▶ H&P Keys
Onset in adolescence; comedones (whiteheads and blackheads), papules, pustules, cysts; face, chest, and back.

▶ Diagnosis
History and physical exam; presence of comedones differentiates from other similar disorders.

▶ Disease Severity
Cosmetic disfigurement; scarring.

▶ Concept and Application
Multiple factors: plugging of hair follicle, increased sebum, bacterial infection, genetics. Topical retinoids promote unplugging of follicles, benzoyl peroxide and antibiotics decrease bacterial colonies.

▶ Treatment Steps
1. Comedonal type: keratolytic (eg, salicylic acid), topical retinoid. For papular–pustular or cystic types, add oral antibiotic (topical if mild disease) and topical benzoyl peroxide.
2. If topical antibiotic ineffective, consider oral antibiotic. If oral antibiotic ineffective, consider hormonal therapy (eg, oral contraceptive).
3. Oral isotretinoin if recalcitrant severe nodulocystic type, acne surgery.

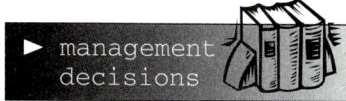

### ACNE VULGARIS

Keratolytics (salicylic acid) and topical retinoids control comedones (beware photosensitivity while using retinoids—sunscreen important), mild soaps minimize irritation. If there is an inflammatory component, add antibiotic, topical (clindamycin, erythromycin, benzoyl peroxide) if mild, oral (tetracycline or derivative, erythromycin) if more severe. If acne is persistent, consider hormonal workup/treatment. Severe cystic acne usually responds well to a course of oral isotretinoin. Need to monitor triglycerides and LFTs.

### 2. Rosacea

▶ H&P Keys
Adult onset, women predominate, associated with flushing; telangiectasia (dilated blood vessels), papules, pustules symmetrically distributed on face (Fig. 2–12); no comedones.

▶ Diagnosis
History and physical exam; may resemble malar erythema of lupus erythematosus.

▶ Disease Severity
Keratitis may be associated.

▶ Concept and Application
Flushing with increase in skin temperature provoked by hot liquids, spicy foods, and alcohol.

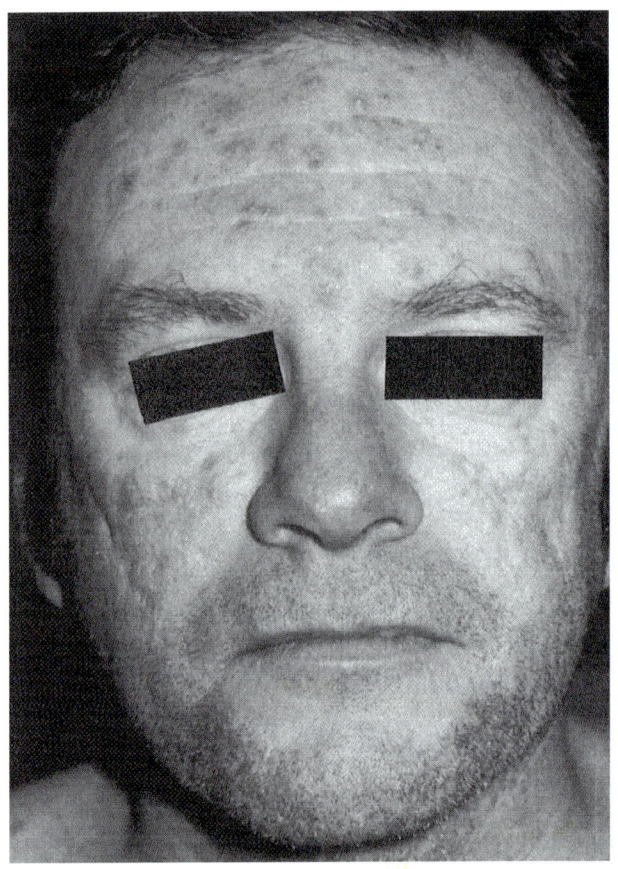

Figure 2-12. Rosacea.

▶ Treatment Steps
1. Reduction or elimination of provoking factors. Topical metronidazole or sulfur lotions.
2. Add oral tetracycline, rarely, isotretinoin.

3. Alopecia Areata

▶ H&P Keys

Localized round or oval patches of hair loss without visible skin inflammation; children or adults; any hair-bearing area can be affected; can be stress provoked.

▶ Diagnosis

History and physical exam, biopsy.

▶ Disease Severity

Can involve entire scalp (alopecia totalis) or entire body (alopecia universalis); associated with other autoimmune disorders (Hashimoto's thyroiditis, vitiligo).

▶ Concept and Application

Autoimmune lymphocytes react against hair follicles, treatment difficult.

▶ Treatment Steps
1. Superpotent topical steroid.
2. If no response, intralesional triamcinolone, consider topical minoxidil, anthralin.
3. Consider referral for psychological counseling.

## V. TUMORS OF THE SKIN

### A. Premalignant and Malignant Neoplasms of Skin

#### 1. Actinic Keratosis (Solar Keratosis)

▶ H&P Keys
Sign of chronic sun damage; light-complected individuals (Northern European); multiple discrete, rough, adherent scaly mildly erythematous patches and plaques on sun-exposed areas.

▶ Diagnosis
History and physical (other signs of sun damage: wrinkling, lentigines, etc.); biopsy.

▶ Disease Severity
May be associated with frank skin cancer (basal or squamous cell carcinoma).

▶ Concept and Application
Chronic sun exposure causes malignant keratinocyte transformation confined to lower layers of the epidermis. Sunscreens are protective.

▶ Treatment Steps
1. Destruction with liquid nitrogen.
2. Excision. Topical 5-fluorouracil or diclofenac for more extensive disease.
3. Surveillance for new lesions, recurrence.

#### 2. Squamous Cell Carcinoma

▶ H&P Keys
Enlarging indurated papule or nodule with variable adherent scale on sun-exposed sites (skin and mucosa) in older people.

▶ Diagnosis
History and physical exam, biopsy.

▶ Disease Severity
May arise from preexisting actinic keratosis (low incidence of metastasis). When occurs de novo, higher rate of metastasis. Tumors on lower lip, particularly, have increased risk of metastasis (Fig. 2–13A). In-situ lesions called Bowen's disease or erythroplasia of Queyrat on the penis.

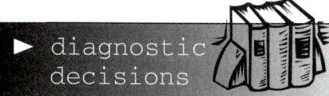

▶ diagnostic decisions

**SKIN CANCERS**

**Actinic keratosis (AK)**
Rough, scaly, faintly erythematous thin plaques on sun-exposed/damaged skin, fair skinned individuals, can progress to invasive squamous cell carcinoma, related to chronic sun exposure, atypical keratinocytes, but not full-thickness.

**Basal cell carcinoma (BCC)**
Dome-shaped pearly papule or nodule with central ulceration and rolled edge, telangiectasias, sun-exposed/damaged skin, most common skin cancer, typically the face, ears and trunk, several variants, eg, pigmented (resembles malignant melanoma) slow growing, metastasis rare, often destructive locally.

**Squamous cell carcinoma (SCC)**
Enlarging scaly papule without sharp borders on sun-exposed/damaged skin, older lesions can ulcerate, locally invasive, may arise in actinic keratoses, chronic ulcers and scars, metastasis more common in de novo lesions and those on lower lip, Bowen's disease is SCC in situ, usually red to brown scaly plaque, anogenital and periungual SCC linked to HPV.

**Malignant melanoma (MM)**
Enlarging asymmetric, variably colored (red, white, blue, black, and brown), large (> 6 mm) patch with irregular borders, may bleed and ulcerate, sometimes pruritic, related to intermittent intense sun exposure, aggressive neoplasm with frequent metastasis, prognosis based on tumor depth.

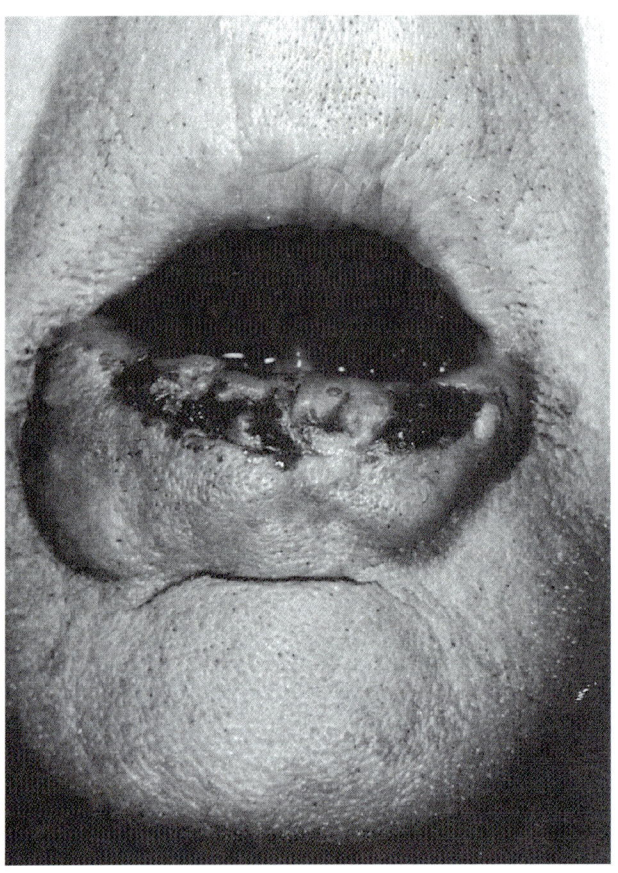

Figure 2–13A. Squamous cell carcinoma of lower lip.

▶ Concept and Application
Numerous factors: sunlight, x-rays, arsenic ingestion, immunosuppression, chronic ulcers, burns, smoking.

▶ Treatment Steps
1. Excision.
2. Surveillance for recurrence, new lesions.

3. Basal Cell Carcinoma

▶ H&P Keys
Slowly growing pearly papule or nodule, often with telangiectasias, on sun-exposed skin (Fig. 2–13B); most common form of skin cancer; lesions often ulcerate (rodent ulcer) and have rolled borders; infiltrate locally and very rarely metastasize.

▶ Diagnosis
History and physical exam, biopsy.

▶ Disease Severity
A sign of chronic sun injury. Variants: pigmented (resembles nodular melanoma), morpheaform (most locally aggressive type), superficial (typically on trunk, may resemble eczematous dermatitis), infiltrative (most likely type to recur after treatment).

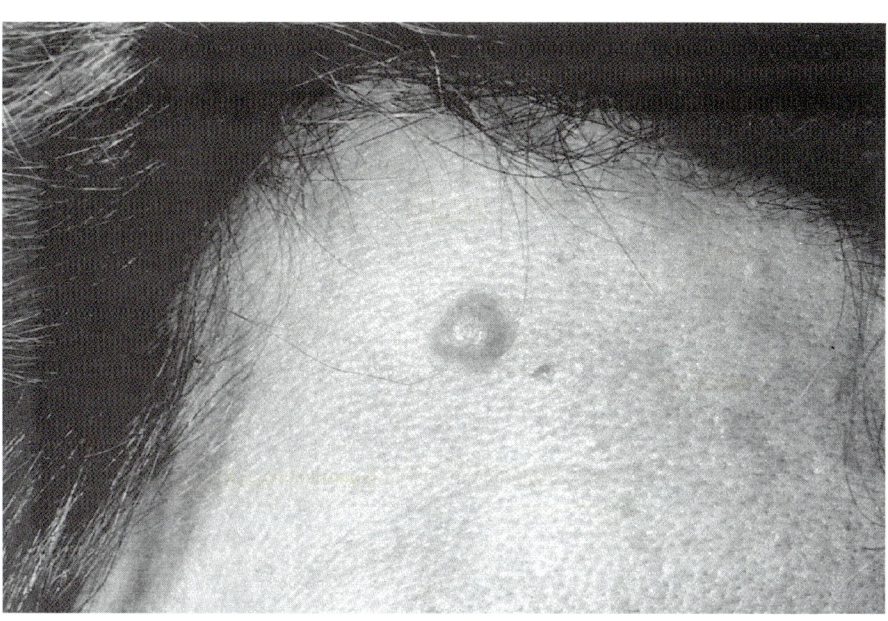

Figure 2-13B. Basal cell carcinoma.

▶ Concept and Application
Malignant tumor of skin related to chronic sun injury.

▶ Treatment Steps
1. Excision, destruction (electrical, freezing).
2. Mohs surgery if cosmetically sensitive site or if morpheiform or infiltrative type.
3. Surveillance for recurrence, new lesions.

4. Malignant Melanoma

▶ H&P Keys

Enlarging, asymmetric, irregularly bordered, variably colored, large (over 6 mm) pigmented patch. Black color is suspicious. Initially is flat (radial growth), then becomes nodular (vertical growth) (Fig. 2-14). May bleed and ulcerate. Family history.

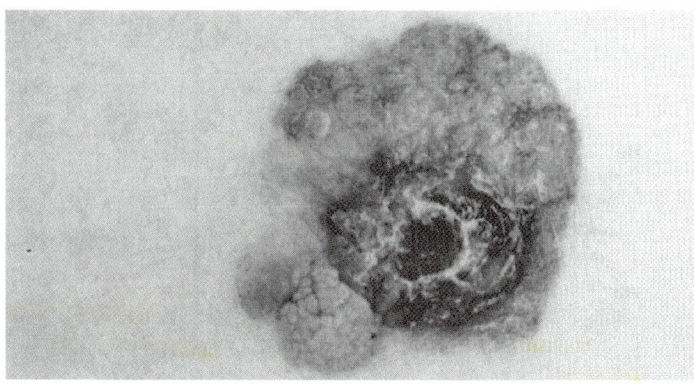

Figure 2-14. Melanoma.

▶ Diagnosis
Excisional biopsy.

▶ Disease Severity
Aggressive tumor with high propensity to metastasize widely. Prognosis related to depth of skin invasion (Clark's and Breslow's levels). Lesions less than 1 mm have good prognosis, greater than 3 mm have poor prognosis.

▶ Concept and Application
Related to intermittent intense sun exposure (blistering sunburns). Higher incidence in white-collar professionals. Can develop from congenital nevi or chronic sun exposure (lentigo maligna). Superficial spreading is most common; nodular is worst prognostically; acrolentiginous (hands, feet, mucosae) is most common in blacks.

▶ Treatment Steps
1. Excision, with surgical margins determined by depth of tumor invasion. Lymph node dissection controversial. INF-α2b indicated for adjuvant therapy in patients with high risk for metastasis.
2. Examination and lab screening for metastasis. Treatment for metastatic disease unsatisfactory.
3. Close monitoring.

**B. Benign Neoplasms**

1. Lipoma

    ▶ H&P Keys
    Single or multiple, rubbery or compressible subcutaneous masses, most often on trunk, posterior neck, or forearms. Angiolipomas are often multiple and painful.

    ▶ Diagnosis
    Physical exam, excisional biopsy.

    ▶ Disease Severity
    Rarely infiltrates into skeletal muscle. May occur in Gardner's syndrome. Midline back lesions can be associated with spinal dysraphism.

    ▶ Concept and Application
    Benign tumor of adipose tissue.

    ▶ Treatment Steps
    1. None if asymptomatic, excision.

2. Melanocytic Nevus

    ▶ H&P Keys
    Pigmented, well-demarcated, symmetric macule (junctional nevus), papule (compound nevus), or flesh-colored papule (intradermal nevus).

▶ Diagnosis
History and physical exam, biopsy.

▶ Disease Severity
Number of nevi correlate with life risk of melanoma; congenital (at birth) nevi often have hair; large type (bathing trunk nevi) have increased risk of malignant transformation.

▶ Concept and Application
A proliferation of melanocytes in skin.

▶ Treatment Steps
None unless melanoma is considered in differential diagnosis. Large congenital nevi should be excised at a young age.

3. Atypical (Dysplastic) Nevus

▶ H&P Keys
Familial or sporadic, large, irregularly bordered, pigmented macules and papules. Family history.

▶ Diagnosis
History and physical exam; biopsy.

▶ Disease Severity
Multiple familial atypical nevi associated with greatly increased risk of melanoma. Lesions themselves are not necessarily precursors.

▶ Concept and Application
Proliferation of melanocytes with varying cytologic atypia.

▶ Treatment Steps
Excision if melanoma is a diagnostic consideration; sun precaution and sunscreens; semiannual complete skin exams.

4. Dermatofibroma (Histiocytoma)

▶ H&P Keys
Firm, pigmented macule or papule that depresses centrally when palpated (dimpling sign). Often on lower leg and preceded by trauma (eg, insect bite).

▶ Diagnosis
History and physical exam, biopsy.

▶ Disease Severity
Multiple lesions may be associated with lupus erythematosus.

▶ Concept and Application
Proliferation of fibrohistiocytes after trauma.

▶ Treatment Steps
None. If cosmetically troublesome, excision.

5. **Hemangioma**

    ▶ **H&P Keys**

    Capillary or strawberry nevus (congenital), cavernous (bluish-purple subcutaneous), senile (red papules on trunk of elderly person).

    ▶ **Diagnosis**

    History and physical exam.

    ▶ **Disease Severity**

    Multiple cutaneous lesions may be associated with internal organ involvement (CNS, GI tract, liver). Large cavernous lesions may be associated with consumption of clotting factors. Kasabach–Merritt syndrome: hemangiomas and thrombocytopenia.

    ▶ **Concept and Application**

    Localized proliferation and dilatation of capillaries.

    ▶ **Treatment Steps**

    1. Capillary hemangiomas may self-involute.
    2. Systemic steroids or surgical/laser treatment for cosmetically disfiguring or deep lesions or lesions that impede vision or eating.

6. **Pyogenic Granuloma**

    ▶ **H&P Keys**

    Rapidly developing, bleeding, bright-red pedunculated papule or nodule (Fig. 2–15). Usually in young people, related to preceding trauma.

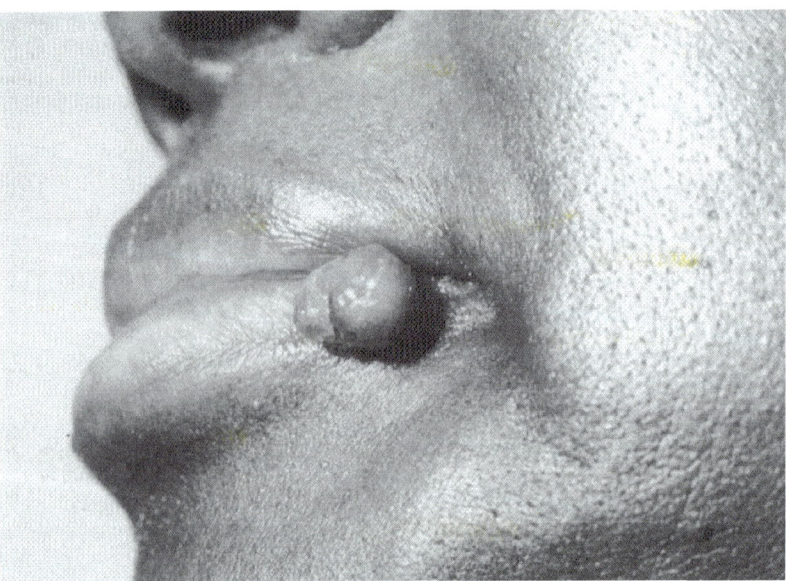

Figure 2–15. Pyogenic granuloma.

▶ Diagnosis
History and physical exam, biopsy.

▶ Disease Severity
None; differentiate from other tumors (melanoma, carcinoma).

▶ Concept and Application
Overproliferation of granulation tissue in response to injury. Drug-induced type (isotretinoin, indinavir).

▶ Treatment Steps
Excision, laser.

7. Blue Nevus

▶ H&P Keys
Blue-black macule or papule; more common on extremity.

▶ Diagnosis
Clinical examination, biopsy.

▶ Disease Severity
None; differentiate from thrombosed hemangioma, tattoo, and melanoma.

▶ Concept and Application
Proliferation of dendritic melanocytes in dermis.

▶ Treatment Steps
Excision.

8. Seborrheic Keratosis

▶ H&P Keys
Most common benign skin lesion. Warty, light to dark brown stuck-on plaques. Usually multiple, in various stages of development (Fig. 2–16).

▶ Diagnosis
History and physical exam, biopsy to confirm or rule out skin cancer.

▶ Disease Severity
Multiple pruritic, eruptive seborrheic keratoses may be sign of internal malignant neoplasm (sign of Leser–Trélat).

▶ Concept and Application
Proliferation of keratinocytes.

▶ Treatment Steps
None, excision if irritated.

C. Follicular Cyst (Epidermal, Pilar, Sebaceous Cyst)

▶ H&P Keys
Slowly enlarging, soft, movable mass. May show punctum. Most common on face or trunk.

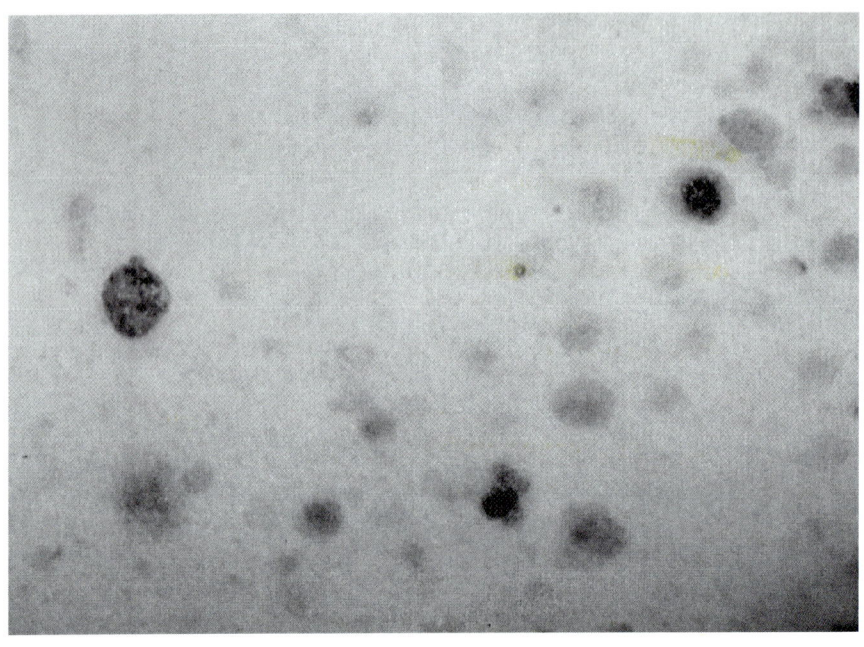

Figure 2-16. Numerous seborrheic keratoses.

▶ Diagnosis
History and physical exam.

▶ Disease Severity
May rupture or become infected and cause pain.

▶ Concept and Application
Follicular occlusion leads to cystic dilatation of follicle. Cyst contains keratin, not sebum.

▶ Treatment Steps
1. Oral antibiotics and/or intralesional corticosteroids if inflamed.
2. Surgical excision ultimately necessary in most cases.

## VI. OTHER CONDITIONS

### A. Acquired Keratoderma (Tylosis)

▶ H&P Keys
Localized or diffuse thickening of skin on palms and soles.

▶ Diagnosis
History and physical exam.

▶ Disease Severity
May be sign of internal malignant neoplasm (esophagus). May appear at menopause (keratoderma climacterium).

▶ Concept and Application
Unknown.

▶ Treatment Steps
1. Lubrication, elimination of aggravating factors.
2. Add keratolytic agents (salicylic acid, urea) if insufficient response.

## B. Decubitus Ulcer

▶ H&P Keys
Four grades, depending on depth of ischemia; most common over bony prominences (sacrum, greater trochanter, ischium, calcaneus, malleolus). Nutritional deficiency, spasticity, compression, loss of cutaneous sensation are contributory factors.

▶ Diagnosis
Clinical exam, roentgenography, culture, biopsy.

▶ Disease Severity
Grades III (into subcutaneous fat) and IV (into underlying muscle) may be associated with osteomyelitis and severe morbidity.

▶ Concept and Application
Prolonged pressure leads to ischemia and cutaneous necrosis.

▶ Treatment Steps
1. Airbed for pressure relief. Treat secondary infection locally with saline/acetic acid soaks, wet to dry dressings.
2. If significant infection present, systemic antibiotics, surgical debridement, skin graft.

## C. Ulcer of Lower Limbs

### 1. Stasis Ulceration

▶ H&P Keys
Minimally painful, superficial, well-demarcated ulcer with red base and variable crust (Fig. 2–17). Typically on medial side of ankle. Associated stasis dermatitis, hyperpigmentation, and varicose veins.

▶ Diagnosis
Clinical exam; biopsy in atypical lesions.

▶ Disease Severity
Multiple or large ulcers may occur; secondary cellulitis.

▶ Concept and Application
Ischemia from venous back pressure, preventing capillary flow.

▶ Treatment Steps
1. Bed rest, leg elevation, hydrocolloid dressings, compression stockings, diuresis.
2. Compression bandage, surgical treatment for varicosities.

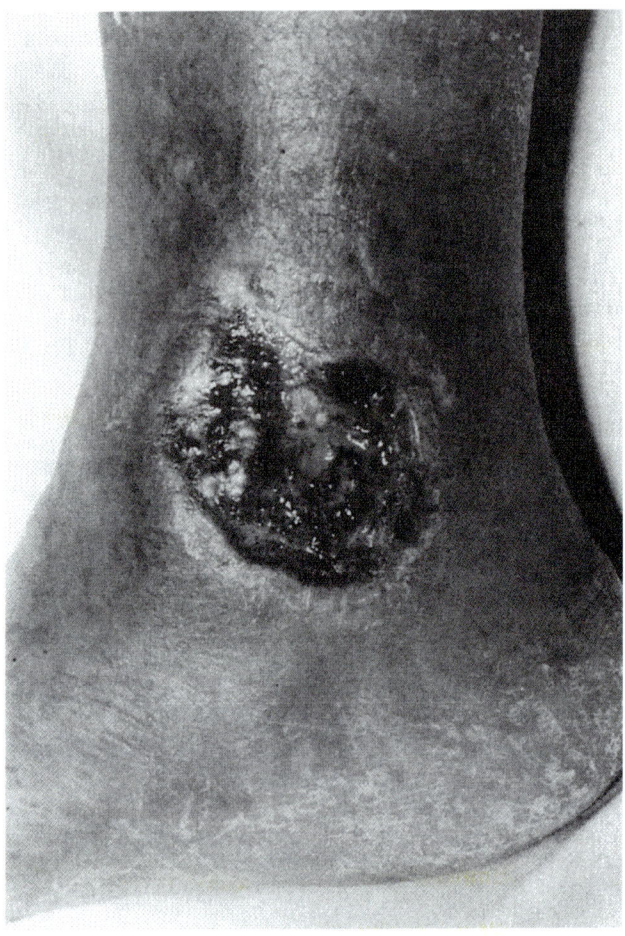

Figure 2–17. Stasis ulcer.

### 2. Arteriosclerotic Ulcer

▶ H&P Keys

Markedly painful, dry, shallow necrotic ulcer on foot or lateral leg. Foot is cold and hypoesthetic. Rest pain, claudication, or other signs and symptoms of atherosclerosis.

▶ Diagnosis

Palpation of peripheral pulses, Doppler studies, arteriography.

▶ Disease Severity

Significant associated large and small arterial disease.

▶ Concept and Application

Chronic obstruction of small and large vessels by atheromas.

▶ Treatment Steps
1. Address underlying disease, smoking cessation, antiplatelet agents, pentoxifylline.

3. **Pyoderma Gangrenosum**

   ▶ H&P Keys
   Painful nodule or pustule that rapidly ulcerates, with a tender, undermined border. Associated with ulcerative colitis, Crohn's disease, arthritis, paraproteinemia, and leukemia.

   ▶ Diagnosis
   History and phyiscal exam, biopsy, rule out associated underlying diseases.

   ▶ Disease Severity
   Lesions may be large and involve sites other than legs. Ulcers usually indicate activity of bowel disease.

   ▶ Concept and Application
   Disturbance in immunoregulation.

   ▶ Treatment Steps
   Systemic steroids, dapsone, local care, treat underlying disease, if any.

D. **Cutaneous Manifestations of Systemic Disease**

   1. **Lupus Erythematosus**

      ▶ H&P Keys
      Three types: acute (systemic), subacute, chronic (discoid) (Fig. 2–18).

      *Acute*—Malar erythema (butterfly rash), Raynaud's phenomenon, oral ulcers, alopecia, vasculitis.

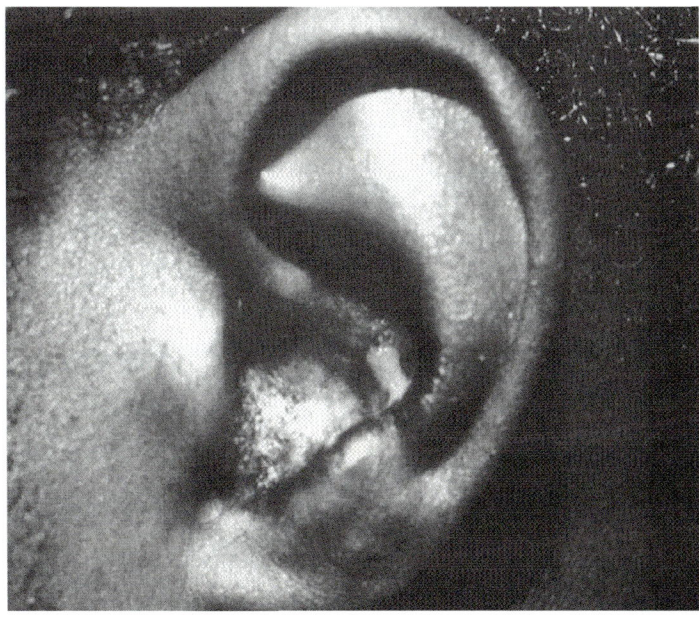

Figure 2–18. Discoid lupus erythematosus of the external auditory canal.

*Subacute*—Annular or polycyclic (resembling tinea or psoriasis), photosensitivity.

*Chronic*—Scarring, red, scaling plaques, primarily on sun-exposed areas. Review of systems check. [discoid lesions]

▶ Diagnosis

History and physical exam; laboratory studies may include: complete blood count, ANA, urinalysis, SMA, Ro (SS-A), La (SS-B); skin biopsy, immunofluorescence.

▶ Disease Severity

Acute may have serious renal or CNS manifestations. Subacute is associated with a low risk of CNS or renal disease. Chronic is usually limited to the skin.

▶ Concept and Application

Autoimmune disease involving vasculature and connective tissue.

▶ Treatment Steps
1. Topical steroids for chronic, systemic and/or antimalarials for acute and subacute, broad spectrum sunscreens.
2. Add intralesional steroids for persistent chronic cutaneous lesions.

2. Dermatomyositis

▶ H&P Keys

Proximal muscle weakness, heliotrope rash (eyelid erythema), Gottron's papules (purple papules on knees and knuckles).

▶ Diagnosis

History and physical exam, creatine phosphokinase (CPK), aldolase, skin and muscle biopsy, electromyogram (EMG).

▶ Disease Severity

In adults may herald internal malignant neoplasms.

▶ Concept and Application

Multisystem disorder with autoantibodies.

▶ Treatment Steps

Topical and systemic steroids, rest, cytotoxic agents.

3. Scleroderma

▶ H&P Keys

Localized: morphea. Diffuse: progressive systemic sclerosis. Latter also associated with Raynaud's phenomenon, dysphagia, masklike face. Skin is tight, woody, bound down.

▶ Diagnosis

History and physical exam, skin biopsy, ANA, anticentromere antibody, Scl-70 (anti-topoisomerase).

► Disease Severity

Progressive systemic sclerosis associated with multisystem involvement: renal, lung, esophagus. Variant: CREST = calcinosis, Raynaud's, esophageal dysfunction, sclerodactyly, telangiectasia. Better prognosis; associated with anticentromere antibody.

► Concept and Application

Unknown etiology. Excessive collagen deposition in skin and other organs.

► Treatment Steps
1. Symptomatic, physical therapy, immunosuppressives. Penicillamine (controversial).

4. Livedo Reticularis

► H&P Keys

Mottled, netlike vascular erythema; aggravated by cold exposure; most common in women under 40 years old.

► Diagnosis

History and physical exam.

► Disease Severity

Associated disease: arteriosclerosis, collagen vascular disease, endocrine disorders, antiphospholipid antibodies, drugs (amantadine).

► Concept and Application

Vasospasm of arterioles.

► Treatment Steps
1. Avoidance of cold exposure, treatment of associated medical conditions.

5. Amyloidosis, Systemic

► H&P Keys

*Specific*—Waxy papules or nodules on face, macroglossia.

*Nonspecific*—Purpura (most common), especially after proctoscopy, alopecia.

► Diagnosis

Exam, biopsy (amyloid stained with Congo red shows apple green birefringence when viewed with polarized light).

► Disease Severity

Systemic organ involvement, associated myeloma.

► Concept and Application

Immunoglobulin-related amyloid deposited in skin and other organs.

► Treatment Steps
1. Symptomatic, melphalan, or prednisone.

6. Behçet's Disease

   ▶ H&P Keys

   *Triad*—Aphthous ulcers, genital ulcers, uveitis.

   *Skin Lesions*—Erythema nodosum, ulcers.

   ▶ Diagnosis
   Clinical exam.

   ▶ Disease Severity
   Associated findings: arthritis, retinal vasculitis, cardiovascular and neurologic effects.

   ▶ Concept and Application
   No known etiology; more frequent in men. Lesions develop at sites of trauma (pathergy).

   ▶ Treatment Steps
   Systemic steroids, colchicine, azathioprine, chlorambucil, cyclophosphamide.

7. Tuberous Sclerosis

   ▶ H&P Keys
   Autosomal dominant, seizures, retardation. Skin lesions: white spots (ash-leaf macule, earliest lesion), adenoma sebaceum (Fig. 2–19), connective tissue nevi (shagreen patch), periungual fibrous tumors.

   ▶ Diagnosis
   History and physical exam, biopsy of adenoma sebaceum.

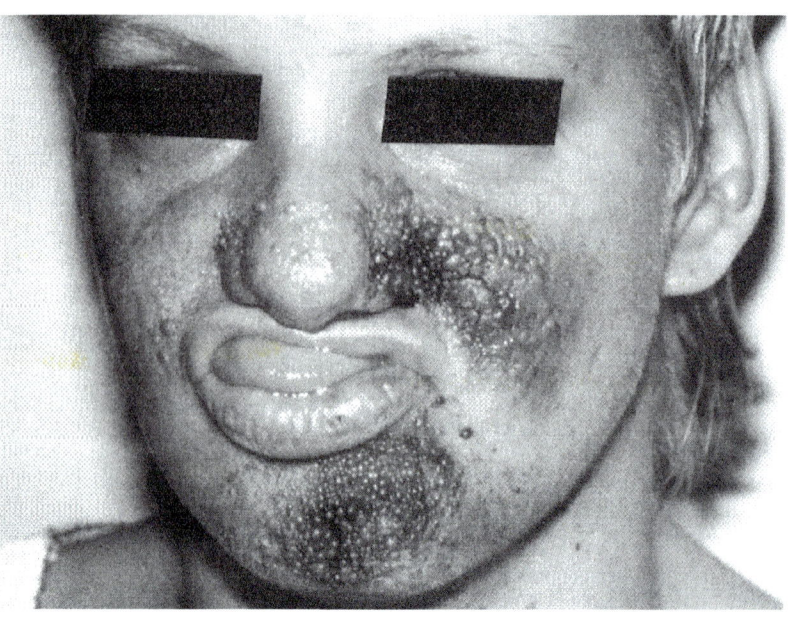

Figure 2–19. Adenoma sebaceum.

▶ Disease Severity
Variable expression. Some patients may show cutaneous features only.

▶ Concept and Application
Genetic multisystem disease.

▶ Treatment Steps
1. Supportive management, MRI of the head to rule out CNS involvement.

8. Necrobiosis Lipoidica

▶ H&P Keys
Yellow-brown atrophic plaques on shins, may ulcerate.

▶ Diagnosis
History and physical exam, biopsy.

▶ Disease Severity
Most cases associated with diabetes.

▶ Concept and Application
Necrosis of the lower dermis, with granulomatous inflammation and vasculitis.

▶ Treatment Steps
1. Topical and intralesional corticosteroids, antiplatelet agents, check glucose.

9. Porphyria Cutanea Tarda

▶ H&P Keys
Photosensitivity, blisters on backs of hands, scars, increased hair growth (werewolf), hyperpigmentation.

▶ Diagnosis
Urine will fluoresce under Wood's light; blood, urine, stool studies for porphyrins; skin biopsy.

▶ Disease Severity
May be hereditary, but induced by hepatitis C infection, ethanol, estrogens, chloroquine, chlorinated phenols, iron. Diabetes in 25%.

▶ Concept and Application
Uroporphyrinogen decarboxylase deficiency.

▶ Treatment Steps
1. Discontinue provoking drugs or chemicals. Liberal use of broad spectrum sunscreen, titanium dioxide/zinc oxide.
2. Phlebotomy and/or anti-malarials.

E. Cutaneous Signs of Internal Malignant Neoplasms
1. See dermatomyositis, sign of Leser–Trélat (seborrheic keratoses), keratoderma (tylosis).

2. Acanthosis nigricans (Fig. 2–20). Velvety brown patches on axillae and neck; associated with GI carcinomas (stomach), lung cancer, as well as obesity, endocrine disease.
3. Sweet's syndrome. Tender, vesicular papules and plaques on face, extremities, and upper trunk; may be associated with leukemia.
4. Cowden's syndrome (multiple hamartoma syndrome). Warty lesions on face (trichilemmomas), gums, hands, and feet; associated with breast cancer, thyroid tumors.
5. Gardner's syndrome (see lipomas). Large epidermal cysts, fibromas, lipomas, osteomas; autosomal dominant; polyps and carcinoma of GI tract.
6. Peutz–Jeghers syndrome. Freckle-like pigmented spots on lips, nose, fingertips; autosomal dominant; hamartomatous GI polyps; low frequency of malignancy.
7. Muir–Torre syndrome. Benign and malignant sebaceous tumors of skin; high incidence of colon cancer; possibly autosomal dominant.
8. Multiple mucosal neuroma syndrome. Multiple neuromas (whitish nodules) on lips and anterior tip of tongue; medullary carcinoma of thyroid, pheochromocytoma, parathyroid adenomas (multiple endocrine neoplasia [MEN] type IIb); autosomal dominant.
9. Glucagonoma syndrome. Necrolytic migratory erythema (erosive, annular, intense erythema) around orifices, abdomen, thighs, and distal extremities; alpha-cell tumor of pancreas.

### F. Nail Signs and Disease
1. Onycholysis. Nail plate lifts off nail bed; associated with trauma, psoriasis, hyperthyroidism.
2. Terry's nails. Proximal two thirds of nail is white; associated with low serum albumin, cirrhosis, congestive heart failure.

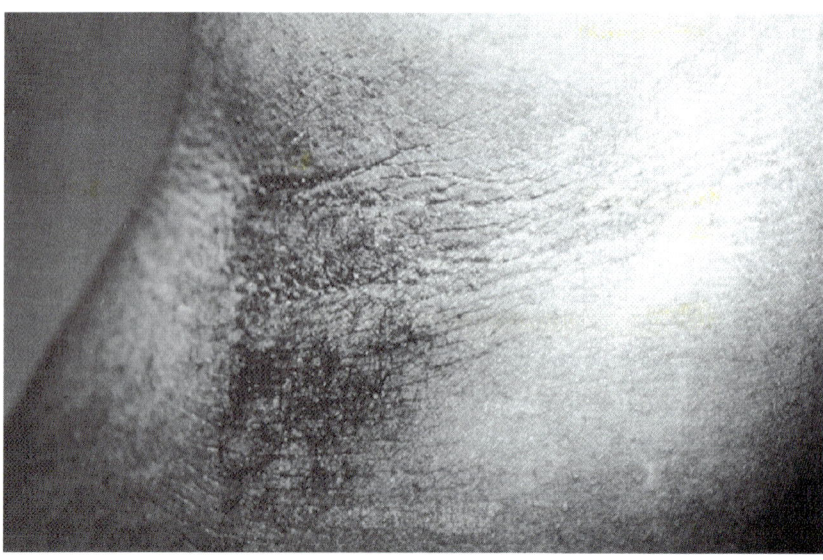

Figure 2–20. Acanthosis nigricans.

3. Splinter hemorrhages. Streaks of blood under distal portion of nail plate; associated with trauma, subacute bacterial endocarditis (SBE).
4. Beau's lines. Horizontal nail depressions (Fig. 2–21); associated with temporary arrest of nail growth from severe illness.
5. Clubbed nails. Overcurvature of nail plate and loss of nail-digit angle; associated with cardiopulmonary disease, cancer.
6. Muehrcke's nails. Two horizontal white stripes; associated with low albumin, nephrosis.
7. Yellow nails. Yellow discoloration of nail plate, no cuticles, associated with lymphedema, pulmonary effusion.
8. Half-and-half nails. White proximal half, distal brown nail; associated with chronic renal failure.

## G. Diseases and Disorders of Newborns

1. Erythema toxicum neonatorum. Pinkish macules, papules, and pustules; self-limited.
2. Port-wine stain (nevus flammeus). Most often on face or neck (stork bite), flat vascular patch; associated with Sturge–Weber syndrome, particularly if it involves the upper eyelid; treatment with laser.
3. Café-au-lait macules. Presence of more than five is associated with neurofibromatosis.
4. Mongolian spot. Blue discoloration of sacrum; common in black races; no clinical significance or treatment.
5. Miliaria. Pruritis red papules from occlusion of sweat duct; aeration is critical; mild topical steroids.
6. Ataxia–telangiectasia. Telangiectasia of bulbar conjunctiva and skin; ataxia, bronchiectasis, IgA deficiency; autosomal recessive.

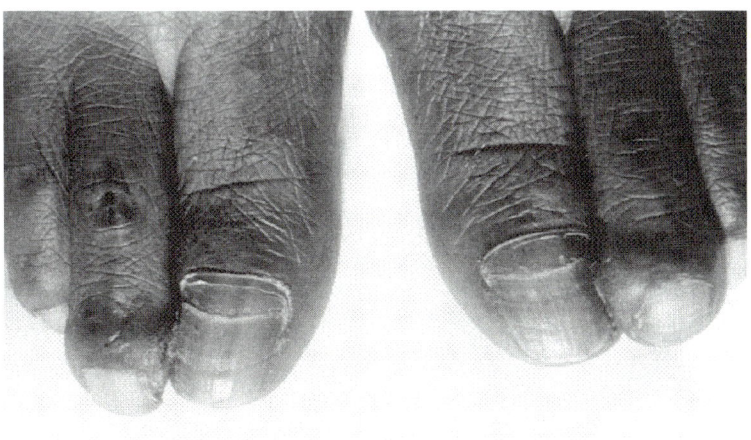

Figure 2–21. Beau's lines (patient had ruptured berry aneurysm 6 months previously).

## BIBLIOGRAPHY

Fitzpatrick TB, et al. *Dermatology in General Medicine*, 6th ed. New York: McGraw-Hill; 2003.

Fitzpatrick TB, et al. *Color Atlas and Synopsis of Clinical Dermatology*, 4th ed. New York: McGraw-Hill; 2000.

Odom RB, James WD, Berger TG. *Andrews' Diseases of the Skin, Clinical Dermatology*, 9th ed. Philadelphia: Saunders; 2000.

# Endocrinology 3

I. **THYROID GLAND DISORDERS / 88**
    A. Hyperthyroidism / 88
    B. Hypothyroidism / 89
    C. Neoplasms of the Thyroid Gland / 91

II. **PARATHYROID GLAND DISORDERS / 91**
    A. Hypercalcemia / 91

III. **PITUITARY GLAND DISORDERS / 92**
    A. Anterior Pituitary / 92
    B. Posterior Pituitary / 94

IV. **ADRENAL GLAND / 95**
    A. Adrenal Insufficiency / 95
    B. Cushing's Syndrome / 96
    C. Hirsutism / 97
    D. Pheochromocytoma / 98
    E. Congenital Adrenal Hyperplasia / 98

V. **CLINICAL LIPOPROTEIN DISORDERS / 99**
    A. Type I Familial Chylomicronemia / 99
    B. Type II Hyperlipoproteinemia / 100
    C. Type III Dysbetalipoproteinemia / 100
    D. Type IV Hyperlipoproteinemia / 100
    E. Type V Hyperlipoproteinemia / 101
    F. Decreased High-Density Lipoprotein / 102
    G. Elevated Lp(a) Lipoprotein / 102

VI. **DIABETES MELLITUS / 102**
    A. Type 1 / 102
    B. Type 2 / 103
    C. Hyperosmolar Hyperglycemic Nonketotic Coma (HHNK) / 104
    D. Hypoglycemia / 105

**BIBLIOGRAPHY / 105**

## diagnostic decisions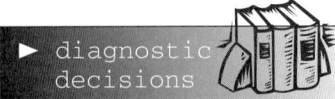

### HYPERTHYROIDISM

**Graves' disease**
Family history of thyroid disease, other autoimmune diseases, diffusely enlarged gland with bruit. Elevated $T_4$, $T_3RU$, suppressed TSH. Increased $I^{123}$ uptake.

**Subacute thyroiditis**
Recent viral illness, painful thyroid. Elevated $T_4$ and $T_3RU$, suppressed TSH. Suppressed $I^{123}$ uptakes.

**Toxic adenoma**
Older age, solitary nodule on exam. Elevated $T_4$, $T_3RU$, and TSH. Single, "hot" nodule on $I^{123}$ scan.

## I. THYROID GLAND DISORDERS

### A. Hyperthyroidism

▶ **H&P Keys**

Most commonly autoimmune etiology (Graves' disease). Can also be toxic adenoma, toxic multinodular goiter, iodine induced or factitious.

Weight loss, palpitations, nervousness, muscle weakness, heat intolerance, dyspnea, increased bowel movements, change in menstrual function, eye symptoms (burning, tearing, diplopia). Family history of thyroid disease.

Thyroid enlargement common, thyroid bruit, proptosis, tremor, tachycardia, hyperactive reflexes, systolic hypertension, pretibial myxedema, onycholysis, proximal myopathy, ophthalmopathy (Fig. 3–1).

Hyperthyroidism in the elderly often presents with apathetic rather than hyperkinetic symptoms. Cardiac manifestations are common (atrial fibrillation, congestive failure).

▶ **Diagnosis**

Elevated levels of total or free thyroxine ($T_4$), triiodothyronine ($T_3$), and resin uptake ($T_3RU$). Suppressed levels of thyrotropin (TSH). Estrogen in pills or pregnancy increases $T_4$ binding globu-

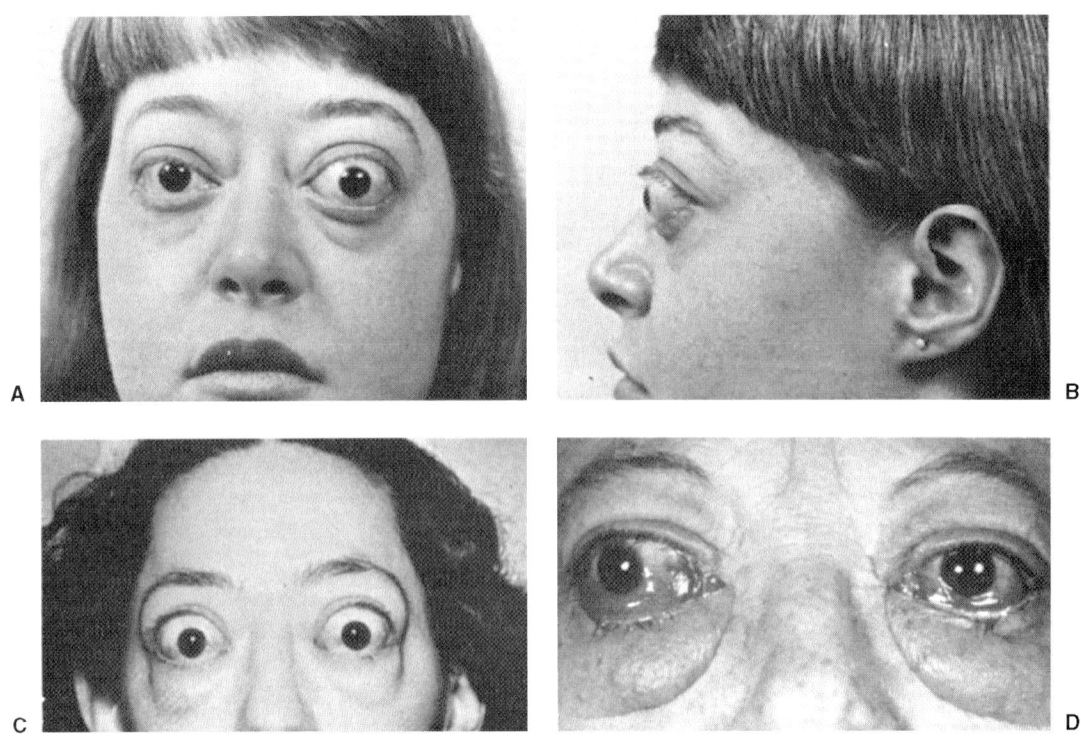

Figure 3–1. Photographs of three patients with ophthalmopathy due to Graves' disease. **A, B.** A young woman with moderate asymmetric proptosis, with marked left eyelid retraction. This patient has few manifestations of ocular inflammatory disease. **C.** A young woman with marked periorbital edema, bilateral lid retraction, and proptosis. **D.** A middle-aged woman with marked infraorbital edema, conjunctival injection and chemosis, and muscle restriction of the right eye, but little proptosis. (Reproduced, with permission, from Felig P. *Endocrinology and Metabolism*, 4th ed. New York: McGraw-Hill; 2001.)

lin: in this situation the $T_4$ is increased and the $T_3$ uptake is decreased. Assay of thyroid antibodies may be performed to exclude Hashimoto's thyroiditis. An iodine ($I^{123}$) uptake and scan can be performed if the diagnosis is not secure or if radioactive iodine therapy is considered.

▶ Disease Severity

Tachyarrhythmias, atrial fibrillation, severe weight loss, mental status change, and fever as in thyroid storm.

▶ Concept and Application

Hypermetabolism and hyperkinesis resulting from autonomous thyroid hormone secretion. Decreased thyroid hormone production with antithyroid drugs and decreased autonomic nervous system hyperactivity with β-blocking drugs.

▶ Treatment Steps

1. β-blockade with propranolol, metoprolol, or atenolol to decrease sympathetic nervous system symptoms.
2. Antithyroid medications, methimazole, or propylthiouracil, especially in women of childbearing age and severe disease.
3. Radioactive iodine ablation if patient older, less severe thyroid disease, or intolerance to antithyroid medications.
4. Surgery if contraindications to medications or radioactive iodine.

## B. Hypothyroidism

▶ H&P Keys

Usually secondary to chronic autoimmune (Hashimoto's) thyroiditis, radioactive iodine therapy, head or neck irradiation, or thyroid surgery. Family history of thyroid disease, fatigue, weakness, cold intolerance, sleepiness, dry skin, hoarseness, constipation, depression, slow mentation, menstrual irregularities, infertility, weight gain.

On physical examination, a firm goiter with multiple nodules (Hashimoto's disease) or a nonpalpable gland; bradycardia; slow, hoarse speech; cool, dry, thick skin; delayed relaxation of deep-tendon reflexes; yellow skin (carotenemia); loss of scalp hair and eyebrows (see Fig. 3–2).

▶ Diagnosis

Elevated level of TSH, low total or free $T_4$ level; triiodothyronine ($T_3$) levels and $I^{123}$ uptake and scans not helpful in diagnosis. Assays for thyroid peroxidase antibodies (previously antimicrosomal antibodies) or antithyroglobulin antibodies to confirm Hashimoto's thyroiditis. If positive, these patients and their families have an increased incidence of other autoimmune diseases such as Graves', pernicious anemia, vitiligo, rheumatoid arthritis, adrenal insufficiency, and premature menopause.

▶ Disease Severity

Mental status: confusion, dementia, stupor, or coma; decreased ventilation and abnormal blood gases; hypothermia, cardiomyopathy, ataxia.

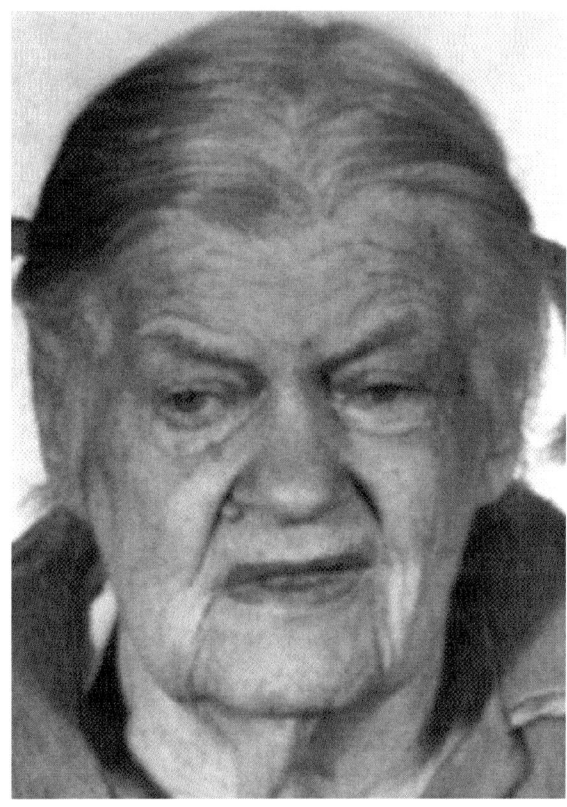

Figure 3–2. Photograph of a patient with hypothyroidism, showing facial puffiness and periorbital edema. (Reproduced, with permission, from Felig P. *Endocrinology and Metabolism,* 4th ed. New York: McGraw-Hill; 2001.)

▶ Concept and Application

Hypometabolic state caused by decrease or lack of thyroid hormone.

▶ Treatment Steps

*Uncomplicated Hypothyroidism*
1. Begin L-thyroxine ($T_4$) replacement at 0.075–0.150 mg daily. Elderly patients should be started on 0.0125–0.025 mg daily.
2. Check TSH level in 6 weeks after any dose adjustment.
3. Avoid concomitant use of cholestyramine, antacids, and iron supplements that interfere with $T_4$ absorption in the gastrointestinal tract.

*Myxedema Coma*
1. Respiratory support.
2. Hydocortisone 100 mg IV every 8 hours; first dose must proceed $T_4$ replacement.
3. L-thyroxine IV 2 mcg/kg load, followed by 100 mcg every 24 hours until respiratory and mental status improve.

## C. Neoplasms of the Thyroid Gland

▶ H&P Keys

Most thyroid nodules are benign. The most common cancer is papillary, followed by follicular, medullary, and the most aggressive, anaplastic (more common in the elderly).

Family history of thyroid cancer, head or neck irradiation as a child, radiation exposure. New-onset hoarseness: indirect laryngoscope needed to rule out recurrent laryngeal nerve involvement. May be a solitary thyroid nodule or a large nodule in a multinodular gland.

▶ Diagnosis

Fine needle-aspiration for histocytopathologic examination. If specimen inadequate, repeat the aspiration. Assay of $T_4$, TSH, and thyroid antibodies to determine if patient has Hashimoto's thyroiditis with a lumpy thyroid. Baseline thyroid ultrasonogram to check nodule size and rule out a cyst. $I^{123}$ thyroid uptake and scan will reveal if the nodule is "cold" (nonfunctioning), or "hot" (hyperfunctioning) and less likely to be malignant. A thyroglobulin level is occasionally helpful as a tumor marker. If elevated, it can be rechecked after surgery, and followed for recurrence of the tumor. Elevated calcitonin levels are seen in medullary thyroid carcinoma.

▶ Disease Severity

Nodule size, distant metastases, hoarseness. Past history of head or neck irradiation. Anaplastic classification.

▶ Concept and Application

None.

▶ Treatment Steps

1. Surgical removal of the thyroid and tumor, along with any obvious nodal involvement.
2. $I^{131}$ ablation of remaining thyroid tissue or metastatic disease.
3. Suppression of the TSH level (to < 0.3 µIU/mL) with exogenous L-thyroxine replacement.

## II. PARATHYROID GLAND DISORDERS

### A. Hypercalcemia

▶ H&P Keys

Family or personal history of hypercalcemia, renal stones, multiple endocrine neoplasia (MEN) type I or II, or malignancy. Many are asymptomatic. Common symptoms: fatigue, lethargy, nocturia, weakness, constipation, depression, or renal colic from kidney stones. History of calcium, vitamin D or vitamin A intake, use of thiazides or lithium.

▶ Diagnosis

Elevation of calcium levels corrected for albumin. Primary hyperparathyroidism will have low levels of phosphorus and normal to

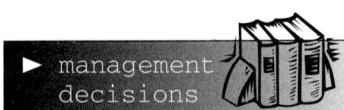

## management decisions

### HYPERCALCEMIA

**Primary hyperparathyroidism**
Surgery indicated if osteoporosis or kidney stones are present; if $Ca^{2+}$ greater than 12 mg/dL, or if patient less than 50 years of age. Familial hypercalcemic hypocalciuria must be excluded prior to surgery.

**Hypercalcemia of malignancy**
Intravenous hydration and furosemide, followed by salmon calcitonin and bisphosphonates. Treatment of the underlying malignancy if possible.

**Vitamin D intoxication**
Removal of Vitamin D source if possible, hydration, glucocorticoids.

---

elevated parathyroid hormone assays (intact PTH assays most reliable). Sestamibi parathyroid scan to localize adenoma or hyperplasia. Suppression of PTH levels in face of hypercalcemia suggests nonparathyroid source. CXR, parathyroid related protein assay in smoker with hypercalcemia. Serum protein electrophoresis to evaluate for multiple myeloma. 1,25 di-hydroxy-vitamin D levels elevated in lymphoma and granulomatous diseases (sarcoidosis, leprosy). $T_4$ and TSH to exclude hyperthyroidism.

▶ **Disease Severity**

Calcium levels greater than 12 mg/dL. Kidney stones, osteoporosis, pancreatitis, lethargy, confusion, stupor or coma.

▶ **Concept and Application**

Overproduction of parathyroid hormone in primary hyperparathyroidism (single adenoma or hyperplasia of all four glands), may be familial (autosomal dominant), part of MEN I, which includes tumors of the pituitary and pancreas (insulinoma, gastrinoma), or MEN II, which includes hyperparathyroidism, pheochromocytoma, and medullary thyroid carcinoma.

In malignancy associated hypercalcemia, production of humoral bone resorbing factors (ie, parathyroid hormone related protein, or direct bone destruction by tumor). Excess vitamin D intake or production.

▶ **Treatment Steps**

*Severe Hypercalcemia*
1. Intravenous hydration with 0.9% (normal) saline solution.
2. Intravenous furosemide to promote calciuresis.
3. Salmon calcitonin subcutaneously every 6–12 hours for rapid lowering of $Ca^{2+}$ level.
4. Intravenous bisphosphonates (pamidronate or etidronate) for prolonged control.
5. Treatment of underlying source.

## III. PITUITARY GLAND DISORDERS

### A. Anterior Pituitary

#### 1. Overproduction Syndromes

▶ **H&P Keys**

Galactorrhea, amenorrhea, infertility (prolactinomas); enlargement of hands, jaw, feet (acromegaly); moon facies, dorsocervical and supraclavicular fat pads, striae (Cushing's disease). May be a nonfunctioning adenoma presenting with visual changes, hypogonadism, fatigue, loss of axillary and pubic hair.

▶ **Diagnosis**

Assays of $T_4$, TSH (rule out primary hypothyroidism, which may elevate prolactin levels). Prolactin level (exclude use of medications that act on the central nervous system and elevate prolactin, eg, phenothiazines).

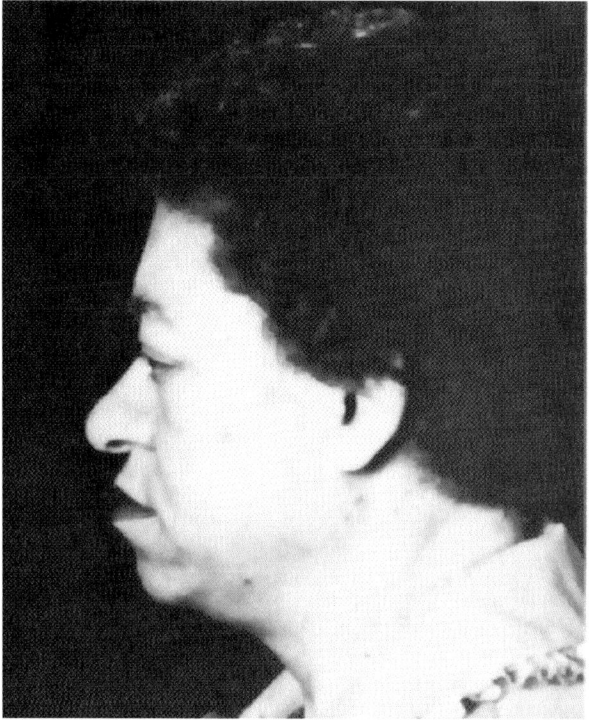 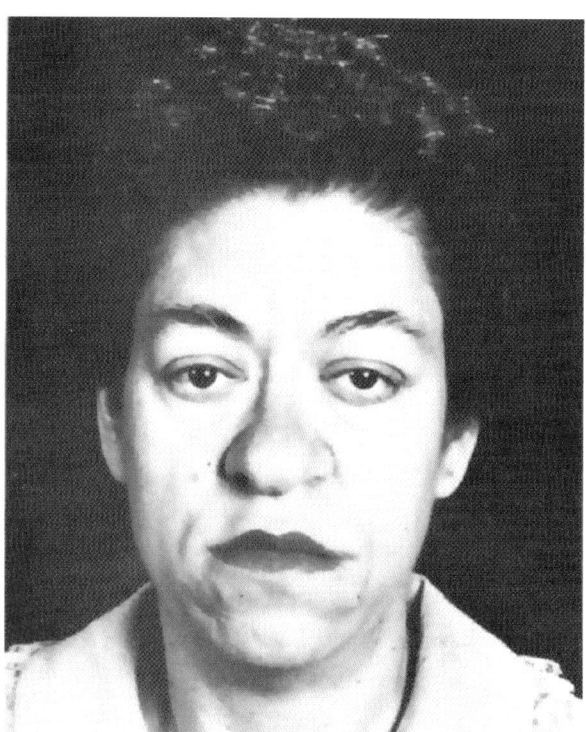

Figure 3-3. Facial appearance of a 43-year-old woman with acromegaly whose disease had been present for 15 years. Soft tissue overgrowth about the eyes, nose, and mouth has resulted in coarsening of the features. Lacrimal overgrowth is evident, as is thickening of the skin folds and the presence of fibroma molluscum (acrochordon). (Reproduced, with permission, from Felig P. *Endocrinology and Metabolism,* 4th ed. New York: McGraw-Hill; 2001.)

Obtain a growth hormone and IGF 1 level (somatomedin C) to evaluate for acromegaly. See Figure 3–3. Corticotropin (ACTH) producing tumors can be screened for with an overnight dexamethasone suppression test (AM cortisol level should be less than 4). Perform a magnetic resonance imaging (MRI) with gadolinium of the pituitary and hypothalamus. Petrosal sinus sampling for Cushing's disease.

▶ Concept and Application

Tumors may be functioning, producing prolactin, growth hormone, corticotropin (ACTH), or TSH. Tumors of the pituitary stalk (craniopharingiomas) may disinhibit prolactin and cause levels to increase. Large tumors can compress the optic chiasm and cause visual disturbance.

▶ Treatment Steps
1. Bromocriptine or cabergoline for prolactinomas and some growth hormone/prolactin producing tumors. Microprolactinomas (< 10 mm) need only medical management.
2. Transsphenoidal surgery for macroprolactinomas with visual changes, and all other tumors.
3. Postoperative radiation therapy for residual tumor.
4. Octreotide for partially treated/recurrent acromegaly.

2. Underproduction Syndromes

▶ H&P Keys

History of prior pituitary surgery or irradiation, history of sinus irradiation, postpartum hemorrhage. Severe headache (acute), inability to breast-feed, fatigue, amenorrhea, sexual dysfunction, testicular atrophy, signs of hypothyroidism, hypotension.

▶ Diagnosis

Measurement of serum $T_4$ and TSH levels. TSH will be low or normal in face of a low $T_4$ level. Measurement of estrogen or testosterone and FSH/LH. Low morning cortisol level, inappropriate adrenal hormone stimulation with insulin or metyrapone challenge. Insufficient stimulation of growth hormone with hypoglycemia. MRI of pituitary with gadolinium showing hemorrhage, necrosis, tumor or granulomatous infiltration (sarcoidosis, tuberculosis).

▶ Concept and Application

Loss of one or more anterior pituitary hormones, leading to insufficiency of end organ hormone production.

▶ Treatment Steps

1. Hydrocortisone replacement with split dosing morning and evening, or long acting glucocorticoid (prednisone, dexamethasone) daily.
2. L-thyroxine replacement; cannot follow TSH levels to determine adequacy of dose, follow free $T_4$.
3. Estrogen replacement (oral or transdermal) or testosterone replacement (intramuscular or transdermal).
4. Growth hormone replacement in children; controversial in adults.

B. Posterior Pituitary

1. Diabetes Insipidus

▶ H&P Keys

Failure to concentrate urine, hypernatremia with thirst, polydipsia, polyuria.

▶ Diagnosis

Measure volume of fluid intake and urine output, serum electrolytes, urine and serum osmolality; water deprivation test.

▶ Concept and Application

Deficiency of vasopressin caused by brain trauma, neurosurgery, sarcoidosis, brain tumors (pinealoma, craniopharyngioma), histiocytosis. Nephrogenic diabetes insipidus (no response to vasopressin) should be ruled out.

▶ Treatment Steps

1. Hydration and normalization of electrolytes.
2. Aqueous vasopressin injections or nasal spray desmopressin (DDAVP). Chlorpropamide in mild cases.

## 2. Syndrome of Inappropriate Vasopressin Secretion (SIADH), Hyponatremia

▶ H&P Keys

Mental confusion. History of cerebrovascular accident, tumor; use of chlorpropamide, phenothiazines; malignancies, pulmonary disease.

▶ Diagnosis

Urine hypertonic to plasma. Exclude adrenal insufficiency, diuretic therapy, nephrosis, cirrhosis, hypothyroidism, compulsive water drinking.

▶ Concept and Application

Inappropriate release of vasopressin causing an inability to dilute urine despite hyponatremia, extracellular fluid expanded without edema.

▶ Treatment Steps

*Acute*
1. 3% saline solution intravenously until Na$^+$ 125 mEq/L.
2. Intravenous furosemide.
3. NSS if further hydration required.

*Chronic*
1. Fluid restriction 800–1,200 mL/day.
2. Demeclocycline.

## IV. ADRENAL GLAND

### A. Adrenal Insufficiency

▶ H&P Keys

Fatigue, weight loss, anorexia, nausea, vomiting, abdominal pain, hyperpigmentation, and volume depletion.

▶ Diagnosis

Electrolyte determination for hyponatremia, hyperkalemia, hypoglycemia. Low morning cortisol level. Cosyntropin (Cortrosyn) stimulation test.

▶ Disease Severity

Hypotension or circulatory collapse, hypoglycemia, hyperkalemia, fever.

▶ Concept and Application

Adrenal gland destruction of autoimmune, infiltrative, or infectious etiology. Underproduction of cortisol.

▶ Treatment Steps

*Acute*
1. Intravenous 5% dextrose/NSS.
2. Intravenous hydrocortisone 100 mg, followed by 100 mg every 8 hours.
3. If diagnosis not secure, IV dexamethasone pending cortisol testing.

*Chronic*
1. Hydrocortisone split dose morning and evening, or long acting glucocorticoid (prednisone, dexamethasone) daily.
2. Florinef started at 0.1 mg daily, dose titrated to normalization of electrolytes and plasma renin activity.
3. Increased glucocorticoid dosing with febrile illness, surgery, or trauma.
4. Increase F and NaCl in hot weather.

## B. Cushing's Syndrome

▶ H&P Keys

Central obesity, violaceous striae > 1 cm wide, general and proximal muscle weakness, easy bruising, dorsocervical and supraclavicular fatty deposition, moon facies, plethora, menstrual irregularities, hirsutism, sexual dysfunction, hyperpigmentation (Fig. 3–4).

▶ Diagnosis

Elevated late afternoon cortisol levels. Baseline 24-hour urinary free-cortisol elevation. Normal or elevated ACTH level. Dexa-

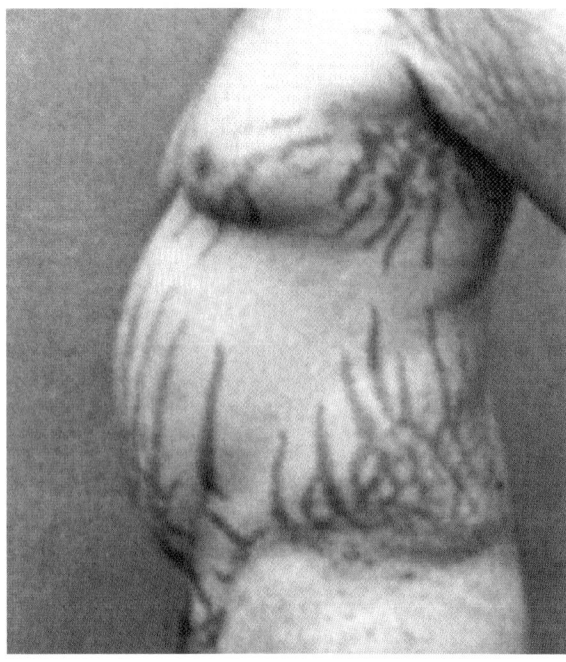

Figure 3–4. Marked striae in a patient with Cushing's syndrome. Reproduced, with permission, from Felig P. *Endocrinology and Metabolism*, 4 ed. New York: McGraw-Hill; 2001.

methasone suppression tests: overnight: 1 mg at 11 PM, serum cortisol at 8 AM; low-dose: 0.5 mg every 6 hours for 48 hours, with 24-hour urine collection for cortisol and 17-hydroxysteroids: high-dose: 2 mg every 6 hours for 48 hours, with 24-hour urine collection for cortisol and 17-hydroxysteroids. Computed tomographic scan (CT) or MRI of pituitary. CT of chest and abdomen. Petrosal sinus sampling.

▶ Disease Severity

Rapidity of symptom onset, hypokalemia, congestive heart failure, paper-thin skin, and osteoporosis.

▶ Concept and Application

Overproduction of cortisol: ACTHproducing pituitary or carcinoid tumor, cortisol-producing adrenal adenoma, and exogenous steroid use.

▶ Treatment Steps

*Acute*
1. Removal of source of excess hormone (transsphenoidal hypophysectomy, adrenal adenectomy, removal of carcinoid tumor).
2. Pituitary irradiation for residual or recurrent pituitary adenoma.
3. Replacement dose steroids until adrenal pituitary axis resumes function.

*Chronic*
1. Ketoconazole, aminoglutethimide, metyrapone or mitotane for nonoperative cases.

## C. Hirsutism

▶ H&P Keys

Age of onset, rate of progression, family history. Terminal hair growth in central location (upper lip, chin, neck, chest), clitoromegaly, male pattern baldness, menstrual irregularities, male body habitus.

▶ Diagnosis

Cosyntropin-stimulated 17-hydroxyprogesterone, and 17-hydroxypregnenolone levels, dehydroepiandrosterone sulfate (DHEAS), testosterone, cortisol levels. Thyroid function tests. CT of abdomen.

▶ Disease Severity

Rapid onset of hair growth, menstrual irregularities, virilization, prepubertal or older age of onset.

▶ Concept and Application

Overproduction of androgens of adrenal or gonadal origin (hyperplasia, tumor, exogenous); hypersensitivity of hair follicles to normal levels of androgens.

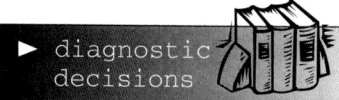

▶ diagnostic decisions

### CUSHING'S SYNDROME

**Cushing's disease**
Basophilic adenoma of pituitary, normal to slightly elevated ACTH, elevated serum/urine cortisol. Suppresses with high dose but not low dose dexamethasone. Unilateral ACTH elevation with petrosal sinus sampling.

**Adrenal adenoma**
Elevated urine/serum cortisol, suppressed ACTH, adrenal nodule on MRI/CT. No suppression with high dose dexamethasone.

**Ectopic ACTH**
Rapid onset symptoms, elevated cortisol levels and ACTH levels. No suppression with low dose dexamethasone, rarely suppressed with high dose. ACTH levels equal bilaterally with petrosal sinus sampling.

▶ Treatment Steps
1. Removal of androgen source if possible.
2. Oral contraceptives.
3. Spironolactone or cyperoterone acetate (contraindicated if chance of becoming pregnant).
4. Replacement hydocortisone if congenital adrenal hyperplasia.
5. Electrolysis, bleaching.

## D. Pheochromocytoma

▶ H&P Keys

Episodes of pallor, palpitations, and headaches; orthostatic hypotension, tachycardia, labile hypertension, panic attacks. Personal or family history of medullary carcinoma of the thyroid, hyperparathyroidism, or other endocrine tumors.

▶ Diagnosis

Supine and standing blood pressures, 24-hour urine collection for catecholamines, metanephrines, and vanillylmandelic acid (VMA); CT of adrenals or MRI of abdomen; methyliodobenzylguanidine imaging.

▶ Disease Severity

Persistent severe hypertension, frequent episodes, increased duration of episodes.

▶ Concept and Application

Tumor of enterochromaffin cells, which produce excessive amounts of catecholamines.

▶ Treatment Steps

*Acute*
1. Phentolamine or nitroprusside for hypertensive crisis.
2. α-Blockade: phenoxybenzamine, (dose adjusted to cessation of paroxysms and hypertension) for 10–14 days.
3. β-Blockade added only after establishment of α-blockade.
4. Surgery to remove tumor.

*Chronic*
1. Phenoxybenzamine.
2. β-Blockers.
3. Metyrosine (catecholamine synthesis inhibitor).

## E. Congenital Adrenal Hyperplasia

▶ H&P Key

Family history of congenital adrenal hyperplasia, dehydration, hypotension, and salt wasting (in infants), ambiguous genitalia, virilization, and hypertension.

▶ Diagnosis

Elevated levels of adrenal androgens, cortisol precursors, or mineralocorticoid precursors (depending on the specific enzyme abnormality).

▶ Disease Severity
Hypotension, salt wasting, failure to thrive in infants; severe genital ambiguity.

▶ Concept and Application
Complete or partial dysfunction of one of the enzymes used in the production of cortisol from cholesterol (21-hydroxylase, 11β-hydroxylase, 17α-hydroxylase, 3β-hydroxysteroid dehydrogenase, or cholesterol side-chain cleavage enzyme). May be due to an absolute or relative absence of the enzyme or abnormal enzyme structure of function. Backup of enzyme substrates causes the clinical sequelae associated with each specific enzyme abnormality.

▶ Treatment Steps

*Acute*
1. Aggressive intravenous fluid repletion.
2. Hydrocortisone 100 mg intravenously every 8 hours.

*Chronic (Infants and Children)*
1. Assignment of gender.
2. Replacement dose steroids (lowest possible dose to ensure adequate hormone concentrations and minimize growth-retarding potential of steroid therapy).
3. Surgical reconstruction of genitalia toward assigned gender.

*Chronic (Adult: Partial Enzyme Blocks)*
1. Glucocorticoids to decrease adrenal androgen production if menstrual irregularities interfere with fertility.
2. Spironolactone for hirsutism (cannot use if pregnancy planned).

## V. CLINICAL LIPOPROTEIN DISORDERS

### A. Type I Familial Chylomicronemia

▶ H&P Keys
Childhood presentation with abdominal pain or acute pancreatitis, eruptive xanthoma, hepatosplenomegaly.

▶ Diagnosis
Increased triglycerides (> 1,000), cloudy plasma, lipoprotein electrophoresis.

▶ Disease Severity
Development of diabetes mellitus, pancreatitis.

▶ Concept and Application
Deficiency of lipoprotein lipase or its cofactor (apo C-II).

▶ Treatment Steps
1. Very low fat diet (< 20 g/d).
2. Supplemental medium-chain triglycerides.
3. Avoidance of alcohol.

## B. Type II Hyperlipoproteinemia

▶ H&P Keys

Premature coronary artery disease (CAD), tuberous and tendinous xanthomas, corneal arcus.

▶ Diagnosis

Lipoprotein measurements with elevated low-density lipoprotein (LDL) alone (type IIa pattern) or elevated LDL and triglycerides (type II b).

▶ Disease Severity

Family history, age of onset of CAD, degree of lipid elevation.

▶ Concept and Application

Three distinct diseases: familial hypercholesterolemia (defect in LDL receptor), familial combined hyperlipidemia (overproduction of apoprotein B100), polygenic hypercholesterolemia.

▶ Treatment Steps
1. Low-fat and low-cholesterol diet.
2. Cholestyramine: will lower LDL (nonabsorbed bile acid sequesterant, not to be used with untreated hypertriglyceridemia).
3. Niacin: will lower both LDL and triglycerides.
4. HMG CoA (hydroxy-methylglutaryl coenzyme A) reductase inhibitors to lower LDL cholesterol.
5. Gemfibrozil: will lower triglycerides primarily, (should not be used with HMG CoA reductase inhibitors).

## C. Type III Dysbetalipoproteinemia

▶ H&P Keys

Obesity, palmar xanthomas, premature CAD.

▶ Diagnosis

Elevated cholesterol and triglycerides; lipoprotein analysis shows elevated very-low-density lipoprotein (VLDL) and intermediate-density lipoprotein (IDL), VLDL-cholesterol and plasma triglyceride ratio below 0.30.

▶ Disease Severity

Presence of premature CAD.

▶ Concept and Application

Abnormality in apolipoprotein E.

▶ Treatment Steps
1. Weight loss.
2. Screen for hypothyroidism.
3. Niacin and/or gemfibrozil.
4. Alcohol avoidance.

## D. Type IV Hyperlipoproteinemia

▶ H&P Keys

May be obese, presence of CAD, gallstones.

▶ **Diagnosis**

Elevated triglycerides, elevated VLDL, decreased high-density lipoproteins (HDL); rule out renal disease and diabetes with appropriate tests.

▶ **Disease Severity**

Premature CAD.

▶ **Concept and Application**

Autosomal dominant inheritance as familial hypertriglyceridemia or familial combined hyperlipidemia.

▶ **Treatment Steps**

1. Low cholesterol, low saturated fat diet.
2. Weight loss.
3. Alcohol and estrogen avoidance.
4. Gemfibrozil or fenofibrate, niacin.

### E. Type V Hyperlipoproteinemia

▶ **H&P Keys**

Obesity, history of pancreatitis, eruptive xanthomas (Fig. 3–5), hepatosplenomegaly.

▶ **Diagnosis**

Elevated triglycerides, cloudy plasma, increased chylomicrons and VLDL.

▶ **Disease Severity**

History of recurrent pancreatitis and/or diabetes.

▶ **Concept and Application**

Multiple molecular defects.

▶ **Treatment Steps**

1. Low-fat diet.
2. Weight loss.
3. Gemfibrozil or fenofibrate, niacin.

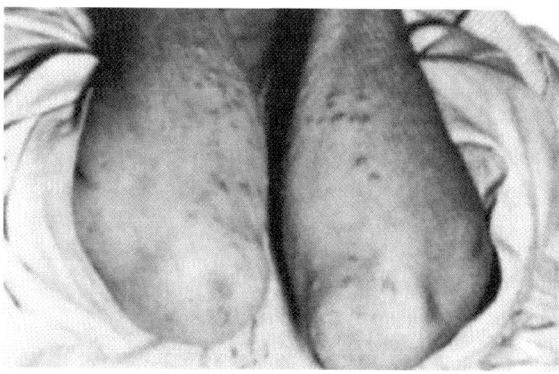

Figure 3–5. Eruptive xanthomas on the arms of a patient with severe hypertriglyceridemia and phenotypic type V hyperlipoproteinemia. (Reproduced with permission from Felig P. *Endocrinology and Metabolism*, 4th ed. New York: McGraw-Hill; 2001.)

### F. Decreased High-Density Lipoprotein

▶ H&P Keys
Often associated with states of increased triglycerides.

▶ Diagnosis
Lipid profile, electrophoresis with low alpha region.

▶ Disease Severity
Presence of premature CAD.

▶ Concept and Application
Multiple defects.

▶ Treatment Steps
1. Coronary risk factor modification.
2. Niacin or gemfibrozil may have some benefit.

### G. Elevated Lp(a) Lipoprotein

▶ H&P Keys
None.

▶ Diagnosis
Electrophoresis.

▶ Disease Severity
Premature CAD, stroke.

▶ Concept and Application
LDL-like particle but with apo B-100 linked to a glycoprotein (apo [a]), which is structurally similar to plasminogen; may be prothrombotic.

▶ Treatment Steps
1. Coronary risk factor modification.
2. High-dose niacin. (Efficacy of drug therapy undetermined.)

## VI. DIABETES MELLITUS

### A. Type 1

Insulin dependent, juvenile onset, ketosis prone. Ten percent of all diabetics are type 1.

▶ H&P Keys
Usually younger patients, before age 20. Weight loss, polyphagia, polydipsia, polyuria, nausea, abdominal pain, and recent infection. Diabetic ketoacidosis (DKA). Thirty percent to 50% concordance rate in identical twins.

▶ Diagnosis
Usually acute or subacute presentation. Blood sugar > 200 md/dL with symptoms. Glucosuria and ketoneuria. Diabetic ketoacidosis (glucose > 300 mg/dL, low bicarbonate, low $Pco_2$, $K^+$ may be high). Serum and urine ketones are elevated. Increased $HbA_{1c}$.

### Disease Severity

DKA, tachycardia, fever, poor skin turgor, lethargy, Kussmaul's respirations (deep, regular, frequent), stupor, coma. Long-term complications of retinopathy, nephropathy, neuropathy, cardiovascular disease, or peripheral vascular disease.

### Concept and Application

Insulin deficiency leading to: increased lipolysis, free fatty acid formation, and ketosis. Glucagon excess, decreased malonyl CoA, and increased ketones. HLA types on chromosome 6 increase risk (HLA-DR3 and HLA-DR4). Viral infection of the pancreas with mumps, coxsackie, rubella may contribute. Autoimmune destruction of the β cells with lymphocytic infiltration. Antibodies to the islet cells are found. Can be associated with other autoimmune disease such as Hashimoto's thyroiditis.

### Treatment Steps

*Diabetic Ketoacidosis*
1. Respiratory support.
2. Intravenous NSS 1–2 L first 1–2 hours, then 150–500 mL/hour until hemodynamically stabilized.
3. K+ replacement if serum K+ normal or low.
4. IV insulin by continuous infusion, initial bolus 10 units followed by 10 units/hour.
5. Monitor blood glucose levels every hour and adjust insulin drip to maintain decrease of 75–100 mg/dL per hour.
6. Change fluids to $D_5NSS$ when serum glucose 250.
7. Continue drip until anion gap normalized.

*Maintenance*
1. Insulin: split mixed regimen (NPH/Regular, lispro, or insulin aspart) before breakfast (two thirds of total daily dose) and dinner (one third of total daily dose). Also can use intermediate acting or long acting insulin 1–2 times daily with lispro or insulin aspart before each meal. Some patients prefer insulin pump.
2. American Diabetes Association (ADA) diet: carbohydrates, 55–60%; protein, 15–20%; fat < 30%. Regular exercise, weight reduction.
3. Monitor blood sugars goal (80–120 before meals, < 180 postprandial). $HbA_{1c}$ goal 7%. (The Diabetes Control and Complications Trial [DCCT] has shown that near normalization of blood sugar helps prevent the retinopathy, nephropathy, and neuropathy).

## B. Type 2

Adult/maturity onset, noninsulin dependent, nonketosis prone. Accounts for 90% of diabetes cases.

### H&P Keys

Family history, obesity, limited exercise, polyuria, polyphagia, polydipsia, blurry vision, weakness, confusion, coma. Usually occurs over age of 40; rapidly increasing prevalence in children and teenagers.

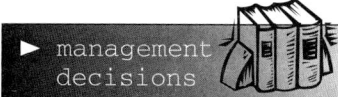

### management decisions

**NEW ONSET DIABETES MELLITUS**

**DKA**
IV hydration; IV insulin continuous infusion; electrolyte management; search for precipitating event.

**HHNK**
IV hydration; search for precipitating event; IV insulin not necessary.

**Type 2, symptomatic, blood sugars > 250–300 mg/dL**
Subcutaneous insulin; meal planning and exercise. Consider switch to oral agents if blood sugar control improves in few months.

**Type 2, symptomatic, blood sugars < 250**
Meal planning and exercise; sulfonylurea or metformin, consider combination therapy if goals not met.

**Type 2, asymptomatic, blood sugars < 200**
Meal planning and exercise. Consider addition of oral agent if blood sugar goals not met.

▶ Diagnosis

Fasting blood sugar ≥ 126 mg/dL on two occasions; 2-hour postprandial blood sugar 200 mg/dL; random glucose 200 mg/dL with symptoms. Exclude secondary causes, eg, Cushing's syndrome, hyperthyroidism, growth hormone excess, steroid use, medications, pancreatitis, cystic fibrosis and pregnancy. $HbA_{1c}$ > 7% consistent with diagnosis.

▶ Disease Severity

Retinopathy, neuropathy, nephropathy/end-stage renal disease, peripheral vascular disease, coronary artery disease. Hyperosmolar hyperglycemic nonketotic coma (HHNK).

▶ Concept and Application

Multiple defects. Patients typically overweight; impaired insulin secretion and peripheral insulin resistance; increased glucose production in the liver and decreased glucose uptake in muscle and adipose tissue.

▶ Treatment Steps

1. ADA diet. Weight reduction as needed. Regular exercise.
2. Diabetes education.
3. Insulin secretagogues (glipizide, glyburide, repaglinide, etc); insulin sensitizers (metformin, pioglitazone, rosiglitazone); acarbose anhydrase inhibitors; insulin.
4. Control of lipid abnormalities: LDL goal < 100.
5. ACE inhibitors for hypertension control or if micro/macro proteinuria present.
6. Yearly dilated ophthalmologic exam.

### C. Hyperosmolar Hyperglycemic Nonketotic Coma (HHNK)

▶ H&P Keys

Usually an elderly patient with infection, MI, or CVA. Lethargy, confusion, coma.

▶ Diagnosis

Blood sugars often > 1,000 mg/dL. Low bicarbonate due to lactic acidosis; ketones normal to minimally elevated. Serum osmolality high. Average fluid deficit is 10 L.

▶ Concept and Application

Decrease water intake/inhibition of thirst mechanism or inability to consume more than deficits. Severe dehydration from osmotic diuresis causing further hyperglycemia and prerenal azotemia. Other causes high-protein tube feedings, peritoneal dialysis, high carbohydrate intake.

▶ Treatment Steps

1. Intravenous hydration with normal saline solution until hemodynamically stable.
2. Evaluate for inciting event (infection, MI, CVA).
3. Decrease to 1/2 NSS or $D_5$ 1/2 NSS as glucose normalizes.
4. Low-dose insulin to control hyperglycema.

## D. Hypoglycemia

### ▶ H&P Keys

Anxiety, sweating, intense hunger, headache, palpitations, blurred vision, irritability, pallor, nausea, diminished mental acuity, convulsions, syncope. Can occur fasting or after eating (reactive). Past history of gastrointestinal surgery, malabsorbtion, hyperparathyroidism, or pituitary tumor. Medications (insulin, sulfonylureas, pentamidine, etc), alcohol consumption. Liver or renal disease.

### ▶ Diagnosis

Blood sugars less than 45 mg/dL in men and less than 35 in women with symptoms that improve with increase in plasma glucose.

Simultaneous measurement of glucose, insulin, C peptide, and urine sulfonylurea metabolites during an episode of hypoglycemia; may need hospitalization for a 72-hour fast. Insulin antibodies can be determined.

### ▶ Disease Severity

Lethargy, coma, seizures, syncope, and death. In diabetes, symptoms may be masked if autonomic neuropathy is present or if the patient is on β-blockers.

### ▶ Concept and Application

Imbalances between hepatic production and glucose utilization. Increased utilization (insulinoma, exogenous insulin, sulfonylureas). Glucose overutilization by other tumors (sarcoma, fibroma, hepatoma, etc). Diminished glucose production from alcoholism, liver disease, adrenal or pituitary deficiency.

### ▶ Treatment Steps

1. Identification and treatment of underlying cause. If decrease production, frequent meals and snacks. Decrease insulin or sulfonylurea dose.
2. If severe (coma, stupor) IV dextrose 50 mL of 50%, the infusion of 10% glucose to keep plasma glucose > 100 mg/dL.
3. Glucagon injection (1 mg), not effective if hepatic glycogen stores are depleted.
4. Surgery for insulinoma or nonpancreatic carcinoma.
5. Diazoxide and octreotide in refractory cases.

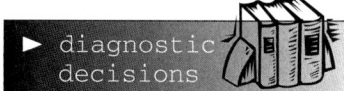

▶ diagnostic decisions

**HYPOGLYCEMIA**

**Insulinoma**
Whipple's triad, blood glucose less than 50 mg/dL, elevated C peptide and insulin levels, negative screen for sulfonylureas.

**Insulin overdose**
Whipple's triad, blood glucose less than 50 mg/dL, suppressed C peptide level, elevated insulin level.

**Sulfonylurea induced**
Whipple's triad, blood glucose less than 50 mg/dL, elevated C peptide and insulin levels, positive screen for sulfonylureas.

## BIBLIOGRAPHY

Bardin CW. *Current Therapy in Endocrinology and Metabolism*, 6th ed. Philadelphia: Mosby–Year Book; 1997.

Braverman LE, Utiger RD, eds. *Werner and Ingbar's The Thyroid: A Fundamental and Clinical Text*, 8th ed. Philadelphia: Lippincott; 2000.

DeFronzo RA. Pharmacologic therapy for Type 2 diabetes mellitus. *Ann Intern Med* 1999;131:281–303.

Degroot LJ. *Endocrinology*, 4th ed. Philadelphia: Saunders; 2000; 1, 2, 3.

Felig P. *Endocrinology and Metabolism*, 4th ed. New York: McGraw-Hill; 2001.

Greenspan FS. *Basic and Clinical Endocrinology*, 7th ed. East Norwalk, CT: Appleton-Century-Crofts; 2003.

Layon JA. *Fluids and electrolytes*. In: *Critical Care*. Philadelphia: Lippincott; 1988.

Lebovitz H. *Therapy for Diabetes Mellitus and Related Disorders*, 2nd ed. Alexandria, VA: American Diabetes Association Inc; 1994.

Mahley RW, Weisgraber KH, Innerarity TL, et al. Genetic defects in lipoprotein metabolism. *JAMA* 1991;265:78–83.

Scanu AM, Lawn RM, Berg K. Lipoprotein (a) and atherosclerosis. *Ann Intern Med* 1991;115:209–218.

Scriver CR. *The Metabolic Basis of Inherited Disease*, 8th ed. New York: McGraw-Hill; 2000.

Speroff L. *Clinical Gynecologic Endocrinology and Infertility*, 5th ed. Baltimore, MD: Williams & Wilkins; 1995.

Thompson JS. *Genectics in Medicine*. Philadelphia: Saunders; 1986.

Wilson J, Foster D, Kronenberg H, Larsen PR, eds. *Williams Textbook of Endocrinology*, 10th ed. Philadelphia: Saunders; 2002.

# Diseases and Disorders of the Digestive System 4

I. **ESOPHAGUS / 109**
    A. Malignant Neoplasms / 109
    B. Gastroesophageal Reflux Disease (GERD) / 110
    C. Motor Disorders of the Esophagus / 111

II. **STOMACH / 114**
    A. Gastric Cancer / 114
    B. Acid-Related Disorders of the Stomach / 115
    C. Disorders of Gastric Motility / 118

III. **SMALL INTESTINE / 120**
    A. Acute Enteric Infections / 120
    B. Celiac Sprue / 124

IV. **COLON / 126**
    A. Invasive Diarrhea / 126
    B. Irritable Bowel Syndrome (IBS) / 126
    C. Colorectal Carcinoma (CRC) / 128
    D. Appendicitis / 132
    E. Inflammatory Bowel Disease (IBD) / 133
    F. Ischemic Bowel Disease / 137
    G. Intestinal Obstruction / 138
    H. Diverticulitis / 138
    I. Constipation / 139
    J. Peritonitis / 140
    K. Familial Mediterranean Fever (Recurrent Polyserositis) / 140

V. **RECTUM / 141**
    A. Malignant Neoplasm of Rectum / 141
    B. Hemorrhoids / 141
    C. Anal Fissure / 142

D. Anorectal Abscess / 142
E. Anorectal Fistula / 143
F. Pilonidal Disease / 144

VI. **GALLBLADDER / 144**
A. Acute Cholecystitis / 144
B. Cholelithiasis / 145
C. Choledocholithiasis and Acute Suppurative Cholangitis / 145

VII. **LIVER / 146**
A. Hepatitis / 146
B. Hepatocellular Carcinoma / 153
C. Hepatic Fibrosis and Cirrhosis / 155

VIII. **PANCREAS / 157**
A. Pancreatic Carcinoma / 157
B. Acute Pancreatitis / 159
C. Chronic Pancreatitis / 161
D. Cystic Fibrosis / 161

IX. **HERNIA / 162**
A. External Hernias / 162
B. Traumatic Hernias of the Diaphragm / 163

X. **ABDOMINAL AORTIC ANEURYSM / 164**

**BIBLIOGRAPHY / 164**

## I. ESOPHAGUS

### A. Malignant Neoplasms

▶ H&P Keys

Symptoms that imply advanced disease include dysphagia, chest pain, weight loss, regurgitation, pulmonary symptoms, and iron-deficiency anemia.

▶ Endoscopy with Biopsy Is Almost Always Diagnostic

▶ Disease Severity (Staging Techniques)
1. Endoscopic ultrasonography (EUS) may be the most accurate technique.
2. Chest and abdominal CT to assess distant organ involvement of liver and lungs.
3. Laparoscopy and thoracoscopy are used increasingly.

▶ Concept and Application

*Epidemiology*—In 1999, 12,000 new cases in the U.S and 12,200 deaths. The incidence is increasing. Mean age of diagnosis is 65 years. Ratio of men to women: 3:1 (Table 4–1). African American men and women have an incidence 3 times greater than Caucasians. Certain countries (China, Iran and South Africa) have a much higher incidence. Outcome is poor with a 10% 5-year survival.

*Etiology*—Squamous cell and adenocarcinoma are the two cell types. Adenocarcinomas are increasing. Among Caucasian males the incidence of adenocarcinoma rose > 350% over the last 20 years.

*Risk Factors*

1. **Squamous Cell Carcinoma**
   - Major risk factors
     1. Alcohol and tobacco
   - Others risk include
     1. Corrosive injury
     2. Chronic vitamin deficiencies (vitamin A, C, iron, riboflavin)

**Table 4-1. GASTROINTESTINAL TRACT CANCERS, ESTIMATED INCIDENCE AND MORTALITY RATES, 1999**

| Organ | New Cases | Male:Female Ratio | Deaths | Male:Female Ratio |
|---|---|---|---|---|
| Esophagus | 12,500 | 3.03 | 12,200 | 3.36 |
| Stomach | 21,900 | 1.67 | 13,500 | 1.41 |
| Small intestine | 4,800 | 1.09 | 1,200 | 1.00 |
| Pancreas | 28,600 | 0.96 | 28,600 | 0.95 |
| Gallbladder/bile ducts | 7,200 | 0.71 | 3,600 | 0.57 |
| Liver | 14,500 | 1.96 | 13,600 | 1.62 |
| Colon and rectum | 129,400 | 0.93 | 56,600 | 0.97 |

Reproduced, with permission, from Landis SH, Murray T, Bolden S, et al. *CA Cancer J Clin* 1999;49:8–31.

3. Esophageal webs (Plummer–Vinson syndrome)
4. Achalasia
5. Human papillomavirus
6. Rubber and asbestosis exposure
7. Tylosis (palmoplantar ketoderma)

2. **Adenocarcinoma**
   - Major risk factors
     1. Alcohol and tobacco
     2. Barrett's esophagus: Barrett's, an intermediate stage between gastroesophageal reflux and esophageal adenocarcinoma, confers a 40 times greater risk of esophageal adenocarcinoma over the general population; median incidence is 1 cancer per 100 years of follow up and increasing.
   - An inverse relationship between *Helicobacter pylori* infection and esophageal adenocarcinoma raises the concern that eradication might confer increased risk for esophageal cancer. However, the newest data imply *H. pylori* as a co-factor in the etiology of adenocarcinoma of the stomach.

▶ Treatment Steps
1. Primary surgical therapy for all with the possibility of cure. Survival correlates with TNM staging. Surgery is offered to less than 40%, and among 85% of these, tumor is found to be at a more advanced stage.
2. Palliation is indicated in most cases to relieve dysphagia, control pain, and assist in nutrition. Expandable metal stents are a promising advance in relieving dysphagia. Debulking therapies include: electrocoagulation, laser photodestruction, laser photodynamic therapy, intra- and extraesophageal radiation, and endoscopic intramural injections of either toxins or chemotherapeutic agents. Chemotherapy includes fluorouracil, cisplatin, and paclitaxel. Combined modalities, including radiation and chemotherapy have shown better results than chemotherapy alone. Chemoradiotherapy followed by surgery provides superior response to surgery alone.
3. Surveillance: Barrett's epithelium longer than 2 to 3 cm (confirmed by histologic identification of intestinal metaplasia) warrants surveillance if there is a potential to prolong life expectancy and treat an early cancer. Surveillance intervals are guided by the degree of dysplasia.

## B. Gastroesophageal Reflux Disease (GERD)

▶ **H&P Keys**

Classic symptoms: heartburn and regurgitation. Heartburn: brought on or made worse by bending, lying flat, stooping, straining, heavy meals, particulary with high fat content, relieved by antacids or acid-suppressing drugs. Other symptoms include upper abdominal pain, bloating, "indigestion" and noncardiac chest pain, sore throat, hoarseness, asthma, dysphonia, chronic cough, globus, and burning tongue. Alarm symptoms: dysphagia, weight loss, iron deficiency anemia, and bleeding suggest severe disease, stricture, or cancer.

▶ Diagnosis

Patients with typical symptoms of GERD (without alarm symptoms) do not require any specific tests initially. Quite often in mild cases, simply giving a trial of a PPI (proton-pump inhibitor) is diagnostic of GERD. Endoscopy reliably demonstrates the presence or absence of erosive esophagitis. However, severity of heartburn correlates poorly with presence or degree of erosive esophagitis. Endoscopy is useful in determining the presence or absence of Barrett's esophagus. A 24-hour pH probe is not routinely recommended. Use to document reflux in patients with atypical symptoms and/or to monitor pharmacologic effect of acid-suppressing therapy. Manometry: prior to elective surgical management.

▶ Pathophysiology

Incompetence of the lower esophageal sphincter (LES) through inappropriate or transient relaxations or through fixed low LES pressure (hypotensive LES). Anatomic disruption of the LES and the crural diaphragm, as occurs with hiatus hernia where two high pressure areas, the LES and the crural diaphragm with an intervening low-pressure area, the intrathoracic hiatal hernia, leads to impaired clearance of gastric acid.

▶ Treatment Steps

1. Initial goals are to relieve symptoms and heal esophagitis. Lifestyle modifications include reduction of dietary fat, weight reduction, smoking cessation, avoidance of large volume meals and alcohol, avoidance of tight-fitting clothes, elevation of the head of bed, remaining upright for q 2–3 hours after eating, and avoidance of reflux-promoting medications.
2. Medications include antacids and antacid/alginate combinations used for short-term symptom relief; and histamine$_2$ receptor antagonists (H$_2$RAs): cimetidine, ranitidine, famotidine, nizatidine, available over the counter, are useful for controlling symptoms in mild grades of GERD. Pharmacologic tolerance to H$_2$RAs may occur. Proton pump inhibitors (PPIs) are effective in relieving symptoms and healing erosive esophagitis and clearly superior to H$_2$RAs. PPIs are taken before food. Some patients require twice daily dosing of PPIs and 70% of those patients have been found to have increased nocturnal reflux acidity. Long-term maintenance treatment is necessary in most patients. There is no evidence that tolerance develops to PPIs. Metoclopramide has no place in treatment because of risks of dystonia or dyskinesia. Laparoscopic antireflux surgery is an alternative for effective long-term management of GERD; however, recent 5-year follow-up postop data has not been encouraging for antireflux surgery.

## C. Motor Disorders of the Esophagus

▶ H&P Keys

Dysphagia, chest pain and reflux symptoms. Ascertain the level of dysphagia:

1. Oropharyngeal dysphagia patients describe food getting stuck in the back of the throat, often with coughing or choking, or nasal aspiration with attempted swallowing.

2. Esophageal dysphagia: patient have difficulty with food getting stuck in the substernal or subxiphoid level, often with odynophagia.

Progressive or intermittent dysphagia evaluation:

1. Progressive implies mechanical obstruction.
2. Intermittent suggests either a motility disorder or a Schatzki ring which is also referred to as the "steakhouse syndrome," ie, sudden difficulty swallowing a piece of meat with dysphagia relieved either spontaneously or with endoscopic removal.

Foods that trigger dysphagia:

1. Progressive obstructive lesions cause progressive dysphagia from large solid foods to soft foods to liquids.
2. Motility disorders have a less predictable progression and may occur with either liquids and/or solids.

▶ Diagnosis

If symptoms suggest oropharyngeal disorder, the first test is cine esophagram or video esophagram. Alternatively, a barium swallow is an appropriate first test.

Esophageal dysphagia: endoscopy to visualize any mucosal or structural abnormality, define strictures, and obtain biopsies. If no obstructive lesions are detected, motility disorders enter the differential diagnosis and esophageal manometry may be helpful (Fig. 4–1).

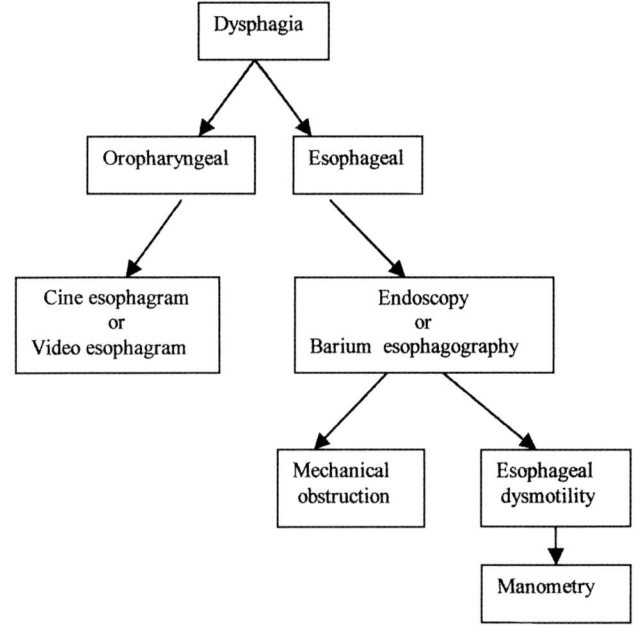

Figure 4–1. Dysphagia.

▶ Concept and Application

Three distinctive disorders of esophageal motor function:

1. Achalasia

   Selective loss of inhibitory vasoactive intestinal peptide (VIP) and nitric oxide (NO) neurons within the LES leads to failure of sphincter relaxation after swallowing.

   Manometric features of achalasia:

   1. Absent or incomplete or inappropriately timed relaxation of the LES upon swallowing.
   2. Simultaneous, low amplitude, nonpropagated contractions in the body of the esophagus.

   Primary achalasia is differentiated from secondary, or carcinoma-related achalasia by endoscopy. Secondary achalasia is caused by carcinoma that infiltrates the LES, typically gastric cardia (most common), breast, prostate, and pancreatic.

   ▶ Treatment Steps
   1. Pharmacological approaches include calcium channel blockers and nitrates, which provide transient, short-term relief.
   2. Botulinum toxin injected directly into the LES at endoscopy provides symptomatic improvement but long-term studies indicate relapse of symptoms and no improvement in esophageal emptying.
   3. Pneumatic dilatation and surgical myotomy are the main therapeutic options and are equally effective. A major advance in therapy is thoracoscopic and laparoscopic approaches to myotomy allowing for minimally invasive Heller myotomy.

2. Diffuse Esophageal Spasm (DES)

   Patients present with intermittent episodes of chest pain and dysphagia.

   Manometric features include episodic or intermittent simultaneous, nonpropagated, and high-amplitude contractions separated by periods of normal esophageal peristalsis. Radiographic features may be absent but a "cork-screw" appearance of the esophagus indicates multiple simultaneous contractions. Radiographic and manometric features can be simulated by gastroesophageal reflux. Therefore, reflux can be considered as one of the causes of "spasm."

   ▶ Treatment Steps
   Symptomatic: nitrates and calcium channel blockers via sublingual administration prior to meals.

3. Scleroderma

   Esophageal manometry is a useful screening test for detection of visceral involvement of scleroderma and mixed connective tissue disorders. Visceral and systemic manifestions may not parallel; severe visceral involvement may occur in patients with relatively minor skin, vasomotor, or connective tissue manifestations.

   Manometric features include low-amplitude aperistaltic contractions and a hypotensive LES. Scleroderma is associated with severe GERD, with progression to advanced esophagitis, stricture, and Barrett's esophagus. These conditions may also develop rapidly with minimal symptoms.

▶ Treatment Steps
1. Aggressive reduction of gastric acid with proton pump inhibitors.
2. Fundoplication is contraindicated in patients with scleroderma with GERD.

## II. STOMACH

### A. Gastric Cancer

▶ H&P Keys

Early symptoms are nonspecific: abdominal pain, dyspepsia, weight loss, early satiety, and anemia. Systemic symptoms suggest advanced disease.

▶ Diagnosis

Endoscopy with biopsy has a 98% accuracy if 8 or more biopsies are taken. Cytology may increase yield. Tumor cells spread through lymphatic and along vascular pathways to liver, lung, bone, and brain. Some gastric tumors in women spread intraperitoneally to involve both ovaries (Krukenberg tumors).

▶ Disease Severity (Staging Techniques)

Endoscopic ultrasound is superior to CT for defining the depth of penetration (T-stage), perigastric lymph nodes, with a limited view of the liver, and it is becoming increasingly available. Abdominal CT +/− laparoscopy to evaluate visceral, peritoneal, liver, and regional and distant lymph nodes (Virchow's node, Sister Mary Joseph's node).

▶ Concepts and Applications

*Epidemiology*—Gastric cancer was the most prevalent cause of cancer mortality in the U.S. prior to 1930. Incidence is steadily declining. In 1999, 21,900 new cases of gastric cancer and 13,500 deaths are estimated (Table 4–1). It remains the second most common cancer in the world and continues in epidemic proportions in Japan, certain parts of Southeast Asia, China, San Marino, and Costa Rica. Overall, 5-year survival is 21%.

*Pathogenesis*—Genetic and environmental factors affect normal gastric mucosa to develop chronic gastritis, gastric atrophy, intestinal metaplasia, dysplasia, and cancer. New data implicates that *H. pylori* may have a causal role as well in gastric cancer.

*Risk Factors*—Environmental (Table 4–2):

- Dietary: Excess dietary salt, decreased fresh vegetables and fruits, nitrites derived from nitrates, smoked foods, and pickled vegetables.
- *Helicobacter pylori* infection.

Other:

- Post-gastrectomy state (two-fold increase risk at 10–20 years), gastric adenomas, and type A gastritis associated with

### 4-2 ENVIRONMENTAL FACTORS ASSOCIATED WITH GASTRIC CANCER

Diet
    Nitrites derived from nitrates
    Smoked foods
    Pickled vegetables
    Excessive salt intake
    Decreased fresh vegetables and fruits
Infection with *H. pylori*
    Chronic gastritis with intestinal metaplasia
Pernicious anemia
    Chronic gastritis with intestinal metaplasia
Subtotal distal gastrectomy (Billroth I, II)

---

pernicious anemia (characteristically seen in persons of Scandinavian and Northern European descent).

### 1. Other Types of Gastric Cancer

**a. Gastric Lymphomas**—These account for 3–5% of gastric cancers and are a common site for extranodal non-Hodgkin's lymphoma. Low-grade gastric mucosa-associated lymphoid tissue (MALT) lymphomas are associated with *Helicobacter pylori* infection. These may regress with eradication of *Helicobacter pylori* infection.

**b. Kaposi's Sarcoma**—Homosexual men with AIDS are affected. It is caused by infection with Kaposi's sarcoma-associated human herpesvirus 8 (HHV-8).

**c. Carcinoid Tumors of the Stomach**—These may be induced by persistent hypergastinemia associated with chronic gastritis or Zollinger–Ellison syndrome patients with multiple endocrine neoplasia-1.

▶ **Treatment Steps**
1. Early detection and surgical removal for both cure and palliation.
2. Chemotherapy is applied for palliation of metastatic disease and as adjuvant therapy to surgery but has no definite survival benefit.
3. New approaches including postoperative intraperitoneal chemotherapy and neoadjuvant protocols designed to downstage tumors preoperatively.

▶ **Screening**
No guidelines exist for screening those at risk in the United States. Endoscopic screening is recommended for some patients who have undergone a partial gastrectomy 15 or more years prior.

## B. Acid-Related Disorders of the Stomach

▶ **H&P Keys**
Periodic epigastric abdominal pain with characteristic pain-free periods lasting days or weeks. Pain is typically intermittent, re-

lieved by antacids or eating. It may awaken a patient from sleep. In the elderly or in patients taking NSAIDs, it may be asymptomatic, or the first presenting sign may be bleeding or perforation.

▶ Diagnosis

*Endoscopy and Biopsy or Upper GI Radiography*—If the diagnosis of gastric ulcer is made radiographically, endoscopy and biopsy are needed to exclude malignancy.

**H. pylori**–*infected Individuals with Asymptomatic Persistent Infections of* **H. pylori**—Only about 15% will develop gastric or duodenal ulcer.

▶ Diagnosis of *Helicobacter pylori*

Endoscopic and nonendoscopic methods for diagnosing *H. pylori* infection include histology, culture, antibody tests, urea breath tests (UBT) and stool tests (Table 4–3). Patients should not receive proton pump inhibitors (omeprazole, lansoprazole, pantoprazole) or antibiotics for 2 weeks prior to undergoing a UBT.

▶ Concept and Application

*H. pylori* and NSAIDs are the major etiologic factors. Eradication of *H. pylori* infection in ulcer patients can provide a permanent cure of the ulcer diathesis.

▶ Treatment Steps

1. Ulcers unrelated to *H. pylori*
   - Long-term acid suppression.
   - Search for a cause (eg, NSAIDs, Crohn's disease, Zollinger–Ellison syndrome) (Table 4–4).
2. Ulcers related to *H. pylori*. (Most ulcer patients have *H. pylori* infection.)
   - All ulcer patients with *H. pylori* should receive treatment for *H. pylori* regardless of whether the ulcer was newly diagnosed or recurrent.
   - *H. pylori*–infected patients taking NSAIDs should also receive treatment for *H. pylori* and, if possible, the NSAIDs are stopped.

## 4-3 DIAGNOSTIC TESTS FOR *H. PYLORI* INFECTION

| Test | | Sensitivity | Specificity | Indications |
|---|---|---|---|---|
| Nonendoscopic | | | | |
|   In-office Ab test | Whole blood | 67–88% | 74–91% | Initial diagnosis |
|   In-office Ab test | Serum | 86–94% | 75–88% | Initial diagnosis |
|   Lab Ab test | ELISA | 86–94% | 78–95% | Initial diagnosis |
|   Stool antigen | | 88–94% | 89–92% | Initial diagnosis and follow-up |
|   Urea breath | | 90–96% | 88–98% | Initial diagnosis and follow-up |
| Endoscopic | | | | |
|   Biopsy urease | | 88–95% | 95–100% | Initial diagnosis and follow-up |
|   Histology | | 90–95% | 98–99% | Initial diagnosis and follow-up |
|   Culture | | 60–95% | 100% | Initial diagnosis and follow-up |

### 4-4 ETIOLOGIES OF GASTRIC AND DUODENAL ULCERS

Most common
    *Helicobacter pylori*
    Nonsteroidal anti-inflammatory drugs
Less common
    Gastric malignancy
    Stress ulceration
    Viral infections (HSV-1, CMV)
Uncommon
    Zollinger–Ellison syndrome
    Drug-induced
    Crohn's diseasee
    *Treponema pallidum*
    Systemic mastocytosis
    Idiopathic (non–*H. pylori*) hypersecretory duodenal ulcer

- *H. pylori* treatment is indicated for all infected patients with a history of duodenal or gastric ulcer, including those with a history of ulcer complication (bleeding, perforation, obstruction).
3. *H. pylori* treatment regimes: See Table 4–5.

▶ Outcomes

**H. pylori–*positive Patients*—**Curing the infection eliminates recurrence of duodenal or gastric ulcers. Reinfection following cure of *H. pylori* is reported in < 2% of adults. True reinfection may be more frequent in underdeveloped countries and among very young children.

**H. pylori—*negative Peptic Ulcer Patients*—**May have a high risk of recurrence and complications.

### 4-5 FDA-APPROVED COMBINATION REGIMENS FOR *HELICOBACTER PYLORI* INFECTION IN PATIENTS WITH PEPTIC ULCER

| Regimen | *H. pylori* Eradication Rate (intent to treat analysis) |
| --- | --- |
| Omeprazole 40 mg or Esomeprazole 40 mg q day + clarithromycin 500 mg tid for 2 weeks, followed by omeprazole 20 mg q day (on esomeprazole 40 mg q day alone for a further 2 weeks) | 64–74% |
| Ranitidine bismuth citrate (RBC) 400 mg bid + clarithromycin 500 mg tid for 2 weeks, followed by RBC 400 mg bid alone for a further 2 weeks | 73–84% |
| Bismuth subsalicylate 525 mg qid + metronidazole 250 mg qid + tetracycline 500 mg qid for 2 weeks; $H_2$-receptor antagonist in standard dose should be started at the same time and continued for a total of 4 weeks | 77–82% |
| Lansoprazole 30 mg bid + clarithromycin 500 mg bid + amoxicillin 1,000 mg bid for 2 weeks | 86% |
| Lansoprazole 30 mg tid + amoxicillin 1,000 mg tid for 2 weeks | 70% |

## C. Disorders of Gastric Motility

▶ H&P Keys

Accelerated emptying of liquids and solids is associated with dumping syndrome. Delayed gastric emptying is associated with postprandial fullness, early satiety, nausea, epigastric discomfort, and vomiting. These symptoms are nonspecific and may also be associated with peptic ulcer disease, mechanical obstruction, and nonulcer dyspepsia.

▶ Diagnosis

Exclude mechanical obstruction with endoscopy or barium radiography (UGI). Scintographic assessment of gastric emptying is a reliable noninvasive study. Solid phase emptying $^{99}$mTc-labeled scrambled eggs is sensitive and specific. $^{13}$C octanoic and $^{13}$C acetate breath tests, recently developed, show reproducibility comparable to scintigraphy and may become an office test of gastric emptying.

▶ Concept and Application

Normal gastric motility ensures trituration of ingested foodstuffs and coordinated delivery of chyme to the small intestine. Disordered gastric motility may result in accelerated or delayed gastric emptying. If gastroparesis is documented, a cause is looked for with the hope of providing specific therapy. Many medications can delay gastric emptying (eg, narcotics, tricyclic antidepressants). Metabolic disorders (diabetes mellitus, hypokalemia, hypothyroidism, hypocalcemia, adrenal insufficiency, uremia) need to be considered. Systemic disorders include scleroderma and hollowvisceral myopathy (Table 4–6).

▶ Treatment Steps

1. The goal of treatment is to correct the underlying motility disorder and provide symptomatic relief. For diabetics, optimize glucose control and correct ketoacidosis and dehydration. In all patients:
   - Avoid medications and dietary factors that may delay gastric emptying.
   - Avoid indigestible solids and fats.
   - Gastroparesis diet (Table 4–7).
   - If dumping is present, separate liquids and solids.
2. Pharmacological: established prokinetic agents include metoclopramide, domperidone, and erythromycin. Metoclopramide use is limited by side effects (dystonia, akathesia, tremor, depression, and extrapyramidal effects). Cisapride has been withdrawn from the U.S. market because of potentially serious drug interactions with drugs that inhibit the cytochrome P450 3A4: ketoconazole, itraconazole, miconazole, troleandomycin, erythromycin, fluconazole, erythromycin, and clarithromycin. Domperidone is not yet available in the U.S. Erythromycin, a motilin agonist, is a potential prokinetic when administered orally as an elixir or intravenously. Its use is limited by tachyphylaxis but is useful for short-term, low-dose therapy.

## 4-6 CAUSES OF DELAYED GASTRIC EMPTYING

Mechanical obstruction
    Pylorus
    Duodenum
    Small intestine
Postgastric surgery
    Vagotomy/antrectomy
    Roux-en-Y
    Fundiplication
Metabolic/endocrine
    Diabetes mellitus
    Hypothyroidism
    Hyperthyroidism
    Adrenal insufficiency
Smooth muscle disorders
    Scleroderma
    Hollow visceral myopathy
Postviral gastroparesis
Medications
    Anticholinergics
    Narcotics
    L-Dopa
    Progesterone, estrogen
    Calcium channel blockers
Chronic mesenteric ischemia
Naturopathic disorders
    Parkinson's disease
    Paraneoplastic syndrome
    Shy-Drager syndrome
    Hollow visceral neuropathy
Idiopathic

## 4-7 GASTROPARESIS DIET

**Step 1 Gatorade and bouillon**
    **Diet:** Patients with severe nausea and vomiting sip small volumes of salty liquids (eg, Gatorade, bouillon), to avoid dehydration. Any liquid ingested should have some caloric content.
    **Goal:** Ingest 1000 to 1500 cc per day in multiple servings.
    **Avoid:** Citrus drinks of all kinds and highly sweetened drinks.

**Step 2 Soups**
    **Diet:** If Step 1 is tolerated, advance diet to include soups with noodles, rice, crackers in small amounts.
    **Goal:** Ingest 1,500 calories per day. Patients who can accomplish this will avoid dehydration and eat enough to maintain their weight.
    **Avoid:** Creamy, milk-based liquids.

**Step 3 Solid food: starches, chicken, fish**
    **Diet:** Starches such as noodles, pasta, potatoes, and rice mix empty easily from the stomach. Solids should be ingested in 6 small meals per day with a MVI.
    **Goal:** Find common foods that the patient finds satisfying without stimulating nausea/vomiting. Gradually, increase the number and variety of foods.
    **Avoid:** Fatty foods, red meats, fresh vegetables, pulpy fibrous vegetables and fruits, foods that require trituration and promote bezoar formation.

Reproduced, with permission, from Koch KL. Clinical approaches to unexplained nausea and vomiting. *Adv Gastroenterol Hepatol Clin Nutr* 1998:3:163–178.

3. For severe, nonresponsive symptoms that compromise nutrition and hydration enteral formulation is given via percutaneous endoscopic gastrostomy (PEG). Enteral feedings are also provided via gastrojejunostomy with a venting gastrostomy (PEJ).

## III. SMALL INTESTINE

### A. Acute Enteric Infections

▶ H&P Keys

*History*—Define onset: abrupt or gradual? Duration: weeks, months, years, or lifelong? Define the pattern and character: loose, watery, large volume, small volume, foul smelling, continuous or intermittent? Is there fecal incontinence? Some individuals complain of diarrhea when their major difficulty is disordered continence. Abdominal pain: presence and character: mild, crampy, diffuse or localized. Identify associated symptoms: nausea, vomiting, headache, fatigue, malaise, anorexia, arthralgias, myalgias, chills and low-grade fever. Ask specific questions regarding:

- Presence of blood
- Weight loss
- Travel
- Food/milk intolerance
- History of gastrointestinal diseases
- Prior evaluations: Review previous evaluations whenever possible
- Abdominal surgery
- Radiation and chemotherapy
- Drug and alcohol use

Identify epidemiological factors, such as travel before the onset of illness, exposure to potentially contaminated food or water, and illness in other family members. Identify aggravating and mitigating factors, such as diet and stress. Consider factitious diarrhea in every patient with chronic diarrhea. Markers of factitious diarrhea include a history of eating disorders, secondary gain, or a history of malingering. Perform a careful review of systems to look for systemic diseases, such as hyperthyroidism, diabetes mellitus, collagenvascular diseases and other inflammatory conditions, tumor syndromes, acquired immunodeficiency syndrome.

▶ Diagnosis

Most acute diarrheal disorders resolve spontaneously and therefore do not need investigation. Get stool culture, O&P, and *C. difficile* toxin when suspicion of bacterial enteritis or parasitic is high. Note the signs of volume depletion, presence of blood, impaired host, and co-morbid disease; and/or diarrhea lasting > 14 days (Table 4–8).

## 4-8 TESTS FOR DIARRHEA

| Test | Comments |
|---|---|
| Stool culture | Not needed in 90% of acute diarrheal illnesses. Although bacterial infection rarely causes chronic diarrhea, it can be excluded by stool culture, including culture on special media for *Aeromonas* and *Pleisiomonas, Yersinia* and *Campylobacter*. *Candida* in stool may cause acute or chronic diarrhea both nosocomial and community acquired, even in immunocompetent individuals. |
| Fecal leukocytes | The presence of white blood cells in the stool suggests an inflammatory diarrhea. This is assessed by Wright's stain or during a stool ova and parasite examination. A latex agglutination test for the neutrophil granule protein lactoferrin may also be useful. |
| Stool lactoferrin | A recently developed latex agglutination test for the neutrophil product lactoferrin is highly sensitive and specific for the detection of neutrophils in stool. |
| Stool ova and parasites | Positive and negative predictive value is dependent on observer skill biopsy may be needed. Special techniques required to detect cryptosporidia and microporidia. |
| Fecal ELISA for *Giardia*-specific antigen | More sensitive and specific for the detection of *Giardia*. |
| Normalization of stool weight with fasting | Common with osmotic diarrhea. |
| Stool weight (g/24 h) | Provides objective data on severity<br>    > 500 common with secretory diarrhea<br>    < 500 common with osmotic diarrhea |
| Stool electrolytes | Use with plasma osmolality to calculate stool osmotic gap[a]<br>    $2(\text{stool }[Na^+] + [K^+]) = {}_p\text{osm}$ common with secretory diarrhea<br>    $2(\text{stool }[Na^+] + [K^+]) < {}_p\text{osm}$ common with osmotic diarrhea |
| Osmotic gap (mOsm/kg)<br>$290 - \{[Na] + [K] \times 2\}$ | Large (> 125 mOsm/kg) in osmotic diarrhea in which nonelectrolytes account for most of the osmolality of stool water.[b]<br>Small (< 50 mOsm/Kg) in secretory diarrhea in which electrolytes account for most of the stool osmolality. |
| Stool *C. difficile* toxin | Toxin B assay is gold standard, requires tissue culture ELISA-based tests detect toxin A, B, or occasionally, both. For highest sensitivity, send three stool samples. |
| Sigmoidoscopy, or colonoscopy with mucosal biopsy | When the differential diagnosis includes ulceration, polyps, tumors, Crohn's disease, ulcerative colitis, amebiasis, microscopic colitis, amyloidosis, granulomatous infections and chronic schistosomiasis and endoscopic biopsy of the proximal small bowel mucosa. A small bowel follow-through examination is preferable to an enteroclysis study for the radiographic evaluation of patients with chronic diarrhea. |
| Upper endoscopy with mucosal biopsy | Useful if small intestinal malabsorptive disorder, such as Whipple's disease, intestinal lymphoma, eosinophilic gastroenteritis, and celiac disease. Aspirate of small intestinal contents for quantitative aerobic and anaerobic bacterial culture is useful if small bowel bacterial overgrowth is suspected. |
| Computerized tomography | Useful in patients with chronic diarrhea when the differential diagnosis includes: chronic pancreatitis or pancreatic cancer, inflammatory bowel disease, chronic infections, intestinal lymphoma, carcinoid syndrome. |
| Stool pH | Values of < 5.6 are consistent with carbohydrate malabsorption. |
| Stool test for cathartics | A panel of tests to detect laxative abuse. Usually includes a test for phenolphthalein (pink color upon alkalization), $Mg^{+2}$, $SO_4$, and $PO_4$. |
| Stool for fat | Performed during the ingestion of a high fat diet. The presence of excess stool fat should be evaluated by means of a Sudan stain or by direct measurement. The presence of excessively large and numerous fat globules by stain or measured stool fat excretion > 14 g/24 h suggests malabsorption or maldigestion. Stool fat concentration of > 8% strongly suggests pancreatic exocrine insufficiency. |
| Fecal occult blood testing | A positive test result suggests the presence of inflammatory bowel disease, neoplastic diseases, or celiac sprue or other spruelike syndromes. |

[a]Na and K are the major cations in fecal fluid. To simplify calculation of the contribution of electrolytes to stool amorality, anions are not directly measured, but assumed to equal the measured cations, hence the doubling of the cation concentration.

[b]Osmolality (mOsm/kg): Measured osmolality of stool water can vary widely and is generally an artifact of the collection process. Because the gut epithelium cannot maintain an osmotic gradient, in vivo stool water amorality is arbitrarily defined as 290–300.

▶ Concept and Application

Infectious agents are a major cause of diarrhea and may cause life-threatening infections in infants, elderly and immunocompromised patients and patients with co-morbid disease.

*Bacterial Pathogens*
- Enterotoxigenic diarrheal pathogens such as *Vibrio cholera* and enterotoxigenic *Escherichia coli* (ETEC) colonize the gut producing toxins that disturb water and electrolyte transport causing high volume, sometimes life-threatening diarrhea not associated with fever, vomiting fecal leukocytes, or blood. Acidosis and hyopokalemia may develop.
- Other communicable bacterial pathogens such as *Campylobacter, Salmonella, Shigella*, and enteroinvasive *E. coli* (EIEC) cause diarrhea by invading and injuring the mucosa. These diarrheal illnesses are associated with high fever, abdominal cramping, bloating, vomiting, and bloody diarrhea. Almost all of these are self-limiting, except *Campylobacter*, which may have a relapsing course.
- Hemorrhagic *E. coli* (EHEC) (*E. coli* 0157:H7) can also cause diarrhea by producing *Shigella*-like toxins, often in food-borne outbreaks of bloody diarrhea associated with undercooked meats and raw milk.
- Enteroadherent *E. coli* (EAEC) infection is a cause of infantile diarrhea.
- Brainerd diarrhea, a chronic idiopathic diarrhea caused by an unknown infectious agent first described in Brainerd County, Minnesota, is also found in travelers.
- Other food-borne bacterial pathogens cause diarrhea via enterotoxin production or by direct cytotoxic effect on the gut. *Staphylococcus aureus*, the most common cause of food poisoning, produces toxins that stimulate intestinal secretion and cause headache, nausea and vomiting. *Bacillus cereus*, from contaminated fried rice, causes severe vomiting and diarrhea. *Bacillus* spp, from contaminated meats, baked goods, and salads, produces predominately diarrhea. *Clostridium perfringens*, causes food poisoning primarily in outbreaks in the fall and winter. *Vibrio parahaemolyticus* is associated with raw or spoiled shellfish and can have a varying presentation of watery diarrhea or dysentery.

*Viral Pathogens*—Rotaviruses and Norwalk virus are major causes of self-limited diarrhea. Both cause watery stools (without fecal leukocytes), with vomiting, abdominal cramps, bloating, low-grade fever and headache. Rotovirus affects children under the age of 2. Norwalk infects older children and adults in epidemic outbreaks of gastroenteritis.

*Parasitic Pathogens*—Helminths and protozoa may cause chronic diarrheal illness particularly in areas with poor sanitation. Helminths that colonize the small bowel and could produce diarrhea and nutrient malabsorption include: *Calilaria philippinesis, Ascaris lumbricoides, Trichinella spiralis, Ancylostoma* (hookworms), and *Strongyloides stercoralis*. Trematodes: Schistosomiasis may cause diarrhea from the inflammatory response to schistosome eggs deposited in the intestine. Protozoa causing diarrhea include: *Cryptosporidia, Amoeba,* and *Giardia lamblia.*

1. Cryptosporidia produces acute, often severe crampy watery diarrhea. Fever is uncommon.
2. Entamoeba histolytic is the only amoebic parasite that causes human disease. Diarrhea is typically mild to moderate, characterized by loose, intermittent stools, occasional blood or mucus, flatulence abdominal cramping.
3. *Giardia lamblia* is a major cause of waterborne diarrhea and travelers' diarrhea. Clinical presentation is variable, ranging from asymptomatic carrier to acute illness (explosive diarrhea, cramps, flatulence, nausea and vomiting) and chronic diarrhea. In children, chronic infection may cause growth retardation.

Yeast and fungi, primarily *Candida albicans* can cause both nosocomial and community acquired chronic diarrhea in immunocompromised and also immunocompetent individuals.

***Diarrhea in Immunocompromised Patients***—*Giardia lamblia* is important in patients with common variable immunodeficiency, AIDS, and IgA deficiency. *Salmonella* and *Shigella* are more frequent and severe in immunocompromised patients. *Legionella* and *Candida albicans* may cause diarrhea in immunocompromised patients. AIDS patients are at particular risk for *Cryptosporidium, Isospora belli, Mycobacterium avium-intracellulare, Microsporidium,* and cytomegalovirus (CMV).

***Noninfectious Diarrheas***—Osmotic diarrhea results from poorly absorbed solutes within the intestinal lumen. Secretory diarrhea is the product of intestinal transport of ions from the epithelial cell into the lumen of the gut, resulting from the interplay among paracrine, immune, neural, and endocrine systems (PINES). "Pure" chronic secretory diarrheas, such as carcinoid and VIPoma [watery diarrhea-hypokalemia-achlorhydria (WDHA), or gastrinoma and medullary carcinoma of the thyroid] are rare.

▶ Treatment Steps
1. Correct the underlying condition.
2. Controlling diarrhea.
3. Replacing fluid and electrolytes, nutrients, vitamins, and minerals. Fluid and electrolyte losses are best replaced with oral rehydration solutions to replace intestinal fluid losses (Table 4–9).
4. Antimotility agents are useful in all except those with dysentery or *C. difficile* infection where risk of mucosal invasion may lead to toxic megacolon.
5. Antibiotic therapy indications: traveler's diarrhea, cholera, pseudomembranous colitis, parasites, and sexually transmitted infections, and in immunosuppressed patients, debilitated patients with malignancy, patients with valvular or vascular prostheses, hemolytic anemia, and those with prolonged or relapsing course.

**4-9 ORAL REHYDRATION SOLUTIONS USED IN DIARRHEAL DISEASES**

| Solution | Na mmol/L | K | Cl | Base | Cho | Osmolality |
|---|---|---|---|---|---|---|
| WHO-ORS | 90 | 20 | 80 | 10 | 111 | 310 |
| Rehydralyte | 75 | 20 | 65 | 30 | 139 | 329 |
| Pedialyte | 45 | 20 | 35 | 30 | 139 | 269 |
| Ricelyte | 50 | 25 | 45 | 34 | — | 260 |
| Sports drink | 20 | 2.5 | 11 | 0 | 111 | 145 |

Reproduced, with permission, from Chang, E. Diarrhea. In: Wilcox, M. ed. *A Core Curriculum in Gastroenterology and Hepatology.*

## B. Celiac Sprue

### ▶ H&P Keys

Common in persons of Western European heritage where prevalence is one in 250. Prevalence in relatives of celiac patients is 15%. Certain disorders are associated with increased prevalence of celiac disease: diabetes mellitus type I, autoimmune thyroid disease, Sjogren's syndrome, microscopic colitis, isolated IgA deficiency, epilepsy, Down's syndrome, dermatitis herpetiformis (a chronic skin condition characterized by recurrent crops of intensely pruritic erythematous papules or vesicles located over the extensor surfaces). All patients with dermatitis herpiformis have gluten enteropathy (Table 4–10).

### ▶ Clinical Presentation

Vague ill health, osteopenia, nonspecific gastrointestinal symptoms such as bloating and indigestion, diarrhea, steatorrhea, weight loss, chronic iron deficiency anemia, osteopenia, hyposplenism with associated red cell abnormalities (Howell–Jolly bodies), and chronic neurologic syndromes including seizures.

### ▶ Diagnosis and Evaluation

Patients with overt generalized malabsorption without obvious cause, small bowel biopsy is the first diagnostic test. Patients with-

**4-10 DISORDERS ASSOCIATED WITH INCREASED PREVALENCE OF CELIAC DISEASE**

Type I diabetes mellitus
Autoimmune thyroid disease
Sjörgren's syndrome
Microscopic colitis
Isolated IgA deficiency
Epilepsy
Down's syndrome
Dermatitis herpetiformis

out overt malabsorption, antibody screening tests are done first. Obtain a panel of IgA and IgG antigliadin (AGA) and IgA endomysial (EMA) antibodies. IgG AGA is not highly specific, but is important in the 5% of patients with celiac disease and IgA deficiency. EMA antibodies are directed to tissue transglutaminase (TTG). TTG antibody ELISA assay may replace EMA antibody testing.

1. A positive antibody screen should be followed up with small bowel biopsy.
2. Consider screening for celiac disease in patients with iron deficiency anemia or osteopenia of uncertain cause and in populations with high prevalence, such as relatives of celiac patients.

▶ Disease Severity

Complications include chronic ulcerative jejunitis, enteropathy-associated T-cell lymphoma, and refractory sprue.

▶ Concept and Application

Ingested gliadins (components of gluten present in wheat, rye, barley and oats) lead to an immunologic reaction in the small bowel mucosa. Most celiac patients have an HLAA-DQ2 subtype or a closely related subtype. These HLA molecule coded by these subtypes elicit a T-cell–mediated immunologic reaction in small bowel mucosa. This leads to mucosal infiltration by chronic inflammatory cells, epithelial cell damage, villous atrophy, and crypt hypertrophy. Damage to the small intestinal mucosa causes a variable degree of malabsorption. Patients can be asymptomatic or have selective nutrient malabsorption (such as iron and calcium) or have severe diarrhea and malnutrition.

▶ Treatment Steps

1. Patient education is important, as celiac disease is a lifelong disorder.
2. Every patient needs education about the physiology of the disease, importance of diet and potential consequences, including anemia, osteopenia, and enteropathy-associated T-cell lymphoma.
3. Refer every celiac patient to a dietician and to a patient support group.
4. Primary treatment is a gluten-free diet.
5. Clinical response to gluten-free diet should be apparent within weeks.
6. Sequential measurements of Indonesia antibody (EMA) are useful for monitoring dietary compliance. EMA levels should fall if gluten is being avoided.
7. Lack of response should prompt a search for inadvertent ingestion of gluten. Other reasons for failure to respond include: incorrect diagnosis, celiac-related pancreatic insufficiency, celiac-related bacterial overgrowth, other dietary intolerances (lactose, fructose, soya, milk protein), and development of small bowel lymphoma (EATCL) or ulcerative jejunoileitis (UJI).
8. Supplemental iron, folate, zinc, vitamin D, calcium.

## IV. COLON

### A. Invasive Diarrhea

▶ **H&P Keys**

Crampy lower abdominal pain, tenesmus, stool bloody or mucoid, volume < 1 L/d; fecal leukocytes are usually seen. History of prior administration of antibiotics suggests *Clostridium difficile* as causative agent. Systemic symptoms may provide a clue to the diagnosis: Hemolytic uremic syndrome (hemolytic anemia, uremia, renal failure and differentiated intravascular coagulation [DIC]) occurs with both *Shigella* and enterohemorrhagic *E. coli*. Reiter's syndrome (arthritis, urethritis, and uveitis) occurs after *Salmonella, Shigella, Campylobacter,* and *Yersinia* infections. Guillain–Barré sydrome occurs after *Campylobacter jejuni* infection.

▶ **Diagnosis**

Stool studies for bacterial pathogens, ova, and parasites, stool cytotoxin assay for *C. difficile*. Proctosigmoidoscopy may show erythema, ulceration, hemorrhage, or pseudomembranes, yellow-white, raised plaques characteristic of pseudomembranous colitis associated with *C. difficile*.

▶ **Disease Severity**

Fever, tachycardia, volume depletion, leukocytosis, abdominal distention, guarding, tenderness, decreased bowel signs, signs of toxemia; development of peritoneal signs suggests progression to toxic megacolon.

▶ **Concept and Application**

Invasive organisms cause histologic damage and may also produce signs and symptoms of systemic infection. Species of *Shigella, Salmonella, Campylobacter, Yersinia, Clostridium,* and *Entamoeba histolytica* produce invasive diarrhea.

▶ **Treatment Steps**

1. Barium enema can make symptoms worse and should be avoided.
2. Oral rehydration in mild disease or intravenous hydration for the more severely ill.
3. Antibiotic therapy with vancomycin or metronidazole for *C. difficile,* ciprofloxacin or trimethoprim–sulfamethoxazole for *Shigella.*
4. Other enteric infections, such as *Campylobacter* and intestinal *Salmonella,* are self-limited and usually don't require antibiotics.
5. Antidiarrheals, which may delay clearance of the pathogen, should be avoided.

### B. Irritable Bowel Syndrome (IBS)

▶ **H&P Keys**

Clinical features are formalized in the "Rome I criteria" (Table 4–11). At least 3 months' continuous or recurrent symptoms of abdominal pain *or* discomfort that is either relieved with defecation, *or* associated with a change in frequency of stool, or associ-

## 4-11 ROME CRITERIA FOR DEFINING IRRITABLE BOWEL SYNDROME

At least 3 months' continuous or recurrent symptoms:
    Abdominal pain or discomfort that is either relieved with defecation, *or* associated with a change in frequency of stool, *or* associated with a change in consistency of stool *and*
Two or more of the following on at least one quarter of occasions or days:
    Altered stool frequency
    Altered stool form (lumpy and hard or loose and watery)
    Altered stool passage (straining, urgency)
    Feeling of incomplete evacuation
    Passage of mucus
    Bloating or feeling of abdominal distention

ated with a change in consistency of stool; and two or more of the following on at least one quarter of occasions or days:

- Altered stool frequency
- Altered stool form (lumpy and hard or loose and watery)
- Altered stool passage (straining, urgency)
- Feeling of incomplete evacuation
- Passage of mucus
- Bloating or feeling of abdominal distention

### ▶ Diagnosis

Identify symptoms complex and the compatible with IBS, associations of symptoms with factors that produce gut hyperactivity, and exclusion of organic cause of symptoms.

### ▶ Evaluation

Use diagnostic tests based on presenting symptoms (diarrhea or constipation). Sigmoidoscopy is helpful to exclude colitis. Mucosal biopsy is used to exclude microscopic or collagenous colitis on histologic examination. CBC, laxative screening, stool ova and parasites, and small bowel radiography. Obtain a detailed dietary history to identify factors that may aggravate or cause symptoms, especially diarrhea and gas-bloat dyspepsia. Dietary factors include lactose, fructose, sorbitol, carbonated beverages, legumes, other gas-producing foods, and caffeinated beverages.

### ▶ Concept and Application

Almost 50% of patients who see American physicians in the United States for bowel symptoms do not have any organic cause for their symptoms. A chronic functional gastrointestinal disorder manifested by abdominal pain and altered bowel habits, which occurs chronically or recurrently at times of life stress, change in diet, menses, and emotional tension.

### ▶ Treatment Steps

1. Establish a good physician–patient relationship.
2. Educate patients about their condition.
3. Emphasize the excellent prognosis and benign nature of the illness.
4. Employ therapeutic interventions centering on dietary modifications, pharmacotherapy, and behavioral intervention.

5. Dietary fiber increases stool bulk, either by water retention or by serving as a substrate for microbial growth in the large intestine. While efficacy of fiber supplements is unproven, a cautious trial of fiber is reasonable as some patients will experience improvement.
6. Pharmacological treatment
   - Synthetic opioids such as loperamine and diphenoxylate are effective in those with diarrhea.
   - Smooth muscle relaxants (anticholinergics and calcium channel blockers) relieve GI symptoms by inhibiting smooth muscle contractions.
   - Tricyclic antidepressants in low doses are advocated for chronic somatic or visceral pain.
   - Selective SSRIs are helpful in patients with a diagnosis of depression, obsessive compulsive disorder, or phobias.
7. Psychological and behavioral therapies: hypnotherapy and psychotherapy are the most effective, cognitive and cognitive–behavioral therapy; relaxation, biofeedback, and combinations of the above may be helpful.

### C. Colorectal Carcinoma (CRC)

The most common GI malignancy in the United States and more common than all others combined. CRC affects women and men equally. The lifetime risk is about 6%. Both incidence and mortality are higher among African Americans than Caucasians.

▶ H&P Keys

Colorectal cancer is considered to arise by a combination of genetic and environmental risk factors with inheritance determining the individual susceptibility. Environmental factors interact with the susceptibility to give rise to the development of small adenomatous polyps, larger adenomatous polyps, and finally cancer. Environmental factors playing an important role in CRC include (Table 4–12):

- Strong risk factors: advanced age, country of birth (North America, Northern Europe vs. Asia, Africa).
- Moderate risk factors: previous adenoma or colon cancer, high red-meat diet and pelvic irradiation.
- Modest risk factors: high fat diet, alcohol, cigarette smoking, obesity, tall stature, cholecystectomy, high sucrose consumption.

Inherited factors are important to the pathogenesis of CRC. Specific genetic syndromes are associated with increases of the hereditary colorectal cancer syndromes below.

*Familial Adenomatosis Polyposis (FAP)*—Characterized by hundreds to thousands of adenomatous polyps, which appear at an average age of 16 years with cancer inevitable at an average age of 39 years. There is the frequent occurrence of polyps in the UGI tract and specific extraintestinal manifestations including desmoid tumors, osteomas of the mandible and long bones, congenital hypertrophy of the retinal pigment epithelium, and soft tissue tumors.

## 4-12 RISK FACTORS FOR COLORECTAL CANCER (CRC) (OTHER THAN FAMILIAL FACTORS)

Strong risk factors (RR > 4.0)
    Advanced age
    Country of birth (North America, Northern Europe vs. Asia, Africa)
    Long-standing ulcerative colitis
Moderate risk factors (RR 2.1–4.0)
    Previous adenoma or colon cancer
    High red meat diet
    Pelvic irradiation
Modest risk factors (RR 1.1–2.0)
    High fat diet
    Alcohol
    Cigarette smoking
    Obesity
    Tall stature
    Cholecystectomy
    High sucrose diet

Adapted, with permission, from: Sandler RS. *Gastroenterol Clin North Amer.* 1996;25:717–736, and Itzkowitz, SH. Gastrointestinal cancer. In Wilcox, C. Mel. Ed. *A Core Curriculum and Self Assessment in Gastroenterology and Hepatology,* Kendall Hunt, Dubuque, Iowa.

*Hereditary Nonpolyposis Colorectal Cancer (HNPCC)*—Previously known as Lynch syndrome or cancer family syndrome, characterized by the development of adenomatous polyps that occur at a younger age and often more advanced pathologic characteristics, compared to the general population. HNPCC kindreds are recognized by three features:

1. At least three first-degree relatives with cancer of the colorectum, endometrium, small bowel, ureter or renal pelvis, and one should be a first-degree relative of the other two.
2. At least two successive generations affected.
3. At least one case diagnosed before the age of 50.

Individuals in the general population may carry familial risk of CRC. Genetic testing is available for identifying affected individuals in families clinically known to have FAP or HNPCC but formal genetic counseling is important before testing is considered (Table 4–13).

*Prevention*—Primary prevention entails lifestyle, dietary, or chemopreventive measures to prevent adenomas and carcinomas from developing. Diet and lifestyle recommendations published by the American Cancer Society and generally endorsed by the National Cancer Institute aim to decrease not just the risk of colorectal cancer but cancer in general. They include:

- Increase daily fiber intake approximately threefold from the present average of 7 grams a day.
- Decrease fat intake to 30% of calories.
- Moderate intake of red meats, salt-cured and smoke-cured meats.
- Five to seven portions of fruits and vegetables a day.
- Eliminate tobacco.

## 4-13 INHERITED FACTORS AND RISK OF DEVELOPING COLORECTAL CANCER (CRC)

| Setting | Lifetime Risk of CRC |
|---|---|
| General population | 6% |
| Familial risk | |
|   One second- or third-degree relative with CRC | ~1.5-fold increase |
|   Two second-degree relatives with CRC | ~2- to 3-fold increase |
|   One first-degree relative with a colonic adenomatous polyp | ~2-fold increase |
|   One first-degree relative with CRC | 2- to 3-fold increase |
|   Two first-degree relatives with CRC | 3- to 6-fold increase |
|   First degree relative with CRC diagnosed < 50 years old | 3- to 6-fold increase |
| Hereditary syndromes | |
|   Familial adenomatous polyposis (FAP) | 100% |
|   Hereditary nonpolyposis colorectal cancer (HNPCC) | 40 to 100% |

Reproduced, with permission, from Itzkowitz, SH. Gastrointestinal cancer, In: Wilcox, C. Mel Ed. *A Core Curriculum and Self Assessment in Gastroenterology and Hepatology*, Kendall Hunt, Dubuque, Iowa.

- Moderate alcohol.
- Regular exercise and weight control.

Chemoprevention (regular use of NSAIDs, particularly aspirin) is associated with a decreased incidence and mortality from sporadic colorectal cancer.

Secondary prevention includes discovering adenomas or early-stage carcinomas and removing them to avert the development of advanced carcinoma. Studies demonstrate the successful detection of earlier stage tumors by screening decreases colorectal cancer mortality. The rationale for colorectal screening: colon cancer is common, curable in its early stages, and asymptomatic in its early stages. Average risk screening for fecal occult blood testing annually and sigmoidoscopy every 5 years, *or* performing colonoscopy every 10 years, or barium enema every 5 to 10 years (Table 4–14). Screening in higher-risk populations include

## 4-14 COLORECTAL CANCER SCREENING GUIDELINES BASED ON FAMILIAL RISK

| Setting | Age to Begin | Test | Interval |
|---|---|---|---|
| General population | 50 | FOBT | Annual |
| | | Sigmoidoscopy *or* | Every 5 years |
| | | Colonoscopy *or* | Every 10 years |
| | | Barium enema | Every 5–10 years |
| First-degree relative with CRC | 40 | Same as general population | Same as general population |
| Two first-degree relatives with CRC or CRC in first-degree relative before age 50 | 40 | Colonoscopy | Every 3–5 years |
| At risk for HNPCC | 25 | Colonoscopy | Every 2 years; annual > 40 |
| | | Genetic counseling/testing | |
| At risk for FAP | 10–12 | Sigmoidoscopy | Every 1–2 years |
| | | Genetic counseling/testing | |

screening/surveillance recommendations for these familial categories, detailed in Table 5–4. Other high-risk individuals include patients with inflammatory bowel disease and those with a history of a colonic hamartomatous polyposis syndrome (juvenile polyposis, Peutz–Jeghers syndrome, serrated polyposis syndrome and other rare syndromes).

### ▶ Diagnosis

Colonoscopy is the preferred examination for patients with positive screening tests (fecal occult blood test, sigmoidoscopy), asymptomatic iron deficiency anemia or colonic symptoms. The goal of colonoscopy is to detect cancer, remove adenomas and in the case of ulcerative colitis, to search for dysplastic lesions that might indicate a higher risk.

### ▶ Disease Severity

Tumor stage is the most important prognostic factor. Determinants of stage are the depth of penetration through the bowel wall and the presence and number of lymph nodes pathologically. Method of staging includes endoscopic ultrasound. It is the staging procedure of choice for rectal cancers to assess depth of invasion and lymph node metastasis. Surgical staging correlates with 5-year survival (Table 4–15). Five-year survival for node negative patients varies from 85% to 95% if the tumor has not penetrated the muscularis propria; and 60–80% if the tumor has penetrated the muscularis propria. With positive nodes, 5-year survival is <60%.

### ▶ Concept and Application

Biologic basis for CRC prevention:

- Most CRC arises from adenomatous polyps.
- Adenomatous polyps are found in 25% of people by age 50 and the prevalence increases to about 50% by age 75.
- Colorectal cancer arises from a series of specific mutations in tumor suppressor genes, oncogenes and DNA mismatch repair genes. The earliest mutation in the progression is in the adenomatous polyposis coli gene (APC—a tumor suppressor gene). Many, if not all adenomas begin with a mutation of the APC gene. After the APC "gatekeeper" gene is lost, other mutations in colon cancer include K-raps, p53, and DCC (deleted in colon cancer) and DNA mismatch repair (MMR) genes.

### 4-15 SURGICAL STAGE AND SURVIVAL

| TNM Stage | AJCC Stage | Dukes' Stage | Five-Year Survival (%) |
|---|---|---|---|
| I | T1–T2, N0, M0 | A, B1 | 85–95 |
| II | T3–T4, N0, M0 | B2, B3 | 60–80 |
| III | Any T, N1–3, M0 | C | 30–60 |
| IV | Any T, any N, M1 | D | 5 |

▶ Treatment Steps

1. Surgery is the mainstay of curative therapy. Surgical therapy is applied to most colorectal cancers, even when metastasis is present, to prevent obstruction or hemorrhage.
2. The value of preoperative CT scans is debated because it usually does not change the surgical approach.
3. Chemotherapy plays an adjuvant and palliative role. Adjuvant chemotherapy, 5-FA, and leukovorin is effective for stage III disease, and possibly stage II disease.
4. Radiation therapy improves outcome of some rectal cancers and is standard therapy for stage II and III rectal carcinomas.
5. CEA is obtained preoperatively for follow-up purposes.
6. Follow-up after resection:
   - Goals include detection of recurrence of the original malignancy and detection of metachronous polyps and cancers.
   - The rationale is that almost all CRC recurrences will occur within 5 years and most will recur within 2 years.
   - The approach is to perform history, physical examination, and CEA every 3 to 6 months for 2–3 years then annually. Colonoscopic surveillance recommendations are identical to those for adenoma follow-up.

### D. Appendicitis

▶ H&P Keys

Typically, the first symptom is upper midline or perimbilical pain. Discomfort develops over several hours and is followed by anorexia, nausea and vomiting. Once the serosal surface of the appendix becomes inflamed, the pain and tenderness shifts to McBurney's point. The usual presentation of periumbilical pain shifting to the RLQ is seen less frequently in older patients, in whom diffuse pain and nonlocalized tenderness are more common. Perforation is suspected if the temperature is > 38°C or if the leukocyte count is greater than 15,000 cells/mm.

▶ Diagnosis

Appendicitis is a clinical diagnosis, supported by carefully selected laboratory studies. Patients with historical features and physical examinations do not need additional diagnostic studies. Immediate surgical exploration is indicated for the following:

- Abnormal gas pattern on abdominal radiographs: right lower quadrant ileus or diffuse small bowel air–fluid levels are seen in 62% of patients with uncomplicated appendicitis, 71% of those with periappendiceal phlegmon, and 97% of those with gangrenous appendicitis or perforation.
- In patients in whom the diagnosis is ambiguous, abdominal sonography may be helpful when the clinical features are ambiguous. CT is a reliable method for differentiating periappendiceal phlegmon from abscess.

▶ Concept and Application

Most common cause of acute abdomen in the United States. About 250,000 appendectomies are performed in the United States annually, with 2000 deaths resulting from complications of the disease. One in 15 develops appendicitis during his or her lifetime. Appendicitis develops as a result of obstruction of the appendiceal lumen by fecalith or appendiceal. Overall perioperative mortality is 0.5%. Fewer than 0.2% of nonperforated patients die. Mortality rises tenfold with perforation. Mortality rises steeply with advancing age. The rate is < 1% for patients < 50, and > 15% for patients > 71 years of age. Septic complications occur with increased frequency in the presence of perforation.

▶ Treatment Steps
1. Emergency appendectomy.
2. In 10% to 20% of patients explored for presumed appendicitis, a normal appendix is found. Mesenteric lymphadenitis, Meckel's diverticulitis, cecal diverticulitis, pelvic inflammatory disease, ectopic pregnancy, and ileitis mimic appendicitis.

## E. Inflammatory Bowel Disease (IBD)

### 1. Ulcerative Colitis (UC)

▶ H&P Keys

Classic symptoms: bloody diarrhea, rectal urgency tenesmus, extracolonic manifestations (uveitis, episcleritis, scleritis, primary sclerosing cholangitis, pyoderma gangrenosum). Among precipitating factors consider NSAIDs, antibiotics, estrogens, smoking cessation.

▶ Diagnosis (Fig. 4–2)
Exclude self-limited colitis:

- Sigmoidoscopy/colonoscopy and biopsy.
- Stool exam for culture/O&P.

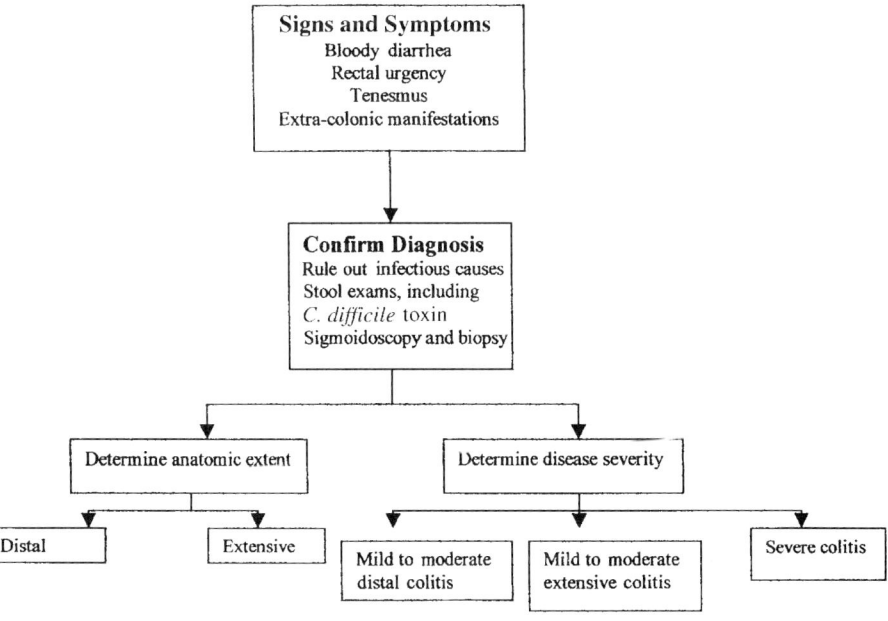

Figure 4–2. Ulcerative Colitis: Diagnosis. Adapted, with permission, from Hanauer SB, Meyers S. Management of Crohn's Disease in Adults. ACG Practice Parameters. *Am J Gastroenterol* 1997;92:559–566.

- Serologic studies—ameba.
- Stool *C. difficile* toxin.

Consider sexually transmitted diseases/AIDS, radiation, ischemia, drugs, gold cleansing agents, "crack," cocaine.

▶ Assessment of Disease Severity

Severity:

- Mild < 4 BMs/day, with or without blood; no toxicity; CBC, ESR/C-reactive protein.
- Moderate > 4 BMs/day without toxicity.
- Severe > 6 bloody BMs/day, toxicity, fever, tachycardia, anemia, leukocytosis, thrombocytosis, elevated ESR/C-reactive protein.

Extent:

- Proctitis.
- Proctosigmoiditis.
- Left colon involvement.
- "Pancolitis" extending proximal to the hepatic flexure.

▶ Concept and Application

Remission can be predicted by the natural history of the individual patient. The longer the remission, the higher likelihood that remission will be sustained. Surveillance colonoscopy at 1- to 2-year intervals after 7 years in patients with extensive disease and after 13 years in patients with left-sided disease.

▶ Treatment Steps

1. Medical therapy goals: induction of remission: defined by (clinical) absence of inflammatory symptoms (eg, no diarrhea, mucoid bloody stool or urgency); (endoscopic) regression of findings consistent with regenerated intact mucosa (eg, absence of ulcers, granularity, or friability; (histologic) absence of inflammatory infiltrate or crypt abscesses.
2. Maintenance of remission.
3. Choice of therapy: Mild-moderate distal colitis: combined oral and topical therapy often achieves prompt response. Oral aminosalicylates sulfasalazine, 5-ASA (Dipentum, Asacol, Pentasa) *and* topical aminosalicylates: mesalamine suppositories, mesalamine enemas, or corticosteroids: hydrocortisone enemas.
4. Extensive colitis: oral aminosalicylates, 5-ASA, oral prednisone: taper once improvement occurs, azathioprine/6MP.
5. Severe colitis: toxic patient refractory to oral medication. Hospital admission for IV corticosteroids—300 mg hydrocortisone or 60 mg methylprednisolone/d) maximum 7–10 days. Failure to improve: surgery. TPN is sometimes needed but not effective in forestalling surgery. Avoid narcotics, antidiarrheals, anticholinergics and antidepressants.
6. Urgent indications for surgery include massive hemorrhage, perforation, toxic megacolon, and failure of maximal medical therapy.

   Nonemergent indications are suspected carcinoma or confirmed dysplasia, growth failure in children, debility and intolerance of side effects of corticosteroids, distal colitis with poor quality of life, intractable extraintestinal complications such as hemolytic anemia and pyoderma gangrenosum.

7. Urgent surgical procedures include subtotal colectomy with Brook ileostomy and Hartmann pouch or mucous fistula.

   Elective procedures are complete proctoctomy (abdominoperineal resection), or ileal pouch–anal anastomosis with rectal mucosal stripping or stapled anastomosis.

2. Crohn's Disease

   ▶ H&P Keys

   Vague and variable manifestations: chronic diarrhea, abdominal pain, weight loss, anorexia, weight loss, fever, recurrent oral aphthous ulcerations, pallor cachexia, abdominal mass or tenderness or history of intestinal obstruction, history of perianal fissures, fistulae, abscesses; extraintestinal manifestations affecting the skin, eyes, joints, growth retardation amount children. Exacerbating factors: infection (respiratory or enteric), cigarette smoking, NSAIDs.

   ▶ Diagnosis

   Exclude: ischemia, neoplasm, infection, drugs and AIDS-related illness.

   Workup: laboratory tests that include CBC, RBC indices, ferritin, $B_{12}$, folate, ESR/C-reactive protein, electrolytes, calcium, magnesium, albumin, prothrombin time, vitamin D, liver chemistries, stool O&P, Culture, *C. difficile* toxin.

   Depending on the site and suspected complication: x-ray of small bowel series, barium enema, CT scan (less often MRI, sonogram, transrectal sonogram, endoscopic ultrasound).

   Colonoscopy to evaluate colonic or anastomotic strictures, monitor recurrences at anastomoses, and surveillance for dysplasia.

   ▶ Disease Severity

   Clinical patterns include inflammatory, stenosing/obstructive, or fistulizing. Systemic manifestations are:

   - Mild to moderate: ambulatory, tolerating symptoms.
   - Moderate to severe: fever, weight loss > 10% of total body weight, pain and tenderness, nausea, emesis, anemia.
   - Severe to fulminant: despite corticosteroids, development of high fever, persistent emesis, signs of obstruction, peritoneal inflammation, cachexia, abscess.

   ▶ Concept and Application

   Entire GI tract is susceptible. Onset is most common among teenagers and young adults with a second peak in the 60s and 70s (usually segmental colonic). Management varies with disease location, severity, and presence of complications.

   ▶ Treatment Steps

   Goal: symptomatic improvement with tolerance of medical therapy. See Figure 4–3.

   1. Mild to moderate disease anticipate 50% response. Oral aminosalicylates sulfasalazine 3–6 g/d, or mesalamine 3.2–4.8

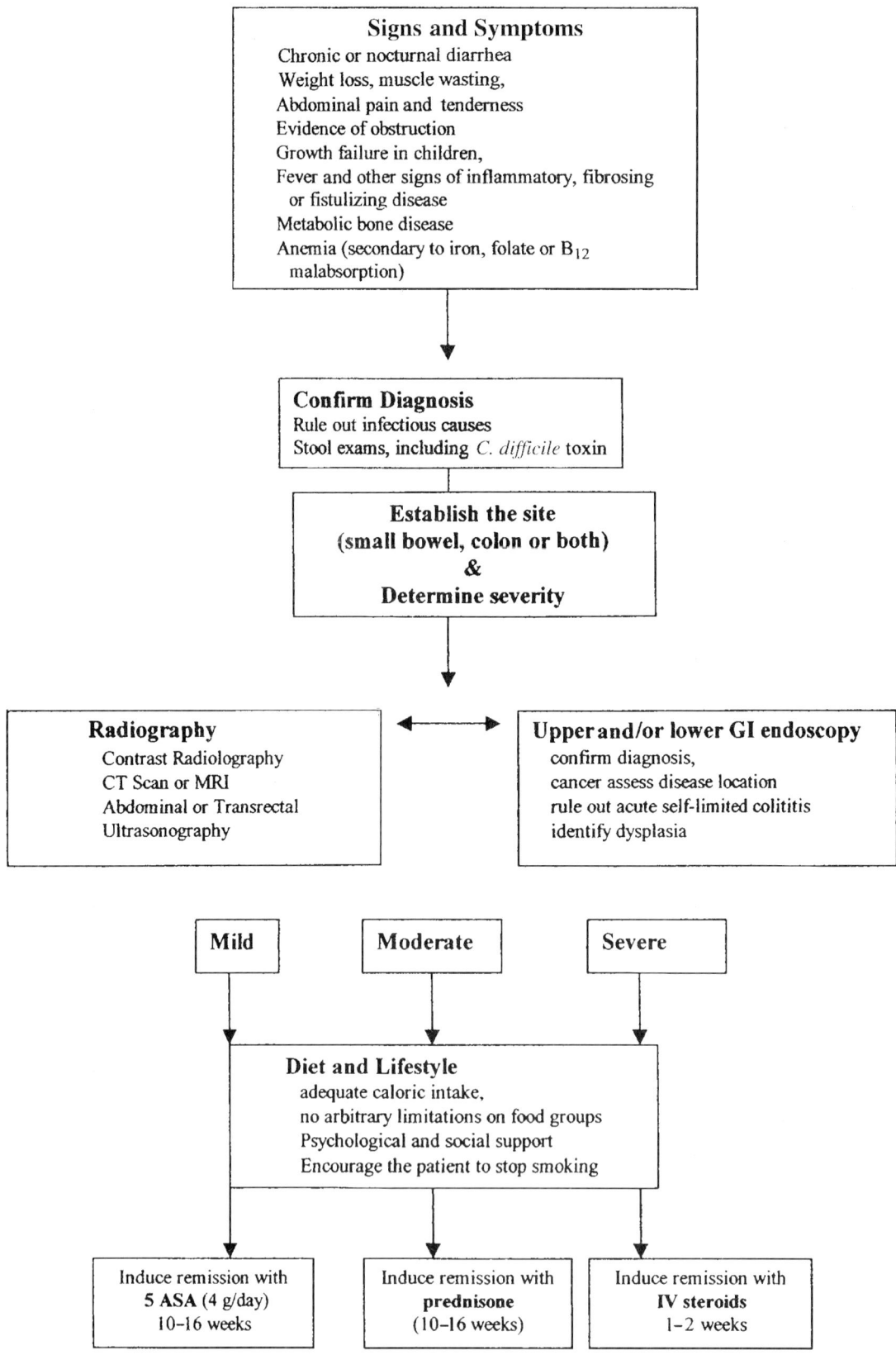

Figure 4-3. Crohn's Disease Management. Adapted, with permission, from Kornbluth A, Sachar DB. Ulcerative Colitis in Adults. ACG Practice Parameters. *Am J Gastroenterol* 1997;92:204–211.

g/d. Antibiotics metronidazole 10–20 mg/kg/d, cipro 500 mg bid. Add proton pump inhibitor for gastroduodenal Crohn's disease. Use topical mesalamine or corticosteroids for distal colonic disease.
2. Moderate to severe disease: Prednisone, 40–60 mg/d until improvement, then taper; treat concomitant infection; nutritional support; azathioprine/6-mercaptopurine.
3. Severe-fulminant disease: hospitalization, IV corticosteroids, antibiotics, surgical consultation for obstruction or progression to abscess, dysplasia, or peritoneal inflammatory findings, tumor necrosis factor alpha (TNFα) for closing enterocutaneous and perianal fistulas, refractory active disease, and maintenance of remission. A new approach today is with use of infliximab, which is excellent for fistula, steroid refractory Crohn's, and maintenance therapy.

## F. Ischemic Bowel Disease

▶ H&P Keys

Typically seen in patients over age 60 with significant cardiac disease; may have history of "intestinal angina," arrhythmias, recent myocardial infarction, previous arterial emboli. Rheumatic heart disease and atherosclerotic heart disease have high risk for ischemic bowel disease. In early occlusive mesenteric ischemia, acute crampy abdominal pain out of proportion to physical findings with spontaneous evacuation and pain with absence of defecatory urge in nonocclusive ischemia. Other signs: vomiting, diarrhea, abdominal distention, hyperperistalsis, tenderness, hematochezia. For thrombotic disease of mesenteric veins, predisposing conditions include peritonitis, abdominal inflammation, trauma, portal hypertension, intraabdominal tumors, coagulopathy, oral contraceptives.

▶ Diagnosis

Hemoconcentration, leukocytosis, elevated amylase levels; abdominal roentgenograms may show "thumbprinting" caused by submucosal hemorrhage and edema; visceral arteriography to exclude acute thromboses.

▶ Disease Severity

Abdominal tenderness, distention, leukocytosis, hemoconcentration, bloody peritoneal transudate, metabolic acidosis (late).

▶ Concept and Application

Four syndromes: acute mesenteric infarctions, ischemic colitis, focal ischemia, and intestinal angina. Infarction results from abrupt arterial occlusion. Nonocclusive ischemia results from poor perfusion. Venous thrombosis has a more insidious course.

▶ Treatment Steps
1. Early intervention for acute occlusive disease of arteries or veins.
2. Treatment for nonocclusive ischemia: bowel rest, fluids, antibiotic therapy resulting in complete resolution in 50%, healing with stricture in 30%, and gangrenous gut requiring resection in 20%.

## G. Intestinal Obstruction

### ▶ H&P Keys
Crampy, spasmodic abdominal pain, vomiting, borborygmi, abdominal distention, obstipation; can develop slowly (months or years) or acutely (over hours). With mechanical obstruction, distress is apparent by extreme restlessness. With ileus, pain is usually less severe. Careful inspection of skin; palpation of umbilicus, lower-trunk inguinal, and femoral areas to detect hernias, intra-abdominal masses, hepatosplenomegaly; rectal and vaginal exam for masses and occult blood. Bowel sounds are infrequent and hypoactive in ileus. In obstruction, bowel sounds become loud, high-pitched, and hyperactive.

### ▶ Diagnosis
Biochemical and hematologic tests including: CBC, levels of amylase, alkaline phosphatase, aspartate aminotransferase, alanine aminotransferase, lactate dehydrogenase; acid–base balance; roentgenographic obstruction series, including plain films of the abdomen to localize the level of obstruction, upright chest film in the lateral and posteroanterior views to detect pneumonia, free air, air-fluid levels. Use barium for retrograde studies but avoid barium if perforation is a possibility. CT scan may be helpful. Endoscopy to visualize and obtain tissue for biopsy from obstructing lesions in the esophagus, stomach, duodenum, rectum, and large intestine.

### ▶ Disease Severity
Fever, rebound tenderness, leukocytosis, unexplained hyperamylasemia.

### ▶ Concept and Application
Most common causes of obstruction in adults are adhesions and hernias in the small bowel and cancer in the colon.

### ▶ Treatment Steps
1. Decompression via nasogastric tube for either obstruction or ileus.
2. Complete obstruction requires urgent surgery to detect strangulation, resect necrotic bowel, and preserve viability of adjacent bowel as soon as preoperative fluid and electrolyte resuscitation and nasogastric decompression are established.

## H. Diverticulitis

### ▶ H&P Keys
Acute diverticulitis commonly manifests with fever, localized left lower quadrant abdominal pain, leukocytosis, and a palpable mass seen, typically, in American patients above the age of 35.

### ▶ Diagnosis
Leukocytosis, roentgenographic obstruction series, ultrasonographic or CT imaging. As the process resolves, colonic evaluation (either colonoscopy or flexible sigmoidoscopy and barium enema) to confirm the diagnosis and exclude other colonic

pathology, eg, Crohn's disease, carcinoma). The risk of perforation in colonoscopy is higher within 4 weeks of resolved diverticulitis.

▶ Disease Severity

Complications include gross perforation and peritonitis: a surgical emergency requiring aggressive resuscitation, broad-spectrum antibiotics, laparotomy, and colonic resection with fecal diversion. Elective resection is indicated after two documented episodes of acute diverticulitis, depending on age, operative risk, and severity. Immunocompromised patients should be treated surgically after one attack due to the higher risks and higher mortality. Chronic diverticulitis is acute diverticulitis complicated by colonic fistula, large bowel obstruction or stricture. Colovesical fistula is the most common fistula. All symptomatic manifestations of chronic diverticulitis are treated surgically by resection and primary anastomosis after resolution.

▶ Treatment Steps

1. Diet and lifestyle: acute uncomplicated diverticulitis bowel rest and antibiotic therapy. Outpatient treatment: clear liquids until symptoms resolve. Inpatient: clear liquids until symptoms resolve; NPO, IV hydration.
2. Antibiotic outpatient regime includes: ciprofloxicin and metronidazole; or trimethoprim–sulfamethoxazole and metronidazole; or trovofloxicin 200 mg/d for 7 to 10 days.

    Inpatient antibiotic regime includes: imipenem, 500 mg q6h; or ticarcillin/clavulinic acid 3.1 g IV q6h; or pipercillin/TZ 3.375 mg IV q6h; or trova, 300 mg IV day, then 200 mg PO q day.

## I. Constipation

▶ H&P Keys

Onset and duration of complaint: constipation present from birth or neonatal period suggests congenital disorder; recent onset demands a workup for organic disorders. Frequency of defecation, defecatory difficulties such as excessive straining, discomfort, sense of incomplete evacuation. Drug history. Careful physical examination with abdominal palpation for distention, retained stool, prior surgical procedures, autonomic dysfunction; anorectal and perineal examination.

▶ Diagnosis

Flexible sigmoidoscopy and barium enema; exclude metabolic and endocrine disorders such as diabetes mellitus, hypothyroidism, hypercalcemia, hypokalemia; exclude muscular collagen vascular and neurogenic disorders. Anal manometry and full-thickness rectal biopsies when Hirschsprung's disease is suspected.

▶ Disease Severity

Colonic transit studies, defecography, and anal manometry for patients with severe constipation who have not responded to simple dietary measures.

▶ Concept and Application

Impairment in large-bowel transit can be a primary motor disorder, in association with a large number of diseases, and a side effect of many drugs.

▶ Treatment Steps
1. Adequate dietary fiber.
2. Behavioral approaches; biofeedback.
3. Discouragement of routine use of laxatives except bulk-forming agents.

## J. Peritonitis

▶ H&P Keys

Severe abdominal pain and rigidity, intercostal breathing, fever, tachycardia, hypovolemia, tenderness on direct and referred palpation, voluntary guarding, tenderness on rectal and pelvic exams, tenderness on percussion, loss of liver dullness, decrease or absence of bowel sounds.

▶ Diagnosis

Leukocytosis with left shift or leukopenia, hemoconcentration, metabolic acidosis, hyperkalemia, paralytic ileus or free air.

▶ Disease Severity

Suppurative peritonitis has abrupt onset and relatively short course with rapid progression. Mortality from fluid shifts, hypovolemia, and septic shock with resultant renal, respiratory, cardiac, and hepatic failure.

▶ Concept and Application

Common causes are intra-abdominal organ disease such as appendicitis, diverticulitis, perforating carcinoma, perforating ulcer, and trauma. Mortality results from fluid shifts and endotoxin that may cause hypovolemia and septic shock.

▶ Treatment Steps
1. Fluid and electrolyte resuscitation.
2. Surgical repair of primary process and removal of debris.
3. Systemic antibiotics with careful monitoring of cardiac reserve via Swan–Ganz catheter, blood pressure, arterial blood gas determination, Foley catheter for recording urine volume, nasogastric intubation to decompress stomach, supplemental oxygen.

## K. Familial Mediterranean Fever (Recurrent Polyserositis)

▶ H&P Keys

Autosomal recessive genetic disorder affects Armenians, Arabs, and Sephardic Jews. Most common manifestation is peritonitis. In 90% the first manifestation occurs at the end of the second decade.

▶ Diagnosis

No specific test. However, a high sedimentation rate could be present. Six diagnostic features: fever, serositis, amyloidosis, ethnic background, family history, and exclusion of other causes. Unless a strong family history is obtained, the diagnosis is often made at laparotomy, where diffuse inflammation of serosal surfaces without other intra-abdominal pathology are seen. No bacteria are cultured. Appendectomy is indicated so that future episodes can be differentiated from acute appendicitis.

▶ Disease Severity

In most patients, the disease is relatively benign. Attacks precipitated by a variety of factors. Complications include amyloidosis, degenerative arthritis, renal vein thrombosis, narcotic addiction.

▶ Concept and Application

Recurring inflammation of any serosal surface including peritoneum, pleura, pericardium, meninges, and synovial membranes.

▶ Treatment Steps

Colchicine treatment may prevent and ameliorate acute attacks and prevent amyloidosis.

## V. RECTUM

### A. Malignant Neoplasm of Rectum

*See* Colorectal Carcinoma.

### B. Hemorrhoids

▶ H&P Keys

Anal discomfort, pruritus ani, fecal soiling, prolapse, bleeding, pain.

▶ Diagnosis

Flexible sigmoidoscopy or colonoscopy. Occult bleeding in the stool requires a complete colonic evaluation, regardless of the presence of hemorrhoids. Hemorrhoids are classified according to their degree of protrusion or prolapse. First-degree bulge into the lumen of the anorectal canal on anoscopy but do not protrude out of the anus. Second-degree hemorrhoids prolapse out of the anus with defecation or straining but reduce to normal anatomic position spontaneously. Third-degree hemorrhoids prolapse out of the anus with defecation or straining and require digital reduction. Fourth-degree are irreducible and are at risk for strangulation.

▶ Disease Severity

Acute, severe bleeding may require transfusion. Chronic bleeding can cause iron-deficiency anemia. External hemorrhoid thrombosis can be extremely painful and must be distinguished from strangulated hemorrhoids, which are larger and more circumferential. Strangulated hemorrhoids cause significant pain and usually have an external and internal component and occur secondary to prolapse, with subsequent lack of blood supply. Progression to gangrene with resultant infection is life threatening.

▶ Concept and Application

Hemorrhoids result from dilatation of the superior and inferior hemorrhoidal veins. Internal hemorrhoids are lined with rectal mucosa and arise from the superior hemorrhoidal cushion above the mucocutaneous junction (dentate line). External hemorrhoids arise from the inferior hemorrhoidal venous plexus below the mucocutaneous junction and are lined by perianal squamous epithelium.

▶ Treatment Steps

1. Thrombosis of external hemorrhoids and mild bleeding of internal hemorrhoids: treat with sitz baths, two to three per day; bed rest to minimize additional thrombosis and swelling; stool-softening agents; topical therapy with anesthetic ointments and witch hazel–impregnated pads.
2. Strangulated hemorrhoids require immediate surgical therapy.
3. Other treatment options include rubber band ligation for third- and fourth-degree hemorrhoids and hemorrhoidectomy for strangulated hemorrhoids.

## C. Anal Fissure

▶ H&P Keys

Severe pain during or after defecation associated with scant, bright red rectal bleeding. Most commonly found in young and middle-aged adults.

▶ Diagnosis

Inspection after spreading the buttocks. Anoscopy difficult without topical anesthesia. Linear tears are perpendicular to the dentate line.

▶ Disease Severity

Can progress to chronic fissure.

▶ Concept and Application

Because elliptical anal sphincteric fibers offer less muscular support posteriorly, 90% occur posterior midline. Lateral tears suggest underlying disease (IBD, proctitis, leukemia, carcinoma).

▶ Treatment Steps

1. High-fiber diet and adequate fluid intake.
2. Topical anesthetic preparations for symptomatic relief.
3. Warm sitz baths to relax the anal sphincter.
4. Chronic fissures (> 6 weeks) usually require surgical therapy.

## D. Anorectal Abscess

▶ H&P Keys

Acute pain and swelling. Pain in absence of swelling with small intersphincteric or pelvorectal abscesses. Sitting, movement, defecation increase pain. Antecedent history of constipation, diarrhea, trauma. Fever, malaise, and purulent foul-smelling drainage are common. Associated medical diseases include diabetes, hypertension, heart disease, IBD, and a neutropenic state as a result of hematologic malignancy.

▶ Diagnosis

Inspection of the perineum reveals redness, heat, swelling and tenderness, drainage from infected crypt orifice. Rectal examination is difficult without anesthesia.

▶ Disease Severity

Delay in making the diagnosis can lead to necrotizing anorectal infection and increases risk of overwhelming sepsis.

▶ Concept and Application

Obstruction, stasis, and infection of anal glands is most common cause. Obstruction may occur as a result of trauma, eroticism, diarrhea, hard stools, and foreign bodies.

▶ Treatment Steps

1. Abscesses require drainage. Superficial abscesses can be drained under local anesthetic in outpatient setting. All others require drainage in the operating room with anesthesia and surgical instrumentation.
2. Antibiotics are not necessary for otherwise healthy patients. Perioperative antibiotics are used for patients with underlying disease such as acute leukemia, valvular heart disease, diabetes.
3. Postoperative management: Inspection to ensure proper healing, sitz baths, analgesia, bulk-forming agents to soften stool.

## E. Anorectal Fistula

▶ H&P Keys

Chronic purulent drainage. Prior history of anorectal abscess. Pain with defecation but not as severe as with anorectal abscess or anal fissure. Perianal skin may be excoriated.

▶ Diagnosis

Inspection of the perineum usually reveals a red, granular papule from which pus is expressed. Anoscopy and sigmoidoscopy to identify primary orifice and proctocolitis.

▶ Disease Severity

Multiple secondary openings suggest either Crohn's disease or hidradenitis suppurativa.

▶ Concept and Application

Primary orifice is at level of dentate line. Secondary orifice is anywhere else on the perineum.

▶ Treatment Steps

1. Anorectal fistula is approached surgically, with postoperative care similar to anorectal abscess.
2. Anorectal disease as a manifestation of Crohn's disease requires special consideration. Metronidazole will heal perineal

Crohn's disease. Discontinuation of therapy is associated with flaring of disease. Remicade may enhance the healing rate of perineal Crohn's and fistulae.

### F. Pilonidal Disease

▶ H&P Keys

Pain, swelling, drainage midline skin lesion of internatal or gluteal cleft seen most commonly in young men.

▶ Diagnosis

Inspection: characteristic midline location. Appearance and lack of communication with anorectum distinguish pilonidal disease from anorectal fistula and hidradenitis suppurativa.

▶ Disease Severity

Acute abscess versus chronic drainage.

▶ Concept and Application

Common acquired lesion of coccygeal skin, possibly induced by local stretching forces. Small skin pits secondarily invaded by hair precede development of draining sinus or abscess.

▶ Treatment Steps

1. Acute pilonidal abscess requires incision, drainage, and hair removal.
2. Chronic draining pilonidal lesions require surgical closure.

## VI. GALLBLADDER

### A. Acute Cholecystitis

▶ H&P Keys

Acute onset of right upper quadrant pain (typically radiating to the right shoulder blade) nausea, vomiting and fever. Murphy's sign: inspiratory arrest elicited when palpating under the liver.

▶ Diagnosis

Laboratory leukocytosis with preponderance of polys and bands. Minor elevations in aminotransferase levels and bilirubin. Ultrasound is the preferred initial screening study. Cholescintigraphy (HIDA, DISIDA) when clinical suspicion is high but ultrasound is normal.

▶ Disease Severity

Secondary bacterial infection can progress to empyema, gangrene, and perforation.

▶ Concept and Application

Most common cause of acute cholecystitis is obstruction of a distended gallbladder with concentrated bile. Acalculus (5% to 10%) occurs in setting of major surgery, critical illness, extensive trauma, and burns.

▶ Treatment Steps
1. Initial: hospitalization, NPO, intravenous hydration and intravenous antibiotics to cover enteric organisms.
2. Definitive: surgical laparoscopic cholecystectomy is the standard approach. Open cholecystectomy done in cases of generalized peritonitic, septic shock, severe coagulopathy, known cancer of the gallbladder, and patients in the third trimester of pregnancy.

## B. Cholelithiasis

▶ H&P Keys

Biliary pain, nausea, and vomiting. Predisposing factors include obesity, oral contraceptives, pregnancy, clofibrate, ileal disease or resection, and genetic factors.

▶ Diagnosis

Ultrasonography has more than 90% sensitivity in diagnosing gallstones.

▶ Disease Severity

Biliary pain lasting for more than 3 hours indicates progression to cholecystitis.

▶ Concept and Application

Cholesterol gallstones constitute 85% of all gallstones. Bile that is supersaturated with cholesterol can lead to formation of cholesterol gallstones.

▶ Treatment Steps
1. Asymptomatic stones require no treatment.
2. Symptomatic gallbladder stones are treated with cholecystectomy.
3. Oral bile acid therapy (Ursodiol) is a treatment option for mildly symptomatic patients with small (< 10 mm) cholesterol stones within a functioning gallbladder.
4. Common bile duct stones, particularly in the elderly and those with comorbid disease are best treated with endoscopic retrograde cholangiopancreatography (ERCP).

## C. Choledocholithiasis and Acute Suppurative Cholangitis

▶ H&P Keys

Biliary pain, involving the central upper abdomen, jaundice, chills and rigors (Charcot's triad), mild hepatomegaly, occasional rebound.

▶ Diagnosis

Leukocytosis with a left shift, mild elevation of serum transaminases and alkaline phosphatase, hyperbilirubinemia, serum amylase level. Ductal dilatation documented by ultrasonography or CT. Lack of dilatation does not exclude obstruction. Gold standard is ERCP for diagnosis and management. Magnetic resonance cholangiopancreatogram (MRCP) and spiral CT provide excellent images of common duct stones and are among available noninvasive alternatives to diagnostic ERCP.

▶ Disease Severity

Progression leads to ascending cholangitis and endotoxemia with shock and liver abscess.

▶ Concept and Application

Gallstones passing into the common duct can lead to acute obstruction, bile stasis, bacterial infection.

▶ Management

Initial resuscitation and stabilization, systemic antibiotics to cover *E. coli, Klebsiella, Pseudomonas,* and enterococci. Removal of obstruction via ERCP, and possible papillotomy, followed by active instrumentation for ductal clearance. If multiple large common-duct stones cannot be removed in one session, temporary drainage must be established via placement of stent or nasobiliary catheter to control biliary sepsis.

## VII. LIVER

### A. Hepatitis

▶ H&P Keys

Pertinent information: age, gender, race, preceding episodes, history of chronic liver disease or cirrhosis, alcohol consumption (Table 4–16), drug and toxin exposure (include herbal as well as "traditional" medications), occupation and work environment, sexual history, immunologic and nutritional status, immunizations, travel history, and family history.

Hepatitis may present with a flulike or serum sickness syndrome, anorexia, malaise, fever, arthralgia, arthritis, rash, and/or angionecrotic edema, with or without jaundice, dark urine, light stools, abdominal discomfort. Nonspecific constitutional symptoms may be present for a short or protracted time.

Physical findings may be subtle or nonexistent. Findings are often reflective of the duration and severity of liver disease and are common to all forms of hepatitis and include jaundice, hepatomegaly (typically mild), lymphadenopathy, ascites, splenomegaly, encephalopathy. Some findings are typically associated with alcoholic liver disease: palmar erythema, Muehrcke's lines and white nails, Dupuytren's contracture, parotid and lacrimal gland enlargement.

1. Viral Hepatitis:

▶ Diagnosis

Use specific tests for viral antigens, viral antibodies and/or nucleic acids (Table 4–17).

- Acute hepatitis A: presence of IgM anti-HAV.
- Acute hepatitis B: presence of IgM anti-HBc and HBsAg.
- Acute hepatitis C: presence of HCV RNA (anti-HCV appears late in course of acute HCV). See Table 4–21.
- Acute Delta coinfection: presence of IgM anti-HBc and IgM anti-HDV or HVD RNA.

## 4-16 CAGE QUESTIONNAIRE

1. Have you tried to **C**ut down on your drinking?
2. Are you **A**nnoyed by criticism of your drinking?
3. Do you feel **G**uilty about your drinking?
4. Do you need an **E**ye opener each morning?

*Scoring:* 1 point for each yes answer. A total of 2 or more indicates a likelihood of underlying alcoholism.

- Acute Delta superinfection: presence of IgM anti-HDV or HDV RNA.
- Acute hepatitis E: IgM anti-HCV and compatible clinical features.

2. **Chronic Hepatitis**
   - Hepatitis A: no chronic state.
   - Hepatitis B: presence of HBsAg, HBeAg, HBV DNA, IgG anti-HBc.
   - Chronic C: presence of anti-HCV ELISA. False positives may be seen in low-risk populations. Confirm with anti-HCV RIBA or HCV RNA.
   - Chronic D: HBsAg and HDV RNA.
   - Hepatitis E: no chronic state.

3. **Alcoholic Hepatitis**

4. **Drug-Induced Hepatotoxicity (See Table 4–18)**

5. **Autoimmune Hepatitis**
   Suspect among women ages 15 to 35 and again at menopause: 40% present with the abrupt onset of illness that can resemble acute viral or toxic hepatitis; 25% have cirrhosis at the time of presentation. The disease is fatal without treatment. History of concurrent autoimmune disease: autoimmune thyroiditis, vasculitis, ulcerative colitis, Grave's disease, vitiligo, insulin-dependent diabetes. Symptoms: fatigue, jaundice, bleeding easy bruisability, right upper quadrant pain. Transaminases range from 200 to 1,000 U/Dl, total serum globulin g-globulin or immunoglobulin G level ≥ 1.5 normal, antinuclear antibodies (ANA), smooth muscle antibodies (SMA), antibodies to liver/kidney microsome type

## 4-17 DIAGNOSTIC SEROLOGY FOR ACUTE VIRAL HEPATITIS

| Serology | | |
|---|---|---|
| Preliminary | Confirmatory | Diagnosis |
| +Anti-HAV | +IgM anti-HAV | Acute hepatitis A |
| +HbsAg | +IgM anti-HBc | Acute hepatitis B[a] |
| +Anti-HCV | +RIBA, HCV RNA | Hepatitis C (acute or chronic) |

[a]Get anti HDV if risk factors.

### 4-18 PATTERNS OF HEPATOTOXICITY

| Type of Reaction | Examples |
|---|---|
| Direct reaction | Acetaminophen, carbon tetrachloride, mushrooms, phosphorus |
| Idiosyncratic reaction | Isoniazid, disulfiram, propylthiouracil |
| Toxic-allergic reaction | Halothane, isoflurane, ticrynafen |
| Allergic hepatitis | Phenytoin, amoxicillin–clavulanate, sulfonamides |
| Chronic hepatitis | Nitrofurantoin, methyldopa |
| Alcoholic hepatitis-like | Amiodarone, valproic acid |

1 (anti-LKM1) titers ≥ 1:80 in adults or ≥ 1:20 in children, antibodies to soluble liver antigen (anti-SLA), antimitochondrial antibodies (AMA).

▶ Concept and Application

Hepatitis, a necroinflammatory process of the liver parenchyma, can be either acute (< 6-month duration) or chronic (> 6-month duration). Acute hepatitis can resolve, progress to hepatic failure, or continue as chronic hepatitis leading to cirrhosis and hepatocellular carcinoma.

A variety of pathogenic mechanisms may cause hepatitis, including viral infection, toxic injury, autoimmune and hereditary disorders.

*Viral Hepatitis*—Can be caused by infection with the hepatotropic hepatitis viruses A–E (HAV, HBV, HCV, HDV, HEV) and the non-A–E viruses. HAV and HEV can cause only acute viral hepatitis. HBV, HCV, HDV causes both acute and chronic viral hepatitis, cirrhosis, and hepatocellular cancer. HDV is dependent on HBV for both survival and replication. HDV induces illness only in the presence of HBV, either by coinfection or superinfection. HEV, an RNA virus, reported in developing nations in areas of poor sanitation after flooding, is similar to HAV but carries a higher mortality, particularly in pregnant women. Non-A–E viral hepatitis has two distinct profiles: (1) a parenteral or community-acquired hepatitis with a

### 4-19 SOME IMPORTANT INDUSTRIAL AND ENVIRONMENTAL TOXIC CAUSES OF HEPATITIS

| Chemical | Uses |
|---|---|
| Arsenic | Pesticides and in production of ceramics, drugs, dyes, fireworks, paint, petroleum, ink, and semiconductors |
| Carbon tetrachloride | Degreasers, fat processors, fire extinguishers, fumigant, insecticides, refrigerants, lacquer, ink propellants, rubber and wax |
| Tetrachloroethylene | Dry-cleaning agent, fumigant, solvent, degreaser |
| Yellow phosphorus | Munitions, explosives, fertilizers, rodenticides, semiconductors, luminescent coatings |

## 4-20 CLINICAL SITUATIONS/SYNDROMES ASSOCIATED WITH HBV INFECTION

|  | HBs Ag | Anti-HBs | Anti-HBc | IgM anti-HBC | HBe Ag | HBV DNA | Anti-HDV |
|---|---|---|---|---|---|---|---|
| Acute hepatitis B | + | – | + | + | + | + | – |
| Chronic hepatitis B | + | +/– | + | –+/– | + | – |  |
| Healthy carrier | + | +/– | + | – | – | – | – |
| Vaccinated | – | + | – | – | – | – | – |
| Recovered HVB | – | + | + | – | – | – | – |
| Acute hepatitis D | + | – | + | + | +/– | +/– | + |
| Chronic hepatitis D | + | – | + | – | +/– | +/– | + |

benign course, and (2) a persistent viral infection that may have a fulminant course.

*Alcohol-induced Liver Injury*—No particular quantity of alcohol is predictive of alcoholic liver disease. The incidence of serious liver disease begins to rise when the daily consumption of alcohol exceeds 60 g/d for men and 20 g/d for women. In addition to habitual alcohol consumption, other factors that predispose to alcohol-induced liver disease include: female gender, race, coexposure to other drugs, coinfection with the hepatotrophic viruses HBV and HCV, nutritional status, and immune dysfunction.

*Drugs*—Drugs causing liver injury can be "predictable," or "direct," hepatotoxins and "unpredictable," or "idiosyncratic," hepatotoxins. Direct hepatotoxins produce injury in a predictable, dose-dependent fashion. Characteristically, direct hepatotoxins produce liver cell necrosis in a predictable region of the hepatic lobule. Idiosyncractic hepatotoxins produce liver injury in an unpredictable manner. The pattern of injury is diffuse and consists of hepatocellular necrosis and/or cholestasis. Some idiosyncratic hepatotoxins are associated with fever, rash, eosinophilia, and autoantibody production. Examples of direct hepatotoxins include acetaminophen and carbon tetrachloride. Idiosyncratic hepatotoxins can be produced by isoniazid and chloropromazine.

## 4-21 CLINICAL SITUATION/SYNDROMES ASSOCIATED WITH HCV INFECTION

|  | Anti-HCV (ELISA) | Anti-HCV (RIBA) | ALT | HCV RNA |
|---|---|---|---|---|
| Acute hepatitis C | =/– | + | Raised | + |
| Chronic hepatits C | + | + | Raised | + |
| HCV carrier | + | + | Normal | + |
| Recovered HCV | + | + | Normal | – |
| False positive | + | – | Normal | – |

***Autoimmune Hepatitis***—Is an inflammation of the liver of unknown cause that is characterized by interface hepatitis (piecemeal necrosis), hypergammaglobulinemia and autoantibodies in serum.

*Hereditary Disorders*
- *Hemochromatosis (HCC),* an HLA-linked autosomal recessive disorder of iron absorption, has a disease prevalence of 1/250. Symptomatic HCC presents with hepatomegaly, well-established hepatic fibrosis and cirrhosis, diabetes mellitus, and hyperpigmentation. AST and ALT may be slightly elevated.
- *Wilson's disease,* an HLA-linked autosomal recessive disorder of copper metabolism, has a disease prevelance of 1/30,000. Young patients (mean age 8–12 years) may present with hepatitis and fulminant hepatic failure.
- *Alpha$_1$-antitrypsin deficiency* is an important cause of neonatal hepatitis and cirrhosis in children and early emphysema in young adults. Fifteen percent to 30% of neonates with conjugated hyperbilirubinemia have alpha$_1$-antitrypsin deficiencies.

▶ Treatment Steps

Treatment for acute hepatitis is primarily supportive care. Basic principles include:

1. Avoidance of potentially liver-damaging circumstances, fluid and electrolyte replacement, ambulation within the bounds of fatigue, a regular or high-protein diet (in the absence of encephalopathy).
2. Follow physical exam and biochemical tests: prothrombin time is the best biochemical indicator of prognosis; also follow bilirubin, ALT, AST twice weekly while values are rising, weekly during the plateau, then at lesser intervals until normalized.
3. Consideration for hospitalization is indicated for severe anorexia, vomiting, changes in mentation and biochemical changes, including a bilirubin value > 15 or 20 mg/dL, persistence hyperbilirubinemia, rapidly falling aminotransferase activity with a rising bilirubin, increasing protrombin time, and other evidence of hepatic failure.
4. *Acute viral hepatitis.* Most individuals with adequate family and medical support are treated in the outpatient setting. Hospitalization for isolation is not required (the period of infectivity precedes symptoms). Immunoprophylaxis (Tables 4–22 and 4–23).
5. *Chronic viral hepatitis B.* Patients with chronic hepatitis B are candidates for therapy if they have evidence of active viral replication (HBeAg or HBV DNA in serum) and raised serum aminotransferases. Patients with decompensated cirrhosis should be treated with extreme caution. The mainstay of therapy of chronic hepatitis B is alpha-interferon (Table 4–24). Because of the side effects associated with interferon (Table 4–25) and relatively low response rates, alternative therapies are emerging. Second-generation nucleoside analog, lamivudine is FDA-approved for hepatitis B.
6. *Chronic viral hepatitis C.* Current standard therapy for chronic hepatitis C is alpha interferon with ribavirin. Ribavirin, a nu-

## 4-22 INDICATIONS FOR HEPATITIS A VACCINATION

Travelers to endemic areas
Military personnel
Special populations where cyclic HAV epidemics occur
Homosexual males
Users of illicit intravenous drugs
Caretakers of the developmentally challenged
Employees of child day care centers
Laboratory personnel handling live HAV
Handlers of primates that may be handling HAV

---

cleoside analog, is administered orally. Ribavirin is well-tolerated except for causing a dose-dependent reversible hemolytic anemia. Ribavirin is also teratogenic and patients must be strongly cautioned against becoming pregnant while being treated with this agent. Also PEG intron alfa 2b (weekly) SQ is used today either alone or with PO Ribavirin.

7. *Drug-induced liver disease.* Discontinue the implicated agent.
8. *Alcoholic liver disease.* Withdrawal of alcohol and substitution of a nutritious diet. Consider hospitalization for individuals with extrahepatic complications of alcohol ingestion (GI bleeding, coexistent infections, fluid and electrolyte abnormalities, pancreatitis, alcohol withdrawal syndromes).
9. *Autoimmune hepatitis.* Responds to prednisone and/or azathioprine. Remission can be induced within 2 years of treatment in > 70%. Relapse is common after withdrawal of drug therapy.

## 4-23 PERSONS RECOMMENDED FOR HBV PROPHYLAXIS (VACCINE OR HBIG OR BOTH)

Preexposure prophylaxis
    Persons with occupational risk, including clients and staff of institutions
    Clients/staff of institutions for developmentally disabled
    Patients on hemodialysis
    Sexually active homosexual men
    Sexually active heterosexual men and women
    Users of illicit injectable drugs
    Recipients of certain blood products, eg, clotting factors
    Household and sexual contacts of HBV carriers
    Adoptees from countries of high HBV endemicity
    Populations with high endemicity
    Inmates of long-term correctional facilities
    International travelers to HBV endemic areas for > 6 months
Postexposure immunoprophylaxis for hepatitis B

| *Type of Exposure* | *Immunoprophylaxis* |
|---|---|
| Perinatal exposure | Vaccination + HBIG |
| Sexual, acute infection | HBIG ± vaccination |
| Sexual, carrier | Vaccination |
| Household contact, carrier | Vaccination |
| Household contact, known exposure | HBIG ± vaccination |
| Infant < 12 months, acute case, primary caregiver | HBIG ± vaccination |
| Inadvertent percutaneous or permucosal | Vaccination + HBIG |

### 4-24 ALGORITHM FOR THERAPY OF HEPATITIS B

Initial evaluation
- Serial ALT, HBsAg, HBeAg, HBV DNA
- Liver biopsy
- Review side effects and expected results
- Verify lack of contraindications

Initial therapy
- Alpha interferon, 5 μ daily or 10 μ three times weekly for 16–24 weeks

Monitor during therapy
- Every 2 to 4 weeks:
  signs and symptoms
  ALT, AST, bili, albumin, CBC + differential
- At 2 and 4 months
  HBeAg, HBsAg, protime, TSH
- Follow up after therapy
- Every 2–3 months
  signs and symptoms
  ALT, AST, bili, albumin, CBC
- At 6 months
  HBsAg, protime, TSH

---

10. *Hemachromatosis*. Requires long-term phlebotomy and chelation therapy.
11. *Wilson's disease*. Requires lifelong copper chelation therapy.

**Prevention**—The health consequences of acute viral hepatitis are reduced by public health measures and immunization.

*HAV*—As the principal mode of transmission is person-to-person, prevention efforts are aimed at sanitation, chlorination, and proper handling of sewerage and identification of individuals at risk. The hepatitis A vaccine, used in Europe since 1991, is now approved by the FDA for use in the United States.

### 4-25 SIDE EFFECTS OF INTERFERON

**Side Effects of Interferon**

Early
    Severe/life-threatening syndrome
        None
    Mild:
        Influenza-like
Late
    Severe/life-threatening
        Severe depression/suicide
        Acute renal failure
        Cardiotoxicity
        Seizures
        Exacerbation of preexisting autoimmune disease (eg, inflammatory bowel disease)
Mild
    Fatigue
    Emotional lability
    Bone marrow suppression

It is indicated for persons traveling to or working in countries with intermediate or high HAV endemicity (countries other than Australia, Canada, Japan, New Zealand and in Western Europe and Scandinavia), military personnel, native peoples of Alaska and areas of the Americas where cyclic HAV epidemics occur: homosexual males; users of illicit intravenous drugs; employees of child day care centers; laboratory workers who handle live HAV; and handlers of primates known to harbor the HAV virus (Table 4–22). Immune globulin (IG) is recommended for children under the age of 2 who are traveling to endemic areas (Havrix is not approved for children of less than 2 years of age) and postexposure, preferably within 2 weeks, for contacts of person with acute hepatitis A.

*HBV*—Despite the development and introduction of the hepatitis B vaccine in the 1980s, the incidence of hepatitis B has actually increased in the United States since 1980. One important reason for the failure of the vaccine has been an inability to reach an estimated 22 million people who are at highest risk. As a result, an expanded vaccination strategy focuses on the universal hepatitis B immunization for newborns, children, and adolescents, including infants born to HBeAg-positive mothers by vaccine plus HBIG within 12 hours of birth.

*HCV*—Development of specific serologic assays has dramatically decreased the dissemination of transfusion-related hepatitis. The residual risk is estimated to be 0.03%. The use of IG for percutaneous exposure to HCV-positive material is not recommended. No vaccine for hepatitis C is available.

*HDV*—No effective vaccine. However, transmission of HDV can be avoided with the hepatitis B vaccine. Carriers of HBsAg are at risk from continued IV drug abuse or sexual promiscuity.

## B. Hepatocellular Carcinoma

▶ H&P Keys

Hepatocellular carcinoma (HCC) has a specific geographic distribution. HCC is common in sub-Sahara Africa, China, Japan, and the Southeast, where it is strongly associated with chronic hepatitis HBV infection and repeated heavy exposure to the mycotoxin aflatoxin B. Intermediate risk for HCC in areas of southern Europe and Japan is associated with HCV infection. In other parts of the world, HCC occurs as a late complication of cirrhosis (particularly alcoholic liver disease and hemachromatosis).

*Clinical Presentation*—Among southern black Africans and Chinese patients, HCC occurs in relatively young (mean age 33 years) and apparently healthy individuals. Typically, the disease is silent in its early stages. Onset of symptoms: abdominal pain, fullness, early satiety, anorexia, and weight loss corresponds to advanced disease. Physical findings include hepatomegaly, hepatic arterial bruit, ascites, splenomegaly, jaundice, fever. Among individuals with cirrhosis, an unexplained deterioration in liver function may be the only clue.

▶ Diagnosis

*Tumor Markers*—In high-incidence geographic regions, serum alpha-fetoprotein (AFP) is the most useful diagnostic test. Most symptomatic individuals (> 75%) from these regions which will have a diagnostic level (> 500 ng/mL) at presentation. In low-incidence regions, the AFP test is far less useful as a single tumor marker. A combination of tumor markers: tumor-associated isoenzymes of gamma-glutamyl transferase (elevated total GGT leads to isoenzyme fractionation) and the abnormal prothrombin, Desgamma-carboxy prothrombin may be abnormal when the AFP is nondiagnostic.

Newer molecular techniques amplify small amounts of tumor-specific gene-transcripts for albumin and alpha-fetoprotein mRNA promise to enhance detection of malignant hepatocytes in circulation.

*Imaging*—In patients with suspected HCC, the combination of arterial phase and portal venous phase CT imaging is superior to conventional dynamic incremental-bolus CT and will detect the majority of tumors. Magnetic resonance (MR) is useful for detecting small (< 5 cm) HCC, differentiating HCC from hemangiomas and evaluating the proximity of HCC to adjacent blood vessels. Dynamic MR is now superior to hepatic arteriography. Ultrasound differentiates a cystic from solid mass but cannot distinguish HCC from other solid lesions. Hepatic scintigraphy has surpassed other imaging modalities.

*Pathology*—A definitive diagnosis depends on histologic appearance. A percutaneous biopsy and/or aspiration cytology or biopsy carries the risk of systemic dissemination or seeding of the tumor and therefore is avoided when the tumor appears resectable.

▶ Disease Severity

Symptomatic HCC carries a poor prognosis. In Africa and China, average survival is less than 4 months from the onset of symptoms. In other geographic regions the course may be somewhat more indolent. Prognosis is more favorable when tumors are detected prior to the onset of symptoms. A high incidence of extrahepatic recurrence and reappearance of tumor in the donor liver after transplantation reflects early hematogenous spread of micrometastases. Recent advances in the use of reverse transcriptase polymerase chain reactions to amplify small amounts of tumor-specific gene transcripts offer promising results to detect small numbers of malignant hepatocytes in peripheral blood.

▶ Concept and Application

HBV and HCV viruses promote mutagenesis indirectly by stimulating necroinflammatory activity in the liver. Emerging evidence indicates that both viruses also have direct oncogenic potential. Geographic differences in the incidence of HCC among populations with comparable dietary aflotoxin B1 exposure may be due to individuals' capacity to detoxify mutagenic metabolites.

▶ Treatment Steps

1. In areas where HBV-related HCC is common, there is some hope that early vaccination will decrease the incidence of HCC. For HCV-related HCC, vaccination remains a distant goal. Parenteral drug abuse and the high incidence of sporadic HCV infection in countries at intermediate risk for HCC offer little hope for reducing the incidence of HCV-related HCC.
2. Dismal results are obtained with all forms of treatment for symptomatic tumors. Newer molecular markers and imaging modalities may increase the detection of small, asymptomatic and potentially resectable HCC in high-risk individuals or populations. Small (< 5 cm) lesions may be resectable when the tumor appears to be confined to one lobe and the remaining liver is noncirrhotic.
3. Liver transplantation is considered for individuals with end-stage liver failure who coincidentally have a small single tumor without vascular invasion or extrahepatic spread.
4. When operative treatment is not an option, dearterialization, embolization, and chemoembolization or injection of alcohol directly into the lesion may reduce the intrahepatic tumor burden.

## C. Hepatic Fibrosis and Cirrhosis

▶ H&P Keys

In its early stages, the process may reverse on withdrawl of the injurious agent (early fibrosis). Persistent injury leads to irreversible scar tissue deposition, increased resistance to blood flow, impaired exchange of nutrients and metabolites, and failure of synthetic function. A gradual and tedious clinical course is typically interrupted by life-threatening complications: bleeding varices, decompensated ascites, peritonitis, or encephalopathy. Alcohol and chronic viral hepatitis B and C are the most common causes. Other etiologies include: drugs and toxins, autoimmune hepatitis, primary biliary cirrhosis, biliary obstruction, heart failure, metabolic and hereditary disorders (hemachromatosis, Wilson's disease, and alpha$_1$-antitrypsin deficiency). Pertinent history includes: alcohol use, risk factors for viral hepatitis, drug and toxin exposure, and family history.

Stigmata suggestive but not necessarily diagnostic of cirrhosis include: jaundice, spider angiomata, palmar erythema, Dupuytren's contracture, digital clubbing, easy bruising, loss of secondary sexual characteristics, skeletal muscle wasting, abdominal hernias, and caput medusae.

▶ Diagnosis

Laboratory tests, imaging studies and liver biopsy screen for the presence, severity, potential causes, and prognosis of liver disease. No single battery of tests is applicable to all patients. The initial battery of biochemical tests, the so-called, liver function tests reflect the following:

- *Synthetic function:* albumin, prothrombin time, coagulation factor levels, lipoproteins.
- *Hepatocellular injury:* aminotransferases (ALT, AST).

- *Cholestasis:* alkaline phosphatase.
- *Excretory function and anion transport:* bilirubin.

Obtain additional tests when specific diagnoses are suspected:

- *Chronic viral hepatitis B and C:* HBsAg, anti-HCV.
- *Autoimmune hepatitis:* ANA, SMA, serum globulins.
- *Primary biliary cirrhosis:* antimitochondrial antibody.
- *Hemachromatosis:* iron, transferrin, ferritin.

Ultrasonography is the noninvasive imaging study of the liver for jaundice, suspected biliary obstruction, and mass lesion. The presence of cirrhosis is suggested by signs of portal hypertension: splenomegaly, ascites, decreased or reversed portal flow (via Doppler measurements). Supplemental diagnostic studies: ERCP, CT, and MR have value for specific situations:

- *Mass lesion:* MR, CT portography.
- *Iron overload and fatty infiltration:* MR.
- *Extrahepatic bile duct obstruction:* ERCP.
- *Bleeding varices:* upper endoscopy, ligation and/or sclerosis.
- *New onset or decompensated ascites:* diagnostic paracentesis.

Liver biopsy plays a central role in the diagnosis of all stages of fibrosis and cirrhosis. Other indications for liver biopsy include otherwise unexplained hepatomegaly and/or liver biochemical abnormalities, documentation of neoplastic disease, assessment of chronic hepatitis, assessment of veno-occlusive disease, and rejection after transplantation.

### ▶ Disease Severity

Severity of cirrhosis is manifested by its clinical consequences: episodes of variceal bleeding, spontaneous bacterial peritonitis, intractable ascites, and poorly controlled encephalopathy. The Child–Turcotte–Pugh scale (Table 4–26) provides a rough measure of prognosis by combining hepatic synthetic function (albumin, prothrombin time), excretory function (bilirubin), and portal hypertension (ascites encephalopathy). Potential candidates for liver transplantation need referral to the liver transplantation

## 4-26 CHILD–TURCOTTE–PUGH SCORE

| | Child–Turcotte–Pugh Score | | |
|---|---|---|---|
| | 1 | 2 | 3 |
| Encephalopathy | None | 1, 2 | 3, 4 |
| Ascites | Absent | Slight | Moderate |
| Bilirubin (mg/dL) | 1–2 | 2–3 | > 3 |
| Albumin (g/dL) | > 3.5 | 2.8–3.5 | < 2.8 |
| Prothrombin time (s. prolonged) | 1–4 | 4–6 | > 6 |
| Total score | | | |
|   1–6 = A | | | |
|   7–9 = B | | | |
|   10–15 = C | | | |

center well before they develop the following signs of decompensation: uncontrolled variceal bleeding, intractable ascites, poorly controlled encephalopathy, and fulminant hepatic failure.

▶ Concept and Application

Fibrosis and cirrhosis are histologic terms that refer to the accumulation of excess extracellular matrix (ECM) within the liver with or without an accompanying inflammatory response. Recent evidence indicates that the ECM has important biologic effects of liver cell function in addition to its well-characterized effects on blood flow.

▶ Treatment Steps

1. *Cirrhotic ascites:* dietary salt restriction, diuretic therapy. Consider large-volume paracentesis, peritoneovenous shunting, transjugular intrahepatic portovenous shunting (TIPS), and liver transplantation for refractory ascites.
2. *Spontaneous bacterial peritonitis (SBP):* cefotaxime is effective for initial therapy. Patients at risk (ascitic fluid protein < 1 g/dL may benefit from norfloxacin prophylaxis, particularly when hospitalized.
3. *Encephalopathy:* correction of any precipitant factors (GI bleeding, infection, electrolyte imbalance), reduction of dietary protein, and decrease in intestinal ammonia absorption of nonabsorbable carbohydrates, especially lactulose.
4. *Acute variceal bleeding:* variceal band ligation, sclerotherapy and/or pharmacologic therapy: somatostatin, octreotide, vasopressin, vasopressin/nitroglycerin. Consider TIPS for failure of urgent endoscopic and pharmacologic therapy.
5. *Prevention of rebleeding:* variceal band ligation, sclerotherapy, nonselective β-blockade (nadalol, propranolol). Consider TIPS, shunt surgery, especially distal splenrenal shunt and small-diameter interposition portacaval graft, for endoscopic and pharmacologic failures.
6. *Liver transplantation:* for all forms of cirrhosis, primary biliary cirrhosis, primary sclerosing cholangitis, biliary atresia, and fulminant hepatic failure.

## VIII. PANCREAS

### A. Pancreatic Carcinoma

▶ H&P Keys

Risk factors for the development of pancreatic cancer include: chronic pancreatitis, hereditary pancreatitis, smoking, a diet high in fat content, and exposure to various chemicals including B-naphthylamine. Earlier studies that reported an association with caffeine appear unfounded.

Most common presenting features are abdominal pain, weight loss, jaundice, and anorexia. With pancreatic head tumors, distended gallbladder (Courvoisier gallbladder) may be palpable. Occasionally, acute pancreatitis or hyperglycemia may be the presenting features. Thromboembolic phenomenon occur in 10% of patients with pancreatic adenocarcinoma.

Tumor markers: carcinoembryonic antigen, CA 19-9 can be helpful (although not diagnostic) when very high.

### ▶ Diagnosis

In patients with suspected pancreatic cancer the goals of the evaluation are (1) to establish the diagnosis, and (2) to determine resectability. Several imaging modalities are useful.

- Biphasic helical CT with thin cuts through the pancreas is the best single imaging study for both diagnosis and staging.
- ERCP: useful for evaluating biliary or pancreatic duct obstruction in the absence of a suspicious mass on CT. When an equivocal pancreatic mass is present, ERCP and brush cytology may support a diagnosis of malignancy. However, when a potentially respectable mass is present, ERCP and biliary decompression does not improve and may worsen outcome after surgery.
- Transabdominal ultrasound provides little in the evaluation of the pancreas. Overlying bowel gas frequently prevents complete and adequate visualization. Transabadominal ultrasound is useful in the evaluation of obstructive jaundice when there is a strong suspicion of choledocholithiasis.
- Endoscopic ultrasonography (EUS) with fine needle aspiration biopsy is the most accurate test to assess resectability. EUS is operator dependent and expertise is not widely available.
- Visceral angiography has largely been replaced by biphasic helical CT at most centers.
- MR cholangiopancreatography is less sentitive than ERCP and does not provide opportunity to obtain tissue brushings. However, because of its noninvasive nature, it may be useful for patients requiring repeat imaging of the pancreatic duct.
- Biopsy: limited indications

A confirming biopsy prior to resection is unnecessary when:

- Clinical suspicion of pancreatic cancer is high
- The cancer is surgically resectable
- The patient is a satisfactory candidate for surgical resection

A confirming biopsy may be needed prior to treatment when:

- The diagnosis of pancreatic cancer is doubtful
- The cancer is not surgically resectable
- The patient is a poor operative candidate
- When tissue diagnosis is needed prior to initiating chemotherapy or radiation therapy.

### ▶ Concept and Application

Tenth most common type of new cancer. In 1998, an estimated 28,6000 new cases occurred in the United States. Frequency is compounded by lethality. Pancreatic cancer accounts of 5% to 6% of the cancer deaths among men and women, making it the 4th leading cause of cancer deaths. Five-year survival between 1986 and 1993 was only 4%. It is the lowest survival rate among all reported sites.

▶ Treatment Steps

Treatment options remain limited. Stage of disease at the time of diagnosis determines optimal treatment.

1. Surgical resection: in the absence of locally advanced or metastasis disease. Adjuvant or neoadjuvant therapy may improve survival.
2. Unresectable disease: more than 75% of pancreatic cancers are unresectable at the time of diagnosis, either because of locally advanced disease or metastatic disease. Treatment goals are palliation of symptoms and treatment of unresected malignancy. Symptoms to be palliated include: jaundice, gastric or duodenal obstruction, and pain.
3. Obstructive jaundice may be palliated endoscopically, radiologically, or surgically. Endoscopic or radiologic decompression methods are associated with lower early complications and shorter hospital stay.
4. Gastric outlet obstruction occurs in 10% to 15% of cases and can be palliated by surgical gastrojejunostomy or the placement of self-expanding metallic stents such as those used for biliary decompression.
5. Pain is a major concern among patients and is present in 90% of those with advanced disease.
6. Transdermal or long-acting narcotics supplemented with shorter-acting agents are used for breakthrough pain. External beam radiation may provide relief. Pain due to obstruction of the pancreatic duct can sometimes be alleviated by endoscopic pancreatic duct stenting. Celiac nerve block provides pain relief in 80% to 90%. Benefit is limited to about 6 months. For many pancreatic cancer patients who are not likely to survive for more than 6 months, the benefit is lasting.
7. Chemotherapy radiation: gemcitabine is the standard treatment for patients with locally advanced or metastatic pancreatic cancer. Patients may also benefit from radiation therapy given with a radiosensitizing agent such as 5-FU. Paclitaxel is currently being studied as a radiosensitizing agent combined with concurrent radiation.

B. Acute Pancreatitis

▶ H&P Keys

Abdominal pain, nausea, vomiting. Patients appear ill, anxious, and restless. Hypotension, tachypnea, tachycardia, hyperthermia or hypothermia, jaundice, mild distention, involuntary guarding in upper abdomen, generalized abdominal tenderness, bowel sounds diminished, basilar atelectasis, pleural effusions, flank and periumbilical ecchymosis (Grey Turner's and Cullen's signs).

▶ Diagnosis

Elevated serum amylase (within 2 to 12 hours, declining over the next 3 to 5 days), elevated lipase (persists 5 to 7 days, can be detected after amylase normalizes), elevated hematocrit, leukocytosis with a leftward shift of the differential, hyperglycemia, hypoalbuminemia, hypocalcemia, prerenal azotemia with elevated blood

> cram facts

### CAUSES OF ACUTE PANCREATITIS

**Obstruction of pancreatic duct**
Choledocholithiasis and microlithiasis
Pancreas divisum with pathologically stenotic minor papilla
Choledochocele
Sphincter of Oddi dysfunction
Pancreatic duct stricture
Ascariasis or clonorchiasis
Pancreatic or ampullary carcinoma

**Toxins**
Ethyl alcohol
Methyl alcohol
Organophosphate insecticides
Scorpion venom

**Drugs**
Antineoplastic
    Azathioprine, 6-mercaptopurine
Antibiotics and antivirals
    Didanosine (DDI)
    Pentamidine
    Sulfonamides
    Tetracycline
    Metronidazole
    Nitrofurantoin
    Erythromycin
Others
    Estrogens (due to hyperlipidemia)
    Furosemide
    5-aminosalicylates
    Sulindac
    Methyldopa
    Cimetidine and ranitidine
    Salicylates

**Metabolic**
Hyperlipidemia
Hypercalcemia

**Infections**
Viral
    CMV
    Mumps
    Hepatitis A, B, C
    Coxsackie B
    Adenovirus
    Epstein–Barr virus
    HIV
Bacterial
    *Mycobacterium* (tuberculosis and MAC)
    *Legionella*
    *Leptospirosis*
    *Mycoplasma*
Parasite
    Ascaris
    Clonorchis
    Cryptosporidiosis
Trauma (including ERCP)
Ischemia
    Postoperative (especially after heart–lung bypass)
    Hypotension
    Vasculitis
Idiopathic
Other
    Posterior penetrating duodenal ulcer
    Cystic fibrosis (usually presents as chronic pancreatitis)

urea nitrogen and serum creatinine, hyperbilirubinemia, and hypertriglyceridemia. Routine roentgenography, ultrasonography, and CT scanning.

### ▶ Disease Severity
Ranson's criteria for prognosis on admission and during initial 48 hours do not predict course or outcome for individual patients.

### ▶ Concept and Application
Biliary tract stone disease and alcohol abuse account for 60% to 80% of cases. Other causes: infections (*Mycoplasma pneumoniae*, mumps, coxsackie, *Ascaris, Opisthorchis*), drugs (azathioprine, thiazide diuretics, sulfonamides), lipid abnormalities, trauma, and ERCP. Most attacks of acute pancreatitis result from injury to the pancreas by digestive enzymes.

▶ Treatment Steps
1. General supportive measures, with meticulous management of fluid, electrolyte, ventilatory and hemodynamic alterations, and parenteral alimentation.
2. Early (within 72 hours) intervention (ERCP) to remove stones from the ductal system improves outcome.
3. Anticipate possible local complications: pseudocyst infection, pancreatic ascites, abscess, blood vessel with or without rupture or thrombosis, bowel necrosis or stricture, esophageal varices, and fistulas.

## C. Chronic Pancreatitis

▶ H&P Keys

Recurrent or persistent abdominal pain, weight loss, steatorrhea, glucose intolerance, epigastric tenderness.

▶ Diagnosis

Plain roentgenogram of the abdomen may show pancreatic calcification. Ultrasonography or CT scan may show enlarged gland, dilated pancreatic duct, or calculi. ERCP is most sensitive and specific test for chronic pancreatitis. ERCP can differentiate chronic pancreatitis from pancreatic carcinoma. Tests of pancreatic exocrine function (secretin, cholecystokinin [CCK], or bentiromide test) for the rare patient with relatively minor ductal changes on ERCP in whom the diagnosis remains in doubt.

▶ Disease Severity

Complications include pseudocyst, pancreatic ascites, fistula, and splenic vein thrombosis. Suspect pseudocyst when a stable chronic pancreatitis patient experiences worsening of abdominal pain.

▶ Concept and Application

Alcohol in Western societies (70% to 80%) and malnutrition worldwide represent major etiologies.

▶ Treatment Steps
1. Avoidance of alcohol, analgesia, enzyme therapy for malabsorption and pain control, especially for patients with non–alcohol-induced chronic pancreatitis.
2. Celiac plexus block.
3. Surgery if all other measures have failed.

## D. Cystic Fibrosis

▶ H&P Keys

Infants fail to gain weight despite vigorous appetite and watery stools. Eighty percent have pancreatic exocrine insufficiency at diagnosis, hypoproteinemia with edema, and "pot belly" on physical examination.

▶ Diagnosis

Sweat electrolytes: sodium and chloride are elevated in sweat in 99%; pancreatic stimulation test with CCK and secretin may confirm diagnosis when sweat test is equivocal; fetal screening and chromosomal analysis to diagnose cystic fibrosis by DNA analysis in the future.

▶ **Disease Severity**

Malnutrition and recurrent pulmonary infections are major concerns. Associated conditions include: Chronic meconium ileus in 15%, distal small-bowel obstruction (meconium ileus equivalent) in older patients, rectal prolapse, intussusception, diabetes mellitus, chronic liver disease, abdominal pain, and recurrent episodes of pancreatitis.

▶ **Concept and Application**

Increased viscosity of exocrine secretions leads to precipitation of exocrine secretions in all exocrine glands (pancreatic acini, intestinal glands, intrahepatic bile ducts, gallbladder, prostate, salivary glands) resulting in impaired pancreatic exocrine secretion, intestinal obstruction, focal biliary cirrhosis, obstructive pulmonary disease, and obstructive lesions of the male genital tract.

▶ **Treatment Steps**

Treatment of malnutrition with adequate caloric intake, balanced diet with vitamin supplementation (vitamins A, D, E, and K), pancreatic enzyme replacement, and $H_2$-blockers to improve maldigestion.

## IX. HERNIA

### A. External Hernias

▶ **H&P Keys**

Pain is derived from mechanical disruption of intestinal transit and tension exerted on the mesentery. Main symptom of groin hernia is an inguinal mass that may appear after activities that increase intra-abdominal pressure. Groin hernias are diagnosed by digital examination, with index finger introduced into inguinal canal through external inguinal ring by depressing the skin.

▶ **Diagnosis**

Examination is performed with the patient standing or in decubitus position. Palpate both sides of the groin and scrotum. Depress the skin of the area to introduce the finger into the inguinal canal through the external inguinal ring. Indirect hernias correspond to the internal inguinal ring. Direct hernias lie more medially. Femoral hernias are palpated inferior to the inguinal ligament.

▶ **Disease Severity**

Hernia is reducible when herniation occurs intermittently and can be reversed spontaneously or by manipulation. An incarcerated hernia cannot be reversed. Sudden onset of pain in a previously asymptomatic hernia suggests compromise of the blood supply of the viscus or strangulation. Colicky abdominal pain, tenderness, nausea, vomiting, increased leukocytosis, and fever indicates bowel obstruction.

▶ Concept and Application

Hernia: protrusion of any viscus from its proper cavity. Herniation occurs as a result of increased intra-abdominal pressure, or decreased resistance of the abdominal wall. Most common hernias are umbilical, incisional, and groin. Groin hernias are classified by the anatomy of the area (indirect inguinal 60%, direct inguinal 30%, femoral 5%, combined 2%).

▶ Treatment Steps

1. Surgical treatment is indicated for healthy patients. Symptomatic hernias in high-risk patients require further consideration. Strangulation and bowel obstruction are the acute complications that require surgical repair. Hernias with small hernial rings such as umbilical and femoral are at greater risk of strangulation.
2. Manual reduction is effective in incarcerated or strangulated hernias of very short duration. Manual reduction is contraindicated when bowel necrosis is suspected or when symptoms have been present for more than 8 hours. A complication of manual reduction is reduction en masse. The hernia is returned to the abdominal cavity, but the bowel and blood supply remain constricted in the hernial sac.
3. Colicky abdominal pain, tenderness, nausea, vomiting, increased leukocytosis, fever, and signs of bowel obstruction demand laparotomy.

## B. Traumatic Hernias of the Diaphragm

▶ H&P Keys

Penetrating or blunt trauma, left upper quadrant pain that may be referred to the left shoulder, followed by nausea, vomiting, central abdominal pain, diaphoresis, respiratory distress.

▶ Diagnosis

Chest roentgenogram shows abdominal viscera in the thorax. Fluoroscopy to evaluate diaphragmatic excursions. Ultrasonography and CT scan are also useful.

▶ Disease Severity

Principal complication is intestinal obstruction, often involving the intra-abdominal viscera more than the intrathoracic.

▶ Concept and Application

Most common injury is a large tear of the diaphragm from the esophageal hiatus to the left costal attachments. Herniated viscera are stomach, spleen, colon, and left lobe of the liver.

▶ Treatment Steps

1. Surgical repair.

## X. ABDOMINAL AORTIC ANEURYSM

▶ H&P Keys

Usually asymptomatic until rupture. Physical examination may reveal a tender, pulsatile mass. Abdominal discomfort, tenderness, ureteral obstruction suggest inflammatory aneurysms. Mycotic aneurysms present as tender enlarging masses.

▶ Diagnosis

Ultrasonography has a sensitivity approaching 100% and is cost-effective for aneurysm detection and sequential follow-up. CT scan is equally effective and should be used when ultrasonography is not possible and precise sizing is required. MRI may be better than either ultrasonography or CT, both for accurate aneurysm measurement and views of relevant vascular anatomy. Chest roentgenogram are done to exclude thoracic aortic aneurysm. Preoperative aortography if visceral, renal, or peripheral vascular disease is suspected. Selective screening of high-risk patients between the ages of 55 and 80: hypertension, aneurysms of femoral or popliteal artery, and family history of abdominal aortic aneurysm.

▶ Disease Severity

Most abdominal aneurysms remain asymptomatic until rupture. Symptoms and complications are related to aneurysm size and expansion rate. Aneurysms smaller than 4 cm have a risk of rupture of about 2%. 25% to 41% of aneurysms larger than 5 cm rupture within 5 years. Risk factors for rupture include initial diameter of the aneurysm, elevated blood pressure, and presence of chronic obstructive pulmonary disease.

▶ Concept and Application

Pathogenesis is multifactorial: genetic predisposition, biochemical alterations of aortic wall, and hemodynamic mechanical factors contributing. Inflammatory reaction can develop around the external calcified layer (inflammatory aneurysms). Mycotic aneurysms can be caused by bacterial or fungal infection and are rare.

▶ Treatment Steps

1. Repair of symptomatic or ruptured abdominal aortic aneurysms and of all symptomatic aneurysms larger than 5 cm.
2. Contraindications to elective aortic reconstruction: myocardial infarction (within 6 months), intractable angina pectoris, severe pulmonary insufficiency with dyspnea at rest, severe chronic renal insufficiency, incapacitating stroke, and life expectancy of less than 2 years.

## BIBLIOGRAPHY

Agrawal NM, Van Kerckhove HEJM, et al. Misoprostol coadministered with diclofenac for prevention of gastroduodenal ulcers: a one-year study. *Dig Dis Sci* 1995;40:1125–31.

Alter HJ, Bradley DW. Non-A, non-B, hepatitis unrelated to the hepatitis C virus (non-ABC). *Sem Liver Dis* 1995;15,1, 110–20.

Baaer DM, Simons JL et al. Hemachromatosis screening asymptomatic ambulatory men 30 years of age and older. *Am J Med* 1995;98:464–68.

Balthazar EJ, Freeny PC, VanSonnenberg E. Imaging and intervention in acute pancreatitis. *Radiology* 1994;193:297–306.

Batey RG, Burns T, et al. Alcohol consumption and the risk of cirrhosis. *Med J Aust* 1992;156:413–16.

Bazzoli F, Fossi S, et al. The risk of adenomatous polyps in asymptomatic first-degree relatives of persons with colon cancer. *Gastroenterology* 1995;109:783–88.

Bond JH, for the Practice Parameters Committee of the ACG: polyp guideline. Diagnosis, treatment, and surveillance for patients with nonfamilial colorectal polyps. *Ann Int Med* 1993;199:836–43.

Cameron AJ, Lomboy CT, et al. Adenocarcinoma of the esophagogastric junction and Barrett's esophagus. *Gastroenterology* 1995;109:1541–46.

Cutler AF, Prasad VM. Long-term follow-up of *Helicobacter pylori* serology after successful eradication. *Am J Gastroenterol* 1996;91:85–87.

deBoer W, Driessen W, et al. Effect of acid suppression on efficacy of treatment for *Helicobacter pylori* infection. *Lancet* 1995;345:817–20.

Desmet VJ, Gerber M, et al. Classification of chronic hepatitis: diagnosis, grading and staging. *Hepatology* 1994;19:1513–16.

DeVault KR, Castell DO, et al. Guidelines for the diagnosis and treatment of gastroesophageal reflux disease. *Arch Int Med* 1995;155:2165–73.

Elton E., Hanauer SB. Review article: the medical management of Crohn's disease. *Aliment Pharmacol Ther* 1996;10:1–22.

Ernst CB. Abdominal aorta in aneurysm. *New Eng J Med* 1993;328:1167–72.

Gallstones and laparoscopic cholecystectomy. *NIH Consensus Statement online* 1992;10(3):1–20.

Hanauer SB. Medical therapy for ulcerative colitis. *Ann Int Med* 1993;118:540–49.

Isaacson PG. Gastrointestinal lymphoma. *Hum Pathol* 1994;25:1020–29.

Lee WM. Drug-induced hepatotoxicity. *N Engl J Med* 1995;333:1118–127.

Liskow B, Campbell J, Nickel EJ. Validity of the CAGE questionnaire in screening for alcohol dependence in a walkin (triage) clinic. *J Stud Alcohol* 1995;56:277–81.

Masuko K, Mitsui T, et al. Infection with hepatitis GB virus C in patients on maintenance hemodialysis. *N Engl J Med* 1996;334;23:1485–89.

*MMWR Morbid Mortal Wkly Rep* 1991.40:1.

Ottinger LW. Current concepts: mesenteric ischemia. *New Eng J Med* 1982;307:535–37.

Owens DM, Nelson DK, Talley NJ. The irritable bowel syndrome: long-term prognosis and the physician–patient interaction. 1995;122:107–12.

Pasricha PJ, Ravich WJ, et al. Intrasphincteric botulinum toxin for the treatment of achalasia. *N Engl J Med* 1995;322:774–78.

Rao SSC, Gregersen H, et al. Unexplained chest pain: the hypersensitive, hyperreactive and poorly compliant esophagus. *Ann Intern Med* 1996;124:950–58.

Rees JH, Soudain SE, et al. *Campylobacter jejuni* infection and Guillain-Barré syndrome. *N Engl J Med* 1995;333:1374–79.

Rosch T, Braig C, et al. Staging of pancreatic and ampullary carcinoma by endoscopic ultrasonography: comparison with conventional sonography, computed tomography, and angiography. *Gastroenterology* 1992;102:188.

Salam I, Katelaris P, et al. Randomised trial of single-dose ciprofloxacin for travellers' diarrhea. *Lancet* 1994;344:1537–39.

Soll AH, for the Practice Parameters Committee of the ACG. NIH consensus conference: medical treatment of peptic ulcer disease. *JAMA* 1996;275:622–29.

Terrault N, Wright T. Interferon and hepatitis C. *N Engl J Med* 1995;332:1509–11.

Toribara NW, Sleisenger MH. Screening for colorectal cancer. *N Engl J Med* 1995;332:861–66.

Valdimarsson T, Franzen L, et al. Is small bowel biopsy necessary in adults with suspected celiac disease and IgA antiendomysium antibodies? 100% positive predictive value for celiac disease in adults. *Dig Dis Sci* 1996;41:83–7.

Warshaw AL, Gu Z, et al. Preoperative staging and assessment of resectability of pancreatic cancer. *Arch Surg* 1990;125:230.

Winawer BJ, Zauber AG, et al. Risk of colorectal cancer in families of patients with adenomatous polyps. *N Engl J Med* 1996;334:82–7.

Wright TL, Perreira B. Liver transplantation for chronic viral hepatitis. *Liver Transplant Surg* 1995;10:471–80.

# Hematology and Oncology 5

I. **ANEMIA / 169**
   A. Iron-deficiency Anemia / 169
   B. Blood-loss Anemia / 169
   C. Folic Acid Deficiency / 170
   D. α-Thalassemia / 171
   E. β-Thalassemia / 171
   F. Vitamin $B_{12}$ Deficiency / 172
   G. Aplastic Anemia / 173
   H. Lead-poisoning Anemia / 174
   I. Anemia of Chronic Renal Disease / 174
   J. Hemolytic Anemia / 175
   K. Anemia of Chronic Disease / 176
   L. Sickle Cell Anemia / 176

II. **MALIGNANT DISEASES / 177**
   A. Acute Myelogenous Leukemia / 177
   B. Acute Lymphocytic Leukemia / 178
   C. Chronic Myelogenous Leukemia / 179
   D. Chronic Lymphocytic Leukemia / 180
   E. Hodgkin's Disease / 181
   F. Low-grade Lymphoma / 182
   G. Intermediate- or High-grade Lymphoma / 183
   H. Multiple Myeloma / 184
   I. Monoclonal Gammopathy of Undetermined Significance / 185

III. **OTHER DISORDERS / 185**
   A. Polycythemia Rubra Vera (Primary Erythrocytosis) / 185
   B. Secondary Erythrocytosis / 186
   C. Transfusion Reactions / 187
   D. Hemophilia A and B / 187
   E. von Willebrand Disease / 188

- F. Vitamin K Deficiency / 189
- G. Lupus Inhibitor / 189
- H. Disseminated Intravascular Coagulation / 190
- I. Antithrombin III Deficiency / 190
- J. Protein C Deficiency / 191
- K. Activated Protein C (APC) Resistance / 191
- L. Idiopathic Thrombocytopenia Purpura / 192
- M. Thrombotic Thrombocytopenic Purpura / 192
- N. Essential Thrombocythemia / 193
- O. Agnogenic Myeloid Metaplasia / 193
- P. Platelet Dysfunction / 194
- Q. Neutropenia / 194

**BIBLIOGRAPHY / 195**

## I. ANEMIA

### A. Iron-deficiency Anemia

▶ H&P Keys

*Etiology*—Menstrual and pregnancy-related losses, iron-deficient diet, chronic gastrointestinal (GI) bleeding, chronic alcohol, aspirin, steroid, or nonsteroidal anti-inflammatory drug (NSAID) use.

*Signs and Symptoms*—Glossitis, spooning of nails, fatigue, weakness, dyspnea, pallor, pagophagia (ingestion of ice).

▶ Diagnosis

Hypochromic, microcytic cells on peripheral smear. Mean corpuscular volume (MCV) and mean corpuscular hemoglobin (MCH) are low; low serum ferritin, low serum iron, increased total iron-binding capacity (TIBC), low percentage of saturation, increased red cell distribution width (RDW), thrombocytosis, and low reticulocyte count. Free erythrocytic porphyrin elevated.

▶ Disease Severity

Absence of iron on bone marrow aspiration (Prussian blue staining).

▶ Concept and Application

Underproduction anemia caused by inability to synthesize heme, which requires iron and porphyrin synthesis. Buildup of free porphyrin in red blood cells is present. May be the result of impaired iron absorption, deficient dietary intake, chronic blood loss, chronic intravascular hemolysis.

▶ Treatment Steps
1. Determine etiology.
2. Begin supplemental oral iron if patient is mildly to moderately symptomatic.
3. Transfuse if patient has any sign of cardiac compromise or is severely symptomatic.
4. Reassess oral replacement in 14–21 days expecting to see a significant reticulocytosis and the hemoglobin corrected by at least half. If it has not, assess compliance and absorption issues.
5. Some patients do not absorb or cannot tolerate oral iron and must receive either transfusion or intravenous supplementation.

### B. Blood-loss Anemia

▶ H&P Keys

*Etiology*—GI bleeding (ulcer disease, gastritis, hemorrhoids, angiodysplasia, polyp, tumor, diverticulum); menstruation; massive hematuria; hemoptysis.

*Acute Symptoms*—Fatigue, pallor, tachycardia, dyspnea, syncope, chest pain.

▶ Diagnosis

Complete blood count (CBC), reticulocyte count, stool guaiac, urinalysis.

*Acute*—Orthostatic changes; normochromic, normocytic anemia; elevated blood urea nitrogen (BUN) secondary to GI bleeding.

*Chronic*—Similar to iron deficiency. Microcytic anemia, low reticulocyte count, low serum iron and transferrin saturation.

▶ Disease Severity

CBC, orthostatic hypotension, tachycardia, chest pain, and level of consciousness.

▶ Concept and Application

Severe blood loss by any mechanism. Hematocrit may not fall if volume loss not repleted.

▶ Treatment Steps

1. Determine etiology.
2. Check for underlying coagulopathy with prothrombin time and partial thromboplastin time.
3. Acute loss requires replacement with blood products (packed red blood cells, fresh frozen plasma, and cryoprecipitate) and IV fluids.
4. Chronic loss can be handled with treatment of the site of bleeding followed by supplemental iron.

## C. Folic Acid Deficiency

▶ H&P Keys

Symptoms of anemia. No neurologic sequelae as in $B_{12}$ deficiency. Nutritional deficiency (lack of green, leafy vegetables, fruit); chronic alcohol use; patients with malabsorption syndromes. Increased losses or increased utilization (dialysis, pregnancy). Chronic hemolytic anemias (ie, sickle cell disease).

▶ Diagnosis

Low serum and red blood cell (RBC) folate levels (serum folate levels quickly correct following one hospital meal therefore RBC folate levels are more accurate but also more difficult to obtain). Macrocytic anemia and hypersegmented neutrophils on peripheral smear. Megaloblastic bone marrow cells. Normal $B_{12}$ level. Increased lactase dehydrogenase (LDH). Increased bilirubin.

▶ Disease Severity

Observable pancytopenia; infertility, skin pigmentation abnormalities. Severe malabsorption syndromes diagnosed by jejunal biopsy. Neural tube defects if folate deficiency present during pregnancy.

▶ Concept and Application

Folic acid absorbed in the proximal jejunum. Folate deficiency leads to diminished thymidylate synthesis and abnormal DNA replication.

▶ Treatment Steps
1. Determine etiology.
2. Replace with oral folic acid 1 mg/day.

### D. α-Thalassemia

▶ H&P Keys

An inherited disorder seen in American blacks and people of Mediterranean or Southeast Asian background. Carrier state (lack of one normal allele) is undetectable and very common. Patients who lack two alleles (called α-thalassemia trait) are usually asymptomatic although they may have a mild microcytic anemia. Patients with deletion of three alleles (hemoglobin [HbH]) have moderately severe hemolytic anemia. Absence of α-chains is incompatible with life.

▶ Diagnosis

Microcytosis on peripheral smear in patients with α-thalassemia trait. Normal iron studies. Low RDW. Elevated RBC numbers. RBC inclusions in patients with HbH and evidence of hemolysis (elevated lactic dehydrogenase [LDH] and bilirubin). Coombs' test is negative. Molecular studies can identify precise abnormalities.

▶ Disease Severity

Hemolytic anemia and splenomegaly in patients with HbH. Hydrops fetalis occurs in homozygotes, in whom no α-globin is produced. Affected fetuses are either stillborn or die shortly after birth.

▶ Concept and Application

Caused by deletion of one or more α-globin genes. Presence or absence of symptoms depends on number of alleles deleted (or mutated). Inadequate production of α-globin leads to precipitation of β-globin (in HbH) or to β4 (beta chain tetramer) formation, which is incompatible with life.

▶ Treatment Steps
1. Establish diagnosis by molecular studies or staining of peripheral blood smear with cresyl blue.
2. Rule out underlying iron deficiency.
3. Symptomatic patients may need periodic transfusions.
4. Prenatal diagnosis can identify fetus at risk for hydrops fetalis.
5. Splenectomy can be beneficial in patients with HbH.

### E. β-Thalassemia

▶ H&P Keys

Most common in patients of Mediterranean background or from equatorial regions of Asia and Africa. Thalassemia minor patients (heterozygotes) usually have asymptomatic mild anemia. Thalassemia major (homozygotes) presents in childhood with symptoms of anemia. Splenomegaly occurs in thalassemia major. Frontal bossing from expansion of marrow cavity and bilirubin gallstones also seen.

▶ Diagnosis

Basophilic stippling and target cells on peripheral smear. Microcytic, hypochromic anemia, elevated RBC number. MCV usually < 75. Hb electrophoresis.

▶ Disease Severity

Severity of disease depends on type of genetic abnormality and amount of HbF present. Some defects result in no β-chain production, others produce a decreased amount of β-chain. Thalassemia minor results in a mild hypochromic microcytic anemia. Elevated hemoglobin $A_2$ ($HbA_2$) on Hb electrophoresis is diagnostic. In thalassemia major, splenomegaly results in shortened RBC survival and at times thrombocytopenia or neutropenia. Serum ferritin to detect iron overload in transfused patients.

▶ Concept and Application

Hereditary anemia resulting from deletion or defective transcription of β-globin genes. Excess α-chains precipitate, causing rapid splenic clearing of RBCs. Frequent transfusions lead to iron overload.

▶ Treatment Steps

1. Transfusions required on a regular basis.
2. Start iron chelation with desferoxamine early to minimize complications of iron overload.
3. Bone marrow transplantation beneficial in thalassemia major.
4. Genetic counseling.

## F. Vitamin $B_{12}$ Deficiency

▶ H&P Keys

Symptoms of anemia (pallor, fatigue, weakness, dyspnea). Neurologic symptoms such as paresthesias, abnormal mental status, ataxia, and premature graying. History of autoimmune or intestinal diseases, such as atrophic gastritis, gastrectomy, sprue, and blind loop syndrome. Dietary deficiency rare.

▶ Diagnosis

Hypersegmented neutrophils (Fig. 5–1), macrocytic, hyperchromic anemia (high MCV). Increased LDH, low serum $B_{12}$

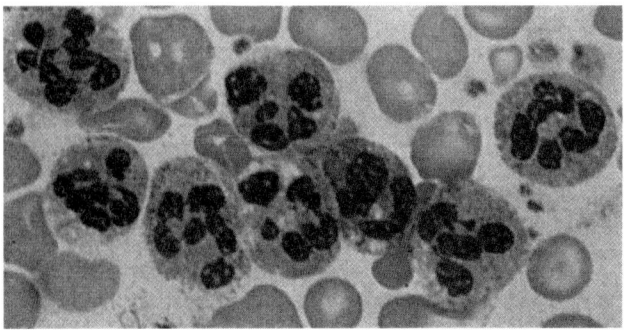

Figure 5–1. Hypersegmented neutrophils associated with vitamin $B_{12}$ deficiency.

level. Document achlorhydria. Perform Schilling test to evaluate cause of pernicious anemia. (Schilling test no longer available in most settings.) Intrinsic factor antibody analysis is now test of choice. Bone marrow, which is not required for diagnosis, shows megaloblastic hematopoiesis with abnormally immature nucleus compared to cytoplasm (nuclear and cytoplasmic dissociation). Complete neurologic exam.

▶ Disease Severity

Serum $B_{12}$ level < 100 pg/mL. Neurologic symptoms consistent with long tract disease, then cerebral dysfunction. No correlation between anemia and neurologic symptoms.

▶ Concept and Application

Body stores of $B_{12}$ last 3–4 years. $B_{12}$ present in animal protein (meats, eggs, milk products). Impaired DNA synthesis, but normal RNA synthesis, induces ineffective erythropoiesis. Defective conversion of propionate to succinyl coenzyme A (CoA) may lead to defective myelin synthesis and patchy demyelination. Absorption of vitamin $B_{12}$ requires secretion of intrinsic factor by the stomach and occurs in the terminal ileum.

▶ Treatment Steps

$B_{12}$ 100 µg given parenterally as a loading dose daily for 5 days, then 100 µg per month for life.

## G. Aplastic Anemia

▶ H&P Keys

Weakness, fatigue, pallor, petechiae, purpura, increased bruising and overt bleeding, fever or evidence of infection. Etiology may be idiopathic, familial (eg, Fanconi's syndrome) or acquired (eg, secondary to radiation, drugs, hepatitis, or autoimmune mechanisms).

▶ Diagnosis

Hypocellular bone marrow. Normal cytogenetics. Decreased reticulocyte count (< 5%). Normochromic and normocytic RBCs. Rule out paroxysmal nocturnal hemoglobinuria with a Ham test (sucrose hemolysis test).

▶ Disease Severity

Severe aplastic anemia defined as two or more of the following: absolute neutrophil count < 500, reticulocyte count < 1%, and platelets < 20,000. Percentage of bone marrow cellularity < 25%.

▶ Concept and Application

Immune suppression of hematopoiesis in most. Some patients have stem cell defect. Associated with benzene, chloramphenicol, parvovirus B19 as well as other drugs and viral infections.

▶ Treatment Steps

1. Determine etiology if possible.
2. HLA-matched bone marrow transplant if patient has a donor.

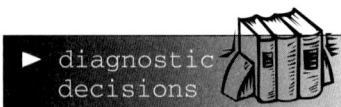

### diagnostic decisions

**ANEMIA**

**Microcytic**

*Iron deficiency*
Menstruating females, chronic GI bleeding, low serum iron, low percent saturation, low ferritin, and high TIBC.

*α- or β-Thalassemia*
African, Mediterranean, or South-East Asian ancestry, normal iron stores.

*Anemia of chronic disease*
Look for chronic inflammatory processes, usually normocytic, low TIBC and elevated ferritin.

**Macrocytic**

*$B_{12}$ deficiency*
Significant body stores, so rarely related to malnutrition. Neurologic changes can precede significant anemia, hypersegmented polys.

*Folate deficiency*
No body stores, so develops more quickly during inadequate dietary periods. Replacement can improve anemia of combined $B_{12}$ deficiency but does not treat the neurologic sequelae. Serum levels inaccurate. If definite proof required, get RBC folate levels.

**Normocytic**

*Acute blood loss*
Should be obvious; transfuse as needed.

*Aplastic anemia*
Fairly acute onset with no gross bleeding; look hard for possible drugs or treatable infections. Avoid transfusions if possible.

*Anemia of chronic renal disease*
Often combined with iron-deficiency; can be seen even in mild chronic renal insufficiency; the patients don't have to be on dialysis.

---

3. If transplant not an option other treatment options include antithymocyte globulin (ATG), cyclosporin, and corticosteroids.
4. Avoid transfusions as much as possible if bone marrow transplant is planned.

### H. Lead-poisoning Anemia

▶ **H&P Keys**

Autonomic neuropathy (abdominal cramps, ileus). Renal dysfunction. Mental status changes. *Etiology:* Ingesting contaminated foods, inhaled particles, pica, lead cookware.

▶ **Diagnosis**

Mild anemia. Peripheral smear: RBCs hypochromic with basophilic stippling. Increased serum lead level.

▶ **Disease Severity**

Encephalopathy or lead levels greater than 70–100 μg/dL.

▶ **Concept and Application**

Inhibition of ALA dehydrogenase leads to denaturing of proteins. Lead limits intestinal absorption of iron.

▶ **Treatment Steps**

1. Remove source of lead.
2. If severe, may require intravenous ethylenediaminetetraacetic acid (EDTA).
3. Mild to moderate intoxication can be treated with an oral medication, succimer.

### I. Anemia of Chronic Renal Disease

▶ **H&P Keys**

Pallor and fatigue. Renal failure patients (not necessarily dialysis dependent).

▶ **Diagnosis**

Low Hb. Low reticulocyte count. Normochromic, normocytic RBCs, Burr cells, and schistocytes on peripheral smear. Increased serum creatinine. Serum erythropoietin level decreased. Iron deficiency, folate deficiency, and blood loss can complicate this disorder.

▶ **Disease Severity**

Development of transfusion dependency.

▶ **Concept and Application**

Decreased erythropoietin production. Iron and folate are lost during dialysis. Increased RBC loss and destruction; decreased RBC survival secondary to azotemia.

▶ **Treatment Steps**

1. Intravenous erythropoietin one to three times per week.
2. Iron and folate replacement.

## J. Hemolytic Anemia

▶ H&P Keys

Hereditary and acquired disorders. Intrinsic enzymatic defects, eg, pyruvate kinase and hexokinase deficiencies. Drug history: glucose-6-phosphate dehydrogenase (G6PD) deficiency leads to episodic hemolysis, after exposure to oxidative stress. Chronic hemolysis can result in splenomegaly. Some hemolytic conditions are secondary to lymphoid malignancies (chronic lymphocytic leukemia, lymphoma) or systemic lupus erythematosus (SLE) whereas others are associated with bacterial (mycoplasma) or viral (infectious mononucleosis) infections. Bilirubin gallstones with chronic hemolysis.

▶ Diagnosis

Elevated reticulocyte count. Coombs' test to determine autoimmune versus nonimmune (positive in autoimmune). Positive Coombs' test: detection of immunoglobulin and/or complement on RBC surface. Increased MCV. Elevated LDH, bilirubin (indirect).

G6PD deficiency: can detect Heinz bodies on peripheral smear, quantitate G6PD in nonacute setting.

Warm antibodies usually IgG: microspherocytes and reticulocytosis on peripheral smear.

Cold antibodies usually IgM: Coombs' test: positive for complement.

Microangiopathic hemolytic anemias (disseminated intravascular coagulation [DIC], thrombotic thrombocytopenic purpura [TTP], malfunctioning heart valve) show evidence of RBC fragmentation (schistocytes, helmet cells). Intravascular hemolysis results in depletion of serum haptoglobin, formation of methemalbumin, urinary hemosiderin, and urinary free hemoglobin if severe.

▶ Disease Severity

Level of Hct, LDH, indirect bilirubin levels. Depletion of haptoglobin, free Hb in urine or serum.

▶ Concept and Application

May be autoimmune (antibody-mediated) or nonimmune (unstable hemoglobin, oxidative stress, as with deficiency of G6PD). Intravascular versus extravascular hemolysis.

▶ Treatment Steps
1. Determine etiology.
2. Transfuse least-incompatible blood if patient requires.
3. G6PD—the primary management is avoidance of oxidative stress, particularly known medications like quinine.
4. Warm antibodies are treated by corticosteroids, less often splenectomy or immunosuppression.
5. Cold antibodies are treated by keeping the patient, especially extremities, warm; steroids and occasionally cytotoxics.
6. Treat underlying disorder.

## K. Anemia of Chronic Disease

▶ **H&P Keys**

Symptoms of underlying disorder (weight loss, anorexia, myalgias, arthralgias).

▶ **Diagnosis**
- Hb rarely < 9 gm/dL
- Normochromic, normocytic anemia
- Normal or increased serum ferritin
- Decreased reticulocyte count
- Serum iron variable
- Decreased TIBC
- Transferrin saturation variable
- Bone marrow: adequate to increased iron stores

▶ **Disease Severity**

Clinical signs of anemia.

▶ **Concept and Application**

Abnormal utilization of iron. Decreased RBC survival. Inadequate production of erythropoietin with respect to anemia.

▶ **Treatment Steps**
1. Treat underlying disease.
2. Subcutaneous erythropoietin, usually weekly.
3. Transfuse if necessary.

## L. Sickle Cell Anemia

▶ **H&P Keys**

Pallor; history of painful crises. Fatigue, tachycardia, leukocytosis, splenic infarctions, renal papillary necrosis, aseptic necrosis, cerebrovascular accident (CVA), priapism, hyposthenuria, bilirubin stones, infections such as pneumonias with encapsulated microorganisms, osteomyelitis with staphylococcus or salmonella. Family history.

▶ **Diagnosis**

Peripheral smear reveals sickle-shaped cells, Howell–Jolly bodies, nucleated RBCs, reticulocytosis, thrombocytosis. HbS on electrophoresis. Prenatal diagnosis by amniotic fluid DNA analysis.

▶ **Disease Severity**

Heterozygous state (sickle cell trait) usually asymptomatic, but a frequent cause of hematuria secondary to papillary necrosis. Homozygous state results in severe hemolytic anemia (Fig. 5–2).

Factors that induce sickling: infection, dehydration, low oxygen tension, low pH, increased serum osmolarity. Microvascular occlusion can lead to ischemia and tissue infarction. This is known as a pain crisis. Aplastic crisis (abrupt halt in erythropoiesis) caused by parvovirus B19 infection.

▶ **Concept and Application**

Point mutation at position 6 of β-globin chains (glutamic acid to valine) allows for polymerization. Amount of Hb in cell impor-

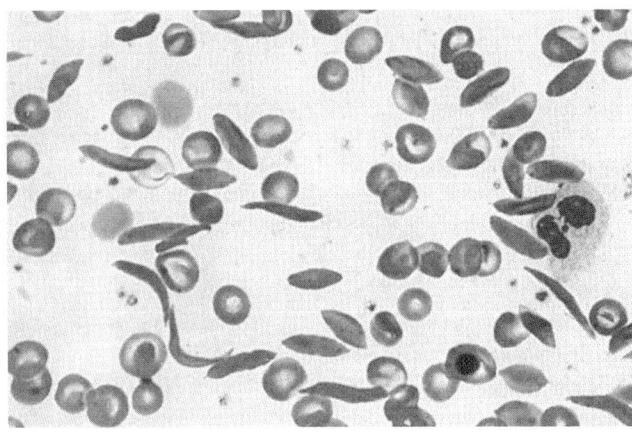

Figure 5-2. Homozygous sickle cell disease.

tant; thus sickle trait plus thalassemia less severe than homozygous sickle cell anemia.

▶ Treatment Steps

### Chronic
1. Folate 1–2 mg PO daily.
2. Pneumovax.
3. Antibiotic prophylaxis in childhood.
4. Genetic counseling.
5. Hydroxyurea helpful in some patients to increase HbF levels and decrease pain crises.
6. Hypertransfusion to suppress Hg S levels.

### Acute
1. Treat pain crises with hydration, adequate analgesia and treatment of inciting event if known.
2. Oxygen if patient hypoxic.
3. Transfuse aggressively or do exchange transfusion for CVA or acute chest syndrome.

## II. MALIGNANT DISEASES

### A. Acute Myelogenous Leukemia

▶ H&P Keys

Fatigue, bruising, petechiae, overt bleeding (eg, menorrhagia), fever or evidence of infection. In certain subtypes of acute myelogenous leukemia (AML) gingival hypertrophy, skin lesions or DIC; modest splenomegaly.

▶ Diagnosis

CBC reveals anemia and thrombocytopenia. White blood cells (WBC) usually elevated with increased blasts or occasionally depressed. Auer rods in some subtypes. Bone marrow is usually hypercellular, positive peroxidase or Sudan black staining, negative

PAS staining. Flow cytometry to determine cell surface markers. Cytogenetic abnormalities include: t(8;21) (M2), t(15;17) (M3), inv16 (M4 with eosinophils). Central nervous system (CNS) involvement can be seen in M4 and M5 subtypes. Spuriously low $Po_2$ (oxygen tension) and serum glucose can be seen with high WBC.

### ▶ Disease Severity
Very high WBCs can cause leukostasis with CNS symptoms or pulmonary syndromes. AML in elderly patients, AML occurring after chemotherapy for other malignancies, and AML developing in a patient with MDS has a very poor prognosis.

*French–American–British (FAB) Classification*—(still in common use but many modifications exist)

- M1: undifferentiated cells
- M2: early differentiated cells, Auer rods
- M3: acute promyelocytic leukemia (APL), large granules, Auer rods
- M4: myelomonocytic leukemia
- M5: monocytic leukemia
- M6: erythrocytic leukemia
- M7: megakaryoblastic leukemia

### ▶ Concept and Application
Failure of myeloid stem cells to differentiate normally leads to progressive accumulation of leukemic blasts. Anemia and thrombocytopenia are due to lack of normal stem cells.

### ▶ Treatment Steps
1. Pathologic diagnosis based on bone marrow biopsy, cytogenetics, and cell typing.
2. Antibiotics if infected.
3. Transfusion of blood products as needed.
4. All-trans retinoic acid (ATRA) for APML (M3). Monitor for DIC. Conventional cytotoxics once induction complete.
5. Allopurinol to prevent urate nephropathy.
6. Monitor for tumor lysis with serum $K^+$, creatinine, and $PO_4$.
7. Treatment usually includes Ara-C and an anthracycline induction followed by 2–4 consolidation cycles.
8. Bone marrow transplant later in appropriate patients.

## B. Acute Lymphocytic Leukemia

### ▶ H&P Keys
Fatigue, anorexia, easy bruising or overt bleeding (petechiae), fever or evidence of infection, lymphadenopathy, splenomegaly, or mediastinal mass. Headache, stiff neck suggest CNS disease. Testicular mass can be seen occasionally.

### ▶ Diagnosis
Hypercellular bone marrow with > 30% blasts. Blasts are often positive for terminal deoxynucleotidyltransferase (TdT), common acute lymphoblastic leukemia antigen (CALLA) (CD10) and PAS; and negative for peroxidase and Sudan black. Flow cytometry to determine cell surface markers. Elevated WBC. Anemia,

thrombocytopenia. Lumbar puncture to rule out CNS involvement. Elevated creatinine, LDH, $PO_4$, $K^+$ predict for tumor lysis syndrome. Philadelphia (Ph) chromosome t(9;22), seen in 10% of children and 30% of adults, confers a poor prognosis. Burkitt's type of acute lymphocytic leukemia (ALL) accompanied by t(8;14) or t(2;8) or t(8;22) involving c-myc oncogene.

▶ Disease Severity

*Favorable Prognostic Factors*—Young age, low WBC, Ph negative, no CNS disease, CALLA positive, rapid induction of remission.

*Subclassifications*—Significant revisions under way—expect more complex terminology soon.

- L1: ALL
- L2: large cells with cleft nuclei
- L3: vacuolated, abundant cytoplasm, Burkitt's type

▶ Concept and Application

Block in differentiation results in the accumulation of immature cells with abnormal function.

▶ Treatment Steps
1. Pathologic diagnosis based on bone marrow biopsy, cytogenetics, and cell typing.
2. Antiobiotics if infected.
3. Transfusion of blood products as needed.
4. Induction chemotherapy usually with vincristine, prednisone, L-asparaginase and an anthracycline.
5. Monitor for tumor lysis.
6. CNS prophylaxis with intrathecal chemotherapy.
7. Maintenance chemotherapy for 2–3 years.
8. Bone marrow transplant in selected patients, second remission.

## C. Chronic Myelogenous Leukemia

▶ H&P Keys

Nonspecific complaints most common; weakness, malaise, weight loss. Left upper quadrant fullness, early satiety and discomfort secondary to splenomegaly. In acute phase of disease, can present like acute leukemia.

▶ Diagnosis

Bone marrow is hypercellular with a marked proliferation of all granulocytic elements, increased eosinophils and basophils, and mild fibrosis. Ph chromosome t(9;22) positive, low leukocyte alkaline phosphatase (LAP) score. Increased WBC (50,000 to 300,000/μL), hyperuricemia, and increased serum $B_{12}$. Normal platelets and no or mild anemia in chronic phase.

▶ Disease Severity

Degree of splenomegaly, percentage of blasts, basophilia and eosinophilia can predict for survival. Presence of cytogenetic abnormalities in addition to Ph chromosome predicts for blastic transformation.

▶ Concept and Application

Myeloproliferative disorder characterized by an abnormal proliferation of myeloid cells without the loss of capacity to differentiate; bcr-abl rearrangement seen in nearly all patients.

▶ Treatment Steps

1. In chronic phase if the patient has an HLA match, bone marrow transplantation should be considered.
2. Hydroxyurea is the preferred, first-line cytotoxic for control of elevated cell counts.
3. IFN-α can produce complete chromosomal responses in some patients.
4. Allopurinol to prevent urate nephropathy if WBC count high.

## D. Chronic Lymphocytic Leukemia

▶ H&P Keys

Usually a disease of elderly patients. Often asymptomatic leukocytosis. Some patients present with lymphadenopathy, hepatosplenomegaly, anemia, or thrombocytopenia.

▶ Diagnosis

Elevated WBC (> 15 000 µL with lymphocytes greater than 60%). Look for kappa/lambda clonal excess or presence of CD5+ CD19+ cells to confirm diagnosis. Chromosomal abnormalities such as 14q+ and trisomy 12 can be seen (Fig. 5–3). Bone marrow is hypercellular and monotonous with diffuse infiltration of small- and medium-size lymphocytes.

Observable autoimmune phenomena (eg, Coombs' test positive, hemolytic anemia). Hypogammaglobulinemia.

▶ Disease Severity

Several staging systems. Rai staging best known:

- Stage 0—lymphocytosis only
- Stage 1—lymphocytosis with lymphadenopathy
- Stage 2—lymphocytosis with splenomegaly
- Stage 3—lymphocytosis with anemia
- Stage 4—lymphocytosis with thrombocytopenia

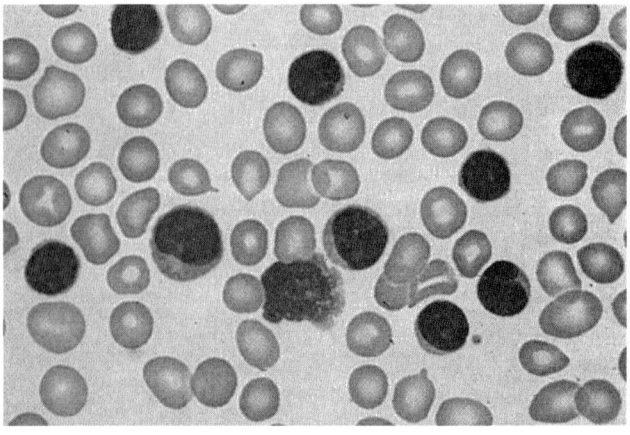

Figure 5–3. Chronic lymphocytic leukemia.

Modified Rai staging:
- Low risk—stages 0 and 1.
- Intermediate risk—stages 2 and 3.
- High risk—stage 4.

Aggressive transformation into large-cell lymphoma, Richter's transformation.

▶ Concept and Application

Monoclonal proliferation of dysfunctional mature β-lymphocytes. More frequent infections due to lack of opsonization.

▶ Treatment Steps
1. Observation for low risk patients.
2. Treat higher risk or symptomatic patients with chlorambucil and prednisone or fludarabine.

## E. Hodgkin's Disease

▶ H&P Keys

Frequently younger patients. Superficial, painless, enlarged "rubbery" lymph nodes (60% to 80% cervical or axillary, nontender), splenomegaly. "B" symptoms: fevers, night sweats, weight loss. Infections associated with depressed cell-mediated immunity. Bimodal peak incidence.

▶ Diagnosis

Lymph node biopsy reveals Reed-Sternberg cells with reactive lymphocytes (Fig. 5–4). Disease spread by contiguous lymph node chains. Initial staging tests include computed tomography (CT) scans of the chest, abdomen, and pelvis, bone marrow aspiration and biopsy. Positron emission tomography (PET) and gallium scans are useful in bulky disease. Laparotomy and lymphangiogram are rarely performed. Nodular sclerosing subtype most common. Lymphocyte-depleted histologic specimens associated with poor prognosis. Mixed cellularity and lymphocyte-predominant tissues offer better prognosis.

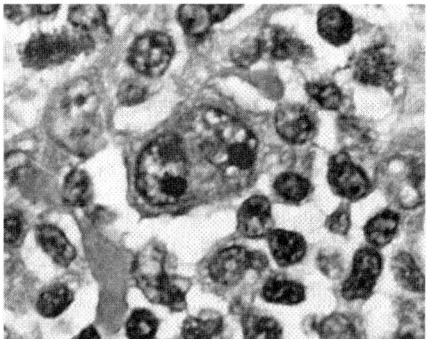

Figure 5–4. Reed–Sternberg cell of Hodgkin's disease.

▶ Disease Severity

*Ann Arbor Staging*
- Stage I: single lymph node group.
- Stage II: multiple lymph node groups on the same side of the diaphragm.
- Stage III: involved lymph node groups on both sides of the diaphragm.
- Stage IV: extranodal disease (bone marrow involvement, liver involvement, lung or skin involvement).

"B" symptoms: fevers, night sweats, and 10% weight loss. Stage A: absence of "B" symptoms. B symptoms are a poor prognostic marker independent of stage.

▶ Concept and Application

Cell of origin is a centroblast (proliferating germinal center cell). Defective T-cell function.

▶ Treatment Steps
1. Staging as outlined previously is critical.
2. Treatment is stage related.
   - Stage IA–IIA: Extended field radiation.
   - Stage IB–IIB: Extended field and chemotherapy or less often total nodal radiation.
   - Stage IIIA/B and IVA/B: Combination chemotherapy.
   - Bulky disease: Radiation and chemotherapy.

Chemotherapy consists of ABVD, though MOPP was the standard for many years. ABVD is Adriamycin (doxorubicin), bleomycin, vinblastine, and dacarbazine. MOPP is mechlorethamine, Oncovin (vincristine), procarbazine, and prednisone.

### F. Low-grade Lymphoma

▶ H&P Keys

Lymphadenopathy usually diffuse and not necessarily contiguous. Splenomegaly can be seen. Extranodal disease (eg, bone marrow) common. Rarely fever, weight loss, night sweats.

▶ Diagnosis

Lymph node biopsy. Bone marrow aspiration and biopsy (bone marrow involvement common). Kappa/lambda clonal excess. Immunoglobulin gene rearrangement. Cytogenetic studies, eg, t(14;18), associated with follicular lymphoma (Fig. 5–5).

▶ Disease Severity

Ann Arbor staging system (see Hodgkin's disease staging). Chest x-ray, CT scans of chest, abdomen, and pelvis. Often stage IV due to bone marrow infiltration. Presence of "B" symptoms, LDH, performance status.

▶ Concept and Application

Clonal proliferation of B-cell lymphocytes, rarely T cells. Can transform into more aggressive lymphoma.

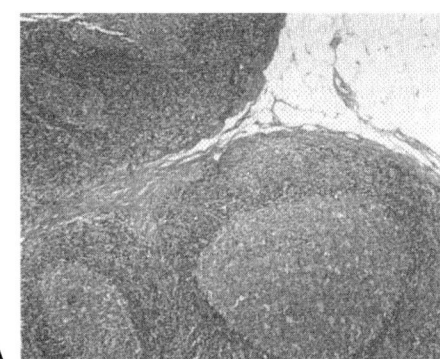 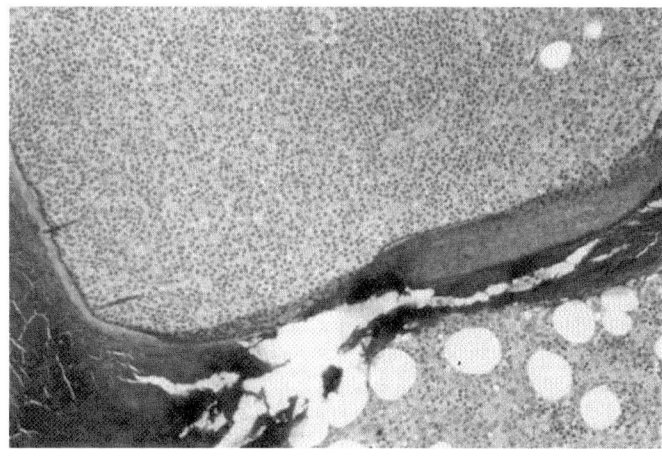

Figure 5–5. (A) A benign lymphoid follicle compared to (B) lymphoma involving the marrow.

▶ Treatment Steps
1. Watchful waiting acceptable if asymptomatic.
2. Treatment for bulky disease, obstruction of vital structures, cytopenias, or autoimmune complications.
3. Treatment options include alkylating agents plus corticosteroids, radiation, fludarabine. Occasional patients require aggressive cytotoxics.

## G. Intermediate- or High-grade Lymphoma

▶ H&P Keys

Lymphadenopathy, splenomegaly. Extranodal disease can be seen. Fatigue, malaise. Rapidly enlarging lymphadenopathy can occur (especially Burkitt's lymphoma). Mediastinal mass can cause symptoms.

▶ Diagnosis

Lymph node biopsy to make diagnosis. Needle biopsy not sufficient. Bone marrow aspiration and biopsy. Spinal tap to rule out meningeal spread especially in lymphoblastic lymphoma. Burkitt's lymphoma associated with Epstein–Barr virus (EBV) and translocation t(8;14), t(2;8) or t(8;22). Increased LDH in aggressive disease. Chest roentgenogram to evaluate mediastinum. CT scans chest, abdomen, and pelvis. PET can be helpful. Testing for HIV. Tumor lysis can be seen with rapidly growing lymphomas (eg, Burkitt's).

▶ Disease Severity

Ann Arbor staging system. Bone marrow involvement or CNS involvement have worse prognosis. Evidence of tumor lysis. Poor prognosis, increased age, large tumor masses, "B" symptoms, bone marrow involvement, increased LDH, poor performance status, HIV associated.

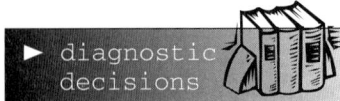

### diagnostic decisions

**LYMPHOMAS**

**Low grade**
Patients are older, often with stage III or IV disease, disease is treatable and the life expectancy is usually many years. Types include: small lymphocytic (same as CLL), plasmacytoid, follicular small cell, and follicular mixed.

**Intermediate grade**
Lots of variability, some behave in more indolent fashions and some are more aggressive. Individual type very important. Types include: follicular large cell, diffuse small cleaved, diffuse mixed, and maybe diffuse large cell.

**High grade**
Often younger patients, aggressive therapy can result in cure. Types include: immunoblastic, lymphoblastic, and Burkitt's.

▶ **Concept and Application**
Most commonly clonal proliferation of B cells. Lymphoblastic lymphoma and cutaneous lymphomas frequently of T-cell origin. Different histologies represent block at different stages of B-cell development.

▶ **Treatment Steps**
1. Staging as outlined previously.
2. Monitor LDH, $PO_4$, creatine for tumor lysis complications.
3. Allopurinol in acute treatment period to prevent urate nephropathy.
4. Intensive combination chemotherapy—CHOP remains the standard. CHOP is cytoxan, doxorubicin, vincristine, and prednisone. Add Rituxamab if CD20+.
5. If CNS involved, intrathecal chemotherapy.
6. Relapsed but still responsive disease can be considered for dose-intense chemotherapy with marrow support.

### H. Multiple Myeloma

▶ **H&P Keys**
Anemia, bone pain, increased susceptibility to infections, fatigue, weight loss, renal insufficiency, altered mental status.

▶ **Diagnosis**
Anemia, hypercalcemia, presence of a paraprotein (or M-component) on serum protein electrophoresis (SPEP), Bence Jones proteins on urine protein electrophoresis (UPEP), lytic bone lesions on skeletal survey, bone marrow with greater than 30% plasma cells. Measure $\beta_2$ microglobulin and serum creatinine. Quantitate amount of immunoglobulin present. Serum viscosity if altered mental status present.

▶ **Disease Severity**
- Stage I: Low tumor burden with Hb > 10 g/dL, normal calcium, IgG < 5 g/dL, IgA < 3 g/dL, urine light chains < 4 g/24 h and normal skeletal survey.
- Stage II: Intermediate tumor burden; patients who are neither stage I or stage III.
- Stage III: High tumor burden and any one of the following: Hb < 8.5 g/dL, serum calcium > 12 mg/dL, IgG > 7 g/dL, IgA > 5 g/dL, urine light chains > 12 g/24 h, or extensive lytic bone lesions. The following subclassification of stages is used:
  A. Creatinine level > 2 mg/dL
  B. Creatinine level ≥ 2 mg/dL

Elevated $\beta_2$ microglobulin at diagnosis reflects a poor prognosis.

▶ **Concept and Application**
Monoclonal proliferation of plasma cells in the bone marrow. Osteoclastic activating factors (possibly interleukins [IL-1, IL-6], tumor necrosis factor [TNF]) responsible for bone lesions. Bone destruction leading to pathologic fractures, pain, hypercalcemia. Patients can develop amyloid deposition over time.

▶ Treatment Steps
1. Manage low stage disease conservatively.
2. Chemotherapy for symptomatic or more advanced disease—melphalan and prednisone or VAD (vincristine, adriamycin, decadron) are common first-line approaches. Thalidomide has recently been approved.
3. Radiation for palliation of localized lesions causing pain.
4. High-dose chemotherapy with bone marrow transplant useful for certain patients.

## I. Monoclonal Gammopathy of Undetermined Significance

▶ H&P Keys
Patients are generally asymptomatic.

▶ Diagnosis
Presence of a para-protein on serum electrophoresis that is monoclonal, usually without suppression of the other immunoglobulins. No other evidence of disease.

▶ Disease Severity
Should be none.

▶ Concept and Application
Monoclonal proliferation of plasma cells in the bone marrow without evidence of organ damage. Levels of paraprotein do not reach significant levels and marrow function is not compromised. 33% of patients will ultimately develop a clear-cut process in a 20-year follow-up period. Of those 33%, 66% will develop multiple myeloma, 12% macroglobulemia, 14% amyloidosis, and 8% another lymphoproliferative disorder.

▶ Treatment Steps
1. Follow the immunoglubulin levels, 3, 6, and 12 months. Yearly follow-up is probably adequate in a patient whose levels are not rising appreciably.
2. Intervene only if process progresses to a definable disease.

## III. OTHER DISORDERS

### A. Polycythemia Rubra Vera (Primary Erythrocytosis)

▶ H&P Keys
Often asymptomatic, diagnosed on routine lab tests. Splenomegaly, early satiety, hypertension, facial plethora, venous thromboses, hemorrhages.

▶ Diagnosis
Increased RBC mass with normal plasma volume key to diagnosis. Erythropoietin levels normal or low. Hypercellular bone marrow. WBC and platelet counts normal or elevated, increased LAP, increased $B_{12}$, low or absent iron stores.

▶ Disease Severity

Degree of Hct elevation determines whole-blood viscosity. Decreased cerebral blood flow. Thromboembolism or life-threatening hemorrhage can occur. Can transform to myelofibrosis or acute leukemia.

▶ Concept and Application

Autonomous proliferation of erythroid progenitors resulting from clonal proliferation of the pluripotent hematopoietic stem cell.

▶ Treatment Steps

1. Phlebotomy combined with hydroxyurea.
2. Maintain Hct at approximately 45%.
3. P32 used occasionally for elderly patients.

## B. Secondary Erythrocytosis

▶ H&P Keys

Spurious erythrocytosis may result from decreased plasma volume. If true erythrocytosis, consider if physiologically appropriate: chronic obstructive pulmonary disease (COPD), right-to-left cardiac shunt, high-affinity Hb, carboxyhemoglobinemia.

Physiologically inappropriate: tumors producing erythropoietin (renal cell, hepatocellular carcinoma, cerebellar hemangioblastomas), renal disease, adrenal cortical hyperplasia, exogenous androgens.

▶ Diagnosis

If true erythrocytosis (increased RBC mass with low plasma volume), no expansion of other cell lines. Erythropoietin level normal or elevated (low in polycythemia vera). Arterial blood gas and determination of oxygen saturation.

▶ Disease Severity

Level of Hct can predict. Hyperviscosity syndrome.

▶ Concept and Application

Sometimes a result of reduced plasma volume (spurious erythrocytosis). It can be a physiologically appropriate response to decreased tissue oxygenation. It can also result from physiologically inappropriate production of erythropoietin or other factors that stimulate erythropoiesis. Higher Hct decreases cerebral blood flow.

▶ Treatment Steps

1. Determine etiology.
2. Correct any factors that can exacerbate or cause erythrocytosis.
3. Supplemental oxygen if needed.
4. Phlebotomy if severe. Hct determined by physiologic needs.

## C. Transfusion Reactions

▶ H&P Keys

Occur minutes to hours or even days after transfusion. Most severe is immunemediated hemolytic reaction: fever, chest or back pain, hypotension, dyspnea, hemoglobinuria, shock. Most common are febrile reactions caused by WBCs present in pRBCs now decreased secondary to common use of WBC filtering by blood banks. Rarely, febrile reactions are due to bacterial contamination.

Patients with IgA deficiency can have anaphylactic reaction: sudden onset, no fever, may have cough, respiratory distress, hypotension, nausea, vomiting, abdominal pain, loss of consciousness, and shock. Delayed hemolytic transfusion reaction results from minor antigen mismatch (not detected by indirect Coombs' test). Posttransfusion purpura results in moderate to severe thrombocytopenia 2–10 days following transfusion of pRBC.

▶ Diagnosis

Stop transfusion and return unit to blood bank. Monitor Hg and Hct, hemoglobinuria, unconjugated bilirubin, serum haptoglobin, LDH, coagulation profile, and renal profile. Repeat ABO, Rh, and compatibility screens. Direct antiglobulin test on posttransfusion blood sample from patient. Check IgA level if anaphylaxis. Culture remainder of blood product.

▶ Disease Severity

Most severe reactions are major hemolytic transfusion reaction or anaphylaxis.

▶ Concept and Application

Major hemolytic transfusion reaction caused by ABO incompatibility (immune-mediated destruction of RBCs after transfusion), often a result of clinical error.

▶ Treatment Steps

1. Stop transfusion.
2. Maintain blood pressure and urine output with IV fluids.
3. For anaphylaxis: epinephrine, diphenhydramine hydrochloride (Benadryl) and glucocorticoids.
4. Antibiotics if bacterial contamination suspected.
5. Premedicate with acetaminophen and use WBC filters to prevent febrile reactions.

## D. Hemophilia A and B

▶ H&P Keys

Hereditary bleeding disorders. Hemophilia A most common. A and B clinically indistinguishable. Frequent episodes of bleeding into joints, muscles, and skin with minimal or no trauma. Can result in chronic arthritis. Easy bruising. Prolonged postoperative hemorrhage. Intracranial hemorrhage can occur.

▶ Diagnosis

Elevated partial prothrombin time (PTT) and low factor VIII or IX level. Normal bleeding time, normal prothrombin time (PT), normal thromboplastin time (TT). Specific assays for factor VIII or IX. 50:50 mixing study demonstrates factor deficiency. Polymerase chain reaction (PCR) analysis for prenatal detection.

▶ Disease Severity

Patients with < 1% factor VIII (or IX) level have severe disease; > 5% factor VIII (or IX) results in mild disease. Clinical history very important in predicting bleeding tendency.

▶ Concept and Application

X-linked recessive bleeding disorder resulting from deficiency of factor VIII (hemophilia A) or IX (hemophilia B).

▶ Treatment Steps

*Mild Hemophilia A*
1. First-line therapy is desmopressin (DDAVP) (stimulates immediate release of VIII:C and von Willebrand factor from endothelial cell stores).
2. Second-line therapy is recombinant human factor VIII or factor VIII concentrate.

*Severe Hemophilia A*
1. Recombinant human factor VIII or factor VIII concentrate.

*Hemophilia B*
1. Desmopressin not effective.
2. Recombinant human factor IX or factor IX concentrates. Factor IX concentrate in more severe cases.

### E. von Willebrand Disease

▶ H&P Keys

Mucocutaneous bleeding, epistaxis, GI bleeding, menorrhagia (can result in iron deficiency). Joint and intramuscular bleeding rare. Posttraumatic, postsurgical, and dental bleeding may be severe.

▶ Diagnosis

(1) Prolonged bleeding time. PTT can be prolonged or normal. (2) Decreased factor VIII:C activity. (3) Decreased ristocetin cofactor on platelet aggregation studies. (4) Decreased von Willebrand factor (vWF). (5) Multimeric analysis.

*Type I*—Generalized decrease in all multimeric forms of plasma vWF.

*Type II*—Selective deficiency of higher-molecular-weight forms. Normal or near-normal levels but dysfunctional.

*Type III*—Markedly decreased plasma and platelet levels of vWF. Autosomal recessive.

*Pseudo von Willebrand Disease*—Abnormal vWF platelet receptor.

▶ Disease Severity

Repeat testing may be necessary to make diagnosis. Hemorrhagic tendency widely variable. Clinical history very important.

▶ Concept and Application

Quantitative or qualitative abnormalities of the vWF protein, which is required for normal attachment of platelets to the endothelium. This interaction critical for normal platelet function. vWF also necessary for normal factor VIII coagulant activity. Autosomal dominant trait with variable presentation.

▶ Treatment Step
1. Establish form of von Willebrand disease.
2. DDAVP for patients with mild disease. This is not useful in most types of patients with type II or any type III.
3. Factor VIII concentrate for moderate to severe disease.
4. Platelets for pseudo von Willebrand disease.

## F. Vitamin K Deficiency

▶ H&P Keys

Inadequate supply (dietary deficiency, antibiotic therapy). Surreptitious ingestion of warfarin anticoagulants. Purpura, ecchymoses, hematuria, or gastrointestinal bleeding.

▶ Diagnosis

Elevated PT, normal PTT unless deficiency is profound, and normal bleeding time. A 50:50 mixing study corrects prolonged PT.

▶ Disease Severity

Coagulopathy results in spontaneous overt bleeding.

▶ Concept and Application

Vitamin K essential for final posttranslational carboxylation of factors II, VII, IX, and X synthesized by GI flora. No bile salt production impairs intestinal absorption and antibiotics destroy gut flora.

▶ Treatment Steps
1. Oral or subcutaneous vitamin K.
2. IV vitamin K rarely indicated.

## G. Lupus Inhibitor

▶ H&P Keys

Usually asymptomatic. Patients may have recurrent thromboembolisms or recurrent miscarriages. Seen in patients with autoimmune diseases, malignancies, AIDS, and otherwise healthy people.

▶ Diagnosis

Elevated PTT that does not correct with mixing studies. PT is normal or slightly elevated. Abnormal platelet aggregation studies. Thrombocytopenia. Positive anticardiolipin antibody or positive antiphospholipid antibody.

▶ Disease Severity

Thromboses such as deep venous thrombosis, pulmonary embolism, or cerebrovascular accident (CVA).

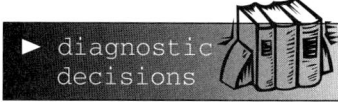

▶ diagnostic decisions

### COAGULOPATHIES

**Prolonged Prothrombin Time (PT)**
1. Vitamin K deficiency: patients on antibiotics, prolonged hospitalizations, poor oral intake.
2. Warfarin (coumadin): related also to a common rat poison.
3. Factor VII deficiency.

**Prolonged Activated Partial Thromboplastin Time (aPTT)**
1. Heparin: check the blood draw site, was it above the IV infusing the heparin, was the sample drawn from a heparinized port?
2. Factor VIII deficiency/inhibitor: deficiency is usually manifest from birth and there is usually a family history, the inhibitor is acquired and occurs later in life.
3. Factor IX deficiency/inhibitor: less common than VIII but the same issues apply.
4. XI, XII, and high molecular weight kininogen (HMWK) deficiency: these are very rare.

**Combined**
1. Hepatic dysfunction.
2. Very severe compromise of the vitamin K dependent factors.
3. Factor V deficiency.
4. Factor X deficiency.
5. Abnormal thrombin.

▶ Concept and Application

Immunoglobulin is directed against lipid components of the platelet membranes and prothrombin activator complex. It interferes with coagulation testing without inhibiting the activity of the coagulation factors; can be seen in SLE but usually occurs in patients with no obvious underlying disorder.

▶ Treatment Steps
1. Therapy not required for asymptomatic patients.
2. Consider prophylactic anticoagulation during hypercoaguable periods, eg, postop, pregnancy.
3. Rare patients need chronic anticoagulation for repeated thrombotic events.

### H. Disseminated Intravascular Coagulation

▶ H&P Keys

Activation of coagulation pathways resulting in both clotting and bleeding tendencies. Diffuse bleeding (IV sites, etc), petechiae, purpura, ecchymoses; may also see evidence of thrombosis. Caused by sepsis, cancers (particularly associated with acute promyelocytic leukemia and adenocarcinomas), tissue damage, and amniotic fluid embolism. Bleeding and thrombotic events can lead to severe organ dysfunction.

▶ Diagnosis

PT and PTT elevated. Low fibrinogen, increased fibrin split products (FSP), decreased factors V and VIII. Presence of D-dimers. Microangiopathic hemolytic anemia with schistocytes on peripheral smear; thrombocytopenia.

▶ Disease Severity

Level of D-dimer formation. Fibrinogen level. PT prolongation. Uncontrolled bleeding leading to death.

▶ Concept and Application

Pathologic activation of coagulation with resultant intravascular generation of excess thrombin. Thrombin activates susceptible coagulation proteins and aggregates platelets, which become trapped in fibrin deposited in the microvasculature. Fibrin stimulates local fibrinolysis. Fibrin strands "clog" microvasculature and induce localized hemolysis.

▶ Treatment Steps
1. Treat underlying disease.
2. Replace clotting factors and platelets as necessary.

### I. Antithrombin III Deficiency

▶ H&P Keys

Family history of thromboembolic disease, recurrent venous thromboembolism (DVTs and pulmonary embolisms [PEs]). Unusual sites for clot formation, eg, mesenteric thrombosis. First episode in second or third decade. Family history of thromboembolic disease.

▶ Diagnosis
Low functional level of antithrombin III. Doppler studies or venograms revealing thromboembolism.

▶ Disease Severity
Arterial thrombosis or life-threatening PE.

▶ Concept and Application
Antithrombin III neutralizes the serine protease coagulation factors IXa, Xa, XIa, XIIa and inhibits thrombin by the formation of stable thrombin-antithrombin complexes. Inherited in an autosomal dominant fashion.

▶ Treatment Steps
1. Treat active thrombosis with heparin; very high doses may be required.
2. Switch to oral anticoagulation as soon as possible.
3. Most patients require lifelong anticoagulation.

## J. Protein C Deficiency

▶ H&P Keys
Positive family history of thromboembolism. Recurrent venous thrombosis. Warfarin-induced skin necrosis. Purpura fulminans in newborns. Arterial thrombosis rare. Acquired protein C deficiency has been reported (liver disease and DIC).

▶ Diagnosis
Normal PT and PTT, bleeding time, decreased protein C level or activity.

▶ Disease Severity
Massive pulmonary embolism, CVA.

▶ Concept and Application
Protein C requires vitamin K for its synthesis and is activated by thrombin on the surface of endothelial cells. Activated protein C acts as an anticoagulant by neutralizing factors Va and VIIIa and by stimulating fibrinolysis. Protein C deficiency predisposes to thrombosis. Inherited as an autosomal dominant trait with variable expression.

▶ Treatment Steps
Long-term oral anticoagulation if patient manifests symptoms.

## K. Activated Protein C (APC) Resistance

▶ H&P Keys
Positive family history of thromboembolism. Recurrent venous thrombosis.

▶ Diagnosis
Mutation of factor V gene, leading to loss of cleavage site (Arg), that is, the site of APC action.

▶ **Disease Severity**
Life-threatening PE, CVA.

▶ **Concept and Application**
APC inactivates Factor Va and VIIIa, reducing clotting tendencies. APC resistance results in increased circulating Factor Va and risk for thrombosis.

▶ **Treatment Steps**
1. Chronic anticoagulation in patients with repeated thrombosis.
2. Aggressive prophylaxis in patients at risk for thrombosis.

## L. Idiopathic Thrombocytopenia Purpura

▶ **H&P Keys**
Easy bruising, epistaxis, menorrhagia, gingival bleeding. Idiopathic thrombocytopenic purpura (ITP) in children has acute onset and is often a self-limited disease that develops after a viral infection, and lasts 5–6 months. Adults have a gradual onset with only 10–15% developing spontaneous remissions. Often ITP is associated with SLE, Hodgkin's disease, chronic lymphocytic leukemia, pregnancy, ulcerative colitis, and infection.

▶ **Diagnosis**
Decreased platelet count. Normal or increased number of megakaryocytes in bone marrow. Peripheral smear often reveals large platelets. These are younger and more effective platelets.

▶ **Disease Severity**
Severity of thrombocytopenia (platelets < 20,000 associated with significant risk of spontaneous bleeding).

▶ **Concepts and Application**
Usually autoimmune. Accelerated platelet destruction in spleen after coating of platelets by IgG autoantibody. Extravascular platelet destruction.

▶ **Treatment Steps**
1. Corticosteroids are first-line therapy.
2. Second-line therapy is variable and includes splenectomy, Win RhoD, danazol, and immunoglobulin.

## M. Thrombotic Thrombocytopenic Purpura

▶ **H&P Keys**
Onset may be fulminant or subacute, single episode or recurring. Mental status changes result of intermittent ischemia. Classic pentad: fever, renal dysfunction, neurologic changes, thrombocytopenia, microangiopathic hemolytic anemia.

▶ **Diagnosis**
Low platelet count, normal or increased number of megakaryocytes in bone marrow, increased LDH, and increased RBC fragments on smear. Elevated BUN and creatinine or proteinuria reflect renal disease. DIC testing is negative. Usually a clinical diagnosis.

▶ Disease Severity
Severity of neurologic symptoms (patients can develop coma), and hemolysis (bilirubin, LDH, reticulocyte count).

▶ Concept and Application
Endothelial damage in microcirculation leads to platelet microthrombi, occlusion of small vessels, and ischemia in tissues. Abnormal vWf multimers.

▶ Treatment Steps
1. Plasmapheresis.
2. If plasmapheresis unavailable, infuse fresh frozen plasma.
3. Treat underlying condition.
4. Corticosteroids usually given unless contraindicated.

## N. Essential Thrombocythemia

▶ H&P Keys
Usually asymptomatic. Neurologic symptoms most common: recurrent or transient headache, visual changes. Episodes of thrombosis, embolism, or hemorrhage can occur.

▶ Diagnosis
Platelet count > 800,000. Bone marrow: increased number of megakaryocytes. Normal Hb level. Mildly increased WBC (15,000 to 30,000). Platelet function testing usually abnormal. Rule out chronic inflammation, iron deficiency.

▶ Disease Severity
Complications infrequent in younger patients. In elderly patients, transient ischemic attack (TIA) most common complication. CNS hemorrhage or CVA secondary to emboli.

▶ Concept and Application
Uncontrolled clonal proliferation of megakaryocytic precursors.

▶ Treatment Steps
1. Anagrelide.
2. Hydroxyurea.
3. Antiplatelet agents (eg, aspirin) for ischemia.

## O. Agnogenic Myeloid Metaplasia

(Other terms include myelofibrosis—a nonspecific term, myelosclerosis, idiopathic myeloid metaplasia).

▶ H&P Keys
Often presents with symptoms of anemia or splenomegaly. Fever, weight loss, fatigue, early satiety, hepatomegaly, lymphadenopathy. Usually disease of elderly patients.

▶ Diagnosis
Anemia, nucleated RBCs, teardrop cells. Bone marrow biopsy shows increased fibrosis, increased megakaryocytes.

▶ Disease Severity

Extent of fibrosis in bone marrow and extramedullary hematopoiesis. Can evolve into acute leukemia.

▶ Concept and Application

Increased type III collagen production. Replacement of normal bone marrow with fibrosis. The reason for this overproduction remains unclear.

▶ Treatment Steps

1. Transfuse as needed.
2. Role of colony stimulators limited.
3. Splenectomy for painful enlargement or refractory cytopenias caused by splenic sequestration.
4. Bone marrow transplant for the rare age-appropriate patient.

P. Platelet Dysfunction

▶ H&P Keys

*Intrinsic*—Congenital defect, easy bruising, epistaxis, menorrhagia with normal platelet count. Petechiae *not* common.

*Extrinsic*—Acquired defect secondary to myeloproliferative disease, uremia, malignancy, or drugs (aspirin, clopidrogel).

▶ Diagnosis

Increased bleeding time. Abnormal aggregation studies.

▶ Disease Severity

Increased risk of postsurgical or posttraumatic bleeding.

▶ Concept and Application

Platelets fail to adhere to endothelium or to aggregate because of a deficiency of surface glycoproteins that bind fibrinogen or vWf. Failure to release platelet storage pool.

▶ Management

1. For congenital platelet dysfunction, trial of desmopressin (DDAVP) or transfuse platelets.
2. For myeloproliferative disease, transfuse platelets.
3. For uremia, dialysis, DDAVP, and occasionally, plasma.
4. Discontinue offending drugs, transfuse platelets if bleeding is significant.

Q. Neutropenia

▶ H&P Keys

Acquired or congenital. Intrinsic or extrinsic abnormalities. Autoimmune neutropenia (Felty's syndrome) is seen as an isolated event and in rheumatoid arthritis and other systemic autoimmune disorders. Cyclic neutropenia: fatigue, decreased appetite, mouth sores that occur every 3 weeks and last 3–4 days. Hepatosplenomegaly. Evidence of infection: mouth sores, sore throat, skin infections, pneumonia, urinary tract infection.

▶ Diagnosis

CBC, follow sequential absolute neutrophil counts (ANCs). Perform bone marrow study to rule out malignancy. If febrile and ANC < 500, obtain cultures and start broad-spectrum antibiotics.

▶ Disease Severity

Fungal infections or sepsis can develop. Agranulocytosis very serious (ANC < 200).

▶ Concept and Application

Cyclic neutropenia results from stem cell defect. Neutrophil-specific antibodies of IgG and IgM subtypes are detected in Felty's syndrome. Infiltration of bone marrow by malignant neoplasm interferes with WBC maturation. Drug-induced marrow suppression often reversible if neutropenia; if agranulocytosis, often irreversible.

▶ Treatment Steps

1. For cyclic neutropenia, chronic granulocyte-colony stimulating factor (G-CSF) is helpful.
2. If possible, treat underlying disorder.
3. If febrile, broad-spectrum antibiotics.

## BIBLIOGRAPHY

Beutler E, Lichtman M, Coller B, et al, eds. *Hematology*. 6th ed. New York: McGraw-Hill; 2000.

Colman RW, ed. *Hemostasis and Thrombosis: Basic Principles and Clinical Practice*. Philadelphia: JB Lippincott Co; 2000.

DeVita V, Hellman S, Rosenberg S, eds. *Cancer: Principles & Practice of Oncology*. 6th ed. Philadelphia: Lippincott-Raven; 2001.

Hoffman R, Benz Jr. E, Shattil S, et al, eds. *Hematology: Basic Principles and Practice*. 3rd ed. New York: Churchill Livingstone; 2000.

Maxwell MW, ed. *Clinical Hematology*. Philadelphia: Lea & Febiger; 1981.

Zucker-Franklin D, ed. *Atlas of Blood Cells: Function and Pathology*. Philadelphia: Lea & Febiger; 1988.

# Immunology and Allergy | 6

I. BRONCHIAL ASTHMA / 198

II. ALLERGIC RHINITIS AND CONJUNCTIVITIS / 200

III. ANAPHYLAXIS OR ANAPHYLACTOID REACTIONS / 202

IV. URTICARIA / 203

V. IMMUNODEFICIENCY / 204
   A. Humoral Immunodeficiency / 204
   B. Cellular (T-cell) Immunodeficiency / 205

VI. HEREDITARY ANGIOEDEMA / 205

VII. ATOPIC DERMATITIS / 206

VIII. CONTACT DERMATITIS / 208

IX. ALLERGIC BRONCHOPULMONARY ASPERGILLOSIS / 209

X. HYPERSENSITIVITY PNEUMONITIS / 210

XI. HYPEREOSINOPHILIC SYNDROME / 211

XII. DRUG ALLERGY / 212

BIBLIOGRAPHY / 214

# I. BRONCHIAL ASTHMA

### ▶ H&P Keys

Chronic or recurrent cough, dyspnea, or wheezing. Prolonged expiration and wheezing with or without use of accessory muscles. Affects > 5% of the population. Incidence, mortality, and hospitalization rates increasing. Allergic (extrinsic) asthma related to exposure to allergens (seasonal pollens such as grasses, trees, and weeds; animal dander, dust mites, and mold). Nonallergic asthma (intrinsic) associated with infection, stress, environmental pollution, exercise, cold air, and in a small percentage of patients, aspirin use.

### ▶ Diagnosis

Pulmonary function studies with a reversible obstructive pattern, positive methacholine challenge, sputum rich in eosinophils, and response to bronchodilator therapy. Chest roentgenogram, total eosinophil count, total IgE, and allergy skin tests. Oximetry and arterial blood gases in acutely ill patients.

### ▶ Disease Severity

*Mild Intermittent*—Symptoms < 2/week, insomnia related to asthma < 3/month, FEV > 80% of predicted.

*Mild Persistent*—Symptoms > 2/week but < 1/day, insomnia > 2/month, FEV > 80% of predicted.

*Moderate Persistent*—Daily symptoms, symptoms affect activity, insomnia > 1/week, FEV > 60% but < 80% of predicted.

*Severe Persistent*—Continual symptoms, limited physical activity, frequent insomnia, FEV < 60% of predicted.

▶ management decisions

## ASTHMA

| Disease | Treatment |
|---|---|
| Exercise-induced asthma | Short-acting $\beta_2$-adrenergic (albuterol)—2 puffs 15 minutes prior to exercise.<br>and/or<br>Cromolyn (Intal)—2 puffs prior to exercise. |
| Mild intermittent asthma | Short-acting $\beta_2$-adrenergic (albuterol)—2 puffs qid, prn. |
| Mild persistent asthma | Add inhaled low to medium potency corticosteroid (Flovent 44 or 110—2 puffs bid). |
| Moderate persistent asthma | Add leukotriene modifier (Singulair 10 mg qd) or long-acting $\beta_2$-adrenergic (Serevent—2 puffs bid).<br>and/or<br>Increase the inhaled corticosteroid dose. |
| Severe persistent asthma | Increase the inhaled corticosteroid dose (Flovent 220—2–4 puffs bid).<br>Add theophylline, nedocromil (Tilade), leukotriene modifier, oral long-acting $\beta_2$-adrenergic or oral corticosteroids. |

▶ Concept and Application

Mast cell mediator release causes inflammatory changes including denudation of airway epithelium, edema, collagen deposition beneath basement membrane, mucus hypersecretion, smooth muscle contraction, and infiltration of neutrophils, eosinophils and Th 2 lymphocytes. Mediators include eosinophil chemotactic factor of anaphylaxis (ECF-A), neutrophil chemotactic factor of anaphylaxis (NCF-A), histamine, leukotrienes, prostaglandins, and platelet activating factor (PAF). Mast cell mediator release involves IgE trigger only in allergic type of asthma.

▶ Treatment Steps

*General*
1. Avoidance of precipitating factors, patient education.
2. Use peak flow meters in moderate and severe persistent asthma.
3. Immunotherapy (allergy injections) can be added as an anti-inflammatory adjunct.
4. Quick-relief medicine is the first step.
5. Add a long-term controller if a quick-relief medicine is necessary more than twice weekly.

*Quick-Relief Medicines*
1. Inhaled short-acting $\beta_2$-adrenergic (Proventil HFA or albuterol solution via nebulizer).
2. Inhaled ipratropium bromide (Atrovent).
3. Subcutaneous epinephrine.
4. Oral corticosteroids.
5. Intravenous corticosteroids.
6. Intravenous aminophylline.
7. Oxygen.
8. Combination inhaled short-acting $\beta_2$-adrenergic and ipratropium bromide (Combivent).

*Long-Term-Control Medicines*
1. Inhaled corticosteroid (Vanceril DS).
2. Inhaled long-acting $\beta_2$-adrenergic (Serevent).
3. Inhaled cromolyn sodium (Intal).
4. Inhaled nedocromil sodium (Tilade).
5. Oral sustained-release theophylline (UniDur).
6. Oral long-acting $\beta_2$-adrenergic (Volmax).
7. Oral leukotriene modifiers (Singulair, Accolate, Zyflo).
8. Combination inhaled corticosteroid and long-acting $\beta_2$-adrenergic (Advair).

*Treatment of Mild Intermittent Asthma*
1. Inhaled short-acting $\beta_2$-adrenergic (Proventil HFA) 2 puffs qid, prn.
2. For exercise-induced asthma, treat with an inhaled short-acting $\beta_2$-adrenergic (as previously) 15–20 minutes prior to exercise and/or Intal 2 puffs, also prior to exercise.

*Treatment of Mild Persistent Asthma*
1. See the treatment of mild intermittent asthma.
2. Add an inhaled corticosteroid (Vanceril) 2 puffs bid, followed by rinsing of the mouth to decrease the incidence of thrush.

*Treatment of Moderate Persistent Asthma*
1. See the treatment of mild persistent asthma.
2. Increase the strength and/or dose of the inhaled corticosteroid (Vanceril DS 2 puffs bid, followed by rinsing of the mouth).
3. Add a leukotriene modifier (Singulair 10 mg qd) and/or a long-acting $\beta_2$-adrenergic (Serevent 2 puffs bid).

*Treatment of Severe Persistent Asthma*
1. See the treatment of moderate persistent asthma.
2. Increase the strength and/or the dose of the inhaled corticosteroid (Flovent 220 2 to 4 puffs bid, followed by rinsing of the mouth).
3. Add an oral sustained-release theophylline (Unidur).
4. Use a home nebulizer to deliver shortacting $\beta_2$-adrenergic therapy (albuterol solution 0.5%, 0.5 cc in 3 cc saline) and/or ipratropium bromide (one vial of Atrovent qid).
5. Tilade 2 puffs qid tapered to bid or Intal 2 puffs tid–qid may be added in the effort to decrease the use of inhaled corticosteroids.
6. Add a short course of oral corticosteroids (prednisone 20 mg bid for 5 days).
7. If short courses of oral corticosteroids are used frequently, then change to alternate-day oral corticosteroids (prednisone 20 mg every other morning). Morning dosing is preferred to minimize side effects involving the hypothalamic–pituitary–adrenal axis.
8. If symptoms are still unstable, resort to oral corticosteroids temporarily on a daily basis (prednisone 20 mg qd) and wean to every other morning dosing.

***Acute Episodes with Respiratory Distress***—Nebulized sympathomimetic (albuterol), oxygen, IV corticosteroids, and in respiratory failure, intubation and mechanical ventilation.

## II. ALLERGIC RHINITIS AND CONJUNCTIVITIS

▶ H&P Keys

Affects 20% of the population. Frequently affects other family members. Itchy eyes, nose, paroxysms of sneezing, pruritus of palate and throat. Postnasal drip, rhinorrhea, anosmia. Associated with serous otitis media, otitis media, or sinusitis. Seasonal symptoms caused by pollen or mold. Perennial symptoms result from exposure to animal dander, house dust mites, mold, and occupational allergens (eg, flour). More common in children than adults. Signs include: swollen bluish turbinates, nasal crease, injected conjunctivae, allergic shiners, allergic salute, and mouth breathing.

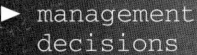 management decisions

### ALLERGIC RHINOCONJUNCTIVITIS

| Severity | Treatment |
|---|---|
| Mild | Avoidance techniques. |
| | Oral antihistamine (Allegra 180 mg qd) with or without a decongestant (Sudafed). |
| | Ocular antihistamines (Naphcon A) or ocular antihistamine/mast cell stabilizer (Optivar) |
| Moderate | Add nasal corticosteroids (Nasonex—2 sprays each nostril qd). |
| | Add immunotherapy (allergy injections). |
| Moderate to severe | Add nasal antihistamine (Astelin—2 sprays in each nostril bid prn) or |
| | Nasal ipratropium bromide (Atrovent 0.03%—2 sprays in each nostril bid prn). |
| Severe | Nasal decongestants (Afrin—1–2 sprays in each nostril bid for 2–3 days). |
| | Oral corticosteroids (prednisone—1–2 mg/kg/day for 5–7 days). |

▶ Diagnosis

Positive allergy skin tests (epicutaneous and/or intradermal tests) or radioallergosorbent test (RAST) assay to suspected allergens. Nasal or conjunctival smear filled with eosinophils. Elevated total IgE.

▶ Concept and Application

Patient develops specific IgE antibodies to offending allergens. IgE binds to mast cells of nasal and conjunctivae mucosa. Environmental allergens trigger mast cell mediator release including ECF-A, NCF-A, histamine, leukotrienes, prostaglandins, and PAF. Eosinophils and neutrophils are found at site of allergic reaction and participate in the inflammatory reaction.

▶ Treatment Steps

1. Avoidance by removal of offending allergen from home (dog, cat), use of an air cleaner, or dustproofing home.
2. Medicines:
   a. Oral antihistamines (Benadryl or Zyrtec) may be added to oral decongestants (Sudafed).
   b. Oral antihistamine/decongestant combination preparations (Allegra D or Claritin D) may be used instead of individual antihistamines and decongestants.
   c. Nasal corticosteroids (Nasonex).
   d. Nasal antihistamines (Astelin).
   e. Nasal ipratropium bromide (Atrovent 0.03%).
   f. Nasal cromolyn sodium (Nasalcrom).
   g. Nasal decongestants (Afrin) should be avoided for extended periods as they may cause rhinitis medicamentosa.
   h. Ocular antihistamines/decongestants (Naphcon A).

i. Ocular mast cell stabilizers (Patanol).
j. Ocular corticosteroids (FML).
k. Oral corticosteroids (prednisone).
3. Desensitization, also known as immunotherapy, to inhaled allergens.

## III. ANAPHYLAXIS OR ANAPHYLACTOID REACTIONS

▶ H&P Keys

Sudden onset of urticaria, angioedema, wheezing, dyspnea, or hypotension. Patients may also have gastrointestinal or uterine cramps. Severe reaction may lead to hypovolemic shock and hypoxemia. Symptoms occur soon after taking a medication (eg, penicillin, aspirin, IV contrast medium), exposure to allergen (food), or following an insect sting. Signs include pallor; cyanosis; diaphoresis; impaired or loss of consciousness; tachycardia; weak or irregular pulse; cold, clammy extremities; tachypnea; or stridor.

▶ Diagnosis

Positive allergy skin tests or RAST assay to offending allergen. IgE-specific antibodies are not identified in anaphylactoid reactions. Other studies include: complete blood count (CBC), total IgE, total eosinophil count, elevated serum tryptase, and urine histamine.

▶ Concept and Application

Mast cells and basophils rich in mediators (ECF-A, NCF-A, PAF, histamine, leukotriene, prostaglandins, etc) suddenly undergo degranulation following exposure to an allergen as a result of specific IgE directed against that allergen or, in the case of anaphylactic reactions, allergens cause mediator release through a non–IgE-mediated mechanism. Mast cell mediator release leads to shifting of intravascular fluid to interstitial tissues and hypotension, and may lead to hives and angioedema. Asthmatic patient will become dyspneic and wheeze.

▶ Treatment Steps

1. Oxygen if cyanosis, dyspnea, or wheezing is present.
2. Trendelenburg position if hypotensive.
3. Epinephrine (1:1000 0.30–0.50 mL SQ or 0.1 mL/kg in children).
4. Tourniquet—place a tourniquet proximal to the site of injection or sting on an extremity, if applicable.
5. Antihistamines (Benadryl IV 1–2 mg/kg up to 100 mg).
6. $H_2$-blockers (cimetidine 300 mg IV).
7. IV fluids through large-gauge line to maintain systolic blood pressure ≥ 100 mm Hg in adults, 50 mm Hg in children.
8. Nebulized $\beta_2$ agonist if there is bronchospasm (albuterol 0.5 cc in 3 cc saline).
9. Corticosteroids (hydrocortisone IV 7–10 mg/kg).
10. Vasopressors (dopamine IV 0.3–1.2 mg/kg/hr).

11. Shock trousers.
12. Intubation and ventilation.
13. Tracheostomy if airway obstruction secondary to airway edema.
14. Prevention of future reaction by avoidance, hyposensitization in cases of insect venom hypersensitivity.

## IV. URTICARIA

### ▶ H&P Keys

Generalized pruritus; hives vary in size from 3–4 mm to giant lesion 10–15 cm in diameter. Usually have central clearing with peripheral erythema. Often associated with angioedema of soft tissues including eyes, lips, and tongue. Lesions leave no permanent changes in the skin and are transient. Acute urticaria: hives occur over a period of < 6 weeks. Chronic urticaria: hives persist for a period > 6 weeks. Hives may be induced by extrinsic agents (eg, drugs such as antibiotics, nonsteroidal anti-inflammatory agents, and opiates; radiocontrast media; and foods such as shrimp, peanuts, and strawberries), physical agents (eg, light, heat friction, pressure, cold, and vibration) and underlying systemic disease (eg, serum sickness, infection, autoimmunity, malignancy).

### ▶ Diagnosis

Complete blood count (CBC), sedimentation rate, antinuclear antibodies (ANA), serum protein electrophoresis (SPEP), urinalysis (UA), liver function tests, TSH, thyroid auto-antibodies, and skin biopsy. Total IgE, allergy tests for suspected allergens.

### ▶ Disease Severity

Mild disease includes intermittent hives responding to antihistamines. Moderate to severe disease includes persistent urticaria that requires corticosteroid treatment or is associated with angioedema of the respiratory or gastrointestinal tracts.

### ▶ management decisions

**URTICARIA**

| Severity | Treatment |
|---|---|
| Mild | One or two antihistamines from different classes (Allegra 180 mg in A.M., Zyrtec 10 mg in P.M.) |
| Moderate | Add $H_2$-blocker (Zantac 150 mg bid). |
| Moderate to severe | Add tricyclic antidepressant (Sinequan 10 mg tid) and/or leukotriene modifier (Singulair). |
| Severe | Add oral $\beta_2$-adrenergic (Volmax 4–8 mg bid) and/or Oral corticosteroids (prednisone 1–2 mg/kg/day). |

▶ Treatment Steps
1. Avoid provocative factors.
2. Antihistamine (hydroxyzine 25–500 mg qid).
3. Additional antihistamine (Allegra 180 mg qd).
4. $H_2$-blocker (Zantac 150 mg bid).
5. Leukotriene modifier (Singulair 10 mg qd).
6. Tricyclic antidepressants in low doses (Sinequan 10–20 mg tid or 30–50 mg qhs).
7. Oral adrenergic (Volmax 4–8 mg bid).
8. Oral corticosteroids (prednisone 1–2 mg/kg/day).
9. Anabolic steroids (stanozolol 1–2 mg bid).
10. Epinephrine (for emergency treatment 1:1000 0.2–0.3 mL SQ or 0.01 mL/kg in children, repeated in 20–30 minutes if needed).

## V. IMMUNODEFICIENCY

### A. Humoral Immunodeficiency

▶ H&P Keys

Recurrent infections including pneumonia, sinusitis, otitis media, and skin infections. Frequent complaints of diarrhea and arthralgia or arthritis. Children may suffer from failure to thrive. Young males may have X-linked agammaglobulinemia. Older children and adults often suffer common variable hypogammaglobulinemia. Patients may have absent lymph nodes, and the physical signs relate to the site of infection. Patients with recurrent bacterial infections usually lack immunoglobulins (humoral immunodeficiency); those with recurrent fungal or viral infection suffer from absent or defective T cells (cellular immunodeficiency).

▶ Diagnosis

CBC, quantitative immunoglobulins (IgG, IgG subclass levels, IgM, IgA), T- and B-cell enumeration, anergy panel, chest and sinus roentgenograms, sweat test, HIV testing.

▶ Concept and Application

Failure of B cells to differentiate into immunoglobulin-producing cells or other defect in immunoglobulin production or secretion. Patients with IgA deficiency often have few symptoms.

▶ Treatment Steps
1. IV gamma globulin (IVIG) 300–400 mg/kg/month to maintain trough serum IgG levels 4 weeks after treatment at > 500 mg/dL.
2. Hyperimmune gamma globulin preparations (eg, zoster immune globulin obtained from immunized donors).
3. Early use of antibiotics in infections.
4. Prevent transfusion reactions. IgA-deficient patients may have anti-IgA antibodies and require blood products depleted of IgA. Similarly, IVIG may cause anaphylaxis, and is not indicated in IgA-deficient patients.

## B. Cellular (T-cell) Immunodeficiency

▶ H&P Keys

Usually affects infants and young children. Patients often suffer from chronic diarrhea, failure to thrive, viral infections, or persistent fungal infections (*Candida*). Patients with combined immunodeficiency (loss of both T-cell and B-cell function) often fail to respond to therapy and die within the first year of life.

▶ Diagnosis

Absence or diminution of T cells or their subsets. Decreased thymus on roentgenography. Diminished evidence of T-cell activity as assayed by the anergy panel or in vitro mitogen-induced lymphoblastic transformation.

▶ Treatment Steps
1. Supportive treatment, use aggressive antibiotic therapy, antifungal therapy.
2. Avoid whole blood transfusions, which may cause a fatal graft versus host reaction.
3. Avoid live virus vaccines (eg, poliovirus, MMR vaccine).
4. Bone marrow transplantation.
5. Fetal thymus transplantation.
6. Lymphokines (eg, aldesleukin—recombinant human interleukin-2).
7. Immunomodulators (eg, filgrastim—recombinant human granulocyte colony-stimulating factor—as adjunctive treatment following immunosuppression).
8. Gene therapy, in selected cases, is being studied.

## VI. HEREDITARY ANGIOEDEMA

▶ H&P Keys

This autosomal dominant inherited disorder is seen in childhood, although an acquired form is seen mostly in adults. Patients develop nonpitting localized subcutaneous or submucosol edema. The face, lips, tongue, and glottal structure are frequently involved. Upper airway obstruction may be fatal. Attacks may be precipitated by mild trauma (eg, dental work). No pruritus is present. Patients do not respond to epinephrine. Gastrointestinal involvement may simulate an acute abdomen.

▶ Diagnosis

$C_1$-esterase inhibitor qualitative levels are depressed. Quantitative levels may be present, but not functional.

$C_1$ levels depressed in the acquired but not the hereditary form. Skin biopsy reveals no inflammatory changes and lacks eosinophilia.

▶ Disease Severity

Severity can vary from episode to episode in an individual patient. Each episode involving the upper airway is potentially life-threatening. Severely affected patients have attacks of angioedema regularly every few weeks, and mildly affected patients may go many months between attacks.

### ▶ Concept and Application

Most commonly is a congenital absence or decrease of the $C_1$-esterase inhibitor levels. The complement cascade is activated without functional $C_1$-esterase inhibitor levels. $C_4$ levels are decreased during asymptomatic periods. $C_1$ and $C_3$ levels are normal. Adult with newly developed disease may have the acquired form, which may be associated with underlying malignant neoplasm.

### ▶ Treatment Steps

1. Supportive therapy during acute attacks (eg, mild analgesics or narcotics, IV fluids, intubation or tracheostomy before critical obstruction occurs).
2. Infusion of $C_1$-esterase inhibitor concentrate has been effective, but not currently available in the United States.
3. Fresh-frozen plasma is not recommended. Some patients may worsen due to the addition of complement components.
4. Attenuated androgens (eg, stanozolol 1–2 mg bid) contraindicated in children who are not fully grown and during pregnancy.
5. ε-Aminocaproic acid (a fibrinolysis inhibitor) may be used in children.
6. Prophylaxis before surgical procedures with fresh-frozen plasma (two units 12–24 hours before the procedure).
7. Epinephrine should not be relied upon.

## VII. ATOPIC DERMATITIS

### ▶ H&P Keys

Atopic dermatitis is a very common chronic pruritic skin disorder seen mostly in infants and children, although it occasionally occurs in adults. The infantile form tends to affect the head but may also present with a symmetrical eczemoid rash involving the extensor surfaces. As the child grows, the rash becomes most prominent in the flexural areas (ie, popliteal fossae, antecubital fossae) and dry skin becomes a prominent feature. Over time, the skin becomes lichenified and often hyperpigmented. Pruritus and scratching may lead to excoriation and infection of eczemoid lesions.

### ▶ Diagnosis

Total IgE is significantly elevated in 80% of patients, often beyond the levels seen in allergic rhinitis or allergic asthma. The total eosinophil count is frequently elevated during acute exacerbations of the rash. Allergy skin tests are usually positive to a wide variety of allergens, as is the RAST assay. However, it is often difficult to correlate these positive allergy tests with the clinical course of this disease.

### ▶ Disease Severity

Although most infants presenting with atopic dermatitis have mild to moderate skin involvement, which can be managed on an outpatient basis, occasionally, affected patients suffer from a generalized eczemoid rash involving much of the body surface. Severely affected patients may become acutely ill and develop generalized erythroderma and infection of their open skin lesions. This latter group require hospitalization, hydration, and intensive topical care as well as systemic antibiotics. On the other hand, mild to moderate cases of atopic dermatitis often respond to antihistamines and topical agents with gradual resolution of their skin rash over a period of years. Some adults diagnosed with atopic dermatitis during childhood continue to have dry skin and occasional hand eczema when they are exposed to irritants.

### ▶ Concept and Application

The mechanism for atopic dermatitis is not well understood. However, most patients are clearly atopic, having high levels of IgE, positive allergy skin tests, and high incidence of allergic rhinitis and conjunctivitis. Paradoxically, these patients may reveal minor defects in their cellular immunity with suppressed delayed hypersensitivity tests, decreased T-suppressor cells (CD8) and an increased ratio of helper (CD4) to suppressor cells. Patients also demonstrate abnormal cutaneous vascular responses. Defects in cellular immunity are demonstrated clinically by patients with atopic dermatitis who contract herpes, which may lead to life-threatening infection.

### ▶ Treatment Steps

1. Identify and eliminate exacerbating factors such as allergens, irritants, and psychosocial stressors.
2. Prevent dryness of the skin by decreasing exposure to hot water and patting the skin dry rather than rubbing vigorously.
3. Moisturize the skin with over-the-counter fragrance-free moisturizers or with prescription agents such as Lac-Hydrin 12% (ammonium lactate). Ointments are more effective than creams, which are more effective than lotions. Apply when skin is wet.
4. Prevent irritation of the skin by wearing loose fitting noncoarse garments, avoiding excessive sweating, and by avoiding irritating soaps.
5. Antihistamines to treat pruritus (eg, hydroxyzine 25–50 mg qid).
6. Antipruritics (eg, Sarna or Zonalon) applied topically.
7. Topical immunomodulator (TIM) agents (Elidel and Protopic) inhibit T-cell–derived cytokines.
8. Topical corticosteroids. Fluorinated agents usually are more effective but have more side effects than nonfluorinated agents.
9. Systemic corticosteroids. Use sparingly due to side effects (eg, prednisone 1 mg/kg/day in divided doses for 5–10 days).
10. Antibiotics to cover *Staphylococcus aureus* if signs of infection are present (eg, dicloxacillin 500 mg qid).
11. Coal tar acts as anti-inflammatory agent (eg, Zetar).

---

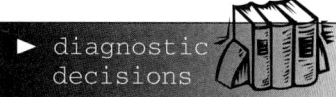

▶ diagnostic decisions

**ALLERGIC DISEASES OF THE SKIN**

**Atopic Dermatitis**
Pruritic, dry lesions may become lichenified and hyperpigmented. Elevated IgE, eosinophil count. Positive immediate allergy to prior skin tests. Skin biopsy is nonspecific.

**Contact Dermatitis**
Pruritic lesions may become lichenified or vesiculate. Positive patch tests within 72 hours. Skin biopsy shows marked infiltration of lymphocytes and macrophages.

**Urticaria**
Transient pruritic hives vary in size from 3 mm to 15 cm, usually with central clearing, often associated with angioedema.

**Hereditary Angioedema**
Nonpruritic nonpitting edema without hives. Skin biopsy reveals no inflammatory changes and lacks eosinophilia. Diminished functional $C_1$-esterase inhibitor level.

12. Wet dressings can promote absorption of topical medications, hydrate the skin, and protect against persistent scratching.
13. Ultraviolet light therapy can be useful for severe atopic dermatitis.
14. Immunomodulatory therapy (thymopentin, interferons, and cyclosporin A) have been used in severe cases.

## VIII. CONTACT DERMATITIS

▶ H&P Keys

Contact dermatitis is an inflammatory reaction of the skin caused by an external stimulis. Inflammation may be allergic or nonallergic (irritant). Nonallergic contact dermatitis is a common occupational skin disease. Most of the skin is simply inflamed as a result of exposure to a nonspecific irritating substance (eg, detergents, solvents, water), which is referred to as irritant dermatitis. Allergic contact dermatitis is related to a delayed hypersensitivity reaction and may be due to a natural exposure to antigens, such as those in poison ivy plants, or may result from exposure to nickel in tools, watches, or jewelry; or allergens in hair dye, rubber products, makeup, or preservatives (parabens) in creams and lotions. Allergic contact dermatitis can occur at any age but is most often seen in adults. The lesions are initially pruritic but with time become lichenified. The location of the rash usually indicates the site of exposure. For example, allergy to a leather dye may cause shoe dermatitis.

▶ Diagnosis

Allergy patch testing to common contact allergens will usually be positive within 72 hours of application. A skin biopsy of the affected skin reveals an intense inflammatory infiltrate characterized by a marked infiltration of lymphocytes and macrophages, which typify a delayed hypersensitivity reaction.

▶ Disease Severity

Acute contact dermatitis such as widespread poison ivy may incapacitate the patient. The lesions are highly pruritic and often blisters, erythema, and edema are noted in acute reactor. Moderate reaction: often limited areas of eczema, which ultimately become lichenified. Dark-skinned patients develop hyperpigmentation at the site of the rash. Once the allergen is identified and eliminated, the rash will gradually resolve. Patients with unavoidable chronic exposure will continue to have a rash even if they receive medication.

▶ Concept and Application

Allergic contact dermatitis is a type IV delayed or cellular allergic reaction. The hapten of the allergen passes into the skin, combining with Langerhans' cells, lymphocytes, and other carrier molecules to form a complete allergen. With repeated allergen exposure, hypersensitivity increases. Lymphocytes release mediators (macrophage inhibiting factor) that recruit macrophages, which attack the allergen and surrounding tissues.

▶ Treatment Steps
1. Avoidance of the precipitating factors.
2. Wet dressings for acute vesiculating dermatitis (eg, Burow's solution, aluminum acetate solution, or aluminum sulfate).
3. Antihistamines to treat pruritus (eg, hydroxyzine 25–50 mg qid). They do not affect the rash.
4. Antipruritics (eg, calamine or Zonalon) applied topically.
5. Topical corticosteroids. Use ointments for thicker lesions; creams or lotions for exudative lesions or intertriginous regions; and lotions or gels for hairy regions such as the scalp.
6. Systemic corticosteroids (especially if lesions are on the face, hands, or other sensitive areas), eg, prednisone 1 mg/kg/day in divided doses for 5–10 days.
7. Antibiotics to cover *Staphylococcus aureus* if signs of infection are present (eg, dicloxacillin 500 mg qid).
8. Ultraviolet light may be considered.

## IX. ALLERGIC BRONCHOPULMONARY ASPERGILLOSIS

▶ H&P Keys

Allergic bronchopulmonary aspergillosis (ABPA) results from a manipulation reaction resulting from the presence of the fungus *Aspergillus fumigatus* present in the bronchial tree of asthmatic patients. Patients typically present with difficult-to-manage bronchial asthma associated with peripheral eosinophilia and high total IgE. Of asthmatic patients, 1% to 2% are affected by ABPA. Approximately 10% of corticosteroid-dependent asthmatics and 6% of patients with cystic fibrosis are also affected by ABPA. Affected patients often have a history of frequent use of or dependence on corticosteroids. At times, patients may complain of fever, general malaise, productive cough, and wheezing. Mucoid impaction may lead to atelectasis. Severely affected patients with pulmonary fibrosis may exhibit signs of chronic hypoxemia, including digital clubbing.

▶ Diagnosis

Total IgE is significantly elevated (> 1,000 IU/mL); elevated total eosinophil count (> 1,000/mm$^3$); positive immediate-type hypersensitivity reaction to *A. fumigatus*. Roentgenograms often reveal transient infiltrates. The presence of central or proximal bronchiectasis and absence of distal bronchiectasis is highly suggestive of ABPA. High-resolution CT (HRCT) is more sensitive and specific in detecting proximal bronchiectasis than plain films. Patients often have significant titers of precipitating IgG antibodies to *Aspergillus*, and *A. fumigatus* may be cultured from sputum of some patients, but a positive culture is not diagnostic. Examination of sputum may identify *A. fumigatus* hyphae and intense eosinophilia.

### ▶ Disease Severity

ABPA may vary from mild to moderate disease, with intermittent flares of asthmatic symptoms that quickly respond to corticosteroids, to severe progressive asthma associated with pulmonary fibrosis, progressive hypoxemia, digital clubbing, and end-stage pulmonary disease. ABPA can be staged as follows: acute, remission, exacerbation, corticosteroid-dependent asthma, and fibrotic.

### ▶ Concept and Application

The mechanism for ABPA is not entirely understood. However, it appears that certain asthmatic patients have a propensity to colonize *A. fumigatus* along their bronchial tree. The fungus does not infiltrate but remains in close proximity to the respiratory mucosa. *Aspergillus* antigens apparently diffuse to the mucosa and elicit a variety of reactions including a type I–IgE reaction as well as a type III or Arthus phenomenon. Specific IgE and IgG antibodies are produced against *Aspergillus*. Eventually, an acute inflammatory reaction ensues, leading to clinical symptoms.

### ▶ Treatment Steps

1. Inhaled short-acting $\beta_2$-adrenergic (eg, albuterol) to treat the asthmatic component.
2. Oral corticosteroids (eg, prednisone 0.5 mg/kg/day initially, then taper to a lower-dose maintenance program) can reduce clinical symptoms with attendant changes, including decreased total IgE and clearing of the chest roentgenogram.
3. Immunotherapy is *not* effective.
4. Antifungal therapy (eg, itraconazole 200 mg bid) has shown promising results.

## X. HYPERSENSITIVITY PNEUMONITIS

### ▶ H&P Keys

Hypersensitivity pneumonitis or extrinsic allergic alveolitis is caused by an immunopathologic reaction involving the alveoli, bronchioles, and surrounding pulmonary tissues resulting from exposure to organic dusts. Allergens causing hypersensitivity pneumonitis may be derived from bacterial (eg, thermophilic actinomycetes in mushroom compost causing mushroom worker's lung), fungi (eg, *Aspergillus* species in moldy tobacco causing tobacco worker's lung), insect proteins (eg, *Sitophilus granarius* in infested flour causing wheat miller's lung), organic chemicals (eg, isocyanates in various industries causing chemical worker's lung), or miscellaneous agents (eg, avian proteins in pigeon droppings causing bird breeder's lung). An acute reaction or insidious chronic disease may occur depending on the concentration and duration of exposure of the allergen. Acute disease is associated with fever, chills, sweats, myalgia, dyspnea, and coughing; symptoms last for hours to days following exposure. Chronic disease usually lacks systemic symptoms, with patients complaining of dyspnea and perhaps cough. Physical examination may reveal bilateral fine rales and signs of hypoxemia. Patients with chronic disease may lack clinical symptoms initially but over time develop symptoms of dyspnea resulting from chronic pulmonary fibrosis and other signs of hypoxemia.

▶ Diagnosis

In part, the diagnosis is based on evidence of the immunologic reaction to the inhaled antigen. Affected patients reveal evidence of the presence of precipitating usually IgG, antibody directed against the offending antigen. ELISA may be used to detect circulating serum antibodies. Pulmonary function tests identify the presence of a restrictive lung disease, decreased diffusing capacity for carbon monoxide (DLCO), and arterial blood gases identify hypoxemia. Chest roentgenogram may be normal initially. However, eventually repeated or prolonged exposure to the antigen will be associated with roentgenologic evidence of interstitial fibrosis. High-resolution CT (HRCT) is more sensitive and specific in chronic disease and reveals scattered, small, rounded opacities. Inhalation challenge is rarely used today because of the potential for serious damage. Bronchoalveolar lavage may reveal IgG and IgA antibodies.

▶ Disease Severity

Hypersensitivity pneumonitis may present as an acute disease associated with fever and elevated white count and sedimentation rates. Within a short time signs, symptoms, and findings resolve. Repeated allergen exposure may lead to subacute episode in which pulmonary functions do not return to normal, and patients with chronic exposure to the allergen will develop irreversible restrictive lung disease and, eventually, end-stage lung disease.

▶ Concept and Application

Type III (immune-complex mediated) and type IV (cell-mediated delayed hypersensitivity) reactions occur to the inhaled organic antigenic matter.

▶ Treatment Steps

1. Avoid offending agent.
2. Inhaled short-acting $\beta_2$-adrenergic (eg, albuterol).
3. Oral corticosteroids (eg, prednisone 60 mg/day for 1 week, tapered slowly).
4. Immunotherapy with the offending antigens is not recommended.

## XI. HYPEREOSINOPHILIC SYNDROME

▶ H&P Keys

Hypereosinophilic syndrome is characterized by high levels of peripheral eosinophilia and pulmonary infiltrates associated with eosinophilic infiltration into tissues and organs. Patients may initially be asymptomatic but over time show symptoms of organ pathology. Organ systems infiltrated with eosinophils are listed in descending order of frequency of involvement: hematologic, cardiovascular, cutaneous, neurologic, pulmonary, splenic, hepatic, ocular and gastrointestinal. Symptoms may include coughing, dyspnea, symptoms of congestive heart failure, abdominal pain, and intravascular clotting abnormalities. Hypereosinophilic syndrome often affects young and middle-aged adult men. The ratio of male to female patients is 9:1.

▶ Diagnosis

Eosinophilia often exceeds 50% of the peripheral white count. The total IgE is not particularly elevated. Bone marrow biopsy reveals an intense myeloid hyperplasia of eosinophils. Biopsy of affected organs (eg, lungs, heart, gastrointestinal tract) reveals an eosinophil infiltrate. The criteria for diagnosis include: eosinophilia of 1,500/mm$^3$ for at least 6 months, tissue eosinophilia as exhibited on biopsy of specific organs, and no other known etiology for eosinophilia.

▶ Disease Severity

Hypereosinophilic syndrome can remain a limited disease with few clinical symptoms and marked primarily by very high eosinophil counts; or vital organs can sustain irreversible damage that ultimately results in the demise of the patient. Cardiac infiltration may lead to a restrictive carditis and congestive heart failure. High leukocyte counts (> 90,000/μL) are associated with a poor prognosis.

▶ Concept and Application

The mechanism for hypereosinophilic syndrome is unknown. It is thought to be related to overactive T-cell secretion of lymphokines, which stimulate the eosinophil line.

▶ Treatment Steps

1. General—treat the affected organ (eg, inhaled bronchodilators if bronchospasm exists, diuretics if there is impaired left ventricular function). No therapy is required if there is no organ involvement.
2. Oral corticosteroids (eg, prednisone 60 mg/day or 1 mg/kg/day).
3. Cytotoxic agents (eg, hydroxyurea and etoposide) if there is significant organ involvement or unresponsiveness to steroids.
4. Interferon-α has shown promising results.

## XII. DRUG ALLERGY

▶ H&P Keys

Drug allergy is an adverse immunologic reaction to an administered medication. The development of drug allergy is influenced by the type of medication, route of administration, frequency of administration, and underlying reactivity of the patient. Patients may suffer adverse drug reactions that are not immunologic in nature and are therefore nonallergic reactions. Examples of nonallergic drug reactions include overdosage, drug side effects, drug-to-drug interactions, and idiosyncratic reactions (eg, primaquine-induced hemolytic anemia in a G6PD-deficient patient. Drug allergies can present as anaphylaxis, urticaria, or angioedema, serum-sickness–like disease, vasculitis, ptomaine disease, drug fever, nephritis, or pathologic cutaneous conditions. Penicillin allergy is quite common and is often IgE-mediated, presenting as urticaria or anaphylaxis. Nonimmunologic reactions simulating drug allergy may occur with mast cell degranulators, such as meperidine hydrochloride (Demerol) and codeine.

▶ Diagnosis

A good temporal correlation between the use of a medication and the onset of typical allergic symptoms (eg, anaphylaxis, urticaria) sets the stage for a diagnosis of drug allergy. However, some supporting evidence of an immunologic reaction is needed to indicate that the origin of the reaction is immunologic. An elevated total or specific IgE, as well as eosinophilia, is supportive of the diagnosis of drug allergy. One of the most commonly diagnosed drug allergies is that of penicillin, confirmed by positive allergy skin test reactions to penicillin major or minor determinants.

▶ Disease Severity

Mild reversible or transient symptoms of drug allergy include cutaneous reactions, including urticaria, angioedema, and various exanthems. With cessation of the medications, symptoms subside without sequelae. On the other hand, drug reactions causing exfoliative dermatitis (eg, sulfa drugs), severe anaphylaxis (eg, penicillin), hepatitis (eg, phenytoin [Dilantin]), pulmonary interstitial fibrosis (eg, nitrofurantoin), interstitial nephritis (eg, methicillin), Stevens–Johnson syndrome (eg, sulfa) in some cases has led to permanent impairment and even death.

▶ Concept and Application

The drug itself or its metabolite is often a low-molecular-weight hapten, which joins with body proteins to become an allergen. IgE-mediated drug reactions usually result in urticaria, angioedema, or anaphylaxis. Autoimmune disease or vasculitis may be a result of a reaction involving immune complexes containing antigen, antibody, and complement, whereas fixed drug eruptions and contact dermatitis appear to be caused by cellular or delayed-hypersensitivity reactions.

▶ Treatment Steps

1. Discontinue the offending medication.
2. Antihistamines to treat pruritus and urticaria.
3. Antipruritics applied topically for maculopapular rashes.
4. Oral corticosteroids are necessary if exfoliative dermatitis, vasculitis, or major organ involvement occurs.
5. Supportive treatment may include transfusions if a hemolytic drug reaction is present or IV fluids if hypotension is noted.
6. Epinephrine subcutaneously is often helpful in acute and severe IgE-mediated reactions.

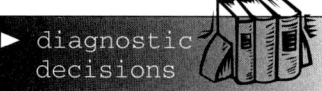

▶ diagnostic decisions

### ALLERGIC DRUG REACTIONS

**Anaphylactic (type I)**
Immediate IgE-mediated anaphylaxis, angioedema, and urticaria. Penicillin is the most common cause of drug-induced anaphylaxis.

**Cytotoxic (type II)**
IgG or IgM antibody against cell surface antigens cause hematologic reactions and nephritis. Drug-induced Coombs'-positive hemolytic anemia and methicillin-induced nephritis are good examples.

**Serum Sickness (type III)**
Immune complex–mediated reaction involving fever, large-joint arthralgias, and multiorgan vasculitis. Drug-induced SLE from hydralazine and procainamide are examples.

**Cell-mediated (type IV)**
Delayed-type hypersensitivity reactions take days to occur. Reactions can range from contact dermatitis if the drug is topical, to drug-induced interstitial nephritis.

## BIBLIOGRAPHY

Braunwald, E. *Harrison's Manual of Medicine.* 15th ed. New York: McGraw-Hill; 2002.

Busse, WW. Advances in Allergic Diseases. *Journal of Allergy and Clinical Immunology* 105(6) (Supplement, Part 2), S593–S644, June 2000.

Tierney, LM. *Current Medical Diagnosis and Treatment.* 41st ed. New York: Lange Medical Books/McGraw-Hill; 2002.

# Injuries, Wounds, Toxicology, and Burns | 7

I. **EPISTAXIS** / 217

II. **CRANIAL INJURY** / 217
    A. Facial Fracture (Frontal Bone, Mandible, Maxilla, Orbits, or Nose) / 217
    B. Skull Trauma or Fracture / 218
    C. Concussion / 219
    D. Subdural Hematoma / 219
    E. Epidural Hematoma / 219
    F. Ocular Injury / 220
    G. Auditory Injury / 220
    H. Epidemiology and Prevention of Ocular and Auditory Injury / 221

III. **CHEST AND ABDOMINAL INJURY** / 221
    A. Rib Cage / 221
    B. Pneumothorax / 222
    C. Hemothorax / 222
    D. Flail Chest / 223
    E. Additional Information / 223
    F. Perforation of Viscus / 223
    G. Pelvic Fractures / 224
    H. Epidemiology and Prevention of Chest and Abdominal Injury / 224

IV. **LACERATIONS** / 225

V. **FOREIGN BODIES** / 225
    A. Eye, Ear, and Nose / 225
    B. Aspiration / 226
    C. Swallowed / 226

VI. **BURNS** / 227
    A. Eye Burns / 227
    B. Thermal Burns / 227
    C. Electrical Burns / 227

VII. **POISONING / 228**
- A. Acetaminophen / 228
- B. Tricyclic Antidepressants / 228
- C. Sedatives / 229
- D. Stimulants / 229
- E. Cocaine / 230
- F. PCP (Phencyclidine) / 230
- G. Alcohol / 230
- H. Solvent Sniffing / 231
- I. Heavy Metals and Arsenic / 231
- J. Carbon Monoxide / 231
- K. Diethyl-m-toluamide (DEET) / 232
- L. Additional Information / 232

VIII. **FRACTURES / 233**
- A. Vertebral Column / 233
- B. Extremities / 233

IX. **SPRAINS AND DISLOCATIONS / 236**
- A. Hands / 236
- B. Ankle / 237
- C. Elbow Dislocation / 237
- D. Shoulder Dislocation or Injury / 237

X. **DROWNING / 237**

XI. **INSECT AND SNAKE BITES / 238**

XII. **ANAPHYLACTIC SHOCK / 239**

XIII. **ADDITIONAL MANAGEMENT INFORMATION / 239**
- A. Traumatic Injury / 239
- B. Shock / 239
- C. Child Abuse, Sexual Abuse, Sexual Assault / 240
- D. Thermal Injuries / 240

XIV. **EPIDEMIOLOGY AND PREVENTION OF SELECTED ACCIDENTS / 241**
- A. Home Accidents / 241
- B. Workplace Accidents / 242
- C. Athletic Accidents / 242
- D. Automobile Accidents and Drunk Driving / 242
- E. Head and Spinal Cord Injury and Whiplash / 242
- F. Drowning / 242
- G. Ingestion of Poisonous and Toxic Agents / 243
- H. Gunshot and Stab Wounds / 243
- I. Thermal Injury / 243
- J. Child, Spouse, and Elderly Abuse / 243
- K. Sexual Abuse and Rape / 244
- L. Fire Prevention / 244
- M. Falls / 244

**BIBLIOGRAPHY / 245**

## I. EPISTAXIS

▶ H&P Keys

Control bleeding with direct pressure by squeezing nostrils or pack nasal passage with cotton soaked in lidocaine and Adrenalin. Remove blood, proceed with a careful exam to pinpoint the source of bleeding. Evaluate history for bleeding disorders and medication.

▶ Diagnosis

If indicated, rule out bleeding disorders (prothrombin time [PT], partial prothrombin time [PTT], platelets), leukemia, and severe liver disease.

▶ Disease Severity

Severe bleeding without a visualized bleeding source is most often posterior. Monitor vital signs including pulse oximetry. Evaluate underlying conditions that exacerbate the bleeding (hypertension, liver disease).

▶ Concept and Application

Anterior bleeding arises from Kiesselbach's plexus; posterior, from external or internal carotids.

▶ Treatment Steps

*Anterior*—Pressure or packing, topical vasoconstrictors, cauterization (silver nitrate, using topical analgesia first).

*Posterior*—Posterior packing, antibiotics, volume resuscitation, if indicated: surgery.

## II. CRANIAL INJURY

### A. Facial Fracture (Frontal Bone, Mandible, Maxilla, Orbits, or Nose)

▶ H&P Keys

History and physical exam, roentgenographic studies, information from witness.

▶ Diagnosis

Primarily includes physical exam and roentgenographic studies. Pain, cerebrospinal fluid (CSF) rhinorrhea, diplopia, deformity, and tenderness suggest fracture.

*Orbital Fracture*—Swelling, difficulty with eye movement, vertical diplopia, and facial emphysema.

*Frontal or Ethmoid*—May have CSF rhinorrhea.

*Nasal Bones*—Deformity, epistaxis.

*Mandible or Maxilla*—Swelling, pain, airway compromise, jaw pain or deformity upon opening or closing the mouth (abnormal occlusion).

▶ **Disease Severity**
Neurologic deficits indicate poorer prognosis. Assess degree of trauma, neurologic status, and associated injuries via physical exam and roentgenograms.

▶ **Concept and Application**
Trauma. Evaluate neurologic status at intervals.

▶ **Treatment Steps**
1. Control of airway and hemorrhage, antibiotics, fracture reduction.

   *Nasal*—Closed reduction for simple fracture, open reduction in severe fracture cases. Always check for septal hematoma: requires immediate ENT consult.

   *Maxillary*—Reduction, interdental wiring (simple fractures), orbital or zygoma wiring and traction (complex fractures).

   *Mandibular*—Internal fixation.

   *Orbital*—Surgery to resupport orbit.

### B. Skull Trauma or Fracture

▶ **H&P Keys**
May be asymptomatic, or pain or swelling, central nervous system (CNS) signs, CSF leak (nose or ears). If CSF in nose or ears or blood in the middle ear, think basilar skull fracture. If ecchymosis behind ear (Battle's sign), think mastoid fracture. With raccoon eyes, think orbital roof or basilar fracture.

▶ **Diagnosis**
History and physical exam, CT scan or roentgenographic exam (remember, basilar fractures may not be evident on roentgenograms).

▶ **Disease Severity**
Frequent neurologic exams. Observe for epidural hematoma with linear fracture across middle meningeal artery.

▶ **Concept and Application**
Skull trauma may result in brain injury, hemorrhage, CSF leak, cranial nerve damage, or meningitis.

▶ **Treatment Steps**
Cardiopulmonary resuscitation (CPR) and ABCs (airway, breathing, circulation), then:

   *Simple Linear (Closed)*—Observation.

   *Compound Linear (Open)*—Antibiotics.

   *Simple Depressed*—Surgical treatment (fragment elevation).

   *Compound Depressed*—Urgent surgical treatment.

## C. Concussion

▶ H&P Keys

Neurologic exam may be normal. History reveals a brief alteration of consciousness. May also have headache, amnesia, nausea, and vomiting.

▶ Diagnosis

History and physical exam (roentgenogram, computed tomography [CT] scan, and magnetic resonance imaging [MRI] are all normal in concussions). Repeated neurologic assessments are important.

▶ Disease Severity

Determine neurologic status, degree of injury.

▶ Concept and Application

Head trauma, resulting in head injury and brief unconsciousness, without physical brain damage, secondary to disruption of the reticular activating system. Condition is the result of brain acceleration or deceleration.

▶ Treatment Steps

Careful observation (neurologic watch).

## D. Subdural Hematoma

▶ H&P Keys

Symptoms may present after brief or prolonged time from injury: lethargy, headache, seizures, and coma. May have dilated ipsilateral pupil.

▶ Diagnosis

History and physical exam, radiography (CT) or MRI.

▶ Disease Severity

Severity determined by neurologic exam and rate of deterioration.

▶ Concept and Application

Trauma resulting in vein or brain tear and hemorrhage under the dura.

▶ Treatment Steps

Surgical (especially in acute subdural), observation in some cases (small amount of bleeding, high-risk patient).

## E. Epidural Hematoma

▶ H&P Keys

Symptoms usually present very shortly after injury: lethargy, headache, seizures, and hemiplegia. May have brief loss of consciousness then return to normal prior to deterioration (lucid interval).

▶ Diagnosis
History and physical exam, radiography (CT) or MRI.

▶ Disease Severity
Evaluate neurologic status.

▶ Concept and Application
Trauma-induced artery tear (middle meningeal artery common). Associated temporal bone fractures are common.

▶ Treatment Steps
Urgent surgery to avoid brain herniation.

## F. Ocular Injury

▶ H&P Keys
May have pain, vision loss, subconjunctival hemorrhage. If light flashes noted, rule out retinal detachment.

▶ Diagnosis
History and physical exam, ophthalmoscopic and slit-lamp exam.

▶ Disease Severity
Evaluate vision. In chemical exposure, prognosis varies with type of agent, duration of exposure, and emergency care provided.

▶ Concept and Application

*Chemicals*—Chemical conjunctivitis, blindness.

*Trauma*—Hyphema, laceration, abrasion.

▶ Treatment Steps

*Hyphema*—(Anterior chamber hemorrhage) ophthalmologist's evaluation needed as soon as possible.

*Chemicals*—Irrigation with normal saline.

*Corneal Abrasion*—Antibiotic ointment, pain control.

*Corneal Laceration*—Eye shield, immediate ophthalmologic consultation.

## G. Auditory Injury

▶ H&P Keys
Swelling, pain, hearing loss, vertigo, and hemorrhage.

▶ Diagnosis
History, physical exam, and audiometric exam, roentgenogram of skull and temporal bone (rule out associated fracture).

▶ Disease Severity
Evaluate trauma to the pinna, external ear canal, and tympanic membrane.

▶ Concept and Application
Trauma.

▶ Treatment Steps

*Tympanic Membrane Perforation*
1. If small, supportive treatment (cotton earplug, systemic antibiotic for infection).
2. If large, surgical treatment.

*Noise-induced Hearing Loss*—No treatment (except hearing aid).

*Additional Information*—Trauma to external ear may cause subperichondral hematoma. Calcified hematoma results in cauliflower ear. Prevent with early drainage.

### H. Epidemiology and Prevention of Ocular and Auditory Injury

*Epidemiology*—Includes blunt ocular trauma (occupational, recreational, environmental), and ophthalmic foreign bodies and lacerations. Auditory injury may affect children (fireworks), teens (high-decibel music), and adults (occupational).

*Prevention*—Involves eye and ear protection along with education.

## III. CHEST AND ABDOMINAL INJURY

### A. Rib Cage

1. Rib Fracture

    ▶ H&P Keys
    Pain following trauma, increased with inspiration and palpation, ecchymosis. Rib roentgenograms may appear negative shortly after injury, yet show a "healing fracture" several weeks later.

    ▶ Diagnosis
    History and physical exam, roentgenographic exam.

    ▶ Disease Severity
    Assess cardiopulmonary status and consider possible trauma in adjacent areas. Rule out pneumothorax if patient remains dyspneic.

    ▶ Concept and Application
    Fracture secondary to trauma. Without trauma, consider pathologic fracture causes.

    ▶ Treatment Steps
    Simple rib fracture: Analgesics, ice initially, injection of local anesthetic (into intercostal nerve) as an option.

## B. Pneumothorax

▶ **H&P Keys**

Dyspnea, chest pain, absent breath sounds, decreased tactile fremitus, hyperresonance. Tachycardia and hypotension may present in tension pneumothorax.

▶ **Diagnosis**

History and physical exam, chest roentgenogram.

▶ **Disease Severity**

Evaluate cardiovascular status, mentation, coexisting problems, oxygenation. Reduced venous return resulting from tension pneumothorax requires urgent treatment.

▶ **Concept and Application**

Air in pleural space, as a result of blunt or penetrating trauma (including iatrogenic trauma). May also be spontaneous, in patients with pulmonary disease, or menses-associated (catamenial).

▶ **Treatment Steps**

*Tube Thoracostomy*—Best treatment if over 50% or recurrent. Use fifth intercostal space, anterior axillary line.

*Small (Under 15%) or Stable Pneumothorax*—Observe.

*Urgent Tension Pneumothorax*—Insert large-bore needle into second intercostal space, mid-clavicular line (MCL).

*Catamenial*—Medication to suppress ovulation.

## C. Hemothorax

▶ **H&P Keys**

Dyspnea, chest pain.

▶ **Diagnosis**

History and physical exam (absent breath sounds), chest roentgenogram.

▶ **Disease Severity**

Evaluate and monitor cardiac and pulmonary status. Prognosis worse in patients with significant preexisting condition.

▶ **Concept and Application**

Trauma or spontaneous. May be iatrogenic (cultural venous pressure [CVP] monitor insertion).

▶ **Treatment Steps**

Large chest tube (32–40 French) with 20-cm water suction.

*Open Thoracotomy*—For persisting hemorrhage or massive initial blood loss. Inadequate hemothorax drainage results in fibrothorax.

## D. Flail Chest

### ▶ H&P Keys
Paradoxic chest wall motion, respiratory distress.

### ▶ Diagnosis
History and physical exam (chest palpation), roentgenographic exam.

### ▶ Disease Severity
Monitor for reduced vital capacity and respiratory distress secondary to multiple fractures.

### ▶ Concept and Application
Respiratory paradox with inspiration, secondary to multiple rib fractures.

### ▶ Treatment Steps
Intubation and positive pressure ventilation with positive end-expiratory pressure (PEEP).

## E. Additional Information

### Pericardial Tamponade Symptoms.
Diminished heart tones, narrow pulse pressure, electrocardiogram (ECG) with low voltage. Also Beck's triad (hypotension, reduced cardiac tones, high central venous pressure [CVP]).

## F. Perforation of Viscus

### ▶ H&P Keys
Abdominal rigidity, pain, peritoneal irritation, reduced or absent bowel sounds, shoulder pain.

### ▶ Diagnosis
History and physical exam, roentgenography, CT scan, diagnostic peritoneal lavage, exploratory laparotomy.

### ▶ Disease Severity
Determined by initial presentation, presence of coexisting medical problems, and baseline condition.

### ▶ Concept and Application
Trauma.

### ▶ Management
Laparotomy and surgical repair.

*Spleen*—Repair or splenectomy.

*Colon*—Repair (resection if severe injury).

*Stomach*—Repair.

▶ Additional Information

*Blunt Abdominal Trauma*—Spleen most often injured.

*Penetrating Abdominal Trauma*—Small bowel most often injured.

*Positive Peritoneal Lavage Criteria*—Red blood count (RBC) over 20,000 (in penetrating injury) or RBC over 100,000 (in blunt injury).

### G. Pelvic Fractures

▶ H&P Keys

Pain, with history of significant injury.

▶ Diagnosis

History and physical exam, roentgenographic studies, CT exam.

▶ Disease Severity

Review roentgenogram. Prognosis worse in elderly and with coexisting medical problems.

▶ Concept and Application

Trauma via falls, motor vehicle accidents, sports injuries, etc, resulting in fracture of innominate bone (ilium, ischium, or pubis), sacrum.

▶ Treatment Steps

1. Depends on multiple factors, with open reduction and internal fixation, traction, and external fixation as choices.
2. Evaluation for coexisting injuries or trauma and treatment accordingly.

*Fracture of Ilium*—Rest.

*Fracture of Anterior Superior Spine*—Surgery.

*Fracture of Sacrum*—Rest and support.

▶ Additional Information

Hemorrhage is the most important complication of pelvic fracture. Angiography with possible embolization may be required for severe, persisting hemorrhage.

### H. Epidemiology and Prevention of Chest and Abdominal Injury

*Epidemiology*—Etiology most often cites motor vehicle accidents. Blunt injury due to occupational injury or falls play a role. Increased incidence of trauma-related abdominal and chest injury in low socioeconomic areas. Pneumothorax and hemothorax, perforation of viscera, and vascular tears are common.

*Prevention*—Involves driver education and vehicle safety modifications for automobiles. Community programs, education, job opportunity, and effective law enforcement reduce the incidence of street crime trauma.

## IV. LACERATIONS

► H&P Keys

Observation; consider both history and source of injury; ascertain tetanus immunization status.

► Diagnosis

History and physical exam.

► Disease Severity

Evaluate neurovascular status and check for associated injuries, fractures, and hypotension.

► Concept and Application

Soft-tissue injury secondary to trauma.

► Treatment Steps

1. Irrigation and debridement, antibiotics if indicated, tetanus toxoid, and primary closure (maintaining minimal wound tension and everting wound edges).
2. Use 1–2% lidocaine for anesthesia (with epinephrine, except for digits and end organs).
3. Remove sutures in 7–14 days. Utilize deep and subcuticular to relieve tension on skin edges. Try to remove facial sutures in 5 days.

► Additional Information

Increased infection is noted with primary closure of human bites.

## V. FOREIGN BODIES

### A. Eye, Ear, and Nose

► H&P Keys

*Ear and Nose*—Asymptomatic or odor, unilateral purulent drainage.

*Eye*—Pain, decreased visual acuity.

► Diagnosis

Physical exam.

► Disease Severity

*Ear and Nose*—Check tympanic membrane, test hearing.

*Eye*—Full ophthalmoscopic exam.

► Concept and Application

*Ear and Nose*—Commonly children.

*Eye*—Often work-related, trauma.

▶ Treatment Steps

*Ear and Nose*—Gentle removal (forceps, irrigation).

*Eye*—Removal of foreign body under local anesthesia. Avoid additional trauma during object removal. Ensure anesthesia is adequate and, in pediatric patient, control movement.

## B. Aspiration

▶ H&P Keys

Wheezing and dyspnea may be present. History of child with object in mouth, reduced cough reflex secondary to anesthesia, disease, etc. Often an abrupt onset of cough or wheezing, dyspnea, and voice change. Most common in children under age 4.

▶ Diagnosis

Chest roentgenogram (opaque foreign body, atelectasis, or unilateral hyperinflation causing mediastinal shift).

▶ Disease Severity

Evaluate degree of respiratory distress.

▶ Concept and Application

Obstruction of trachea or bronchi by a foreign body.

▶ Treatment Steps

Removal via bronchoscopy.

▶ Additional Information

*Epidemiology*—Children are a high-risk group.

*Prevention*—Includes identification and management of high-risk patients (postop, sedated, or overdosed, with nasogastric [NG] tube, with neuromuscular disorders), reduction of gastric acidity (ranitidine [Zantac], etc). In children: avoidance of grapes, hot dogs; checking toys and objects for small parts, and maintaining alertness. Peanuts are the most frequently aspirated object in children. Instruction in the Heimlich maneuver.

## C. Swallowed

▶ H&P Keys

Sudden onset of gagging, pain, and choking.

▶ Diagnosis

Indirect laryngoscopy, roentgenography, including barium swallow.

▶ Disease Severity

Observation and evaluation for esophageal perforation.

▶ Concept and Application

Increased frequency with motility disorders, stricture, and children results in lodged foreign body. Most common location is at the cricopharyngeus muscle.

▶ Treatment Steps

Endoscopic removal. Identify location (above or below GE sphincter). Observe. If perforation, antibiotics are given to avoid mediastinitis. Do not give meat tenderizer for obstruction by meat.

## VI. BURNS

### A. Eye Burns

See Ocular Injury section on page 220.

### B. Thermal Burns

▶ H&P Keys

Assess degree of burn depth, determine etiology (thermal, chemical, etc), duration of exposure, and emergency or home treatment rendered.

▶ Diagnosis

History and physical exam.

▶ Disease Severity

Erythema minor (first degree). Blisters (split thickness; second degree). Pain (first and second degree). No pain (third degree).

▶ Concept and Application

Burns result in thermal skin and tissue injury. Total epidermis destruction with partial dermis destruction is typical of second-degree burns. Total epidermis and dermis destruction is noted in third-degree burns.

▶ Treatment Steps

Removal of patient from source of burn, CPR, cooling burn, cleaning and debridement of burn, fluids (Ringer's initially), determination of area of burn, full history and physical exam, antibiotics, tetanus toxoid, grafting. For minor burn: loose gauze wrap on nonadhering dressing. For severe burns: CPR and airway control, fluid replacement (monitoring CVP and output), NG tube, pain and sepsis control (morphine), surgical treatment (grafting, etc).

▶ Additional Information

Rule of nines to estimate burn extent: Each leg is 18%, each arm is 9%, body front is 18%, back is 18%, head is 9%, groin 1%.

### C. Electrical Burns

▶ H&P Keys

Look for an entry or exit wound (high-voltage, lightning). Massive tissue and bone destruction may be noted. Patients may be comatose and in cardiac arrest.

▶ Diagnosis
History and physical exam, serial arterial blood gases (ABGs), and hematocrit.

▶ Disease Severity
Prognostic factors include duration of electrical contact, amount of grounding present, path of the current, and amount of moisture present (moisture lowers skin resistance).

Massive tissue necrosis may precede infection, rhabdomyolysis. Assess and monitor cardiac and pulmonary status. Persisting myoglobinuria indicates significant muscle injury.

▶ Concept and Application
Direct electrical tissue trauma.

▶ Treatment Steps
1. Removal of patient from source safely, CPR, fluids and electrolyte treatment, cleaning and debridement of burns, surgical evaluation (fasciotomy, amputation), tetanus toxoid.
2. Significant fluid replacement may be required.
3. Monitoring for arrhythmias.
4. Silver sulfadiazine cream may be employed topically.

## VII. POISONING

### A. Acetaminophen

▶ H&P Keys
Nausea and vomiting and diaphoresis.

▶ Diagnosis
Serum acetaminophen level.

▶ Disease Severity
Plot acetaminophen level on Rumack–Matthew normogram to define risk. Monitor vital signs; may have hepatic failure or hepatic necrosis (jaundice, abnormal liver functions, right upper abdominal pain).

▶ Treatment Steps
1. Activated charcoal. Consider gastric lavage if < 1 hour from time of ingestion. Ipecac used in children only if < 1 hour from time of ingestion.
2. Antidote is acetylcysteine (Mucomyst).

### B. Tricyclic Antidepressants

▶ H&P Keys
Transient hypertension, then hypotension, tachycardia, arrhythmias, conduction blocks, seizures, anticholinergic symptoms (dry mucosa or skin, urinary retention).

▶ Diagnosis

History and physical exam, ECG (wide QRS). Blood levels not routinely available as stat test.

▶ Disease Severity

Increasing serum levels correlated with increasing risk (seizures, arrhythmias). Monitor mentation, cardiac status, respiratory rate and exchange.

▶ Treatment Steps
1. Gastric lavage, activated charcoal, NG tube suction.
2. Sodium bicarbonate to correct acidosis.
3. Physostigmine, phenytoin (Dilantin) for seizures.

## C. Sedatives

▶ H&P Keys

Lethargy, confusion, coma, hypotension, respiratory depression, disconjugate eye motion.

▶ Diagnosis

History and physical exam, urine drug screen, blood drug level available.

▶ Disease Severity

Coma scale, respiration depression. Length of time since ingestion and history of amount ingested may assist in severity determination.

▶ Treatment Steps
1. Control of airway, activated charcoal (if patient awake), cautious gastric lavage.
2. Supportive care.

## D. Stimulants

▶ H&P Keys

Euphoria, dilated pupils, hypertension, tremors, tachycardia, hyperactivity, psychosis, hyperthermia, seizures, anxiety, nausea and vomiting.

▶ Diagnosis

History and physical exam (tremor, increased bowel sounds, etc).

▶ Disease Severity

Determined by amount ingested (peak effects 1 to 2 hours after ingestion), coexisting medical problems, cardiac status.

▶ Treatment Steps
1. Supportive (treatment of hypertension, seizures, arrhythmias), charcoal.
2. Emesis may cause seizures.

### E. Cocaine

▶ **H&P Keys**

Agitation, hyperthermia, hypertension, cardiac arrhythmia, tachycardia, seizures, pulmonary edema.

▶ **Diagnosis**

History and physical exam, urine drug screen.

▶ **Disease Severity**

Assess by history, cardiac status.

▶ **Management**

Supportive treatment, control of airway, monitor core temperature.

### F. PCP (Phencyclidine)

▶ **H&P Keys**

Nystagmus, blank stare, psychosis, lethargy, incoordination, violent behavior, self-destructive behavior.

▶ **Diagnosis**

History and physical exam, uring drug screen. May have elevated creatine phosphokinase and myoglobinuria.

▶ **Disease Severity**

Physical exam.

▶ **Treatment Steps**

Control of airway, activated charcoal, supportive therapy.

### G. Alcohol

▶ **H&P Keys**

*Methanol*—Blurry vision, headache, vomiting.

*Ethanol*—Incoordination, diplopia, drunkenness.

▶ **Diagnosis**

History and physical exam, blood alcohol level. May have elevated triglycerides, uric acid, and γ-glutamyl transferase (GGT).

▶ **Disease Severity**

Assess history, impact on the individual and the family, and clinical picture (withdrawal, abnormal lab tests, hepatic function).

▶ **Treatment Steps**

*Methanol*—Antidote (ethanol), sodium bicarbonate, detoxification, and rehabilitation.

*Ethanol*
1. Supportive care, airway protection/control.
2. Prevention includes continued support (AA meetings) and medication (disulfiram).

## H. Solvent Sniffing

▶ H&P Keys

Gastrointestinal (GI) irritation, CNS symptoms. Skin injury.

▶ Diagnosis

History and physical exam.

▶ Disease Severity

Assess duration and frequency of abuse; neurologic exam.

▶ Treatment Steps

Supportive treatment, control of airway, oxygen.

## I. Heavy Metals and Arsenic

▶ H&P Keys

GI symptoms, arrhythmia, CNS symptoms, skin bronzing, cyanosis, delirium, Mees' lines, renal failure, vomiting, garlic odor.

▶ Diagnosis

History and physical exam, roentgenogram of abdomen (arsenic, lead, and iodides may be radiopaque), anemia, hematuria.

▶ Disease Severity

Assess by clinical exam (neurologic, cardiac, and pulmonary status).

▶ Treatment Steps

Emesis, gastric lavage, dimercaprol (BAL), 3–5 mg/kg IM q 4–6 h.

▶ Additional Information

*Lead*—Vomiting, lethargy, blue gum line; lavage, then use edetate calcium disodium (EDTA calcium).

*Mercury*—Give milk, gastric lavage, then dimercaprol. Chelators such as edetate calcium disodium (EDTA calcium), penicillamine, and dimercaprol (BAL) may be used for treatment of heavy metal toxicity.

## J. Carbon Monoxide

▶ H&P Keys

Headache, confusion, nausea, dyspnea, clumsiness, cyanosis, or cherry-red skin.

▶ Diagnosis

History and physical exam (cyanosis), elevated blood carboxyhemoglobin.

▶ Disease Severity

Chronic exposure associated with parkinsonism.

▶ Treatment Steps
1. Removal from source, 100% oxygen.
2. Hyperbaric oxygen (if available) for comatose patients.

### K. Diethyl-*m*-toluamide (DEET)

▶ H&P Keys
CNS symptoms, seizures, coma, hypotension, GI irritation.

▶ Diagnosis
History and physical exam.

▶ Disease Severity
By clinical exam (neurologic status, time since exposure, degree of exposure).

▶ Treatment Steps
Emesis, gastric lavage.

### L. Additional Information

1. Other Poisonings

   *Iron*—Symptoms include diarrhea, abdominal pain, and bloody stools. Gastric lavage, parenteral deferoxamine.

   *Aspirin*—Causes respiratory alkalosis and metabolic acidosis. Patient may be hyperventilating, diaphoretic, and report tinnitus.

   *Theophylline*—Look for tremor, nausea and vomiting, and metabolic acidosis. Blood drug level can be checked.

   *Narcotics*—Pinpoint pupils, hypotension; administration of naloxone hydrochloride (Narcan).

   *Barbiturates*—Respiratory depression, hypotension; supportive care, charcoal, and alkalinization of urine.

2. Selected Antidotes
   Folic acid for methyl alcohol poisoning. D-Penicillamine for copper poisoning. Protamine sulfate for heparin overdose. Latrodectus antivenin for black widow spider bites.

3. Drugs Visible on Roentgenogram
   Heavy metals, phenothiazines, iodides, and chloral hydrate.

4. Poisoning Management Overview
   1. Airway, breathing, circulation: history and physical exam; lab studies; gastric lavage and emesis; antidote after lavage; supportive care; laboratory workup.
   2. Avoid ipecac with caustic ingestion and in somnolent patient.
   3. If antidote available, cautious use of charcoal in addition. Used primarily in children.

## VIII. FRACTURES

### A. Vertebral Column

▶ H&P Keys
Pain, neurologic abnormalities.

▶ Diagnosis
History and physical exam, roentgenographic exam, CT exam.

▶ Disease Severity
Neurologic status, serial evaluations.

▶ Concept and Application
Vertebral body fracture (wedging, body fracture), articular process fracture, transverse process fracture.

▶ Treatment Steps

*Simple Compression Fracture*—Brace (some advocate surgical intervention, especially in young individual).

*Initial Cervical Spine Treatment.*
1. Airway control with cervical spine protection, assess and support breathing, control shock and hemorrhage.
2. For unstable fracture or progressing neurologic deficit, cranial traction followed by surgical internal fixation.
3. Most other simple spinal fractures are treated with bracing or casting, with surgical intervention reserved for progressive neurologic symptoms.

### B. Extremities

#### 1. Tibia

▶ H&P Keys
Pain when pressure applied to the tibia.

▶ Diagnosis
History and physical exam, roentgenogram.

▶ Disease Severity
Determine severity via roentgenogram, coexisting medical problems.

▶ Concept and Application
Trauma.

▶ Treatment Steps

*Tibial Shaft*—Closed reduction and cast or internal fixation with intramedullary rodding.

*Medial Tibial Condyle*—Open reduction and internal fixation (ORIF).

*Lateral Tibial Condyle*—External reduction.

2. **Fibula**

   ▶ **H&P Keys**
   Pain and swelling, with retained ability to walk.

   ▶ **Diagnosis**
   History and physical exam, roentgenographic exam.

   ▶ **Disease Severity**
   Rule out coexisting ankle injury.

   ▶ **Concept and Application**
   Trauma.

   ▶ **Treatment Steps**
   Walking cast or boot, followed by therapy.

3. **Femur**

   ▶ **H&P Keys**
   Pain, swelling, deformity.

   ▶ **Diagnosis**
   History and physical exam, roentgenographic studies.

   ▶ **Disease Severity**
   Evaluate for coexisting medical problems, hypotension.

   ▶ **Concept and Application**
   Usually significant trauma. With children, rule out child abuse.

   ▶ **Treatment Steps**

   *Femoral Neck*
   1. ORIF vs. long-term traction (usually in immobile patients).
   2. *Complications* of femoral neck fractures include avascular necrosis and nonunion of fracture.

4. **Radius**

   ▶ **H&P Keys**
   Pain, reduced elbow-joint motion.

   ▶ **Diagnosis**
   History and physical exam, roentgenographic studies.

   ▶ **Disease Severity**
   Check neurovascular status.

   ▶ **Concept and Application**
   Fall on hand common.

   *Colles' Fracture*—Fall on extended wrist, fracture of distal radius and ulnar styloid (volar angulation and dorsal displacement).

   *Smith's Fracture*—Fall on flexed wrist (dorsal angulation and volar displacement).

▶ Treatment Steps

*Radial Head*
1. Hemarthrosis aspiration and mobilization if simple.
2. Surgical (ORIF) if complete or displaced fracture.

*Distal Radius Undisplaced*—Cast 4–6 weeks, therapy.

5. Ulna

▶ H&P Keys
Pain, swelling, deformity.

▶ Diagnosis
History and physical exam, roentgenogram.

▶ Disease Severity
Check neurovascular status.

▶ Concept and Application
Trauma.

▶ Treatment Steps

*Undisplaced*—Closed or open reduction.

*Displaced*—ORIF.

*Greenstick Radial or Ulnar Fractures in Children*—Complete the break, then cast.

6. Humerus

▶ H&P Keys
Pain, swelling.

▶ Diagnosis
History and physical exam, roentgenographic studies.

▶ Disease Severity
Evaluate neurovascular status.

▶ Concept and Application
Trauma.

▶ Treatment Steps

*Humeral Shaft or Distal Humerus*—Reduction (traction), then splint and sling.

*Surgical Neck of Humerus*
1. Avoid immobilization, instead gentle range of motion.
2. ORIF for displaced tuberosity fracture.

▶ Additional Information

*Childhood Medial or Lateral Epicondyle Fractures*—If without displacement, splint elbow at 90°. With any displacement, ORIF.

## IX. SPRAINS AND DISLOCATIONS

Sprains involve ligament injury; strains affect muscle; dislocations affect joints.

### A. Hands

#### 1. Distal Interphalangeal (DIP) Sprain

▶ H&P Keys

Pain, difficulty with joint flexion or extension.

▶ Diagnosis

History and physical exam, roentgenographic exam.

▶ Disease Severity

Evaluate strength and range of motion.

▶ Concept and Application

DIP joint injury or sprain, resulting in possible flexor–extensor tendon disruption.

▶ Treatment Steps

Symptomatic (if able to bend or extend joint).

▶ Additional Information

*Mallet Finger*—Tendon disruption, with loss of joint extension. Treat with splinting in hyperextension or surgery.

#### 2. Proximal Interphalangeal (PIP) Dislocation

▶ H&P Keys

Pain. Displaced digit and motion loss.

▶ Diagnosis

History and physical exam. Roentgenogram to rule out fracture.

▶ Disease Severity

Examine for neurovascular status.

▶ Concept and Application

Injury secondary to hyperextension, trauma.

▶ Treatment Steps

Flexion splint 2 weeks.

▶ Additional Information

*PIP Sprain*—Splint if a hyperextension injury or collateral ligament sprain (flexion splint). Extensor slip tear-splint in hyperextension.

#### 3. Metacarpal Phalangeal (MCP) Sprain

▶ H&P Keys

Sprained finger or thumb MCP joint resulting in pain and motion loss.

▶ Diagnosis
History and physical exam, roentgenographic exam.

▶ Disease Severity
Evaluate for pinch, laxity of thumb ligaments. Use of hand contingent on adequate thumb strength.

▶ Concept and Application
Trauma, often hyperextension.

▶ Treatment Steps
Splint.

▶ Additional Information

*Gamekeeper's Thumb*—MCP joint of thumb sprained, affecting the ulnar collateral ligament. If suspected requires immobilization of thumb and urgent hand surgeon consultation.

### B. Ankle

#### 1. Lateral Ankle Pain
Injury to anterior talofibular ligament. May also include injury to fibulocalcaneal and posterior talofibular ligaments.

#### 2. Medial Pain
Deltoid ligament injury.

▶ Treatment Steps
1. RICE (rest, ice, compression, elevation).
2. Nonsteroidal anti-inflammatory drugs (NSAIDs).
3. Ankle splint for second-degree sprain; cast for third-degree sprain.

### C. Elbow Dislocation
Check vascular and neurologic status; if urgent reduction indicated, splint.

### D. Shoulder Dislocation or Injury
Anterior-inferior dislocation most common (in young patients).

▶ Treatment Steps

*Dislocation*—Urgent reduction (slow traction or reduction under anesthesia). Other dislocations include posterior and inferior.

*Mild Sprain*—Prevent external rotation for 6 weeks; sling.

## X. DROWNING

▶ H&P Keys
Wheezing, tachypnea, vomiting, pulmonary edema, unconsciousness, shock, and cardiac arrest.

▶ Diagnosis

History and physical exam, chest roentgenogram, ABGs, ECG.

▶ Disease Severity

Consider duration of immersion, patient's baseline medical status, water temperature, timing of rescue measures, cardiac and pulmonary status, electroencephalogram (EEG).

▶ Concept and Application

Dry (laryngospasm) or water-induced asphyxia results in hypoxia and brain damage.

▶ Treatment Steps

1. Urgent CPR and 100% oxygen.
2. Remember to continue CPR in hypothermic or prolonged cold-water submersion victims.

## XI. INSECT AND SNAKE BITES

▶ H&P Keys

*Insect Bite*—Mild erythema to anaphylaxis and hypotension.

*Snake Bite*—Pain, swelling, hemorrhage, weakness, disseminated intravascular coagulation (DIC), possible systemic signs (lethargy, vomiting, shock).

▶ Diagnosis

History and physical exam. Leukocytosis and coagulation disorders.

▶ Disease Severity

Assess cardiac and pulmonary status. Consider patient's age and preexisting medical problems, time since envenomation, location of bite (trunk has worse outcome than extremity), snake size (larger worse), and emergency treatment received.

▶ Concept and Application

*Insects*—Hymenoptera species commonly.

*Snakes*—In United States, pit vipers (copperhead, rattlesnake, water moccasin) are responsible for poisonous bites and are toxic to cardiac, vascular, and hematologic systems.

▶ Treatment Steps

*Insect Bite*—Remove stinger, ice, diphenhydramine hydrochloride (Benadryl).

*Anaphylaxis*—Epinephrine (1:1000 0.3 mL SQ), antihistamines, prednisone.

*Snake Bite*—Tourniquet, antivenin.

▶ Additional Information

*Black Widow Spider* (**Latrodectus mactans**)—Red hourglass pattern on abdomen, bite results in muscle spasm and cramping. First, clean wound, give tetanus toxoid, muscle relaxant, antivenin.

*Brown Recluse Spider* (**Loxosceles reclusa**)—Violin design on back; possible skin necrosis; treat by cleaning wound and tetanus toxoid.

## XII. ANAPHYLACTIC SHOCK

Systemic severe IgE-induced allergic reaction.

▶ H&P Keys

Hypotension, urticaria, dyspnea, tachycardia, vascular collapse, pruritus.

▶ Diagnosis

History (onset of symptoms in seconds to minutes) and physical exam.

▶ Disease Severity

Assess cardiac and pulmonary systems. Prognosis worse without early intervention.

▶ Concept and Application

Mast cell and basophils release histamine, platelet-activating factor (PAF), and arachidonic acid.

▶ Treatment Steps
1. CPR and control airway.
2. Epinephrine (1:1000 0.3 to 0.5 mL SQ or 1:10,000 0.5–1 mg slow IV administration if in shock), diphenhydramine hydrochloride (Benadryl), fluids, dopamine, inhaled β-agonists, β-agonists, corticosteroids, oxygen.

## XIII. ADDITIONAL MANAGEMENT INFORMATION

### A. Traumatic Injury

Administer CPR, control airway, treat urgent problems (large pneumothorax, hemorrhage, etc), administer oxygen, insert IV line, give fluids and medications, obtain history and physical exam, roentgenographic and lab studies.

### B. Shock

Administer CPR, control airway, obtain history and physical exam, administer fluids (caution with cardiogenic shock, check CPV and output), administer vasopressors (dopamine), get lab studies, administer: corticosteroids, diuretic (protects kidneys), buffers, antibiotics (septic shock).

## C. Child Abuse, Sexual Abuse, Sexual Assault

History and physical exam, medical treatment, documentation of evidence and appropriate reporting, psychologic evaluation and support, separation from danger (child abuse), and long-term care plan.

## D. Thermal Injuries

### 1. Frostbite

▶ H&P Keys

Tissue cold and hard without feeling.

▶ Diagnosis

History and physical exam; affected area may be white (superficial injury) or firm and frozen (deep injury).

▶ Disease Severity

Duration of exposure, prior presence of peripheral vascular disease or other medical problems.

▶ Concept and Application

Tissue damage as a direct result of thermal trauma. Skin and tissue damage from ice crystal formation. May be superficial or deep. Line of demarcation may develop.

▶ Treatment Steps

Rapid rewarming after body core temperature warming, tetanus toxoid, possibly antibiotics, surgical evaluation, amputation.

### 2. Hypothermia

▶ H&P Keys

Reduced core temperature (under 35°C), lethargy, coma, hypotension, confusion, miotic pupils.

▶ Diagnosis

History and physical exam, core temperature at or below 95°F (35°C), ECG (Osborne wave, elevated J-point; bradycardia; arrhythmias), flat EEG, metabolic acidosis.

▶ Disease Severity

Assess duration of exposure, age (mortality much worse in the elderly), emergency treatment rendered, and preexisting medical problems. Worse prognosis with lower temperatures.

▶ Concept and Application

Reduced core temperature from cold exposure resulting in decreased cardiac output, hypotension.

▶ Treatment Steps
1. CPR, core rewarming (heated oxygen), warming blankets, volume expansion.
2. Monitor ABGs, electrolytes, and rule out sepsis.

▶ Additional Information

*Hypothermia Complications*—DIC, pneumonia.

*Hypothermic Death*—Never declare dead unless patient rewarmed to 98.6°F.

3. Heatstroke

▶ H&P Keys

Confusion, elevated core temperature with or without diaphoresis, tachycardia, hypotension, hot skin, and headache.

▶ Diagnosis

History and physical exam, core temperature high, combined with CNS signs.

▶ Disease Severity

Assess cardiovascular status. Worse prognosis with significant pre-existing disease.

▶ Concept and Application

Tissue injury from elevated temperature, with children and elderly at most risk.

▶ Treatment Steps

Urgent cooling (water spray, fans, ice packs).

▶ Additional Information

*Heat Cramps*—Cramps from salt depletion; skin cool; give fluids and salt, keep cool.

*Heat Exhaustion*—Salt and water loss; nausea, weakness, headache, thirst; give fluids and salt, keep cool.

*Complications of Heatstroke*—DIC, rhabdomyolysis, acidosis.

## XIV. EPIDEMIOLOGY AND PREVENTION OF SELECTED ACCIDENTS

### A. Home Accidents

*Epidemiology*—Involves all age groups and consists of a wide variety of hazards (electrical, thermal, poisoning, and trauma).

*Prevention*—Includes education, preventive planning (bicycle helmets, toy and playground equipment checks, removal of dangerous objects, obstacles, etc).

### B. Workplace Accidents

*Epidemiology*—Includes increased risk groups (meatcutters and packers, steelworkers, etc), along with all employees.

*Prevention*—Includes both education and exercise of precautions (eye shield, hearing protection, hard hats, steel-tip shoes, etc) and elimination of dangerous materials, practices, and procedures.

### C. Athletic Accidents

*Epidemiology*—Includes home, school, recreational, and professional accidents. Impact and type of injuries are multiple, including falls, trauma, thermal injury, sprains and strains, fractures, concussions, contusions, and death.

*Prevention*—Includes education, correction of both training and performance errors (spearing in football), providing protective equipment of correct fit.

### D. Automobile Accidents and Drunk Driving

*Epidemiology*—Includes all ages of society, with increased risk for both teenagers (drunk and reckless driving) and the elderly (visual impairment, cognitive functioning, and reaction time). Increased risk is associated with motorcycle and three-wheel all-terrain vehicle use.

*Prevention*—Includes education (driving, using seat belts, avoidance of drugs and alcohol), reduced speed limits, better roads, improved roadway markings and median barriers, and abutment protection. Numerous other factors play a role, such as larger-size vehicles, air bags, collapsible steering wheel, and padded dash regulations. Drunk driving prevention includes both education and modification of drinking age, along with effective legal deterrents (fines and jail terms).

### E. Head and Spinal Cord Injury and Whiplash

*Epidemiology*—Includes motor vehicle accidents (the major cause of these injuries), falls, child abuse, occupational and trauma-induced accidents.

*Prevention*—Includes education, safety devices (automotive: air bags, seat and shoulder belts, padded dashboards, headrests; work: hard hats, etc), and behavior modification (avoidance of high-risk activities or behavior). Appropriate emergency care may prevent permanent neurologic sequelae (sandbag, head stabilization).

### F. Drowning

*Epidemiology*—Involves children most often.

*Prevention*—Centers on education (parents and children), swimming instruction, water and boating safety, dangers of hyperventilation, dangers of drug and alcohol use, and CPR training. Recognition of high-risk patients (epilepsy, syncope, divers, children, etc).

### G. Ingestion of Poisonous and Toxic Agents

*Epidemiology*—Includes accidental overdose in both children and adults and work and environmental toxicology and suicide in adolescents and adults.

*Prevention*—Includes education, awareness and labeling of dangerous substances, prevention of child access (keeping medication and toxins locked and in unaccessible locations, "childproof" containers), and easy access to emergency advice and treatment. Importance of home supply of ipecac.

### H. Gunshot and Stab Wounds

*Epidemiology*—Demonstrates an increasing rate of violent crime and increasing use of handguns and automatic weapons. Elevated level of crime in poor socioeconomic areas. Impact includes an ever-increasing utilization of medical emergency facilities, financial burden on the medical insurance system, and morbidity and mortality, including innocent bystanders.

*Prevention*—Includes education, gun control, control of alcohol and drug use and abuse, law enforcement, and society efforts to diffuse inner-city neglect.

### I. Thermal Injury

*Prevention*—Key points include education (increased heat disorders with alcohol; cystic fibrosis patients; dehydration; dark, nonbreathable clothing; use of antipsychotics and diuretic; high-humidity days) and need for increased fluid intake and gradual heat acclimatization. Skin protection and early recognition of symptoms in frostbite and hypothermia patients is critical. Increased awareness for high-risk patients (elderly and children, alcohol and drug abusers, CNS disease, and sepsis) is important.

### J. Child, Spouse, and Elderly Abuse

*Epidemiology*—Suggests that susceptible abuse victims include children, spouses, and the elderly. Impact is significant as a frequent society malady with great morbidity, mortality, and possible permanent psychologic impact. Difficulty in obtaining accurate numbers of cases involved because of sensitivity of the subject and reluctance of many abused individuals to tell their stories.

*Prevention*—Physician and family education to obtain early diagnosis and screen for potentially abusive parents (observe and evaluate mother for postpartum depression). High index of suspicion may be required. Past medical history (abusers may have been abused themselves as children).

### K. Sexual Abuse and Rape

*Epidemiology*—Suggests that adolescents and young children are at risk for sexual abuse (usually by family member).

*Prevention*—Includes early recognition by health care workers, and education. Rape prevention includes patient education (how to avoid being a target) and self-defense.

### L. Fire Prevention

*Prevention*—Includes education (not smoking in bed, proper storage of flammables, etc), home precautions (smoke detectors and fire extinguisher, fireplace glass screen, fire safety plan, escape route, upkeep of electrical systems, etc).

### M. Falls

*Epidemiology*—Affect children, elderly, and adults (workplace injury, seizure-disorder patients, alcoholics) and are a frequent cause of accidental death. Significant morbidity and mortality associated with hip fractures.

*Prevention*—For children includes child-proofing the house, covering sharp corners, window locks, stair gates, and control of obstacles. For the elderly, medical and family assessment for need of cane, walker, or wheelchair; medical treatment or control of contributing illness (Parkinson's disease, visual impairment, anemia, stroke, etc).

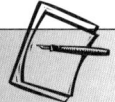

▶ on rounds

---

#### POISONING SYMPTOMS AT A GLANCE

- Carbon monoxide: Headache, confusion, cyanosis, cherry-red skin
- DEET: CNS symptoms
- Iron: Diarrhea, abdominal pain, bloody stools
- Theophylline: Tremor, nausea, vomiting
- Aspirin: Respiratory alkalosis, metabolic acidosis, hyperventilation, tinnitus
- Stimulants: Dilated pupils, euphoria, hypertension, tremor
- Cocaine: Agitation, hyperthermia, hypertension, arrhythmia
- PCP: Nystagmus, blank stare, violent behavior, incoordination
- Acetaminophen: Nausea and vomiting
- Sedatives: Lethargy, confusion, coma, hypotension
- Heavy metal and arsenic: GI symptoms, CNS symptoms, skin bronzing

# BIBLIOGRAPHY

Ballenger JJ. *Diseases of the Nose, Throat, Ear, Head, and Neck.* 14th ed. Philadelphia: Lea & Febiger; 1991.

Behrman RE. *Nelson Textbook of Pediatrics.* 16th ed. Philadelphia: WB Saunders Co; 2000.

Birnbaum JS. *The Musculoskeletal Manual.* 2nd ed. Orlando, FL: Academic Press Inc; 1986.

Bryson PD. *Comprehensive Review in Toxicology.* 2nd ed. Rockville, MD: Aspen Publishers Inc; 1989.

Cailliet R. *Neck and Arm Pain.* 3rd ed. Philadelphia: FA Davis Co; 1991.

D'Ambrosia RD. *Musculoskeletal Disorders, Regional Examination and Differential Diagnosis.* 2nd ed. Philadelphia: JB Lippincott Co; 1986.

Dreisbach RH. *Handbook of Poisoning: Prevention, Diagnosis and Treatment.* 13th ed. Norwalk, CT: Appleton & Lange; 2001.

Goldfrank LR, Flomenbaum NE, Lewin NA, et al, eds. *Goldfrank's Toxicologic Emergencies.* 7th ed. Stamford, CT: Appleton & Lange, 2002.

Hardy JD. *Textbook of Surgery.* 2nd ed. Philadelphia: JB Lippincott Co; 1988.

Rockwood CA. *Fractures in Adults.* 3rd ed. Philadelphia: JB Lippincott Co; 1991; 1, 2.

Tierney L. *Current Medical Diagnosis and Treatment.* New York: McGraw-Hill, 2003.

Turek SL. *Orthopaedic Principles and Their Application.* 4th ed. Philadelphia: JB Lippincott Co; 1984; 1, 2.

Upton AC. Environmental medicine. *Med Clin North Am.* Philadelphia: WB Saunders Co; 1990.

# Infectious Disease 8

I. **HUMAN IMMUNODEFICIENCY VIRUS INFECTION AND THE ACQUIRED IMMUNE DEFICIENCY SYNDROME / 248**
   A. Human Immunodeficiency Virus Infection / 248
   B. *Pneumocystis carinii* Pneumonia / 252
   C. Cytomegalovirus (CMV) Infection / 253
   D. Tuberculosis / 254
   E. Disseminated *Mycobacterium avium-intracellulare* Complex / 255
   F. Toxoplasma Encephalitis / 256
   G. Cryptococcal Infection / 257
   H. Herpes Simplex Virus / 258

II. **SEXUALLY TRANSMITTED DISEASES / 259**
   A. Gonorrhea / 259
   B. Chlamydia / 260
   C. Syphilis / 260
   D. Chancroid / 262
   E. Pelvic Inflammatory Disease / 262
   F. Epididymo-orchitis / 263
   G. Genital Herpes / 263

III. **OTHER INFECTIOUS DISEASES / 264**
   A. Infectious Mononucleosis / 264
   B. Varicella (Chickenpox) / 265
   C. Measles (Rubeola) / 265
   D. Mumps / 266
   E. Rubella (German Measles) / 266
   F. Lyme Disease / 267

**BIBLIOGRAPHY / 268**

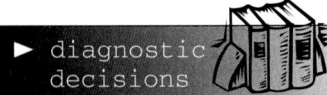
## diagnostic decisions

### HIV DIAGNOSIS—FACTORS LEADING TO SUSPICION

**Risk Factors**
Sexual contact, sharing needles, unscreened blood or blood products, maternal/fetal.

**Clinical Features Before Developing Opportunistic Infection**
Weight loss/wasting, fatigue, adenopathy, diarrhea, oral lesions, cognitive deficits.

**Opportunistic Infections**
*Pneumocystis carinii* pneumonia, *Mycobacterium avium* complex infection, toxoplasmosis, cryptococcal meningitis, unexplained thrush or esophageal candidal infection.

**Unexplained "Normal Infections"**
Tuberculosis, syphilis, severe pneumococcal disease, histoplasmosis.

**Malignancies**
Kaposi's sarcoma, lymphoma, Hodgkin's disease.

## I. HUMAN IMMUNODEFICIENCY VIRUS INFECTION AND THE ACQUIRED IMMUNE DEFICIENCY SYNDROME

### A. Human Immunodeficiency Virus Infection

▶ H&P Keys

Human immunodeficiency virus (HIV) infection is acquired by sexual transmission, direct blood contact, or from mother to child. About 4–6 weeks after exposure to HIV, an acute mononucleosis-like illness lasting for 1–2 weeks consisting of fever, malaise, lymphadenopathy, rash, headache, arthralgias, or myalgias occurs in most but not all people. Following primary infection, there is an asymptomatic period of variable duration. There is active viral replication and reduced immune function during this period. Ultimately, the patient may develop systemic complaints such as sweats, weight loss, diarrhea, and/or an opportunistic infection (see individual descriptions of common opportunistic infections [OIs] for clinical clues) or malignant disease associated with the HIV-related immunosuppression. Without treatment, rate of progression of disease is highly variable, with an average period of 10 years from HIV infection to acquired immune deficiency syndrome (AIDS).

▶ Diagnosis

HIV serologic testing (enzyme-linked immunosorbent assay [ELISA], Western blot test) is indicated for work-up of unexplained symptoms or for those at risk. Further work-up in the HIV-positive patient has three elements: (1) tracking immune function (CD4+-positive T-lymphocyte count [CD4+]); (2) following viral burden (quantitative viral RNA levels or branched chain DNA [b-DNA]); (3) general tests such as complete blood count (CBC), chemistry (including liver tests), VDRL or rapid plasma reagin (RPR), purified protein derivative (PPD), hepatitis B serology, cytomegalovirus (CMV) serology, toxoplasmosis serology, Pap smear. Viral load measurements help to predict the initial rate of progression to AIDS and to select, maintain, and modify effective antiretroviral therapy.

▶ Disease Severity

Association between development of OIs and absolute (normal = 800–1,200) or percentage (normal = 55–70%) CD4+. As CD4+ declines, risk of OI increases substantially. With CD4+ > 800, risk of OI very small; CD4+ 200 to 500, increasing risk for *Mycobacterium tuberculosis, Histoplasma, Cryptococcus;* CD4+ < 200, risk for *Pneumocystis carinii* pneumonia (PCP); CD4+ < 100, increasing risk for Toxoplasma, CMV, *Mycobacterium avium* complex (MAC). OIs associated with the majority of AIDS deaths. Classification of HIV infection modified to include CD4+ as marker for HIV-related immunodeficiency (Table 8–1). Categorization is based on clinical conditions associated with HIV infection and CD4+ count. Clinical category A includes acute primary infection, asymptomatic HIV infection, and persistent generalized lymphadenopathy (PGL). Conditions in category B include bacillary angiomato-

### 8-1 1993 REVISED CLASSIFICATION SYSTEM FOR HIV INFECTION AND EXPANDED AIDS SURVEILLANCE CASE DEFINITION FOR ADOLESCENTS AND ADULTS[a]

| CD4+ T-cell Categories | Clinical Categories | | |
|---|---|---|---|
| | (A) Asymptomatic, Acute (Primary) HIV or PGL | (B) Symptomatic, not (A) or (C) Conditions | (C) AIDS-Indicator Conditions[b] |
| 1. ≥ 500/μL | A1 | B1 | C1 |
| 2. 200–499/μL | A2 | B2 | C2 |
| 3. < 200/μL AIDS-indicator T-cell count | A3 | B3 | C3 |

[a]Persons with the AIDS-indicator conditions (category C) as well as those with CD4+ T-lymphocyte counts < 200/μL are reportable as AIDS cases.
[b]See text AIDS case definition.
PGL, persistent generalized lymphadenopathy.

sis, oropharyngeal candidiasis, persistent vulvovaginal candidiasis, cervical dysplasia or carcinoma in situ, constitutional symptoms (fever or diarrhea for more than 1 month), hairy leukoplakia, herpes zoster (more than two episodes or more than one dermatome), idiopathic thrombocytopenic purpura (ITP), listeriosis, pelvic inflammatory disease (PID), or peripheral neuropathy. Category C includes the clinical conditions listed in the AIDS surveillance case definition (Table 8–2). All patients in clinical category C as well as all with a CD4+ < 200 meet the case definition of AIDS. People with a high HIV viral load are at increased risk for

### 8-2 CONDITIONS INCLUDED IN THE 1993 AIDS SURVEILLANCE CASE DEFINITION

- Candidiasis of bronchi, trachea, or lungs
- Candidiasis, esophageal
- Cervical cancer, invasive
- Coccidioidomycosis, disseminated or extrapulmonary
- Cryptococcosis, extrapulmonary
- Cryptosporidiosis, chronic intestinal (> 1 mo duration)
- Cytomegalovirus disease (other than liver, spleen, or nodes)
- Cytomegalovirus retinitis (with loss of vision)
- Encephalopathy (HIV-related)
- Herpes simplex: chronic ulcer(s) (> 1 mo duration), or bronchitis, pneumonitis, or esophagitis
- Histoplasmosis, disseminated or extrapulmonary
- Isosporiasis, chronic intestinal (> 1 mo duration)
- Kaposi's sarcoma
- Lymphoma, Burkitt's (or equivalent term)
- Lymphoma, immunoblastic (or equivalent term)
- Lymphoma, primary, of brain
- *Mycobacterium avium-intracellulare* complex of *M. kansasii*, disseminated or extrapulmonary
- *M. Tuberculosis*, any site (pulmonary or extrapulmonary)
- *Pneumocystis carinii* pneumonia
- Pneumonia, recurrent
- Progressive multifocal leukoencephalopathy
- *Salmonella*, septicemia, recurrent
- Toxoplasmosis of brain
- Wasting syndrome caused by HIV

disease progression. Initiation or modification of antiretroviral therapy may be dictated based on these results.

### ▶ Concept and Application

The etiologic agent of AIDS is the human retrovirus, HIV. The CD4+-positive T lymphocyte is the primary target of infection because of the CD4+ surface marker. Loss of CD4+ T lymphocytes results in progressive impairment of the immune response. There is a wide spectrum of disease, from asymptomatic infection to life-threatening illness, caused by OI or cancer. HIV binds CD4+ cells and then fuses with the membrane to enter the cell. The virus uncoats, and reverse transcriptase transcribes viral RNA into DNA, which is integrated into the host chromosome. The latent virus reactivates, DNA is transcribed into RNA, viral proteins are synthesized, and new virus is assembled (mediated by HIV protease) budding from the cell membrane. Antiviral chemotherapy may be aimed at any point in the viral life cycle. Reverse transcriptase (nucleoside, nucleotide, and nonnucleoside reverse transcriptase inhibitors) and protease (protease inhibitors) are the only viral targets thus far utilized in antiretroviral therapy. Our knowledge concerning HIV viral dynamics and host CD4+ dynamics has recently expanded markedly. The HIV viral load is quite high during initial infection and then, after approximately 3 months, falls to a steady-state level. These steady-state levels vary considerably from person to person (approximately $10^2$ to $10^6$ HIV RNA copies/mL). The CD4+ count also falls during acute HIV infection and then rebounds to a steady-state level. We now appreciate that even during the so-called latent phase of infection when the HIV viral load and CD4+ count appear stable, there is tremendous daily turnover of both HIV and CD4+. Understanding these dynamics has important treatment implications. The high mutational rate of HIV, occurring constantly, has greatly influenced the rapid acceptance of combination therapy in an effort to escape or delay antiretroviral resistance. The initial steady-state HIV load has predictive value for the rapidity of disease progression. People with very high viral load are at risk for rapid progression, whereas those with very low viral burden may be long-term nonprogressors. The HIV viral load has also important implications for monitoring and modifying antiretroviral therapy (see Treatment Steps). Some AIDS-indicator conditions are caused directly by HIV infection (AIDS encephalopathy, wasting syndrome [cytokine dysregulation], enteropathy, nephropathy).

### ▶ Treatment Steps

1. The antiretroviral armamentarium has expanded markedly.
2. There are four classes of antiretroviral agents approved for use in the United States. There are five nucleoside reverse transcriptase inhibitors, including zidovudine (AZT, ZDV, Retrovir), didanosine (ddI, Videx), zalcitabine (ddC, Hivid), stavudine (d4T, Zerit), lamivudine (3TC, Epivir), and abacavir (Ziagen). There are six HIV protease inhibitors approved, including saquinavir (Invirase, Fortovase), ritonavir (Norvir), indinavir (Crixivan), lopinavir/ritonavir (Kaletra), atazanavir (Zrivada), and amprenavir. There are three nonnucleoside re-

verse transcriptase inhibitors currently available, nevirapine (Viramune), delaverdine (Rescriptor), and efavirenz (Sustiva). Tenofovir (Viread) is a nucleotide reverse transcriptase inhibitor. Fusion inhibitors should be available soon as an injectable anti-retroviral agent.

3. Immune modulation (eg, interleukin-2) is an intriguing option under study.
4. Therapy of HIV infection is based on CD4+ count, HIV RNA level, and clinical status. The optimal time to initiate antiretroviral is unknown and remains an area of controversy. Most would initiate antiretroviral therapy in symptomatic HIV disease, in asymptomatic individuals with a CD4+ of < 500, and in asymptomatic persons with a CD4+ of > 500 but with a high viral load and/or a rapidly declining CD4+ count.
5. Preferred initial antiretroviral regimens include nucleoside combinations such as AZT/3TC in combination with a protease inhibitor such as nelfinavir or a nonnucleoside agent such as efavirenz. Another approach is a combination of two protease inhibitors such as indinavir and ritonavir. The specific agents may be determined by the exposure history of the source (if known) or by patient preference vis-à-vis dosing schedule, side effects, etc. Twice-a-day regimens are preferred over multiple-times-a-day approaches. Once-daily treatment would be even better. The total number of pills can be reduced by using combination tablets. Once-a-day regimens are also available and seem to have a high rate of compliance.
6. Changes in recommended regimens are frequent and drug combinations and dosages must be reassessed frequently as new information is available. The minimal decrease in HIV RNA indicative of effective therapy is > 0.5 log decrease. The goal level of HIV RNA after initiation of treatment is undetectable or at least < 400 copies/mL. However some patients who are clinically stable and are tolerating their medications may be able to meet a less rigorous goal. A return of the HIV RNA level to within 0.3–0.5 log of the pretreatment value suggests drug treatment failure and the need to modify therapy. Such modifications can be based on in vitro susceptibility testing (preferred) or on clinical judgment.
7. New drugs should not be added one at a time since this favors the gradual emergence of resistance.
8. HIV RNA measurements should be obtained at baseline, 3–4 weeks after initiating or changing therapy, and every 3–4 months along with CD4+ counts.

*Health Maintenance*—Pneumococcal vaccine, hepatitis B vaccine (if seronegative) and annual influenza vaccine should be given. (See comments in the specific OI section for prophylaxis recommendations for PCP, MAC, etc.) Those patients who are able to restore near-normal immune function can generally stop their prophylaxis for OI. It is important to note that during the restoration of immune function, some patients will experience some apparent exacerbation of symptoms related to OIs. Counseling and HIV testing should be offered to all pregnant women. Anti-retroviral therapy administration and cesarean section delivery have been documented to reduce significantly perinatal transmission of HIV. The risk of neonatal acquisition of HIV is below 5%. Postexposure prophylaxis for health care workers may reduce the probability of HIV transmission. The Centers for Disease Control and Prevention has published recommendations for this indication depending on the type and source of the exposure. Combination prophylaxis with ZDV, 3TC, and indinavir has been recommended.

## B. *Pneumocystis carinii* Pneumonia

▶ H&P Keys

The most common AIDS defining illness in the United States. Usually presents with subacute shortness of breath and dry cough (median symptom duration before presentation is 4 weeks).

▶ Diagnosis

Usually develops when CD4+ < 200. Arterial blood gas: hypoxemia, increased A-a gradient. Chest radiograph usually shows bilateral infiltrates. Definitive diagnosis by demonstrating organism in pulmonary specimen (induced sputum, bronchoalveolar lavage [BAL], biopsy). Cysts commonly visualized with silver stain, trophozoites with Giemsa stain.

▶ Disease Severity

Mild disease (patient may be candidate for oral, outpatient therapy): $Po_2$ > 70 mm Hg, able to take oral medication, reliable follow-up. More severe hypoxemia and tachypnea are poor prognostic features.

▶ Concept and Application

*P. carinii* has now been shown to be a fungus, albeit quite distinct from all other fungi implicated in human infection. Infection with *P. carinii* can occur early in life but rarely causes disease in the normal host. HIV-related immunosuppression, severe malnutrition, lymphopoietic malignancy, and organ transplantation allow *P. carinii* to cause disease.

▶ Treatment Steps
1. Mild disease may be treated orally; severe disease is treated parenterally.
2. Drug of choice is considered to be trimethoprim–sulfamethoxazole (TMP-SMZ).
3. Alternative agents include pentamidine, dapsone and trimethoprim, clindamycin and primaquine, atovaquone, or trimetrexate and leucovorin.
4. Duration of therapy is usually 21 days. For nonventilated patients with more severe disease (room air $Po_2$ < 70, A-a gradient > 35 mm Hg), a short course of adjunctive corticosteroids is recommended at the inception of treatment.

*Health Maintenance*—Primary PCP prophylaxis is recommended for all HIV-infected individuals with a CD4+ < 200. Secondary prophylaxis is indicated for all with a previous episode of PCP. Drug of choice is TMP-SMZ with alternatives, including dapsone with or without trimethoprim or pyrimethamine,

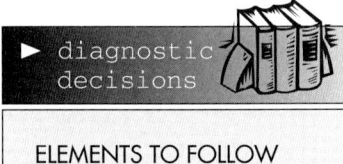

**ELEMENTS TO FOLLOW IN HIV INFECTED ADULT**

**Clinical**
Weight loss, sense of well-being, cognitive function, functional status new infection, new malignancy.

**Laboratory—Immune**
CD4+ absolute count, CD4+/CD8+ ratio, skin test reactivity.

**Laboratory—Virologic**
Level of HIV RNA (by PCR of b-DNA), genotypic.

aerosolized or IV pentamidine, or clindamycin and primaquine. People receiving active treatment for toxoplasmosis need not take PCP prophylaxis. For people with stable increase in CD4+ cells above 250/mm$^3$, prophylaxis can be discontinued.

## C. Cytomegalovirus (CMV) Infection

▶ H&P Keys

CMV infection is the most common viral OI in advanced AIDS. The most common infections are retinitis, gastrointestinal (GI) tract (colitis, esophagitis), and systemic (viremia associated with wasting syndrome). Ocular complaints include "floaters," decreased vision, or blindness. Ophthalmoscopic exam is diagnostic. Colitis is associated with persistent diarrhea and crampy abdominal pain. Esophagitis presents with odynophagia. Wasting syndrome consists of significant weight loss with fever or diarrhea.

▶ Diagnosis

CMV retinitis diagnosed by ophthalmoscopic exam revealing exudates and inflammatory changes following a vascular distribution. Isolation of CMV from other body sites confirms the ophthalmoscopic impression. CMV colitis or esophagitis is diagnosed by endoscopy revealing edema, erythema, erosions, and hemorrhage. Cytomegalic inclusions seen on histopathologic exam are diagnostic. CMV may be recovered from buffy coat blood culture in some patients with the wasting syndrome.

▶ Disease Severity

The severity of CMV retinitis often is dictated by the anatomic location of lesions. Macular involvement severely affects vision; optic nerve involvement may cause blindness.

▶ Concept and Application

CMV infection is common in the general population, but significant disease is rare in the normal host. HIV-related immunosuppression allows for reactivation of latent viral infection or severe progressive new infection. Shedding of virus in urine, saliva, or blood documents viral presence but does not prove disease.

▶ Treatment Steps

1. For patients with symptomatic infection or proved retinitis, a two-step approach to therapy is recommended.
2. Induction therapy is given with either ganciclovir or foscarnet for an average of 14–21 days.
3. Both drugs effectively suppress retinitis but cannot cure infection.
4. Maintenance therapy must be given lifelong to prevent recurrence.
5. Patients who can suppress HIV to the point of regaining significant immune function (evidenced by rising CD4+ counts over 200) may be able to stop therapy.
6. Efficacy of either agent for disease other than retinitis is less well documented, but these drugs are often used for CMV gastrointestinal disease.

7. Neutropenia or thrombocytopenia with ganciclovir and renal insufficiency and electrolyte disturbance with foscarnet are frequently dose limiting.
8. Long-term maintenance therapy with ganciclovir is associated with a risk of emergence of ganciclovir resistance, dictating treatment with foscarnet.
9. Cidofovir is available for the treatment and maintenance therapy of CMV retinitis in patients with AIDS. Because of its long half-life, cidofovir is given once weekly for therapy and every other week for maintenance. Pharmacokinetics may allow for outpatient induction and maintenance without long-term IV access. Nephrotoxicity and neutropenia have limited the initial enthusiasm for this therapy, and the role of cidofovir is still being clarified.
10. Oral valganciclovir is also approved for maintenance/preventive therapy of CMV retinitis. It is much better absorbed than oral ganciclovir but it is very expensive.
11. Ganciclovir intraocular implants are effective, but without systemic therapy there is a risk of disease in the contralateral eye or of systemic disease.

***Health Maintenance***—Oral valganciclovir is available as prophylaxis for CMV disease in AIDS.

### D. Tuberculosis

▶ H&P Keys

In the mid-1980s there was a resurgence of tuberculosis (TB) in the United States, with many of the cases present in HIV-infected individuals. This is now leveling off and actually decreasing again. Symptoms are usually pulmonary in nature or may reflect extrapulmonary disease. The most common extrapulmonary sites are peripheral lymph nodes and bone marrow. Other extrapulmonary sites include bone and joint, urine, liver, spleen, GI mucosa, and cerebrospinal fluid (CSF). TB may present as wasting syndrome. TB in early HIV infection tends to be similar to disease in non–HIV-infected patients. TB in later-stage HIV disease is more commonly atypical.

▶ Diagnosis

Pulmonary TB often occurs at a CD4+ of 250 to 500; extrapulmonary TB more commonly occurs at a lower CD4+, often < 200. Skin testing with PPD may be unreliable because of skin test anergy but should be done as it poses no increased risk. Chest roentgenography may show typical nodular infiltrates, with or without cavitation (apical lung fields most common), or more atypical lesions. Isolation of *M. tuberculosis* from pulmonary or other sites is diagnostic.

▶ Disease Severity

Though response to therapy is often good, the prognosis for AIDS patients with tuberculosis is worse because of overall reduced patient survival. Mortality rates are higher and median survival time shorter in the AIDS patient. Disseminated or extrapulmonary disease is more common with advanced immunodeficiency.

▶ Concept and Application

HIV-related immunosuppression increases the frequency and severity of TB disease. The HIV-infected person is at risk for developing active disease from a new exposure as well as from reactivation of previously acquired, inactive disease. Furthermore, people with prior resolved TB can become reinfected when their immunity is severely depressed by HIV.

▶ Treatment Steps

1. A minimum treatment course of 9 months is recommended in AIDS patients.
2. In patients without previous treatment for TB and living in an area where drug resistance is low, a four-drug regimen (isoniazid [INH], rifampin, pyrazinamide, and ethambutol) is recommended for initial treatment.
3. In patients with a history of previous TB treatment, contact with multidrug-resistant TB, or living in an area with frequent drug resistance, five or more initial anti-TB drugs are indicated.
4. These regimens consist of the standard four drugs **plus** ofloxacin, ciprofloxacin, or streptomycin or other second-line anti-TB drugs.
5. Even with these regimens, the likelihood of response for documented multi-resistant TB is disappointing.
6. Direct observed therapy (DOT) should be used whenever possible with susceptible or resistance TB.

*Health Maintenance*—Twelve months of isoniazid is indicated for all HIV-infected people with a positive PPD. A 2-month course of rifampin and pyrazinamide is also effective but may be more toxic.

### E. Disseminated *Mycobacterium avium-intracellulare* Complex

▶ H&P Keys

Disseminated MAC is the most common systemic opportunistic bacterial infection in patients with AIDS. MAC most commonly causes lymphadenopathy and disseminated infection. Persistent fever and significant weight loss are common. Other associated symptoms include chronic diarrhea or malabsorption and abdominal pain. Lymphadenopathy, organomegaly, or an abdominal mass may be present.

▶ Diagnosis

Abnormal liver tests, anemia, and leukopenia are common. Diagnosis requires isolation of the organism from blood or tissue (bone marrow, lymph node, or liver are commonly positive).

▶ Disease Severity

There are a tremendous number of organisms present in the blood and tissues of AIDS patients with disseminated MAC. Despite the number of organisms, most patients remain asymptomatic until late-stage disease. Survival without therapy is only about 4 months, although MAC is seldom the *cause* of death.

▶ Concept and Application

MAC is ubiquitous in the environment and acquisition in AIDS is thought to result from ingestion or inhalation of organisms. MAC is minimally virulent and rarely cause disease in the immunocompetent host. The immune dysfunction in AIDS allows for disseminated infection. Disseminated MAC almost always occurs when the CD4+ is < 100, usually when the CD4+ is < 50.

▶ Treatment Steps

1. MAC is resistant to most antituberculous agents.
2. Effective therapy has been shown to sterilize blood cultures and reduce the symptoms associated with infection, such as fever and night sweats. Not all patients enjoy a complete response.
3. Current recommendations for therapy include either clarithromycin or azithromycin with ethambutol.
4. Sicker patients should receive one or more additional drugs from among rifabutin, ciprofloxacin, and amikacin.
5. Therapy is continued for life or until immune reconstitution has occurred.

*Health Maintenance*—Prophylaxis is indicated for HIV-positive patients with a CD4+ of < 100, as it appears to reduce disseminated MAC by approximately 55% to 85%. In order of decreasing efficacy, azithromycin **plus** rifabutin, clarithromycin, azithromycin, and rifabutin, are all approved for MAC prophylaxis. The combination regimen is the least tolerated and most expensive. There is a risk of emergence of resistance with a macrolide regimen, potentially risking a loss of efficacy if a therapeutic regimen is needed.

F. Toxoplasma Encephalitis

▶ H&P Keys

*Toxoplasma gondii* is the most common cause of latent central nervous system (CNS) infection in AIDS patients. Toxoplasma encephalitis is a multifocal process, often involving the brain stem or basal ganglia, with associated neurologic abnormalities that may include focal deficit, change in reflexes or sensation, ataxia, or decreased cognition.

▶ Diagnosis

Patients with toxoplasma encephalitis are usually seropositive, but this test can be unreliable. Computed tomographic (CT) scan or magnetic resonance imaging (MRI) will typically reveal multifocal disease. Clinical, serologic, and imaging studies lead to a presumptive diagnosis for which empiric therapy is often prescribed. Definitive diagnosis requires visualization of the organism in brain tissue. CSF tests are important but PCR is promising.

▶ Disease Severity

Brain biopsy for definitive diagnosis usually is reserved for patients who are seronegative, have atypical radiologic imaging (single lesions), or do not improve on empiric therapy.

▶ Concept and Application

Serologic evidence suggests that up to one third of the U.S. population has been infected with toxoplasma. Reactivation of a latent infection generally occurs when the CD4+ is < 100. Up to one third of seropositive AIDS patients may ultimately develop toxoplasma encephalitis. The immunosuppression associated with AIDS allows for the release of tachyzoites from tissue cysts, resulting in necrotic foci of infection.

▶ Treatment Steps

1. The initial 6 weeks of therapy commonly consists of pyrimethamine, sulfadiazine, and folinic acid.
2. Response rates (at least partial improvement) are quite high, approximately 85%. Response is usually fast—failure to respond in a week casts significant doubt on the diagnosis.
3. Clindamycin may replace sulfadiazine in the sulfa-allergic patient.
4. Chronic maintenance, often at reduced dose, is required life long to prevent relapse.

*Health Maintenance*—There is evidence that trimethoprim–sulfamethoxazole used for PCP prophylaxis may also be effective prophylaxis for toxoplasma encephalitis. Conversely, most toxoplasma therapy also functions as good PCP prophylaxis.

## G. Cryptococcal Infection

▶ H&P Keys

Cryptococcal infections are the most common disseminated fungal infections in patients with AIDS. *Cryptococcus* may involve the lungs, skin, blood, bone marrow, prostate, and genitourinary tract, but more than one half of the time it causes meningitis. The symptoms of cryptococcal meningitis are often subacute and nonspecific. The most common symptoms are fever and headache, with nausea, vomiting, and mental status changes occurring less frequently. Classic symptoms of meningismus, neck stiffness, and photophobia are uncommon.

▶ Diagnosis

Serum cryptococcal antigen may be used to screen patients with nonspecific symptoms. CSF cryptococcal antigen allows for the most rapid diagnosis of cryptococcal meningitis, and culture is the standard confirmatory test. The India ink exam is usually positive in patients with AIDS but is less sensitive than antigen tests or cultures.

▶ Disease Severity

Mental status changes and very high serum or CSF cryptococcal antigen titers are associated with poor prognosis.

▶ Concept and Application

*Cryptococcus neoformans* is an encapsulated yeast commonly found in soil and associated with bird feces. Disease is acquired by inhalation and primarily infects the lungs. The humoral and cell-mediated immune defects in AIDS predispose to dissemination.

▶ Treatment Steps
1. Standard acute therapy includes an approximate 2-week course of amphotericin B with or without flucytosine. Ideally, the CSF should become culture negative.
2. Some patients with mild disease may be able to start with fluconazole.
3. All patients receive lifelong maintenance therapy to prevent relapse unless they achieve immune reconstitution.
4. Fluconazole is preferred for maintenance therapy.
5. Maintenance may be stopped if immune restoration has been achieved.

## H. Herpes Simplex Virus

▶ H&P Keys

Herpes simplex virus (HSV)-1 and HSV-2 may cause ulcerative lesions at a variety of sites including orolabial, genital, anorectal, and esophageal ones. Lesions are characterized by pain and vesicle formation, followed by ulceration. Crusting and epithelialization may be delayed but resolves without scarring. Regional lymphadenopathy may be present. Esophagitis is associated with retrosternal pain and dysphagia. In the most severe cases ulcers can persist and expand without anti-viral therapy.

▶ Diagnosis

The diagnosis of mucocutaneous HSV should be confirmed with HSV culture. Cultures are fairly inexpensive and rapid. Esophagitis requires endoscopy, with histopathologic and culture confirmation.

▶ Disease Severity

Severity depends on the site of infection and degree of immunosuppression.

▶ Concept and Application

Most AIDS patients have previously been infected with HSV and have latent infection in nerve root ganglia. Latent HSV often reactivates in the immunocompromised patient and can cause severe, prolonged disease.

▶ Treatment Steps
1. Usual therapy consists of oral or parenteral acyclovir until the lesions are healed.
2. Many patients will relapse after initial therapy and will require repeated therapy, followed by long-term maintenance.
3. Long-term maintenance therapy with acyclovir is associated with a risk of development of acyclovir resistance, dictating therapy with other agents such as foscarnet.
4. Topical acyclovir is of very limited utility and can be messy.
5. Valacyclovir is also effective but there have been rare cases of TTP in people with immune problems who get high doses of valacyclovir.

## II. SEXUALLY TRANSMITTED DISEASES

### A. Gonorrhea

▶ H&P Keys

Uncomplicated gonococcal infections include urethritis, cervicitis, anoproctitis, and pharyngitis (pelvic inflammatory disease [PID] is discussed separately). Urethritis in men causes discharge and dysuria, whereas women report only dysuria. Cervicitis is generally asymptomatic. Pharyngitis generally causes no symptoms, but erythema and exudate may be present on exam. Anoproctitis may be associated with pain, and discharge may also be present. Disseminated gonococcal infection resulting from bacteremia may cause petechial or pustular skin lesions, tenosynovitis, septic arthritis, and occasionally, hepatitis, endocarditis, or meningitis.

▶ Diagnosis

Specific diagnosis is made by recovery of *Neisseria gonorrhoeae* from discharge, blood, or other body fluid. Therapy for uncomplicated disease is often empiric (without benefit of culture).

▶ Disease Severity

Of the uncomplicated gonococcal infections, pharyngitis is the most difficult to cure and dictates more specific therapy than does anal or genital infection (see Treatment Steps, below). Hospitalization may be advisable for initial therapy of disseminated infection.

▶ Concept and Application

It is estimated that 1 million new infections with *N. gonorrhoeae* occur each year in the United States. Most infections in men produce symptoms for which they seek medical care, though often not before transmitting the disease. Many infections in women produce minimal or no symptoms and medical care is delayed until serious complications such as PID occur. PID may cause tubal scarring, resulting in infertility or ectopic pregnancy.

▶ Treatment Steps

1. Coinfection with chlamydia is common in people treated for gonococcal infections.
2. Treatment for gonorrhea should include therapy that is effective against *C. trachomatis* (see chlamydia Treatment Steps recommendations).
3. Resistance to penicillin and tetracycline largely dictates current treatment regimens. Recommended regimens for uncomplicated gonorrhea include ceftriaxone, cefixime, ciprofloxacin, or ofloxacin, all as a single dose, plus a regimen effective against *Chlamydia*.
4. Ceftriaxone or ciprofloxacin should be used for pharyngeal disease.
5. Many additional antibiotics are effective for uncomplicated gonorrhea, including spectinomycin (intramuscular only), a number of second- and third-generation cephalosporins (oral and parenteral), and all the fluoroquinolones.

6. The initial treatment of disseminated gonococcal infection consists of a parenteral cephalosporin (ceftriaxone, cefotaxime, ceftizoxime) or spectinomycin.
7. After clinical improvement, oral therapy with cefixime or ciprofloxacin is given to complete a week of treatment.

*Health Maintenance*—Persons treated for gonorrhea should be screened for syphilis by serologic testing. Sex partners should be referred for treatment. Safer sex is encouraged and evaluation for HIV may be appropriate for many of these patients.

## B. Chlamydia

### ▶ H&P Keys
*C. trachomatis* causes urethritis and cervicitis (PID is discussed separately). Urethritis is characterized by mucoid or purulent discharge and dysuria. Cervicitis is characterized by yellow endocervical exudate.

### ▶ Diagnosis
Nonculture tests for chlamydia are reliable and much more available and sensitive than cultures. Combined tests, eg, ligase chain reaction, for gonorrhea and chlamydia.

### ▶ Disease Severity
As with gonococcal disease, chlamydial infection may go untreated in the female patient and result in tubal scarring, infertility, or ectopic pregnancy.

### ▶ Concept and Application
*C. trachomatis* is an obligate intracellular parasite of columnar or pseudostratified cells. The incidence of chlamydial infection is higher than that of gonorrhea.

### ▶ Treatment Steps
1. Coinfection with the gonococcus is common in patients treated for chlamydial infection.
2. Treatment for chlamydia should include therapy effective for gonococcal infection (see Gonorrhea Treatment Steps recommendations).
3. Recommended regimens for chlamydial urethritis or cervicitis include doxycycline or azithromycin.
4. Alternatives include ofloxacin or erythromycin.
5. These antibiotic therapies (with the exception of ofloxacin, which is active against gonorrhea) should include an antigonococcal regimen.

*Health Maintenance*—Sex partners should be referred for evaluation and treatment. Safer sex is encouraged.

## C. Syphilis

### ▶ H&P Keys
Patients may seek treatment for signs or symptoms of primary infection (ulcer at the site of infection), secondary infection (rash, mucocutaneous lesions, adenopathy), or tertiary disease (cardiac,

neurologic, ophthalmic, auditory, or gummatous lesions). Patients with latent infection may be identified by serologic testing.

▶ Diagnosis

Darkfield exam and direct fluorescent antibody tests of exudates or tissue allow the diagnosis of early syphilis. Presumptive diagnosis may be made serologically with a nontreponemal test: eg, RPR, confirmed with a treponemal test: eg, fluorescent treponemal antibody absorption (FTA-ABS). Neurosyphilis can be diagnosed with CSF tests. At a minimum this would include a VDRL (which is diagnostic of neurosyphilis when positive), cell count, protein, and glucose. About one half of the patients with neurosyphilis will have a positive CSF VDRL. Patients with primary, secondary, or latent syphilis need not undergo CSF exam unless there are: neurologic or ophthalmic signs or symptoms, other evidence of active disease (aortitis, gumma, iritis), treatment failure, HIV infection, or therapy not involving penicillin is planned. The CSF results can be difficult to interpret in the presence of HIV infection because even an asymptomatic person with HIV can have minor CSF cell count and protein abnormalities that mimic the changes of neurosyphilis. The VDRL test is still very useful in this setting.

▶ Disease Severity

Patients are staged and treated according to clinical signs and symptoms (see above) or the duration of latency. Patients with latent disease for < 1 year are considered to have early latent disease, whereas others have late latent syphilis or syphilis of unknown duration. The duration or intensity of therapy is largely dictated by stage. The titer of the nontreponemal test correlates with disease activity.

▶ Concept and Application

Syphilis is a systemic disease caused by *T. pallidum*. Although CSF invasion in primary or secondary syphilis is common, few patients develop neurologic disease when treated appropriately.

▶ Treatment Steps

1. Patients with primary, secondary, and early latent syphilis are treated with one 2.4 mouse units IM injection of benzathine penicillin.
2. Nonpregnant penicillin-allergic patients can be treated with a tetracycline for 2 weeks. This is less satisfactory than penicillin and needs closer follow-up.
3. Patients with late latent and tertiary syphilis are treated with three weekly 2.4-MU IM injections of benzathine penicillin G.
4. Four weeks of a tetracycline offers alternative therapy.
5. Neurosyphilis is treated for 10 to 14 days with high-dose penicillin. Even patients with documented penicillin allergy should be considered for penicillin desensitization.
6. All patients require follow-up serologic testing (CSF if appropriate) to monitor response.
7. Although data are incomplete, HIV-infected patients are generally treated as above (although some recommend more intense treatment than is dictated by stage).

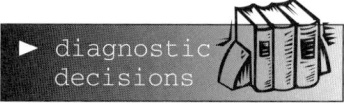

### GENITAL ULCER DISEASE

**Syphilis**
Clean, painless, usually single ulcer; large nodes.

**Chancroid**
Dirty, ragged, painful ulcer; large nodes.

**Lymphogranuloma Venereum**
Small ulcer, large nodes, "groove sign" between the inguinal and femoral nodes.

**Herpes Simplex**
Multiple painful, clustered vesicles or ulcers; variable nodes.

*Health Maintenance*—Sex partners should be referred for evaluation, although transmission occurs only when mucocutaneous lesions are present (uncommon after the first year). Patients should be considered for HIV testing.

### D. Chancroid

▶ H&P Keys

One or more painful genital ulcers, often in association with tender inguinal lymphadenopathy. Inguinal adenopathy may be suppurative.

▶ Diagnosis

Special cultures not readily available. Diagnosis probable with clinical signs and no evidence of syphilis or HSV.

▶ Disease Severity

In extensive cases, scarring may occur despite successful therapy.

▶ Concept and Application

Chancroid is caused by *Haemophilus ducreyi* and is endemic in many areas of the United States. It is a well-established cofactor for HIV transmission.

▶ Treatment Steps

1. Azithromycin or ceftriaxone single-dose therapy and 7 days of erythromycin are all successful.
2. Alternatives include 7 days of amoxicillin/clavulanate or 3 days of ciprofloxacin.

*Health Maintenance*—Patients should be tested for HIV infection.

### E. Pelvic Inflammatory Disease

▶ H&P Keys

PID represents a spectrum of upper genital tract inflammatory disorders, including endometritis, salpingitis, tubo-ovarian abscess, and pelvic peritonitis. Minimal clinical criteria for diagnosis of PID include lower abdominal tenderness, adnexal tenderness, and cervical motion tenderness. Fever and cervical discharge may be present.

▶ Diagnosis

Evidence of cervical infection with *N. gonorrhoeae* or *C. trachomatis* may be present. Endometritis on endometrial biopsy, tubo-ovarian abscess on ultrasound exam, or laparoscopic evidence is more definitive.

▶ Disease Severity

Patients with mild disease may be considered for outpatient therapy. Initial hospitalization is recommended if: diagnosis is uncertain, abscess is suspected, pregnancy or HIV infection is present, patient is unable to tolerate oral medication, or compliance or follow-up are in question.

▶ Concept and Application

PID is caused by sexually transmitted organisms such as *N. gonorrhoeae* or *C. trachomatis,* as well as genital tract flora such as anaerobes Enterobacteriaceae and group B streptococcus.

▶ Treatment Steps

1. Outpatient regimens include cefoxitin plus probenecid or a third-generation cephalosporin plus 14 days of doxycycline or ofloxacin plus either clindamycin or metronidazole for 14 days.
2. Common parenteral regimens include cefoxitin or cefotetan plus doxycycline or clindamycin plus gentamicin.

   *Health Maintenance*—Sex partners should be referred for evaluation and treatment.

## F. Epididymo-orchitis

▶ H&P Keys

Unilateral testicular pain and tenderness and palpable swelling of the epididymis are common.

▶ Diagnosis

Culture for *N. gonorrhoeae* and *C. trachomatis* and urine culture.

▶ Disease Severity

Failure to improve within 3 days requires reevaluation and consideration of hospitalization.

▶ Concept and Application

In men under 35 years of age, epididymo-orchitis is caused by gonococcal or chlamydial infection. Nonsexually transmitted disease associated with urinary tract infection caused by enteric bacilli is more common in men over 35 years of age.

▶ Treatment Steps

1. Treatment of sexually transmitted epididymo-orchitis includes therapy for both chlamydia and gonorrhea.
2. Single-dose ceftriaxone and 10 days of doxycycline or of ofloxacin are recommended.

   *Health Maintenance*—Sex partners should be referred for evaluation and treatment.

## G. Genital Herpes

▶ H&P Keys

Groups of painful vesicles that progress to shallow ulcerative lesions prior to crusting and healing. Commonly seen on external genitalia and on the cervix. Systemic symptoms such as fever, headache, and myalgias are not uncommon with initial episodes.

▶ Diagnosis

Viral culture for HSV.

▶ Disease Severity

Most infected persons never recognize signs of genital herpes; some have symptoms during the initial episode and then never again. A minority of infected persons have recurrent genital lesions.

▶ Concept and Application

Genital herpes, usually caused by HSV-2, is a recurrent disease without cure. Serologic evidence suggests that 30 million people in the United States have been infected.

▶ Treatment Steps

1. Acyclovir and similar drugs such as valacyclovir and famciclovir speed recovery from initial episodes or recurrences and can be used to suppress recurrent disease.
2. Therapy cannot eradicate latent virus.

## III. OTHER INFECTIOUS DISEASES

### A. Infectious Mononucleosis

▶ H&P Keys

Fever, sore throat, lymphadenopathy, splenomegaly. Headache, myalgias, sweats, anorexia, and abdominal pain may also be present.

▶ Diagnosis

Atypical lymphocytosis, positive test for heterophile antibody (positive Monospot or Mono-Diff test), positive serology for Epstein–Barr virus (especially IgM antibody to viral capsid antigen [VCA-IgM]).

▶ Disease Severity

Complications of infectious mononucleosis include hemolytic anemia (positive Coombs' test), thrombocytopenia, granulocytopenia, splenic rupture rarely, neurologic problems (e.g. Guillain–Barré syndrome), myocarditis, or pericarditis.

▶ Concept and Application

Infectious mononucleosis is an acute, self-limited infection predominantly occurring in children and young adults and caused by the herpesvirus, Epstein–Barr virus (EBV). Usual course of illness is 2–4 weeks.

▶ Treatment Steps

1. There is no specific therapy for EBV infection.
2. Corticosteroids are occasionally prescribed for severe tonsillitis with airway compromise, severe hemolytic anemia or thrombocytopenia, neurologic complications, myocarditis, or pericarditis.

## B. Varicella (Chickenpox)

### ▶ H&P Keys

Erythematous, maculopapular lesions that rapidly become vesicular and then pustular. The lesions then crust and heal. Spread of the rash is centripetal.

### ▶ Diagnosis

Positive Tzanck preparation for multinucleate giant cells and isolation of varicella-zoster virus (VZV).

### ▶ Disease Severity

Varicella is occasionally complicated by pneumonia, encephalitis, or Reye's syndrome. Infection in the compromised host often includes severe skin disease and dissemination to visceral organs.

### ▶ Concept and Application

Varicella, or chickenpox, is caused by the herpesvirus VZV. Varicella is the primary infection in the nonimmune host, whereas zoster (shingles) is a reactivation of latent virus. Transmission of infection is very efficient from 1 day before skin lesions appear to approximately 5 days after onset.

### ▶ Treatment Steps

1. The use of acyclovir in a usual episode of varicella, though approved, is controversial except in pregnancy.
2. Acyclovir therapy is routinely used for disseminated disease, CNS involvement, and pneumonia (zoster is discussed in Chapter 2).
3. Acyclovir not likely to be effective if use is delayed beyond 3–4 days following onset of symptoms.

*Health Maintenance*—Vaccine for VZV is indicated for everyone older than 1 year without a history of clinical varicella. The duration of protection remains to be determined. Zoster-immune globulin is given to seronegative immunosuppressed patients exposed to varicella.

## C. Measles (Rubeola)

### ▶ H&P Keys

Malaise, fever, coryza, conjunctivitis, and cough are accompanied by the rash. Koplik's spots appear on the buccal mucosa prior to appearance of the rash and then rapidly fade. The exanthem begins as an erythematous maculopapular eruption behind the ears, on the forehead at the hairline, and on the upper neck. Spread of the rash is centrifugal. The rash begins to fade at 3 days and typically lasts 1 week.

### ▶ Diagnosis

Viral isolation is not readily available. Diagnosis based on the clinical picture. Serologic proof of infection may be obtained (significant rise in antibody titer).

▶ Disease Severity

Pulmonary involvement is not uncommon and accounts for 90% of measles deaths. Encephalitis may occur (may be autoimmune rather than viral infection).

▶ Concept and Application

Highly contagious disease producing a distinct clinical syndrome after a 10- to 14-day incubation period.

▶ Treatment Steps
1. No specific therapy for measles.

   *Health Maintenance*—Routine immunization is highly recommended. Two doses of vaccine are needed for maximal protection.

## D. Mumps

▶ H&P Keys

Prodromal symptoms include anorexia, malaise, headache, myalgias, and fever. Orchitis or meningitis may occur before parotitis and may be the sole manifestation of disease. Typically, the disease is characterized by pain and swelling in one or both of the parotid glands. Sublingual and submaxillary glands are frequently involved.

▶ Diagnosis

Diagnosis based on clinical manifestations. Definitive diagnosis established by viral culture (not readily available) or serologic methods.

▶ Disease Severity

Complications of mumps occur more frequently in the older patient and include meningoencephalitis and other CNS manifestations, orchitis, oophoritis, pancreatitis, thyroiditis, arthritis, and myocarditis.

▶ Concept and Application

Acute contagious viral disease with typical incubation period of 14–24 days.

▶ Treatment Steps
1. No specific therapy.

   *Health Maintenance*—Routine immunization highly recommended.

## E. Rubella (German Measles)

▶ H&P Keys

Prodromal symptoms may include low-grade fever, headache, malaise, anorexia, mild conjunctivitis, coryza, pharyngitis, or cough. The rash (varyingly pruritic), lasts 1–5 days and typically begins on the face and behind the ears, spreading downward.

▶ Diagnosis

Diagnosis based on clinical manifestations. Serologic testing or viral isolation (not readily available) confirms the diagnosis.

▶ **Disease Severity**

Usually mild disease with few complications, although more common in adults. Arthralgias and arthritis occur most frequently. Other rarer complications include thrombocytopenia, myocarditis, Guillain–Barré syndrome, encephalitis, and optic neuritis.

▶ **Concept and Application**

Common childhood viral illness with a typical incubation period of 14–21 days.

▶ **Treatment Steps**

1. No specific therapy.

    *Health Maintenance*—Routine immunization highly recommended; goal is to prevent congenital rubella syndrome. Immunization *during* pregnancy is not recommended but has not been shown to be harmful.

## F. Lyme Disease

▶ **H&P Keys**

Lyme disease is associated with a variety of clinical manifestations. Classically, the disease has been divided into three stages:

Stage 1. Erythema migrans.
Stage 2. Neurologic or cardiac involvement.
Stage 3. Arthritis or subtle neurologic complaints.

As Lyme disease does not progress in an orderly manner from stage to stage, there is greater clinical utility in determining whether the infection is localized or disseminated and whether it is acute or chronic. Current therapy is largely based on this determination. Erythema migrans (EM) is an expanding, annular, erythematous skin lesion at the site of tick attachment that clears centrally. Systemic symptoms often occur with EM and correlate with systemic dissemination. There may be secondary skin lesions. Nervous system manifestations early in Lyme disease include meningitis, cranial neuritis, and painful radiculopathy. Chronic nervous system manifestations are more difficult to prove as being related to Lyme disease but may include anything in the range from subtle changes in cognitive function to significant focal abnormalities. The peripheral nervous system may also be involved. Cardiac involvement is manifested as varying degrees of heart block, myopericarditis, and possibly, cardiomyopathy. If untreated, nearly one half of patients will develop arthritis, mainly affecting large joints such as the knee. Only a minority of patients progress to chronic arthritis. Some people with late-stage Lyme disease can have persistent neurologic complaints including forgetfulness, fatigue, and mild cognitive impairment.

▶ **Diagnosis**

The diagnosis is based on the clinical manifestations, with EM being most useful. Serologic evidence is supportive but not standardized. CSF (including serology) is examined with suspected CNS disease.

### ▶ Disease Severity

Given the wide variety of acute and chronic manifestations of Lyme disease, severity must be assessed individually. The response to therapy of chronic manifestations is often not as good as that observed with acute manifestations.

### ▶ Concept and Application

Lyme disease is caused by the spirochete *Borrelia burgdorferi*. Ixodes ticks are the principal vector throughout the world. Though reported from most of the states, the majority of Lyme disease occurs in three regions; coastal areas in the Northeast, upper Midwest, and the far West, corresponding to the distribution of the tick vector. Primary reservoirs for the tick include the white-footed mouse and other small rodents. The larval, nymphal, and adult ticks feed on progressively larger animals, with the adult tick favoring the white-tailed deer. Transmission to humans occurs during feeding and requires attachment for at least 24 hours.

### ▶ Treatment Steps

1. EM, Bell's palsy, mild cardiac disease, and early arthritis are treated with oral doxycycline or amoxicillin.
2. More serious CNS disease, more serious cardiac disease, and chronic arthritis are treated with parenteral ceftriaxone or penicillin G.
3. A single 200-mg dose of doxycycline can abort infection but only a small minority of tick bites transmit *B. burgdorferi*.

   ***Health Maintenance***—One may attempt to limit tick exposure and the risk of Lyme disease by using repellents, reducing exposed skin, and promptly removing any attached ticks.

## BIBLIOGRAPHY

Gorbach SL. *Infectious Diseases*. 2nd ed. Philadelphia: WB Saunders Company; 1997.
Mandell GL. *Principles and Practice of Infectious Diseases*. 5th ed. New York: Churchill Livingstone Inc; 2000.
Murray PR. *Manual of Clinical Microbiology*. 7th ed. Washington, DC: ASM Press; 1999.
Yu VL. *Antimicrobial Therapy and Vaccines*. Baltimore: Williams & Wilkins; 1999.

# Musculoskeletal and Connective Tissue Disease 9

I. **INFECTIONS** / 271
   A. Osteomyelitis / 271
   B. Septic Arthritis / 271
   C. Lyme Disease / 272
   D. Gonococcal Tenosynovitis / 272

II. **DEGENERATIVE DISORDERS** / 273
   A. Degenerative Joint Disease; Arthralgia / 273
   B. Low Back Pain / 274
   C. Lumbar Disk Disease / 275
   D. Disorders Secondary to Neurologic Disease / 276

III. **INHERITED, CONGENITAL, OR DEVELOPMENTAL DISORDERS** / 276
   A. Congenital Hip Disorders / 276
   B. Legg–Calvé–Perthes Disease / 277
   C. Slipped Capital Femoral Epiphysis / 278
   D. Intoeing / 278

IV. **METABOLIC AND NUTRITIONAL DISORDERS** / 279
   A. Osteoporosis / 279
   B. Gout / 280
   C. Rickets / 280

V. **INFLAMMATORY OR IMMUNOLOGIC DISORDERS** / 281
   A. Polymyalgia Rheumatica / 281
   B. Lupus Arthritis / 281
   C. Polymyositis–Dermatomyositis / 282
   D. Rheumatoid Arthritis (Juvenile, Adult) / 283
   E. Ankylosing Spondylitis / 283
   F. Bursitis / 284
   G. Tendinitis / 285
   H. Fibromyalgia / 285

VI. **NEOPLASMS / 286**
- A. Osteosarcoma / 286
- B. Metastases to Bone / 286
- C. Pulmonary Osteoarthropathy / 287

VII. **OTHER DISORDERS / 288**
- A. Shoulder–Hand (Frozen Shoulder) Syndrome / 288
- B. Dupuytren's Contracture / 288
- C. Carpal Tunnel Syndrome / 288
- D. Paget's Disease of Bone / 289
- E. Eosinophil Granuloma / 290

VIII. **ACUTE OR EMERGENCY PROBLEMS / 290**
- A. Effusion of Joint / 290
- B. Spinal Stenosis / 291
- C. Contusions / 292
- D. Fractures and Dislocations / 292
- E. Other Orthopedic Emergencies / 299

**BIBLIOGRAPHY / 300**

## I. INFECTIONS

### A. Osteomyelitis

▶ H&P Keys

More common in children, may be triggered by trauma, usual seeding is hematogenous. Presents with refusal to bear weight or move joint or extremity. Fever usually present.

▶ Diagnosis

White blood cell count (WBC), erythrocyte sedimentation rate (ESR), blood cultures. Radiographs may show soft-tissue swelling early, followed by periosteal elevation and finally bone infarct and involucrum. Bone scan shows focal increased activity. MRI shows marrow changes and soft tissue involvement early in course of disease.

▶ Disease Severity

Clinical evaluation following a change in ESR may be useful, and C-reactive protein.

▶ Concept and Application

In children, osteomyelitis is usually hematogenous. Seeding occurs in the small arterioles of the metaphysis where there is sluggish blood flow. Infection elevates pressure, creating pain. Pus lifts the periosteum and may cause cortical necrosis, resulting in a sequestrum. The most common organism is *Staphylococcus aureus*, except in neonates, where *Streptococcus* B is most common. From 6 months to 5 years *Haemophilus influenzae* is the most common.

▶ Management

Aspiration is useful to recover organisms for antibiotic selection. Blood cultures may substitute if positive. IV antibiotics, followed by oral medication after temperature normalized for 6 weeks or until ESR normal. Immobilization for symptomatic relief. Surgical debridement for refractory cases with involucrum and sequestra.

### B. Septic Arthritis

▶ H&P Keys

Pain, erythema, joint effusion, and soft-tissue swelling. Refusal to bend joint or bear weight in children.

▶ Diagnosis

Joint aspirate, high white count > 50,000 suspicious, > 100,000 presumptive of infection pending culture results of infection. Polymorphonuclear leukocytes predominate. High peripheral WBC, elevated ESR.

▶ Disease Severity

Coexisting morbidity predisposes to infection (chronic disease, cancer, drug abuse, immune deficiency).

▶ Concept and Application

*H. influenzae* most common in children under 5 years old, *S. aureus* in children over 5 years old, gonococci in adults and adolescents. In children, joint may be seeded from area of contiguous osteomyelitis.

▶ Treatment Steps

1. In children, hip joint requires early surgical drainage to prevent joint destruction.
2. Adults may be treated with serial aspiration, following the WBC in the fluid.
3. If no response (fall in WBC count in synovial fluid), surgical debridement, often arthroscopically.
4. IV antibiotics, followed by oral antibiotics.

### C. Lyme Disease

▶ H&P Keys

Variable presentation: joint effusions, arthralgia, myalgia, fatigue, occasional cardiac arrhythmia, central nervous system (CNS) involvement (Bell's palsy, headaches). May have characteristic rash, erythema chronicum migrans ("bull's-eye" rash).

▶ Diagnosis

Joint aspirates negative by culture, radiographs normal, serologic testing: enzyme-linked immunosorbent assay (ELISA) screen confirmatory Western blot.

▶ Disease Severity

Cardiac and CNS symptoms.

▶ Concept and Application

Disease caused by *Borrelia burgdorferi*, a spirochete borne by the deer tick (*Ixodes dammini*). The disease occurs in three stages: rash, neurologic symptoms (neuritis, neuropathy, encephalopathy), arthritis. Immune complexes and cryoglobulin accumulate in the synovial fluid and tissues of the host.

▶ Treatment Steps

1. Treatment with oral doxycycline 100 mg bid or amoxicillin 2 g/d for 3–4 weeks.
2. Recalcitrant cases: IV ceftriaxone (Rocephin) 2 g/d for 6 weeks.

### D. Gonococcal Tenosynovitis

▶ H&P Keys

Acute loss of joint motion with fusiform swelling of digit. Erythema, redness, fever, migratory polyarthritis, multiple arthralgia.

▶ Diagnosis

Diagnosis confirmed by aspiration and culture (Gram stain showing intracellular gram-negative diplococci. Radiographs normal.

▶ Disease Severity

Multiple-location presentation.

▶ Concept and Application
Presentation of systemic gonococcal infection.

▶ Treatment Steps
Penicillin G or ceftriaxone.

## II. DEGENERATIVE DISORDERS

### A. Degenerative Joint Disease; Arthralgia

▶ H&P Keys
Eighty percent of adults 65 years and older demonstrate radiographic signs of osteoarthritis (OA). Signs and symptoms are usually localized. If diffuse symptoms exist, collagen vascular disease should be considered. Pain occurs after use and is relieved with rest; in later stages, rest pain and night pain may be present. Crepitation occurs with passive motion and may be associated with pain. Joint enlargement from osteophyte and synovial hypertrophy is present late.

▶ Diagnosis
Characteristic radiographic findings are joint-space narrowing, subchondral bony sclerosis, marginal osteophyte formation, subchondral cyst formation. Laboratory findings are normal.

*Differential Diagnosis*—Roentgenographic findings of OA of the hands are also seen with seronegative inflammatory arthritis. OA of the hip may be avascular necrosis or pigmented villonodular synovitis. OA of the knee may be meniscus pathology, osteochondritis dessicans, or a sequela of septic arthritis, osteonecrosis.

▶ Disease Severity
Disease severity is a clinical diagnosis with severe restriction of activities of daily living. Radiographs may be normal early, weight-bearing films demonstrate joint-space narrowing. Osteophyte formation with sclerosis and cyst formation occur late.

▶ Concept and Application
Disease is characterized by progressive loss of articular cartilage, followed by formation of new bone and cartilage at the joint margins (osteophyte). Incidence increases with age, obesity, repetitive occupational activities (coal miners, jackhammer operators, etc). The pathology of OA reflects the damage to the joint and reaction of the surrounding tissues. There is an increase in water content of the cartilage, with increased proteoglycan synthesis. As the disease progresses, the joint surface thins and becomes fibrillated. Appositional bone growth in the subchondral region leads to the sclerosis seen on radiographs. With further decrease progression clefts, and fractures of the subchondral plate occur, with the formation of subchondral cysts. Growth of bone and cartilage at the joint margins form osteophytes. Synovitis and joint effusions may be present.

▶ Treatment Steps
1. Protection of the joints from excessive force and chronic overuse. Supportive splints, unloading braces, shoe wedges, and the use of ambulatory aids (cane, crutches, walker) are protective.
2. Avoidance of repetitive impact loading (jumping, running) in lower-extremity OA. Weight loss is beneficial. Physical therapy to increase joint motion and strength is beneficial.
3. Drug therapy consists of analgesics (acetaminophen), aspirin, and nonsteroidal antiinflammatory drugs (NSAIDs). Narcotics should be used only as short-term measures. Intra-articular corticosteroid may be helpful in the management of acute flares. Intra-articular injections of high-molecular weight hyaluronic acid preparations may be used in knee arthritis. Nutriceuticals—glucosamine and chondroitin sulfate may slow the course of disease progression.
4. Surgery is reserved for cases in which conservative therapy fails. Options include arthroscopic lavage and debridement if mechanical signs are present, osteotomy to realign mechanical axis, arthroplasty, or fusion.

## B. Low Back Pain

▶ H&P Keys

Predisposing factors include age 30–50, repetitive movements such as lifting, pulling, bending, and twisting. Exposure to chronic vibration and prolonged sitting. Personal behavior (sedentary lifestyle, cigarette smoking, poor posture, emotional stress, obesity).

*Etiologic Factors*—Acute or chronic muscle, tendon, or ligamentous strain, lumbar disk herniation, degenerative changes of the spine, facet joint dysfunction, metabolic conditions that result in mechanical failure (osteoporosis).

▶ Diagnosis

Radiographs show age-related changes. Disk space narrowing, marginal osteophytes, facet joint sclerosis, and hypertrophy resulting in foraminal narrowing may be present. Magnetic resonance imaging (MRI), computed tomographic (CT) scan not necessary for initial evaluation; indicated when symptoms persist with radicular neurologic symptoms.

▶ Disease Severity

Physical evaluation, with loss of spine motion in all planes. Perivertebral muscle spasm. The presence of radicular pain below the knee suggests neurologic involvement (eg, disk disease).

▶ Concept and Application

Back pain is usually a self-limiting condition resulting from an acute strain or repetitive overload. The resulting inflammation and pain of ligaments, muscles, and tendons creates the short-term disability. Treatment addresses the cause of the overload and the underlying inflammation.

▶ Treatment Steps
1. Short period of rest (3–5 days).
2. Treatment of muscle spasm with ice massage and lumbar support.
3. Acetaminophen or NSAIDs for anti-inflammatory effect.
4. Major treatment is education in proper body mechanics to prevent recurrence.
5. Muscle strengthening for the back and abdomen, combined with a flexibility program, complete the treatment.
6. Aerobic fitness is beneficial in preventing recurrence.

## C. Lumbar Disk Disease

▶ H&P Keys

Low-back pain with radiation below the knee; leg pain is usually greater than back pain. Ten percent of backaches are related to some sort of nerve root irritation. Altered sensation, pins and needles, numbness may be present in the lower extremity. Pain increases with coughing, sneezing. Weakness may be present. Central disk may cause bilateral symptoms. Signs of limited spine motion, antalgic gait, sciatic list. Hip and knee flexed with standing, extended with sitting, absent or diminished reflexes, diminished sensation in a dermatome pattern. Positive tension signs with straight leg raising or sitting root tests.

▶ Diagnosis

Radiographic evaluation may demonstrate disk space narrowing or may be normal. CT scan and MRI allow visualization of the disk and neural elements. Electromyogram (EMG) will show changes only after several weeks of symptoms.

▶ Disease Severity

Dense paresthesias with complete motor loss are signs of severe nerve root impingement. Progressive loss of motor function and sensation an indication for early surgical intervention. Loss of bowel and bladder function (cauda equina syndrome) requires emergency treatment with surgical decompression of the neural elements to prevent permanent dysfunction.

▶ Concept and Application

Nuclear material bulges, protrudes, or extrudes from the disk space to put pressure on the ligaments and nerve roots. Molecular changes in the disk with aging alter the structural properties of the disk and the annulus fibrosis that contains the disk. The disk loses water and becomes dry and friable, decreasing its ability to withstand axial loads. With sudden loading or repetitive loading in flexion and rotation, disk material is extruded beyond the confines of the annulus, resulting in the neurologic symptoms.

▶ Treatment Steps
1. Early intervention with a short period of bed rest 3–5 days, in conjunction with anti-inflammatory medication and ice.
2. This is followed by mobilization with back rehabilitation exercises.

3. Sixty percent of patients obtain relief in 4 weeks, 90% in 3 months, 96% in 6 months.
4. Surgical intervention is required for progression of symptoms and for those who are unresponsive to conservative management.

### D. Disorders Secondary to Neurologic Disease

▶ H&P Keys

Stroke, diabetes, muscular dystrophy, cerebral palsy, neuropathies all have musculoskeletal consequences.

▶ Diagnosis

Physical examination of joint motion and muscle balance. Examination for altered sensation. Painless swelling and joint deformity may be present with Charcot's joint arthropathy.

▶ Disease Severity

Clinical evaluation. Radiographs show progressive joint destruction and loss of position.

▶ Concept and Application

Neurologic conditions that alter muscle strength, balance, and protective sensation have musculoskeletal manifestations. Increased spasticity after stroke creates flexion deformities of the affected joints because of the increased strength of flexor over extensor musculature. This may result in functional problems, such as thumb-in-palm deformity, equinus deformity, gait abnormality. The loss of protective sensation and proprioceptive sensation as a result of neuropathy from diabetes leads to Charcot's arthropathy (painless destruction of a joint) as well as problems of skin ulceration from excess pressure (dropped metatarsal heads).

▶ Treatment Steps

1. Protective splinting to prevent contractures and physical therapy to preserve joint motion may prevent surgical intervention.
2. For severe muscle imbalance, corrective surgery with release and weakening of the flexors or augmentation of the extensors with muscle transfers may be required.
3. Protection of insensate joints with bracing and full-contact orthotics may delay or prevent joint destruction.
4. Patient education in skin care.

## III. INHERITED, CONGENITAL, OR DEVELOPMENTAL DISORDERS

### A. Congenital Hip Disorders

▶ H&P Keys

Congenital hip dislocation (CDH) is a serious condition if not diagnosed and treated in the first weeks of life. Girls are affected eight times more often than boys. Diagnosis is made by clinical exam at the time of birth. Backward and forward pressure on the femur in full flexion and abduction can demonstrate the femoral head moving in and out of the acetabulum.

▶ Diagnosis

Radiographs are not helpful because the femoral head is not calcified until at least 10 weeks of age. Ultrasonography of the hip is the diagnostic procedure of choice in the first weeks of life.

▶ Disease Severity

Delay in diagnosis gravely affects prognosis and treatment. If diagnosis delayed until 12–18 months as walking begins demonstrating a limp and rolling gait, surgery will only achieve a useful hip but one that will not be normal.

▶ Concept and Application

Risk factors include family history of dislocations, breech presentation at birth. Every birth should be screened for CDH.

▶ Management

*Treatment at Birth*—Treatment with splint or harness (Pavlik) to hold the hips in an abducted and forward-flexed position. Reduction is confirmed with radiographs and possibly arthrogram. Worn for 12 weeks.

*Treatment at 2 Months*—Managed with traction and plaster immobilization.

*Treatment at 12 Months*—Surgery is indicated to achieve a stable joint. Hip is never normal, however.

## B. Legg–Calvé–Perthes Disease

▶ H&P Keys

Painful hip in child ages 2–11. Child with limp.

▶ Diagnosis

X-ray may be normal in early disease. Later x-rays will demonstrate increased femoral head density or subarticular fracture line.

▶ Disease Severity

Age is key to prognosis: Presentation after age 8 represents a poor prognosis.

▶ Concept and Application

Noninflammatory self-limiting deformity of the weight-bearing surface of the femoral head secondary to avascular necrosis of the femoral head. Increased incidence with a positive family history, low birth weight, and abnormal birth presentation.

▶ Treatment Steps

1. Maintenance of the sphericity of the femoral head is most important factor for obtaining a good outcome.

2. Treatment is to first obtain normal range of motion with bed rest, traction.
3. This is followed with bracing or surgery to contain the femoral head in the acetabulum until revascularization and ossification occurs.

### C. Slipped Capital Femoral Epiphysis

▶ H&P Keys

Presents as groin pain or as knee pain. Limp may be present with displacement. With complete displacement leg may be shortened and externally rotated.

▶ Diagnosis

Radiographic images, especially a lateral, are essential for showing displacement.

▶ Disease Severity

Degree of displacement determines residual problems. Significant displacement may result in the development of avascular necrosis. Chondrolysis may occur with the resultant osteoarthritis.

▶ Concept and Application

Adolescents with complaints of hip or knee pain should be considered to have a slipped capital femoral epiphysis. Occurs through the growth plate or epiphysis of the femoral neck during the adolescent growth spurt and is more common in boys than girls. The slip is probably caused by a weakening of the epiphyseal structures by hormonal changes of adolescence. Most often occurs in gynecoid boys.

▶ Treatment Steps
1. Slight to moderate displacement should be treated with percutaneous pinning to prevent further slip.
2. Manipulation may disturb the blood supply and create avascular necrosis.
3. For gross displacement, it is better to accept the deformity and correct it after growth has been completed with an osteotomy.

### D. Intoeing

▶ H&P Keys

Patient presents with an intoed gait. May complain of falling and tripping over feet.

▶ Diagnosis

No diagnostic studies are necessary.

▶ Disease Severity

Clinical evaluation of degree of intoeing.

▶ Concept and Application

There are three causes of intoeing: (1) anteversion of the femoral neck, (2) metatarsus adductus, and (3) outward-curved tibiae (tibial torsion). Femoral anteversion allows for greater internal rotation of the hip than external rotation and is the major cause of intoeing. The condition corrects itself as growth continues. Most instances are corrected by age 10.

▶ Treatment Steps
No treatment other than reassurance is needed.

## IV. METABOLIC AND NUTRITIONAL DISORDERS

### A. Osteoporosis

▶ H&P Keys
Progressive loss of height. Spontaneous, multiple vertebral body compression fractures. Development of thoracic kyphosis. Fractures of the hip and wrist. May complain of bone pain in the axial skeletal or in the long bones of the lower extremity. History of multiple stress fractures.

▶ Diagnosis
Plain radiographs may show osteopenia. Increase in medullary/cortex ratio of 2:1. Bone densitometry; single photon absorptiometry, dual energy x-ray absorptiometry (DEXA), quantitative CT scan have technical limitations. DEXA is the most sensitive of the monitoring techniques. Complete lab evaluation should consider thyroid, parathyroid, and renal disease; hematologic disorders; and malignant disease.

▶ Disease Severity
Loss of axial skeletal height, multiple compression fractures with thoracic kyphosis. Multiple fractures of hips, wrists, ribs, ankles. Recurrent stress risks.

▶ Concept and Application
Decrease in bone mineral content leading to spontaneous fractures of the spine, hip, and wrist. Commonly postmenopausal women, other risk factors include hereditary, drug use (steroids, heparin, thyroid), nutritional factors, activity (sedentary), cigarette smoking, alcohol. Disuse osteoporosis results when bones are not stressed normally, eg, paralysis, prolonged bed rest or immobilization, space flight.

▶ Treatment Steps
Best treated with prevention, low-dose estrogen replacement in menopausal women. Calcitonin and bisphosphonates block bone resorption. Adequate intake of oral calcium and vitamin D are essential for prevention and treatment (400 IU/d of vitamin D and 1,500 g/d calcium. Fluoride causes increases in bone density, but the bone is more brittle. Weight-bearing exercise helps prevent development and progression of osteoporosis. Alendronate 70 mg/wk or 10 mg/d or residronate 35 mg weekly is effective in the treatment of osteoporosis, but with a high rate of gastrointestinal side effects.

## B. Gout

### ▶ H&P Keys
Acute onset of painful, swollen, erythematous joints, deposition of crystals in soft tissue, tophi. Attacks may be preceded by trauma, alcohol, drugs, surgical stress, or acute medical illness. Great toe commonly involved; ankle, knee, tarsal bone may be affected.

### ▶ Diagnosis
Aspiration of joint fluid for birefringent crystals. Always send for culture and sensitivity.

### ▶ Disease Severity
Polyarticular attacks, soft-tissue tophi formation, joint destruction, associated renal failure.

### ▶ Concept and Application
Tissue deposition of monosodium urate crystals from supersaturated extracellular fluids. Recurrent attacks of severe articular and periarticular inflammation: gouty arthritis. Accumulation of crystalline deposits in the soft tissue: gouty tophi. Renal impairment: gouty nephropathy. Causes: overproduction, 10%; underexcretion, 90%. Dehydration as a result of trauma, surgery, diuretics may precipitate attack.

### ▶ Treatment Steps
1. Treatment with anti-inflammatory medications, indomethacin (Indocin) 50 mg tid or colchicine.
2. Aspiration and identification under polarized light microscopy diagnostic with birefringent crystals.
3. If attacks reoccur, treatment with allopurinol is helpful.
4. Intra-articular steroids effective if oral medication is not tolerated or contraindicated as in patients on anticoagulants or with chronic renal insufficiency.

## C. Rickets

### ▶ H&P Keys
Brittle bones with ligamentous laxity, flattening of the skull, enlargement of the costal cartilages (rachitic rosary), dorsal kyphosis, bowing of long bones.

### ▶ Diagnosis
Radiographic evaluation: transverse radiolucent lines ("Looser's lines"), physeal cupping and widening. Laboratory evaluation: calcium levels are normal with low phosphate and high alkaline phosphatase levels.

### ▶ Disease Severity
Clinical evaluation: long-bone bowing, rachitic rosary.

### ▶ Concept and Application
Decrease in calcium and/or phosphorus affecting the mineralization of the epiphyses of long bones. Histology: Widened osteoid

seams, distortion of the zone of maturation with poorly defined zone of provisional calcification. There are four causes for rickets:

1. Vitamin D deficiency resulting from inadequate diet or lack of exposure to sunlight.
2. Malabsorption of calcium secondary to steatorrhea.
3. Renal osteodystrophy caused by renal abnormality that affects the metabolism of vitamin D.
4. Hypophosphatemia resulting from defect in renal tubule (vitamin D–resistant rickets).

▶ Treatment Steps
1. Vitamin D produces rapid improvement.
2. Residual long-bone deformities may require surgical correction.
3. Vitamin D–resistant rickets requires treatment with phosphate replacement and vitamin $D_3$.

## V. INFLAMMATORY OR IMMUNOLOGIC DISORDERS

### A. Polymyalgia Rheumatica

▶ H&P Keys
Occurs in men and women over 60, and occurs twice as often in women. Patients complain of abrupt onset of pain affecting the shoulders, neck, upper arms, lower back, and thighs. Morning stiffness and gelling are predominant features. Physical examination reveals only tenderness and restriction of motion.

▶ Diagnosis
Radiographs are normal. Rheumatoid factor and antinuclear antibodies (ANA) are normal, ESR is elevated. Diagnosis is by history and response to treatment with prednisone.

▶ Disease Severity
Elevated ESR, clinical impairment of activities.

▶ Concept and Application
Common syndrome of older patients, characterized by stiffness and pain in neck, shoulders, and hip lasting at least 1 month. Inflammation is present without joint destruction.

▶ Treatment Steps
1. Responds rapidly to low-dose prednisone.
2. If response is not seen in 1 week, diagnosis should be questioned.
3. Start prednisone 10 to 20 mg/d with taper to 5–7.5 mg/d.
4. Therapy may continue for longer than 1 year.

### B. Lupus Arthritis

▶ H&P Keys
Disease of young females 14–40, with a 5:1 female-to-male ratio. The acute arthritis may involve any joint but usually involves the

small joints of the hand, wrists, and the knee. It may be persistent and chronic or migratory. Soft-tissue swelling and effusion are mild. Fatigue, rash, and fevers are common.

▶ Diagnosis

Clinical symptoms of morning stiffness, myalgia, arthralgia. Serologic testing: 95% of ANA are positive.

▶ Disease Severity

Articular complaints are usually mild and reversible. They can become fixed deformities if untreated. Disease activity, however, can severely impair renal function and cause pulmonary and cardiac involvement. Neuropsychiatric manifestations may also be present. Increased tendency for thrombosis.

▶ Concept and Application

Autoimmune disease characterized by the production of autoantibodies to components of the cell nucleus. Pathologic findings are manifested by inflammation, vasculitis, and immune complex deposition disease (lupus kidney). Lupus arthritis is a polyarthritis characterized by low-grade synovitis without joint destruction. Joint distention may cause ligamentous laxity of the metacarpal phalangeal (MCP) and proximal interphalangeal (PIP) joints of the hand with resulting instability and deformity (swan-neck deformity, ulnar deviation of the fingers) without articular erosions.

▶ Treatment Steps

Treatment consists of periods of rest, avoidance of sun exposure, NSAIDs, hydroxychloroquine and corticosteroids and other immunosuppressants such as cyclophosphamide, azathioprine, and methotrexate. Splinting may preserve function in weakened joints. Methotrexate is used in recalcitrant disease.

## C. Polymyositis–Dermatomyositis

▶ H&P Keys

Complaints of proximal hip weakness, with difficulty on stairs and getting out of cars. Arm symptoms with difficulty lifting above the horizontal. Physical examination will show diffuse symmetric muscle wasting and weakness. Affected muscles may be sore to palpation. Gait may be slow and wide based.

▶ Diagnosis

Clinical presentation of symmetric proximal muscle weakness. Elevated serum creatine kinase, aldolase, lactic dehydrogenase, and transaminase. Characteristic EMG abnormalities. Autoantibodies may be present. Muscle biopsy.

▶ Disease Severity

Involvement may extend to the heart, gastrointestinal tract, lungs, peripheral joints.

▶ Concept and Application

This disease is an idiopathic inflammatory myopathy characterized by proximal limb weakness.

▶ Treatment Steps
1. High-dose corticosteroid medication is the initial treatment.
2. Graded exercise after inflammation is controlled restores some strength and range of motion.
3. Methotrexate or azothioprine is used in patients not responding to corticosteroid.

### D. Rheumatoid Arthritis (Juvenile, Adult)

▶ H&P Keys

Characteristically presents with morning stiffness with symmetric painful swelling in the small joints in young women ages 15 to 35. It may involve other joints not seen in OA such as elbows, shoulders, ankles, hips, and spine. Fatigue may be present.

▶ Diagnosis

Radiographs show juxta-articular erosions around the small joints of the hands and feet. Positive rheumatoid factor (RF), elevated ESR, and anemia are usually present.

▶ Disease Severity

Functional impairment in activity of daily living. Systemic involvement of other organ systems such as the lung, heart, skin, eye, gastrointestinal and genitourinary systems is possible.

▶ Concept and Application

Etiology is unclear but is related to cell-mediated immune response (T cells) that incites an inflammatory response, initially against soft tissue and later cartilage, with subsequent bone loss secondary to periarticular bone resorption. Lymphokines and other inflammatory mediators initiate the cascade that leads to cartilaginous destruction.

▶ Treatment Steps
1. Aimed at controlling the inflammation with acetaminophen, NSAIDs, antimalarial immunosuppressives (such as methotrexate, azathioprine, leflunomide CellCept, and anti-TNF agents). Corticosteroids may be used to improve patient functional levels.
2. Methotrexate, leflunomide (ARAVA), and anti-inflammatory drugs are also used. Severely affected joints can be protected with splints and braces to prevent destruction.

### E. Ankylosing Spondylitis

▶ H&P Keys

Common in young men aged 15–30. Presents with complaint of diffuse low backache without radicular symptoms. Profound morning stiffness. Usually a rapid response to anti-inflammatory medication. May have painless or painful effusions of large joints.

▶ Diagnosis

History and physical examination are most important. Restriction of chest expansion and spine flexion. Elevated ESR. May be HLA-B27-positive. Radiographs of the sacroiliac joints show the earliest changes of sacroilliitis. Later, the spine films demonstrate progressive ankylosis.

▶ Disease Severity
Restriction of spine motion, chin-on-chest deformity, restriction of chest expansion.

▶ Concept and Application
An inflammatory disease of the spinal joints and sacroiliac joints. If left untreated, there can be complete loss of spinal motion from the occiput to the coccyx. Treatment is to preserve motion through exercise and control inflammation with medication.

▶ Treatment Steps
1. Initial flair is treated with rest and anti-inflammatory medication.
2. Mobilization and flexibility exercises are started as the inflammation is controlled.

## F. Bursitis

▶ H&P Keys
Soft-tissue swelling that may be either painful or nonpainful, usually over a bony prominence. Swelling may occur spontaneously or as a result of trauma or an inflammatory disease (gout, rheumatoid arthritis).

▶ Diagnosis
Clinical evaluation. Additional evaluation for underlying inflammatory diseases. Radiographs to evaluate for bony prominences and soft-tissue calcifications.

▶ Disease Severity
Clinical evaluation.

▶ Concept and Application
Bursae form wherever two tissue planes move in opposite direction or where tissues travel over a bony protuberance. Normal bursal locations are in the subacromial space of the shoulder, over the olecranon of the elbow, and over the tibial tubercle, and in the prepatellar space. This normal structure allows skin and tendon and muscle to slide over each other easily. If the bursa becomes infected, injured, or inflamed, fluid will accumulate in the bursa and produce visible swelling. Fibrinous loose bodies may also be formed in the bursa. After the inflammation subsides, adhesions and fibrosis may occur in the bursa, resulting in crepitation and, sometimes, pain.

▶ Treatment Steps
1. Avoidance of repetitive motions and trauma will prevent bursal inflammation.
2. Treatment of any underlying collagen vascular disease or crystalline arthritis will control the bursal swelling.
3. Acute treatment consists of rest, ice, anti-inflammatory medication. Aspiration to identify crystals or elevated WBC and bacteria may be required.

4. The use of protective padding, elbow and knee pads, can prevent recurrence.
5. Surgical excision is sometimes needed if the size or the location interferes with activities of daily living.

## G. Tendinitis

▶ H&P Keys

Pain over tendon or at tendon insertion. May be acute in onset or as a result of repetitive overload, often seen after a sudden change in activity or sporting activity.

▶ Diagnosis

Physical signs of localized inflammation with point tenderness over the tendon. Weakness may be present secondary to pain.

▶ Disease Severity

Functional assessment of impairment.

▶ Concept and Application

Tendinitis is an inflammation of the tendon secondary to overload. This may be due to acute overload with partial tearing of the tendon or as a result of repetitive stress. A sudden change in activity or sporting activity that exceeds the body's reparative capabilities will result in an "overuse" tendinitis.

▶ Treatment Steps
1. Local treatment with ice massage and oral NSAIDs.
2. Splinting to restrict motion and rest injury zone.
3. Restoration of normal motion through a gentle stretching program followed by strength exercises and endurance training.
4. Return to sport and activity is gradual.
5. Assessment of work activity and sport intensity with adaptation of program will prevent recurrence. Training and equipment must also be adapted to prevent recurrence.

## H. Fibromyalgia

▶ H&P Keys

Patients present with diffuse achiness, stiffness, fatigue, associated with multiple areas of clinical tenderness. Seventy-five percent are female, with an age distribution of 20–60 years. Pain tends to be localized to axial locations such as the neck and lower back. The upper trapezius is a common location of pain. On physical examination tenderness is present with moderate pressure. Common locations: occiput, trapezius, supraspinatus at ridge of scapula, lower back, lateral epicondyle.

▶ Diagnosis

Clinical examination makes the diagnosis. Laboratory evaluation to exclude collagen vascular diseases (ESR, RF, ANA, CBC) and infectious causes (Lyme disease). Thyroid function tests are also valuable.

▶ Disease Severity

Clinical examination.

▶ Concept and Application

Etiology is unknown; fatigue is felt to be due to sleep disturbances, with loss of rapid eye movement (REM) sleep patterns. Highly correlated with abnormal sleep patterns.

▶ Treatment Steps

1. Patient education and reassurance.
2. Aerobic exercise is more beneficial than stretching alone.
3. NSAIDs are not effective as single agents but are effective in conjunction with bedtime dose of amitriptyline or cyclobenzaprine.

## VI. NEOPLASMS

### A. Osteosarcoma

▶ H&P Keys

Most common in second and third decade of life. Presents often as a painless mass. Found after rather minor trauma on routine radiograph.

▶ Diagnosis

Radiographs are diagnostic: demonstrate increased radiodensity with areas of radiolucency and permeative destruction and soft-tissue extension. Elevated periosteum (Codman's triangle) may be present. Bone scans and MRI will show extent of lesion and skip lesions.

▶ Disease Severity

Extent of disease with involvement of multiple compartments.

▶ Concept and Application

A malignant tumor of bone characterized by the production of osteoid directly from a malignant spindle cell stroma. The knee and proximal humerus are the most commonly affected locations. Early diagnosis is difficult because of the disease's painless nature. Secondary osteosarcomas can arise from Paget's disease of bone and post–radiation therapy fields.

▶ Treatment Steps

1. Adjunctive chemotherapy pre- and postoperatively profoundly improves survival.
2. Limb salvage surgery may be offered to those patients who are good responders, with 95% tumor necrosis. Otherwise, amputation and prosthetic fitting is the treatment of choice, with the best survival and lowest recurrence rates.

### B. Metastases to Bone

▶ H&P Keys

Presentation is usually with pain or with a pathologic fracture.

▶ Diagnosis

Radiographs demonstrate lytic and blastic lesions. Lesions involving > 50% of the cortex or that are > 2.5 cm in diameter are at risk for spontaneous fracture. Bone scanning sensitive for detection of early metastatic disease. MRI will show accurately extent of metastatic tumor involvement of bone. Alkaline phosphatase is usually elevated.

▶ Disease Severity

Lesions > 2.5 cm in diameter or > 50% of the cortex are at risk for spontaneous fracture and should be prophylactically stabilized.

▶ Concept and Application

Metastatic tumors are the most common malignancies of bone. Spread to bone can be either arterial or venous. Classically, lytic lesions are found in the axial skeleton and long-bone diaphyses and usually multiply. Most common lesions are breast, prostate, lung, kidney, and thyroid. Prostate and breast metastases are typically blastic. The most common metastases in children are Wilms' tumor and neuroblastoma.

▶ Treatment Steps

1. Radiation therapy is often helpful to control the pain and metastatic activity. Adenocarcinoma of lung does not respond to radiation therapy.
2. For impending fractures, stabilization with load-sharing devices (intramedullary rods) is preferred. For collapse of bony support of joint surfaces, replacement arthroplasties may be useful procedures if survival is expected beyond 6 months.

## C. Pulmonary Osteoarthropathy

▶ H&P Keys

Clubbing of the fingers is the characteristic feature. In some patients, especially those with malignant lung tumors, severe bone pain may be present. Obtain family history of clubbing.

▶ Diagnosis

Physical feature of bulbous deformity of the digits (clubbing). Periostitis and thickening of the bones is present radiographically.

▶ Disease Severity

Clinical evaluation; evaluate for occult pulmonary tumor, especially if long-bone pain is present.

▶ Concept and Application

Disease characterized by excessive proliferation of skin and bones at the ends of the digits (clubbing).

▶ Treatment Steps

1. An NSAID is useful in controlling the pain of the periostitis.
2. Occult malignant tumor of the lung must be ruled out.

## VII. OTHER DISORDERS

### A. Shoulder–Hand (Frozen Shoulder) Syndrome

▶ H&P Keys

Decreased range of motion in the shoulder often painful. May be associated with minor trauma. Associated with diabetes, hypothyroidism, surgery; and higher in females.

▶ Diagnosis

Diagnosis is clinical; arthrogram will show decreased joint-space volume.

▶ Disease Severity

Clinical evaluation of functional loss of shoulder motion.

▶ Concept and Application

Adhesive capsulitis of the shoulder. Inflammatory condition with fibrosis and loss of normal joint space secondary to capsular contracture.

▶ Treatment Steps
1. Institution of early, aggressive range-of-motion exercises.
2. Adjunctive treatment with NSAIDs and ice.
3. May take 1 year to resolve. Surgical releases and manipulation are reserved for nonresponders to physical therapy.

### B. Dupuytren's Contracture

▶ H&P Keys

Patients are usually males older than 40, of Northern European ancestry, with a family history of the condition. Alcohol, smoking, diabetes, and seizures are contributory. Forty percent are bilateral. Ulnar digits are more commonly involved.

▶ Diagnosis

Clinical evaluation.

▶ Disease Severity

Interference with hand function, inability to get the fingers out of the palm of the hand.

▶ Concept and Application

Proliferative fibrodysplasia of the palmar subcutaneous tissue. Myofibroblast proliferation and increased type III collagen. Leads to progressive contracture from these nodules and cords of tissue.

▶ Treatment Steps
1. Surgical intervention for deformities of > 30–45° of the MCP or of any PIP involvement.

### C. Carpal Tunnel Syndrome

▶ H&P Keys

Patients usually complain of night symptoms with paresthesias in the median distribution (the front of the thumb, index and long finger, and the radial half of the ring finger). May have weakness of pinch with thenar atrophy late in the disease process.

▶ Diagnosis

Other causes (thyroid disease, diabetes, pregnancy, amyloidosis) need to be excluded. Physical examination is usually diagnostic. Diminished sensation in the median nerve distribution. Positive Tinel's sign of the carpal canal. Positive Phalen's test. Nerve conduction velocity delays across the carpal ligament.

▶ Disease Severity

Progressive median nerve dysfunction with loss of two-point discrimination and weakness of thumb adduction. Thenar atrophy.

▶ Concept and Application

The median nerve and common flexors pass through a common tunnel in the wrist, bounded volarly by the transverse carpal ligament. Any process that decreases the volume of the canal will compress the median nerve and create symptoms.

▶ Treatment Steps
1. Primary treatment is rest with a cock-up resting splint.
2. Injection of hydrocortisone may be effective.
3. Surgical decompression for those not responding to conservative treatment.
4. Treatment of underlying disease process.

## D. Paget's Disease of Bone

▶ H&P Keys

The most common sites are the spine, pelvis, skull, femur, tibia. In most cases patients are asymptomatic. However, disease becomes clinically present with pain, progressive deformity, compression of neurologic structures, pathologic fractures.

▶ Diagnosis

Laboratory evaluation: increased alkaline phosphatase, increased urinary hydroxyproline excretion. Radiographic appearance: initial lesion is a focal area of radiolucency (osteoporosis circumscripta of the skull). In the long bones, resorption is characterized by an advancing wedge of radiolucency. Attempts at repair create sclerotic-appearing bone with thickening of the cortex.

▶ Disease Severity

The major complication of Paget's disease is sarcomatous transformation. This occurs in less than 1% of cases. Presents with severe pain and extremely elevated serum alkaline phosphatase activity. Increased local circulation in hypervascular bone can create high-output congestive heart failure. Paget's fracture risk due to brittle bones. Increased bone density results in early osteoarthritis of surrounding joints. Spinal stenosis may occur with Paget's involvement of the spine.

▶ Concept and Application

Disorder of unknown etiology characterized by excessive bone resorption followed by excessive bone formation. Creates classic lamellar mosaic bone pattern.

▶ Treatment Steps

1. In most instances no treatment is necessary because of the paucity of clinical symptoms.
2. In symptomatic patients, NSAIDs may suppress the discomfort. Calcitonin administered subcutaneously may decrease pagetoid bone activity. Etidronate will decrease bone resorption.
3. With irreversible joint destruction, total joint arthroplasty offers relief of pain. Spinal decompression (laminectomy) for stenosis.

### E. Eosinophil Granuloma

▶ H&P Keys

May present as progressive back pain, more often in the thoracic spine. Common locations: pelvis, femur, and spine. First and second decade of life. Lytic-appearing lesion characteristic. Periosteal thickening is common.

▶ Diagnosis

Classically, may cause vertebral flattening (vertebra plana), lytic lesions in long bones.

▶ Disease Severity

Lesions that compromise the structural integrity of long bones or cause neurologic compromise.

▶ Concept and Application

Bracing in children may be necessary to prevent progressive kyphosis.

▶ Treatment Steps

1. Treatment consists of observation (many lesions heal spontaneously), low-dose radiation for neurologic deficits.
2. Curettage or excision may be indicated for persistent lesions.

## VIII. ACUTE OR EMERGENCY PROBLEMS

### A. Effusion of Joint

▶ H&P Keys

Swelling of the joint either spontaneous in onset or posttraumatic. Physical examination reveals loss of the normal joint contours and possibly a restriction in motion.

▶ Diagnosis

Aspiration of the joint classifies the fluid as noninflammatory (WBC < 2,000/mm$^3$), inflammatory or infectious (WBC > 100,000/mm$^3$). Evaluation for crystals is essential to differentiate gout and pseudogout. Culture and Gram stain are needed to rule out infection. A bloody effusion with the history of trauma is suggestive of a severe injury, either a fracture or ligament injury; 85% of hemarthroses of the knee are anterior cruciate injuries.

▶ **Disease Severity**
High WBC indicate infectious etiologies until proven otherwise. They demand prompt treatment, or rapid joint destruction can occur as a result of proteolytic enzymes produced by the bacteria.

▶ **Concept and Application**
Any synovium-lined joint can have an effusion. The effusion is the production of excess synovial fluid in response to an inflammatory event. This event can be trauma, as in a hemorrhagic effusion, or inflammatory, as in gout or rheumatoid arthritis, or an infection.

▶ **Treatment Steps**
1. Management depends on the etiology of the effusion.
2. Treatment of the inflammatory condition with oral anti-inflammatory medications or intra-articular steroids.
3. Infectious effusions are treated with serial aspirations or surgical drainage in combination with antibiotics.
4. Traumatic effusions resolve with rest, but treatment must address the injury pattern.

## B. Spinal Stenosis

▶ **H&P Keys**
Elderly patients with complaints of back and buttock pain. Pain is made worse with walking and descending stairs and relieved only with prolonged rest. If activity continues, paresthesia and weakness may develop. Pain is increased with hyperextension of the spine and relieved with forward flexion of the spine. Sensory changes are described as water or candle wax dripping down the leg.

▶ **Diagnosis**
Radiographs often show degeneration of the facet joints. CT scan is best noninvasive test for bony stenosis. MRI underestimates the degree of stenosis. Myelogram and postmyelogram CT are useful to fully define the disease, especially stenosis of the lateral recesses of the neural foramina.

▶ **Disease Severity**
Clinical impairment of activities with neurogenic claudication. Pain increased with any activity that causes hyperextension of the spine. Acute trauma in the presence of stenosis may cause catastrophic neurologic symptoms with paraplegia and cauda equina symptoms and demands prompt surgical decompression.

▶ **Concept and Application**
The maturing of the skeleton results in degenerative changes involving the disk margins and facet joints. The bony overgrowth constricts the nerve roots. This may be exacerbated by ligamentous thickening and diskogenic protrusions.

▶ Treatment Steps
1. Adjustment to the limitations of the disease in conjunction with anti-inflammatory medications, ice or heat, and an exercise program.
2. If symptoms are severely disruptive to the patient, surgery (laminectomy) to decompress the nerve roots will give relief. Fusion may be required if facetectomies are needed to decompress the neural elements.

### C. Contusions

▶ H&P Keys
Contusions are a result of direct trauma. Localized erythema and swelling are present with palpable tenderness. There may be loss of adjacent joint motion if swelling is pronounced.

▶ Diagnosis
Diagnosis is by history and clinical examination. Radiographs rule out fracture or late myositis ossificans.

▶ Disease Severity
Clinical loss of function of the joint and affected extremity define severity. Large hematomas and contusions to a large area of the muscle mass will produce greater disability. Myositis ossificans, or calcification of the muscle, is a late sequela of a severe contusion or a result of repetitive contusions to the same muscle before primary healing has occurred or early application of heat.

▶ Concept and Application
Contusions are a result of direct trauma. Following the trauma there is local damage to blood vessels and muscle. As bleeding and swelling continue, there is increased muscle stiffness and loss of joint motion. Secondary agents of inflammation produced as response to the local tissue trauma produce the ache and stiffness that characterize the early period after a contusion.

▶ Treatment Steps
1. Treatment consists of ice and compression to control the swelling and bleeding.
2. Adjunctive use of NSAIDs is useful in controlling the secondary inflammation.
3. Early therapy is provided to restore painless range of motion, followed by flexibility and strengthening exercises.
4. Return to activity is allowed when there is full, painless range of motion and strength equal to the unaffected extremity.

### D. Fractures and Dislocations

#### 1. Cervical Spine

▶ H&P Keys
Fractures of the cervical spine are caused in four ways: (1) flexion, (2) extension, (3) vertical compression, and (4) rotation.

*Flexion Injuries*—Are the most common and usually involve the lower cervical spine. May be associated with compression of the vertebral body, rupture of the supraspinous ligament, dislocation of the posterior facets.

*Extension Injuries*—Are generally less serious than flexion, with the most common being fractures of the odontoid; hyperextension injuries can result in damage to the anterior spinal artery, with the resultant anterior spinal artery syndrome. The hangman's fracture or fracture of the pedicles of C2 and spondylolisthesis of C2 on C3 results from hyperextension during falls.

*Vertical Compression*—Axial loading injuries cause vertical compression and result in fractures of the atlas or burst fractures.

▶ Diagnosis

Radiographs: anterior-posterior (AP), lateral, oblique, open-mouth odontoid view are the standard views. Flexion and extension lateral radiographs evaluate instability. CT scan and MRI are useful in determining the geometry of fracture fragments and evaluating the degree of cord compression.

▶ Disease Severity

Disease severity is based on clinical findings of neurologic compromise.

▶ Concept and Application

The pattern of injury is dependent on the mechanism of injury. Treatment is based on decompression of the neurologic elements and stabilization of the spine either surgically or with bracing.

▶ Treatment Steps
1. Treatment is stabilization of the unstable elements with surgery or bracing.
2. For neurologic compromise, prompt intervention to decompress the neural elements and stabilize the bony and ligamentous structures.

2. Thoracic Spine

▶ H&P Keys

Usually, high energy is necessary to produce these injuries unless significant osteoporosis is present. The pattern of injury depends on the position of the axis of flexion and direction of the force at the time of injury. These result in compression fractures, burst fractures, flexion–distraction injuries (seat belt), and fracture dislocations.

▶ Diagnosis

Radiographic evaluation with plane roentgenograms is usually adequate for thoracic fractures. CT scan is beneficial to define fracture geometry and neurologic compromise.

▶ Disease Severity

The degree of bony compression, displacement, and neurologic compromise defines the severity of the injury.

▶ Concept and Application

Compression fractures are common on falls from heights and falls onto the backsides by elderly osteoporotic patients. The injury occurs at the thoracic–lumbar junction where the thoracic kyphosis and lumbar lordosis meet. This results in loading forces on the anterior aspect of the vertebral body, with the resulting vertebral wedge fractures. Burst fractures are caused by pure axial loading and cause retropulsion of material, resulting in cord compromise with neurologic symptoms. The rapid deceleration injury of the seat-belted passenger results in the flexion–distraction fracture with a splitting of the vertebral body; displacement can be significant. Fracture dislocations are a result of a combination of flexion, compression, and rotation.

▶ Treatment Steps

1. Compression fractures of < 50% are usually treated with a short period of rest with supportive bracing and restorative exercise.
2. For those > 50%, surgical stabilization may be indicated.
3. Persistent back pain may occur after even minor compression injuries.
4. Burst fractures associated with neurologic symptoms require operative stabilization and may require decompression.
5. Fracture dislocations often result in paraplegia; early operative stabilization will allow for early rehabilitation.

3. Lumbar Spine

▶ H&P Keys

Mechanism of injury is usually flexion or a combination of flexion and rotation. Pain is present of the posterior elements of the spine, and neurologic compromise may be present. Compression fractures are caused by pure axial loading. Differentiating between cord and root lesion is essential for prognosis.

▶ Diagnosis

Radiographs (AP, lateral, oblique), CT scan.

▶ Disease Severity

Based on level of neurologic compromise.

▶ Concept and Application

The cord ends at L1 and therefore only the lower motor and sensory nerves are involved in this injury. There is greater room in the lumbar spine for displacement, and therefore greater displacement is necessary before neurologic compromise is present. The neurologic picture cannot be determined until spinal shock has passed, as exhibited by the return of the bulbocavernous reflex.

▶ Treatment Steps

Serial monitoring of the neurologic status and early stabilization and decompression of compressed neural elements provide for the best outcomes.

## 4. Closed Fracture of Hand Phalanges

▶ H&P Keys

Fractures are usually caused by twisting or angular forces. With fracture, there is loss of ability to use the hand fully, with associated pain and swelling. The location of the swelling and pain, as well as the pattern of altered motion, will suggest which of the phalanges has been injured. Loss of extension at the distal interphalangeal (DIP) joint is characteristic of a mallet finger or avulsion of the distal insertion of the extensor tendon onto the base of the distal phalanx and is the result of a sudden violent hyperflexion injury. Fractures of the phalanges may also present with acute angular deformities or rotation deformities, often seen with spiral fractures. Fractures of the distal phalanx are usually a result of a crushing blow.

▶ Diagnosis

Clinical examination correlated with biplanar radiographs is usually diagnostic.

▶ Disease Severity

Intra-articular comminution is associated with poor function outcomes. Spiral fractures may result in rotation residuals if great care is not taken in the treatment of the fracture. Fractures of the distal phalanx often result in injuries to the nail bed, which can result in nail deformities if not anatomically repaired.

▶ Concept and Application

Fractures of the phalanges are caused by sudden, violent blows to the hand. They result in loss of joint function and angular deformities, accentuated by the pull of the tendons that act across the injured joints.

▶ Treatment Steps
1. Mallet fingers are treated with hyperextension splinting. Phalangeal fractures can be treated with splinting and buddy taping. Care must be taken to ensure flexion at the MCP and gentle flexion of the PIP to prevent loss of motion secondary to contraction of the collateral ligaments seen with prolonged splinting in full extension.
2. When there is loss of articular congruency, open reduction or percutaneous pinning is indicated. Unstable fracture geometries also require surgical stabilization.
3. Distal phalangeal fractures that involve the nail bed require repair of the nail bed with suture.

## 5. Fracture of Neck of Femur

▶ H&P Keys

In the adolescent and early adult, femoral neck fractures occur as a result of high-energy accidents. In the elderly they may occur with relatively minor trauma secondary to osteoporosis. Fractures may occur as a result of a direct fall on the greater trochanter or from a rotational force along the shaft of the femur. Symptoms include groin pain, inability to bear weight with the hip held in mild adduction and external rotation. The pain is exaggerated by motion, especially rotation of the hip. In an impacted fracture in the elderly, the symptoms may consist of groin pain only with ambulation; the pain may be referred to the knee or thigh.

▶ Diagnosis

AP and lateral radiographs usually confirm the diagnosis. In the elderly with groin pain and osteopenia, CT and a bone scan may be necessary to confirm the diagnosis.

▶ Disease Severity

Displaced fractures of the femoral neck have a high rate of complications, with delayed unions and the development of avascular necrosis of the femoral head from disruption of blood supply to the femoral head by the circumflex vessels. In the young patients with axial loading fractures, posttraumatic chondrolysis may also be a complication. Even with minimal displacement, avascular necrosis and collapse of the femoral head may occur.

▶ Concept and Application

Femoral neck fractures should be considered in any elderly patient with groin pain. In younger patients, the diagnosis should be considered with high-energy trauma and associated groin pain. Displaced fractures of the femoral neck disrupt the blood supply to the femoral head and result in avascular necrosis.

▶ Treatment Steps

1. In young patients, the fracture of the femoral neck should be promptly reduced and internally fixed.
2. In the elderly, impacted and nondisplaced fractures may be pinned in situ. Because of the osteopenia, the fixation hardware may fail and require revision to a joint replacement. Displaced fractures in the elderly should be treated with hemiarthroplasty or total hip arthroplasty if degenerative arthritis is present.

6. Fractures of the Foot and Leg

▶ H&P Keys

Fractures are a result of trauma but may also occur as a result of repetitive stress that results in a stress fracture. Fractures usually present with acute pain and swelling. Ecchymosis develops secondary to the fracture hematoma. Inability to bear weight, or pain exacerbated with weight bearing is usually present. Obvious angular deformity may be present with severely displaced fractures.

▶ Diagnosis

Radiographs are usually diagnostic. AP and lateral films are standard. Special views are necessary to evaluate the ankle (mortise view) and the foot (oblique views) to fully assess the injury pattern. The mortise view evaluates whether there has been injury to the syndesmosis with widening of the ankle mortise. The oblique foot views evaluate Lisfranc's joint. Injury to this region is often missed with plain radiographs. When pain is present only with activity and there is no history of trauma, bone scan may be necessary to evaluate for a stress injury. The most common locations for stress fractures in the foot and leg are the metatarsal, tibia, and fibula.

### ▶ Disease Severity
The location and the degree of comminution and displacement are predictive for rates of healing and complications of stiffness and lost joint motion. The distal third of the tibia is notorious for slow bony union, with a high percentage of delayed unions or nonunions. The fifth metatarsal in the diaphyseal region is also prone to nonunion, especially if weight bearing is allowed. Lisfranc's joint at the base of the second metatarsal is another region for complications following injury, with late arthritis and stiffness often present.

### ▶ Concept and Application
Fractures of the lower extremity require definition of their location and fracture geometry to ensure proper treatment.

### ▶ Treatment Steps
Fractures of the lower extremity require immobilization for adequate healing. This may be provided with casting, fracture bracing, or internal fixation with plates and screws or intramedullary devices. Principles of treatment are restoration of joint congruity and bony length with correction of angular and rotation deformities.

## 7. Dislocations and Separations

### ▶ H&P Keys
Any joint may suffer a dislocation. A dislocation occurs when a violent force applied to the joint results in the disruption of the supporting ligamentous structures. Pain is usually present, with ecchymosis over the injured ligamentous structures. Joint deformity and loss of motion may be present if the joint does not reduce spontaneously. There is joint instability with stress testing and a sense of insecurity with weight bearing.

### ▶ Diagnosis
Radiographs are used to show displacement or associated fractures. Stress testing of ligamentous supports confirms damage to and instability of the joint.

### ▶ Disease Severity
The residuals of joint dislocation depend on the joint injured. Hip dislocations have a high rate of complication with avascular necrosis. Dislocations of the knee may result in arterial injury to the popliteal vessels and loss of perfusion to the lower leg. Shoulder dislocations may result in injuries to the axillary or musculocutaneous nerves and persistent instability of the shoulder. Dislocations of Lisfranc's joint may result in persistent pain stiffness and ambulatory dysfunction.

### ▶ Concept and Application
Joint dislocations are serious injuries. They result when the forces that are applied to the joint exceed the ligaments' ability to with-

stand the stress. Instability occurs as a result of the loss of the passive restraints provided by the ligaments. The displacement of the normal joint structures may result in secondary injury to adjacent structures. Chronic instability may be a result of the injury.

▶ Treatment Steps
1. Rapid reduction of the dislocation and assessment of secondary injury patterns are the mainstays of treatment.
2. Fracture bracing and early protected motion programs may be useful in decreasing the morbidity associated with prolonged immobilization with rigid casting.
3. Operative repair is indicated for irreducible dislocations and for stabilization of grossly unstable joints.

8. Rotator Cuff Syndrome

▶ H&P Keys

Rotator cuff insufficiency may occur as an acute event after a fall into the shoulder. The injury usually occurs when the extremity is extended to break the fall and the weight of the body is suddenly applied to the tendon while it is under tension. The injury may result in sudden loss of shoulder function with inability to abduct the shoulder. The tear may occur by attrition in the older patient, with gradual deterioration of shoulder strength. Immediate symptoms are pain and swelling in the shoulder region. Pain may be increased with passive motion. There is weakness in shoulder abduction. Pain may be increased in activity above the horizontal and with resistance to abduction. There may be a positive drop arm test, with inability to hold the arm at the horizontal against any resistance.

▶ Diagnosis

Radiographs may be normal or may show superior migration of the humeral head, impinging on the inferior surface of the acromion. In an acute injury, the humeral head may be low in the glenoid fossa secondary to intra-articular hematoma. Arthrography and MRI will define the magnitude and location of the tear.

▶ Disease Severity

The degree of symptoms depends on the magnitude of the tear. Partial or small tears may result in only minimal dysfunction and present with the predominant feature of pain. Larger tears will result in loss of shoulder strength. Long-standing cuff tears will result in cuff arthropathy, arthritis characterized by a high-riding humeral head impinging on the acromion, with glenohumeral arthritis.

▶ Concept and Application

Rotator cuff tears may occur as a sudden failure or as a result of slow attrition. Loss of balance in the musculature of shoulder results in altered mechanics of the shoulder. The humeral head migrates superiorly and may herniate through the hole in the cuff to impinge on the acromion. The altered mechanics result in the late development of glenohumeral arthritis.

▶ Treatment Steps
1. Initial treatment is with ice, rest, and antiinflammatory medications.
2. As the pain of the acute injury subsides, rehabilitation is started to increase strength in the cuff and restore muscle balance. If the shoulder does not improve with rehabilitation, surgery is indicated for repair of the cuff.
3. In young patients and those who require overhead strength in the shoulder, early surgical repair is advised. Decompression of the subacromial space by partial acromionectomy is indicated to decrease the compressive forces on the shoulder.
4. In older patients with irreparable tears, symptomatic relief may be obtained with debridement of the cuff and rehabilitation.

### E. Other Orthopedic Emergencies

Other orthopaedic emergencies include compartmental syndrome, cauda equina syndrome, joint infections, open fractures, fractures and dislocations with vascular involvement.

1. Compartmental Syndrome

   A rise in the interstitial compartment pressures as a result of bleeding or soft-tissue swelling that prevents the perfusion of the compartment. Presents first with severe pain, which increases with passive stretch of the compartment. Diagnosis with intracompartmental pressure assessment. Greater than 30 mm Hg warrants surgical decompression.

2. Cauda Equina Syndrome

   Progressive loss of lower-extremity function, with loss of bowel and bladder control. Secondary to pressure on the cauda equina. Requires immediate surgical decompression.

3. Joint Infections

   Painful inflammation with pain on passive motion of the joint. Serial aspiration or surgical lavage is needed promptly to prevent the destruction of the joint by chondrolytic enzymes.

4. Open Fractures

   Fractures in which the bone is exposed through the skin surface either from within or without. Grading is dependent on the size of the wound and zone of injury and the degree of soft-tissue contamination. The greater the zone of injury and the greater the degree of contamination, the greater the increase in risk of infection and limb loss.

5. Vascular Compromise Following Fracture and Dislocation

   Fractures and dislocations that cause loss of perfusion require prompt attention, with reduction usually restoring blood flow. Angiography is necessary if pulses are not restored. Knee dislocations mandate an angiogram because of the high rate of intimal injury to the popliteal artery and late thrombosis and subsequent limb loss.

▶ on rounds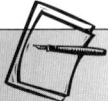

### MUSCULOSKELETAL DISORDERS, FOCUS ON INFLAMMATORY/IMMUNOLOGIC CONDITIONS

#### Polymyalgia Rheumatica
- Women over age 60, more common in women
- Pain in the shoulders, neck, upper arms, low back, thighs; morning stiffness, gelling
- X-rays are normal, RF and ANA are normal, ESR is elevated
- Treat with prednisone

#### Ankylosing Spondylitis
- Common in men ages 15–30
- Low back pain, profound morning stiffness
- Elevated ESR, may be HLA-B27 positive, sacroiliitis on x-ray.
- Treat with anti-inflammatory medication

#### Rheumatoid Arthritis
- Women ages 15–35
- Symmetric painful swelling in the small joints, morning stiffness, fatigue; may affect elbows, ankles, hips, spine, and shoulders
- X-rays positive for erosions, positive RF, elevated ESR, anemia
- Treat with acetaminophen, NSAIDs, antimalarial, gold, penicillamine and immunosuppressives

#### Lupus Arthritis
- Females 14–40 (5:1 female/male ratio)
- Acute arthritis most often affecting the small joints of the hand, wrists, and knee
- ANA positive in 95%
- Treatment includes NSAIDs and corticosteroids

#### Polymyositis–Dermatomyositis
- Symmetric proximal hip weakness, symmetric muscle wasting, weakness, slow gait, muscle tenderness to palpation
- Elevated serum creatine kinase, aldolase, LDH and transaminase; EMG abnormalities, may have autoantibodies
- Treat with corticosteroids or methotrexate

## BIBLIOGRAPHY

Ball GV. *Clinical Rheumatology*. Philadelphia: WB Saunders Co; 1993.
Cailliet R. *Neck and Arm Pain*. 3rd ed. Philadelphia: FA Davis Co; 1991.
Callen JP. Cutaneous manifestations of collagen vascular disease and related conditions. *Med Clin North Am*. Philadelphia: WB Saunders Co; September, 1989.
Connolly JF. *The Management of Fractures and Dislocations: An Atlas*. 3rd ed. Philadelphia: WB Saunders Co; 1997.
D'Ambrosia RD. *Musculoskeletal Disorders*. 2nd ed. Philadelphia: JB Lippincott Co; 1986.
Dieppe PA. *Atlas of Clinical Rheumatology*. Philadelphia: Lea & Febiger; 1986.
Enneking WF. *Musculoskeletal Tumor Surgery*. New York: Churchill Livingstone Inc; 1983.
Morrissy RT. *Pediatric Orthopedics*. 5th ed. Philadelphia: JB Lippincott; 2001; 1, 2.
Niwayama G, Resnick D. *Diagnosis of Bone and Joint Disorders*. 2nd ed. Philadelphia: WB Saunders Co; 1988.
O'Donoghue DH. *Treatment of Injuries to Athletes*. 4th ed. Philadelphia: WB Saunders Co; 1984.
Pettid, FJ. *Practical Orthopedics*. 5th ed. Mosby; 2000.
Turek SL. *Orthopedics: Principles and Their Application*. 4th ed. Philadelphia: JB Lippincott Co; 1984; 1, 2.

# Neurology 10

I. **INFECTIOUS DISEASES OF THE CENTRAL NERVOUS SYSTEM** / 303
   A. Viruses / 303
   B. Meningitis / 306
   C. Abscesses / 308
   D. Spirochetes / 309

II. **NEUROMUSCULAR DISORDERS** / 310
   A. Carpal Tunnel Syndrome / 310
   B. Guillain–Barré Syndrome (Acute Inflammatory Demyelinating Polyneuropathy) / 311
   C. Myasthenia Gravis / 312
   D. Myopathies and Dystrophies / 313

III. **NUTRITIONAL AND METABOLIC DISORDERS** / 313
   A. Vitamin $B_{12}$ Deficiency / 313
   B. Thiamine Deficiency / 314
   C. Metabolic Encephalopathy / 315

IV. **PAROXYSMAL DISORDERS** / 315
   A. Seizures / 315
   B. Trigeminal Neuralgia / 316
   C. Headaches / 317

V. **CEREBROVASCULAR DISORDERS** / 318
   A. Ischemic Thrombotic Strokes / 318
   B. Cardioembolic Strokes / 320
   C. Intracerebral Hemorrhage / 321
   D. Subarachnoid Hemorrhage / 321
   E. Venous Thrombosis / 322

VI. **TOXIC DISORDERS** / 323
   A. Heavy Metals / 323
   B. Medications / 324

**VII. NEOPLASMS / 325**
    A. Glioblastoma / 325
    B. Meningioma / 326
    C. Metastases / 326

**VIII. DEGENERATIVE DISEASES / 327**
    A. Alzheimer's Disease / 327
    B. Amyotrophic Lateral Sclerosis / 328
    C. Parkinson's Disease / 328
    D. Huntington's Disease / 329

**IX. TRAUMA / 330**
    A. Subdural Hematoma / 330
    B. Epidural Hematoma / 330
    C. Contusion / 331

**X. DEMYELINATION / 331**
    A. Multiple Sclerosis / 331

**XI. SPINE DISEASE / 333**
    A. Spinal Stenosis / 333
    B. Radiculopathy / 333

**XII. SLEEP DISORDERS / 334**
    A. Sleep Apnea / 334
    B. Narcolepsy / 335

**XIII. DEVELOPMENTAL DISORDERS / 335**
    A. Tay–Sachs Disease / 335

**DEFINITIONS / 336**

**BIBLIOGRAPHY / 338**

## I. INFECTIOUS DISEASES OF THE CENTRAL NERVOUS SYSTEM

### A. Viruses

#### 1. Human Immunodeficiency Virus (HIV)

▶ **H&P Keys**

Risk factors include blood transfusion, needle sharing, unsafe sex; presentations include: headache and fever (meningitis) 1%, progressive dementia with impaired saccadic eye movements (15% to 20%), paraparesis (myelopathy) 20%, pain and numbness (neuropathy) 30%, focal deficits in central nervous system (CNS), lymphoma, toxoplasmosis, or progressive multifocal leukoencephalitis (PML).

▶ **Diagnosis**

HIV antibodies by enzyme-linked immunosorbent assay (ELISA) (if positive confirm with Western blot); magnetic resonance imaging (MRI) of affected area to exclude mass lesion in myelopathy, dementia, or focal deficits; cerebrospinal fluid (CSF) for pleocytosis; cultures in meningitis; CSF protein and electromyography (EMG) and nerve conduction velocities (NCV) in neuropathy; vitamin $B_{12}$ level.

▶ **Disease Severity**

CD4+ count under 200 associated with severe immunosuppression and opportunistic infections; viral load > 100,000 copies/mL correlate with CD4+ decline and clinical progression; dementia, myelopathy, lymphoma, and PML carry poor prognosis.

▶ **Concept and Application**

Etiology of dementia and myelopathy unknown; direct invasion in meningitis; reduced immunocompetence in toxoplasmosis, lymphoma, neuropathy, or PML.

▶ **Treatment Steps**
1. For parenchymal mass lesion, pyrimethamine and sulfadiazine for 2 weeks, biopsy if not better.
2. Radiation for CNS lymphoma.
3. Amphotericin for fungal meningitis.
4. IV IgG if neuropathy is demyelinating; otherwise biopsy to rule out specific infectious or vasculitic etiologies.
5. Pain treatment with tricyclic antidepressants, gabapentin, lamotrigine, carbamazepine.
6. For dementia treatment protocols include reverse transcriptase and protease inhibitors.
7. Vacuolar myelopathy has no specific therapy.

#### 2. Herpes Simplex Virus (HSV)

▶ **H&P Keys**

In the CNS usually presents with encephalitic symptoms including clouding of consciousness, aphasia, fever, headache, seizures; exam denotes aphasia, hemiparesis, nuchal rigidity, confusion, and variable somnolence.

► Diagnosis

Brain computed tomography (CT) shows edema and hemorrhage in the temporal lobe and orbitofrontal cortex; MRI demonstrates areas of high signal intensity on T-weighted images; electroencephalogram (EEG) shows periodic epileptiform discharges (PLEDs) (Fig. 10–1), CSF has increased protein and mild lymphocytic pleocytosis and, at times, xanthochromia; polymerase chain reaction (PCR) of CSF is helpful for the diagnosis; biopsy makes definitive diagnosis.

► Disease Severity

Sequelae directly related to duration of disease prior to therapy; often fatal if not treated; age greater than 30 associated with poor prognosis.

► Concept and Application

Virus accesses brain by reactivation from fifth cranial nerve; direct invasion causes necrosis, hemorrhage, edema; sporadic occurrence.

► Treatment Steps

1. IV acyclovir when diagnosis suspected.
2. Biopsy of lesion, but therapy should not be delayed while waiting for biopsy.

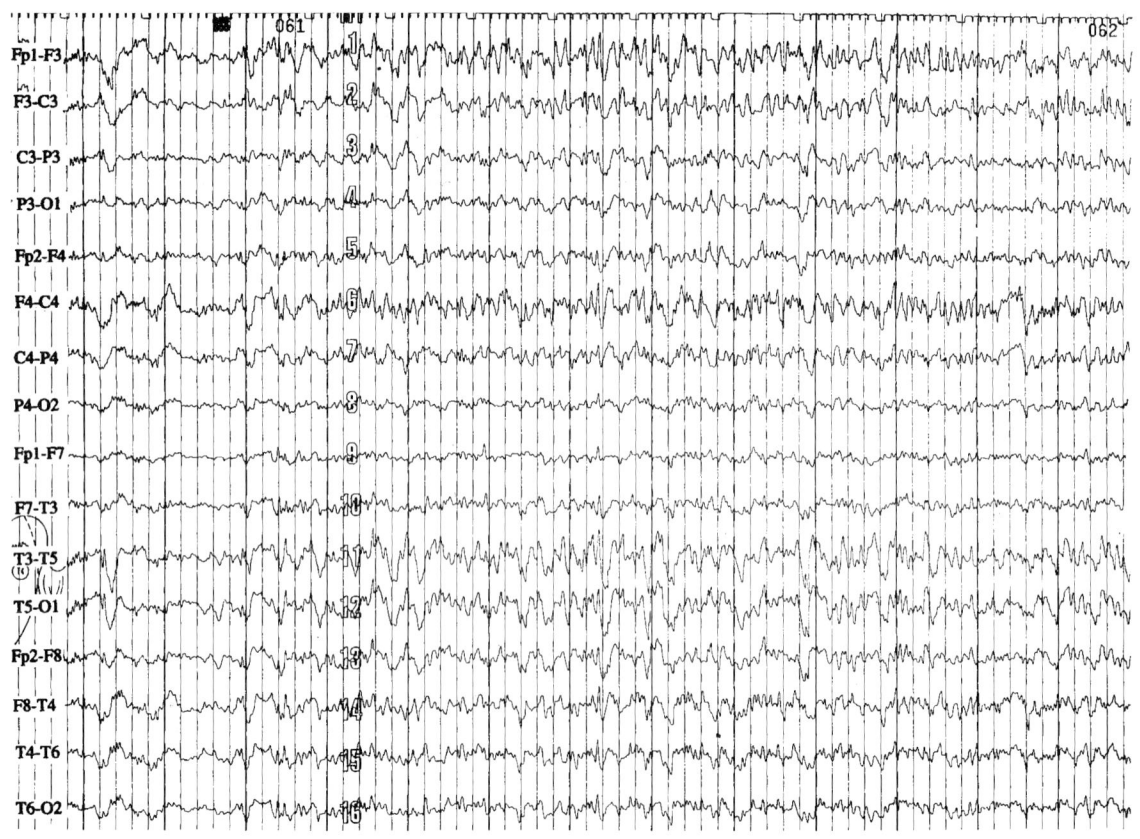

Figure 10–1. Electroencephalogram with periodic lateralizing epileptiform discharges escalating to electrographic seizure in a patient with herpes encephalitis.

3. Anticonvulsants for seizures.
4. Supportive care.

### 3. Spongiform Encephalopathy (Creutzfeldt–Jakob Disease)

▶ **H&P Keys**

Middle-aged patient with rapidly progressive change in behavior, intellectual function, and emotional responses, followed by startle myoclonic jerks, ataxia, and dysarthria. Stupor and coma follow.

▶ **Diagnosis**

Blood and CSF are usually normal. Detection of 14-3-3 proteinase inhibitor in CSF has proven useful in difficult cases. When advanced, EEG shows 1 to 2 cycles per second triphasic sharp waves superimposed on a depressed background occasionally occuring in synchrony with myoclonic jerks. Brain biopsy shows spongiform changes in the cortex, which is diagnostic. Immunoblot analysis of frozen brain tissue homogenates reveal the presence of prion protein.

▶ **Disease Severity**

Invariably fatal; mode of transmission unclear; may be transmissible iatrogenically; familial cases associated with mutations in prion protein gene.

▶ **Concept and Application**

The etiology is still unclear. Probably caused by abnormal prion protein, but transmissible.

▶ **Treatment Steps**

1. No treatment available.

### 4. Poliomyelitis

▶ **H&P Keys**

Fever, anorexia, vomiting, followed in a week with asymmetric painful paralysis that involves any or all limbs and bulbar muscles; no sensory findings or levels.

▶ **Diagnosis**

CSF shows lymphocytic pleocytosis; viral cultures of feces; EMG and NCV show denervation of motor nerves.

▶ **Disease Severity**

Bulbar presentation, if severe, causes respiratory and vasomotor instability, leading to death in 25% of these cases.

▶ **Concept and Application**

Neurotropic virus affects anterior horn cells in spinal cord and motor nuclei of brain stem; also hypothalamus and thalamus.

▶ **Treatment Steps**

1. Supportive, including mechanical ventilation and physical therapy.
2. May develop postpolio syndrome in 20–40 years, manifested by progressive weakness and fatigue.
3. Immunization with attenuated virus is now universal.

5. Rabies

   ▶ H&P Keys

   Rabid animal bite followed by anxiety, overactivity, difficulty swallowing fluids (hydrophobia) progressing to dysphagia, facial spasm, and seizures in 2 to 8 weeks; death occurs 4 to 10 days later.

   ▶ Diagnosis

   Obtain infected animal brain when bite occurs, test for Negri bodies.

   ▶ Disease Severity

   Lack of prior immunization is the largest risk factor for poor outcome.

   ▶ Concept and Application

   Viral particles seen as eosinophilic cytoplasmic inclusions (Negri bodies) throughout CNS.

   ▶ Treatment Steps
   1. If the animal is rabid, treatment of patient with human rabies immunoglobulin or duck embryo vaccine (to offer passive immunity while active develops).
   2. If symptoms occur, supportive care.

B. Meningitis

   1. Aseptic

      ▶ H&P Keys

      Preceding upper respiratory infection, exanthem, exposure to rat excreta; headache, fever, photophobia, nuchal rigidity.

      ▶ Diagnosis

      CT scan to rule out abscess; CSF examination shows pleocytosis, predominantly lymphocytic, mild protein elevation, normal glucose; negative bacterial cultures and Gram's stain; acute and convalescent viral titers helpful.

      ▶ Disease Severity

      Usually benign course, without sequelae; decreased mentation; focal neurologic signs, seizures suggest concurrent encephalitis and worse outcome.

      ▶ Concept and Application

      Meningeal infection with virus, most often enterovirus or mumps virus; initial infection with Lyme disease, HIV, leptospirosis, and syphilis may present similarly.

      ▶ Treatment Steps
      1. Supportive management.

   2. Bacterial (Septic)

      ▶ H&P Keys

      History of sinusitis, ear infection, epidemic meningitis, pneumonia; presents with headache, fever, photophobia, seizures, nuchal rigidity, and obtundation; suspect meningococcus with petechial rash, pneumococcus with pneumonia or sinus infection in adults, *Haemophilus influenzae* with similar symptoms in children.

▶ Diagnosis

Negative CT of head (if timely); CSF pleocytosis up to 10,000, mainly neutrophils; low (< 40% of serum) glucose; protein elevation; positive bacterial cultures and Gram's stain; positive bacterial antigens if partially treated; positive blood cultures in 60%; elevated CSF pressure (200 mm/$H_2O$).

▶ Disease Severity

Coma, focal neurologic signs, signs of herniation, seizures bear poor prognosis and may suggest abscess formation; sequelae and outcome directly related to time of institution of therapy.

▶ Concept and Application

Pyogenic infection of meninges with prominent vascular changes (small to medium arteritis).

▶ Treatment Steps
1. Blood culture; CT of head, lumbar puncture (LP).
2. Do not delay antibiotics for LP or LP for CT; cefotaxime in adults and children over 3 months; ampicillin and cefotaxime in neonates and infants.
3. Steroids may lessen hearing loss in children.
4. Supportive care.

3. Fungal

▶ H&P Keys

Progressive dementia, headaches, nuchal rigidity, lack of fever, cranial nerve involvement, often immunosuppression or history of lymphoma or other malignant disease; exposure to birds; suspect *Cryptococcus* in the immunosuppressed, mucormycosis in diabetics.

▶ Diagnosis

CSF with predominantly lymphocytic and monocytic pleocytosis; positive cryptococcal antigen and positive India ink in cryptococcal meningitis; positive fungal cultures in weeks.

▶ Disease Severity

Hydrocephalus; arteritis, thrombosis, and infarction of the brain.

▶ Concept and Application

Granulomatous meningitis composed of fibroblasts, giant cells, and necrosis.

▶ Treatment Steps
1. Amphotericin B along with antifungal agents (fluconazole, itraconazole).
2. Supportive care.

### 4. Tuberculous (TB)

▶ H&P Keys

Positive purified protein derivative (tuberculin) (PPD) in 75%; fever, malaise, headache; development of nuchal rigidity, decreased mental status, confusion, dementia, lower cranial nerve involvement.

▶ Diagnosis

Chest roentgenogram; PPD; CSF shows lymphocytic pleocytosis, elevated protein (often to several hundreds), low glucose (normal in 30%), positive acid-fast bacillus (AFB) stain or immunofluorescence; cultures take several weeks and often require multiple LPs.

▶ Disease Severity

Residual deficits depend on onset of therapy in relation to stage of disease; obtundation, seizures, hydrocephalus, or focal signs indicate poor prognosis.

▶ Concept and Application

Caseating granulomas surrounded by epithelioid cells, lymphocytes, and connective tissue; exudate results from fibrin, lymphocytes, and areas of caseation necrosis; exudate spreads along pial vessels and invades underlying brain.

▶ Treatment Steps
1. Isoniazid can cause peripheral neuropathy and seizures.
2. Daily addition of pyridoxine; addition of rifampin and pyrazinamide; use of streptomycin when resistance is suspected.
3. Careful observance for liver toxicity.
4. Use of steroids for treatment of all cases of TB meningitis.
5. Treatment of increased intracranial pressure; hydrocephalus treated with ventriculoperitoneal shunt.

## C. Abscesses

▶ H&P Keys

History of sinus, ear, periodontal, pulmonary, or head wound infection, endocarditis; suspect congenital heart disease in children; presents with focal severe headache, nausea and vomiting, seizures; focal signs dependent on location.

▶ Diagnosis

MRI or CT with contrast of affected area shows ring-enhancing lesion with edema, mass effect, "daughter lesion"; LP shows "aseptic" pleocytosis but is usually not necessary and may be contraindicated because of possible herniation.

▶ Disease Severity

Untreated cases produce major disability or death; mortality rate in treated cases is 30%; 50% suffer neurologic sequelae.

▶ Concept and Application

Focal infection of brain parenchyma, usually without meningitis; encapsulated with central necrotic material and pus; solitary 75% of the time; usually caused by anaerobes or microaerophilic organisms, most commonly anaerobic streptococci or bacteroides.

▶ Treatment Steps

1. Biopsy using stereotaxic CT guidance.
2. Steroids for management of intracranial pressure.
3. Mechanical hyperventilation and $P_{CO_2}$ of $< 30$ may be needed if severe.
4. Anticonvulsants for seizures.
5. IV antibiotics include penicillin and metronidazole if pathogen is unknown; vancomycin for methicillin-resistant staphylococci and third-generation cephalosporin for gram-negative bacteria.

## D. Spirochetes

### 1. Lyme Disease

▶ H&P Keys

History of tick bite in about 50% of patients; history of erythema chronicum migrans in about 60% of patients; influenzalike symptoms; can present as an aseptic meningitis; weeks to months later neurologic involvement will happen in 15% of the cases; most common neurologic presentation is one of meningoencephalitis with cranial or peripheral neuritis; chronic symptoms include encephalopathy and axonal neuropathy; peripheral nervous system presentation include Bell's palsy, mononeuritis multiplex, myositis, and peripheral neuropathy.

▶ Diagnosis

Lyme titers by ELISA, confirmed by Western blot; perform CSF examination in all neurologic cases; typical CSF abnormalities include mononuclear cell pleocytosis as high as 3,000 and increased protein level up to 400; check for intrathecal production of Lyme-specific antibodies, cultures and PCR testing in equivocal cases.

▶ Disease Severity

Myelitis-causing quadriparesis, seizures, and dementia have infrequently been described but are likely to leave sequelae. Radiculoneuritis is commonly reported in Europe but rare in United States.

▶ Concept and Application

Arthropod-borne infection. *Borrelia burgdorferi* is a spirochete inoculated into humans by the *Ixodes* or deer tick; endemic in northeastern United States.

▶ Treatment Steps

1. Treat erythema migrans or Bell's palsy with oral doxycycline or amoxicillin for 30 days; for any other neurologic symptoms or conditions, treat with IV ceftriaxone 2 g daily for 14 days.
2. Corticosteroids are used in failure to respond to antibiotics.

## 2. Neurosyphilis

▶ **H&P Keys**

Sexually transmitted; develops a painless chancre in genital region; subsequently patient might complain of headaches, stiff neck, nausea, or vomiting that resolve within days to weeks and evolve within 6 to 12 years into a meningovascular disease with cerebrovascular accidents; within 15 to 20 years a progressive mental dissolution including dementia, dysarthria, myoclonic jerks, seizures, hyperreflexia, and Argyll–Robertson pupils (general paresis); another presentation within the same time frame is tabes dorsalis, which includes the development of ataxia, lightning pains, urinary incontinence, and absent reflexes with impaired vibratory and position sense, Argyll–Robertson pupils (90% of cases).

▶ **Diagnosis**

Examine CSF for cells, protein, and Venereal Disease Research Laboratory (VDRL) test; treat those patients who have a positive VDRL or rapid plasma reagin (RPR) test and whose past antibiotic therapy cannot be confirmed as adequate or have not had antibiotic therapy; CSF picture often consists of lymphocytic pleocytosis, elevated protein, and positive VDRL. Oligoclonal bands, IgM antibodies, and PCR may increase diagnostic sensitivity.

▶ **Disease Severity**

Most late symptoms of neurosyphilis are unpredictable and often unresponsive to treatment with penicillin; intraparenchymal gumma can develop in HIV-infected patients and behave like mass lesions.

▶ **Concept and Application**

Syphilis is due to a treponemal disease that invades the CNS within 3–18 months of inoculation with the organism; after this time, the chances of CNS infection are markedly reduced to a total of 1% if the CSF remains negative after 5 years.

▶ **Treatment Steps**

1. Treatment of choice is IV penicillin G 4,000,000 U q4h for 14 days.
2. IV therapy should be started in the hospital because of possible Jarisch–Herxheimer reaction.
3. Lancinating pain treated with anticonvulsants; neuropathic joints treated with bracing.
4. CSF examination repeated every 3–6 months; cells should clear first, then protein, then VDRL.

## II. NEUROMUSCULAR DISORDERS

### A. Carpal Tunnel Syndrome

▶ **H&P Keys**

Nocturnal pain or numbness in first three digits of the hand, weakness on thumb opposition, wrist pain with rare shoulder pain; exacerbation with repetitive motion of wrist; positive Tinel's sign at median nerve at the wrist.

▶ Diagnosis

Wrist roentgenograms show bony deformities; MRI wrist demonstrates focal compression of median nerve; EMG and NCV will show focal median nerve conduction velocity slowing at the wrist, axonal loss; depending on history, check for diabetes, rheumatoid arthritis, Lyme disease.

▶ Disease Severity

Severe atrophy of thenar muscles, marked thumb opposition weakness, permanent pain or numbness of first three digits, absent sensory early and later, motor potentials on nerve conduction of the median nerve.

▶ Concept and Application

Compression of median nerve with intussusception of node of Ranvier or traumatic injury of nerve by repetitive motion; diabetes, amyloidosis, acromegaly, hypothyroidism, sarcoidosis, rheumatoid arthritis, and pregnancy increase risk of syndrome.

▶ Treatment Steps

1. Mild cases will respond to wrist splint.
2. Recurrence of pain or numbness will respond to steroid injection.
3. Surgery offers excellent results in over 90% of cases of well-demonstrated carpal tunnel syndrome.
4. Reduction of repetitive activity.
5. Modification of work environment.

## B. Guillain–Barré Syndrome (Acute Inflammatory Demyelinating Polyneuropathy)

▶ H&P Keys

Progressive ascending weakness a few weeks after an upper respiratory or gastrointestinal illness or surgery; back discomfort in 60%; no sensory level; areflexia; distal, but may be proximal, progressive weakness mainly in the legs; no fever on presentation; very symmetrical; maximum evolution of disease in 2 weeks in 50% of patients, in 4 weeks in 90% of patients.

▶ Diagnosis

CSF with high protein but less than 10 white blood cells (WBCs) (50 in HIV patients); slowing of conduction velocities to conduction block on EMG and NCV studies; check for Lyme, HIV, urine porphyrins, hepatitis; culture stools for *Campylobacter jejuni*. GM1, Gd1a and GD1b myelin glycolipid antibodies in CSF support the diagnosis.

▶ Disease Severity

Poor prognostic indicators include severe tetraparesis, hyperacute onset, assisted ventilation, low nerve amplitudes on EMG and NCV (suggesting axonal involvement and likely to result in prolonged sequelae), and abnormal phrenic nerve studies; autonomic instability may increase morbidity.

▶ Concept and Application

Proximal and later distal segmental demyelination with inflammatory cell infiltration in nerve.

▶ Treatment Steps

1. Plasmapheresis in first week for quickly progressing cases (inability to stand) or ventilator dependence.
2. Supportive care.
3. Recent evidence favors intravenous immune globulin (IVIG) as treatment.
4. Corticosteroids are not helpful.

## C. Myasthenia Gravis

▶ H&P Keys

Diplopia, ptosis; symptoms worsen at end of day; young females; elderly males; demonstrable fatigue on examination, such as worsening of ptosis on prolonged upward gaze.

▶ Diagnosis

Dramatic improvement with IV edrophonium chloride (Tensilon) (test double blind); positive antibodies to acetylcholine receptors (80% in generalized, only 50% in ocular myasthenia); decrement of motor nerve potential with repetitive stimulation; may need single-fiber analysis; thoracic MRI for thymic abnormalities (hyperplasia in 85%, thymomas in 10–15%).

▶ Disease Severity

Bulbar weakness increases risk of aspiration; low pulmonary vital capacity indicates respiratory compromise; thymoma requires surgery.

▶ Concept and Application

Antibodies that block or permanently bind to the acetylcholine receptors; presumably resulting from autoimmune reaction possibly triggered by or cross-reactive with thymic acetylcholine receptors; this leads to disturbance in the neuromuscular synaptic transmission and decreased muscle excitation.

▶ Treatment Steps

1. Acetylcholinesterase inhibitor increases available acetylcholine.
2. Corticosteroids reduce the immunologic process; other immunosuppressants are used in severe cases.
3. Thymectomy, although controversial, can eliminate the need for medications in some cases or reduce the doses in others.
4. Acute worsening is best treated by discontinuation of medications and ventilatory support.
5. Plasmapheresis is useful for short periods to hasten improvement.

### D. Myopathies and Dystrophies

▶ H&P Keys

History of progressive proximal weakness in most cases; myalgias and cramps are more the exception than the rule; weakness is noted raising arms overhead and in related activities, or getting up from a chair; myotonic dystrophy will show myotonia on percussion of small muscles (eg, tongue); Duchenne's dystrophy shows calf muscle enlargement.

▶ Diagnosis

Creatine kinase (CK) is elevated in most cases of myopathy and muscular dystrophy; EMG and NCV demonstrate small, brief (myopathic) motor unit potentials and normal nerve conduction velocities; muscle biopsy is diagnostic in most cases; metabolic myopathies may require biochemical studies; ischemic exercise test is abnormal in some glycogen metabolic myopathies because of the inability to utilize energy substrate; electrocardiogram is needed for high incidence of cardiac abnormalities.

▶ Disease Severity

Severe weakness could be associated with respiratory compromise; high CK might cause myoglobinuria and renal failure in metabolic myopathies; many myopathies associated with life-threatening cardiac abnormalities; swallowing and respiratory difficulties could result in death.

▶ Concept and Application

Duchenne's dystrophy is the result of lack of dystrophin (muscle fiber surface membrane protein resulting in disturbance of structural integrity of sarcolemma); a severe inflammatory process of the muscle results in polymyositis; other myopathies are the result of metabolic derangements (McArdle's), protein serine-threonine kinase enzyme defect (result of triple nucleotide repeats expansion) in myotonic dystrophy, or intrinsic sarcomere dysfunction (congenital myopathies).

▶ Treatment Studies

1. Appropriate genetic studies facilitate diagnosis and genetic counseling along with prenatal diagnosis.
2. Corticosteroids in polymyositis and Duchenne's dystrophy; anticonvulsants in myotonic dystrophy to reduce cramps.
3. Orthoses and ambulatory aides might be helpful in activities of daily living.

## III. NUTRITIONAL AND METABOLIC DISORDERS

### A. Vitamin $B_{12}$ Deficiency

▶ H&P Keys

Painful dysesthesias in feet and hands followed by difficulty ambulating; ataxia, leg weakness, spasticity, changes in mentation, visual loss.

▶ Diagnosis

Vitamin $B_{12}$ levels can be obtained in most laboratories; because neurologic presentation does not necessarily parallel the hematologic picture, a high level of suspicion is needed; a few cases may have "normal" levels, and these may require measurement of methylmalonic acid and homocysteine, both of which are elevated in $B_{12}$ tissue deficiency.

▶ Disease Severity

Progressive leg weakness and spasticity leading to the need for ambulatory aids; in general symptoms lasting more than 3 months are unlikely to revert; the etiology for the deficiency should be established.

▶ Concept and Application

White matter degeneration of the spinal cord and occasionally of the brain; changes begin in the posterior column of the lower cervical segment and spread downward, forward, and laterally.

▶ Treatment Steps
1. Initial management is emergent.
2. Daily $B_{12}$ (1,000 mg) is needed in the first 7 days to replete stores. Subsequently, needs are supplied by 1,000 mg of $B_{12}$ monthly.

## B. Thiamine Deficiency

▶ H&P Keys

Usually undernourished alcoholics, but sometimes patients with gastric carcinoma or hyperemesis gravidarum, who present with ataxia of gait, gaze palsies or nystagmus, and mental confusion (Wernicke's encephalopathy); ocular abnormalities might include nystagmus that could be both horizontal or vertical, weakness or paralysis of conjugate gaze, or weakness of the external rectus muscle, which is always bilateral; the ataxia is one of stance and gait with no evidence of tremor, and the confusion could present as a global confusional state, stupor, and coma or as a hallucinatory state with overactivity; Wernicke's encephalopathy might progress to an amnesic syndrome with severe short-term memory impairment and confabulation (Korsakoff's psychosis).

▶ Diagnosis

CSF is almost always normal; blood pyruvate may be elevated; red blood cell (RBC) transketolase activity is markedly reduced, but the diagnosis remains a clinical one.

▶ Disease Severity

Transition to the Korsakoff state heralds poor outcome, even with therapy; other symptoms are likely to improve with treatment; concurrent septicemia, pneumonia, and liver disease result in about 15% mortality rate.

▶ Concept and Application

Thiamine deficiency results in necrotic lesions of the mamillary bodies, periaqueductal region, thalamus, hypothalamus, and floor of the fourth ventricle.

▶ Treatment Steps
1. Administer IV thiamine 50 mg and IM 50 mg initially; and IM 50 mg daily subsequently until normal diet is resumed.
2. Avoid glucose infusion prior to thiamine administration.
3. Provide supportive care.
4. Evaluate for infections and other conditions.

### C. Metabolic Encephalopathy

▶ H&P Keys

Progressive clouding of consciousness in general without any focal symptomatology; history of medication overdose, infections, anoxia, hypo- or hyperglycemia, renal insufficiency, liver disease, alcohol intoxication; examination demonstrates normal pupillary reactions with small pupils, normal oculovestibular responses, normal corneal responses, and no focal deficits in a mentally obtunded patient.

▶ Diagnosis

CT of the head is used to rule out mass lesions in patients with focal neurologic deficits (hypoglycemia, hypoxia, azotemia, and hepatic encephalopathies might cause focal neurologic signs); EEG to rule out nonconvulsive status epilepticus or postictal state; drug screen and metabolic parameters including sodium, glucose, oxygen, $Pco_2$; chest roentgenogram and urinalysis (UA) to rule out infections.

▶ Disease Severity

Prolonged hypoxia or hypoglycemia may result in permanent neurologic injury; ventilatory support might be needed in many instances of coma; fever should raise suspicion of meningitis or abscess.

▶ Concept and Application

Usually reversible; nonstructural injuries resulting in generalized cerebral dysfunction.

▶ Treatment Steps

Correction of metabolic derangement.

## IV. PAROXYSMAL DISORDERS

### A. Seizures

▶ H&P Keys

History of abrupt stereotypic transitory loss or alteration of consciousness with or without involuntary movements; short or no warning (aura); confusional state after recovery of consciousness; bowel and bladder incontinence and tongue biting may happen, usually accompanied by bodily injuries; physical examination usually normal after the event; may have upgoing toes and abnormalities of tone immediately at the end of the episode; if witnessed, the event can start focally in one limb, with automatism or behavioral manifestations or generalized increase or decrease in tone; brief alteration of consciousness without postictal confusion happens in absence seizures in children.

▶ Diagnosis

CT or MRI of brain to rule out irritative lesion (stroke, tumor, abscess); routine EEG might be diagnostic in 20% or less of patients; prolonged EEG monitoring might be necessary in difficult cases; single photon emission computed tomography (SPECT) and positron emission tomography (PET) studies helpful in epileptogenic focus localization; diagnosis remains a clinical one; cardiac evaluation might be needed to rule out convulsive syncope in selected cases.

▶ Disease Severity

Seizures, although most often idiopathic, can be the presentation of otherwise treatable conditions such as brain tumors, abscesses, arteriovenous malformations; repeated seizures during the day might result in severe functional and social disability along with bodily injuries; the disease carries a number of social limitations with it; status epilepticus markedly increases morbidity and mortality.

▶ Concept and Application

Usually caused by an irritative lesion capable of causing abnormal neuronal discharges that can spread and perpetuate themselves.

▶ Treatment Steps

1. Treatment depends on seizure type.
2. When no seizures, patients respond best to valproic acid.
3. Generalized and partial seizures respond to phenytoin, valproate, zonisamide, lamotrigine, topiramate, tiagabine, carbamazepine, and levetiracetam.
4. Febrile seizures do not require chronic anticonvulsant therapy.
5. Refractory cases may require surgery or vagal nerve stimulator placement.
6. Status epilepticus (continuous seizure activity lasting more than 20 minutes or multiple seizures without interictal recovery) are medical emergencies requiring immediate use of IV benzodiazepines followed by IV phenytoin or valproic acid and, if necessary, barbiturate coma with mechanical ventilation.

### B. Trigeminal Neuralgia

▶ H&P Keys

Brief, sharp, lancinating pain mainly in the third or second division of the fifth cranial nerve. Precipitated by touch, cold, or chewing.

▶ Diagnosis

Normal neurologic exam; if abnormal, consider other conditions such as posterior fossa mass lesion; beware of young multiple sclerosis (MS) patients with similar symptoms; any neurologic abnormality should cause a prompt investigation of the posterior fossa with CT or MRI for cerebellar pontine angle tumors, tumors of the fifth nerve, and MS.

▶ Disease Severity

The condition is a painful disease that results in no permanent sequelae to the patient if untreated; however, the pain is severe enough to have caused some patients to commit suicide.

▶ Concept and Application

The specific etiology is unknown, but may involve arterial ectasia with nerve compression in some cases.

▶ Treatment Steps

1. Medical management is highly satisfactory; oral carbamazepine is usually started at the beginning (75% response rate) refractoriness may require the addition of baclofen, gababenten, lamotrigine, or amitriptylene.
2. Monitoring for dizziness, unsteadiness, bone marrow suppression with carbamazepine.
3. Acute confusional state and seizures may occur with abrupt discontinuation of baclofen.
4. Microvascular decompression of the nerve might result in long-standing relief.

## C. Headaches

▶ H&P Keys

History of intermittent or persistent head pain with or without associated vegetative symptoms; migraines are usually unilateral, pulsating headaches and if classic are associated with visual scotomata; hemisensory disturbances; nausea and vomiting; and photo-, phono- and osmophobia; cluster headaches are retro-orbital, occurring in the adult smoker associated with lacrimation; ipsilateral Horner's syndrome usually lasts 90 minutes, may occur at the same time of the day; tension headaches are chronic, bandlike headaches with no other symptomatology; examination should be normal.

▶ Diagnosis

CT or MRI of the head to rule out intracranial mass lesion; early generalized, pulsating headaches might mean nocturnal hypoxemia and may require oximetry; LP should be done on patients with nuchal rigidity or fever; sinus roentgenography should be done on patients with percussion tenderness.

▶ Disease Severity

Headaches might be the initial and sole presentation of intracranial lesions such as brain tumors, abscesses, hydrocephalus, and other space-occupying lesions (Fig. 10–2); otherwise, these are benign conditions.

▶ Concept and Application

Migraine is a familial disorder characterized with abnormal cerebral and intra- and extracranial vascular reactivity; chronic tension headaches are secondary to self-perpetuating muscle tension; cluster headaches could be paroxysmal parasympathetic discharges through the superficial petrosal nerve.

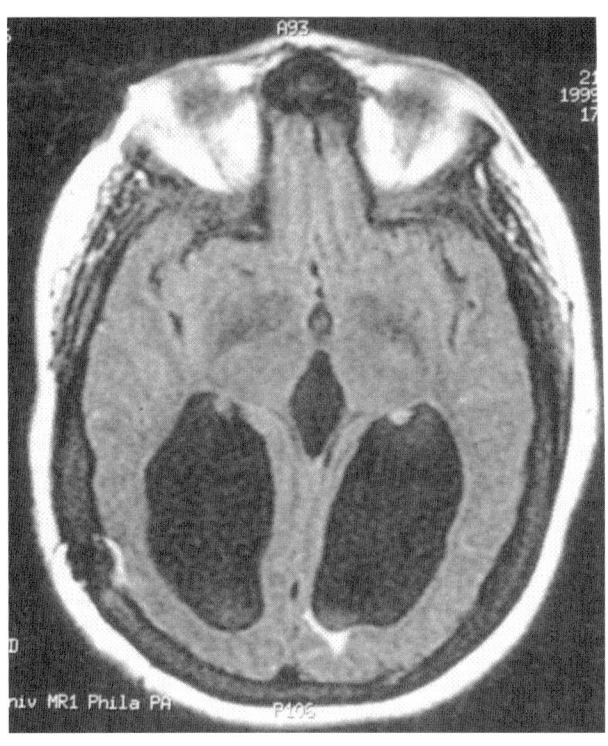

Figure 10-2. T1-weighted MRI image of acute obstructive hydrocephalus revealing dilated third and lateral ventricles.

▶ Treatment Steps
1. Abortive therapy can be provided by means of nonsteroidal anti-inflammatory drugs (NSAIDs).
2. 5HT1B and 5HT1D agonists (sumatriptan, zolmitriptan, rizatriptan, faoratriptan, and naratriptan) are highly effective migrainous attack abortive agents except in patients with known vascular disease or hypertension.
3. Migraine prophylaxis can be achieved by using β-receptor blockers, valproic acid, topiramate, tricyclic antidepressants, riboflavin, magnesium supplementation.
4. Cluster headaches respond well acutely (over 70% of cases) to oxygen inhalation.
5. Ergotamine orally and intranasal lidocaine can provide abortive therapy as well.
6. Prophylaxis is achieved by oral corticosteroids or verapamil.

## V. CEREBROVASCULAR DISORDERS

### A. Ischemic Thrombotic Strokes

▶ H&P Keys

Predisposing risk factors include diabetes, hypertension, hypercholesterolemia, smoking, elevated homocysteine and C-reactive protein; acute onset of fixed neurologic deficit, usually while sleeping; possible prior history of short-lived deficits or unilateral visual loss (transient ischemic attacks); contralateral hemiparesis and aphasia in middle cerebral or carotid distribution; contralateral leg and shoulder weakness in anterior cerebral territory; dense visual field cut in posterior cerebral territory.

▶ Diagnosis

CT or MRI of head to further localize lesion and exclude bleeding (Fig. 10–3); carotid noninvasive or magnetic resonance angiogram (MRA) study to assess for stenosis; blood count and chemistry for risk factors; antinuclear antibodies (ANA), sedimentation rate, RPR, coagulation factor deficiency studies, homocysteine, C-reactive protein; arteriography in young individuals.

▶ Disease Severity

Large clinical or radiologic deficits correlate with large areas of infarction and have increased risk of edema and herniation or hemorrhagic conversion; rehabilitation is also limited.

▶ Concept and Application

Predisposing factors reduce resilience of large arteries; atherosclerosis at branching and curves of cerebral arteries cause stenosis with subsequent embolization or narrowing of lumen (Fig. 10–4). Migraines and oral contraceptives increase risk of infarction.

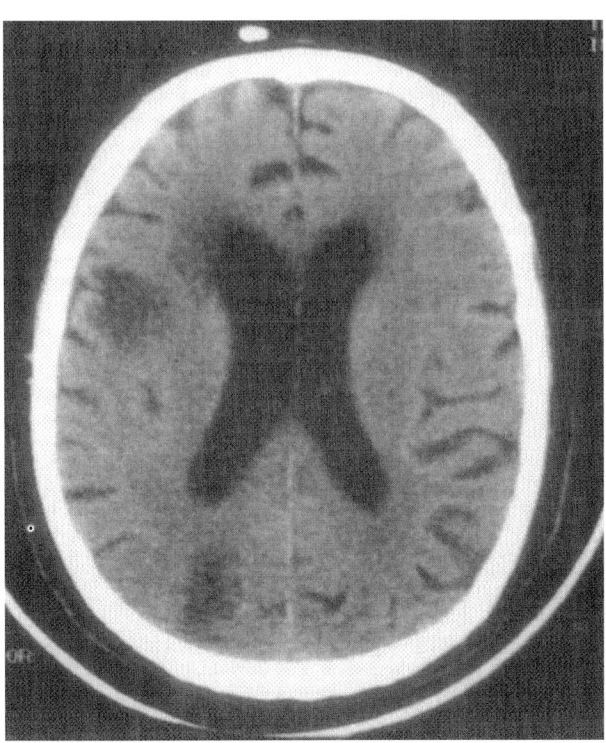

Figure 10–3. CT scan demonstrating right frontal and occipital infarcts in a patient with carotid artery thromboembolism.

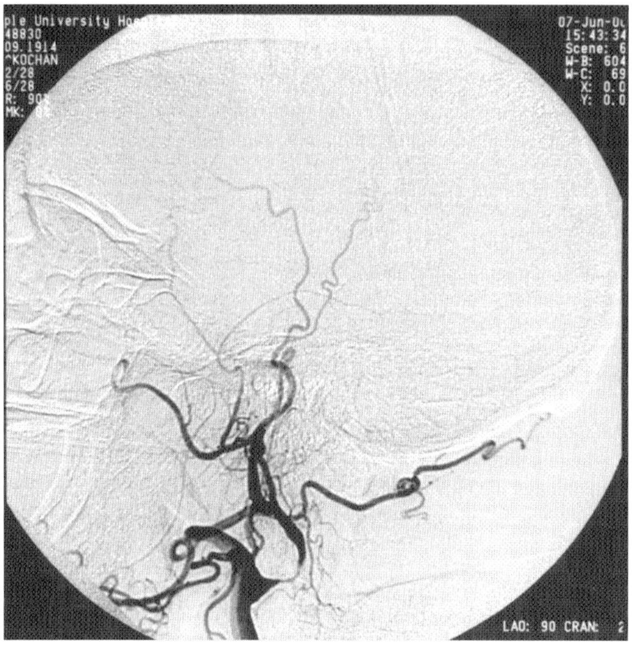

Figure 10–4. Digital subtraction carotid angiogram revealing large atherosclerotic plaque in the common carotid artery extending to internal and external carotid branches.

▶ Treatment Steps
1. Includes reduction of risk factors, management of stroke complications, secondary prevention with antiplatelet or anticoagulant agents.
2. Surgery in carotid arteries if stenosis over 70%.
3. Discontinuation of oral contraceptives.
4. Physical therapy.
5. Periodic follow-up for recurrences.

## B. Cardioembolic Strokes

▶ H&P Keys

History of rheumatic fever, cardiac dysrhythmias; abrupt onset; hemorrhagic strokes, or multifocal distribution. Evidence of cortical signs including aphasia, seizures, more than one arterial distribution in addition to findings similar to thrombotic strokes.

▶ Diagnosis

CT or MRI of head, ECG, transthoracic and transesophageal echocardiogram if ECG is normal and suspicion for cardiac source still high, Holter monitor, blood cultures if endocarditis suspected.

▶ Disease Severity

Embolic strokes tend to be larger and more commonly hemorrhagic, higher incidence of edema with mass effect and seizures increase morbidity and mortality.

▶ Concept and Application

Sources of embolization include atrial fibrillation (with or without valvular disease), prosthetic valves, endocarditis, left ventricular hypokinesis or thrombus, cardiac tumors (myxomas).

▶ Treatment Steps
1. With the exception of myxoma and recent heart attack, long-term anticoagulation is needed.
2. Anticoagulation with heparin can be started within a few hours if stroke is not too large or there is no hemorrhage.
3. Switch to warfarin (Coumadin) when therapeutic and follow International Normalized Ratio (INR) recommendations depending on cause of stroke.

## C. Intracerebral Hemorrhage

▶ H&P Keys

Usually, history of uncontrolled hypertension or coagulation deficits, sudden apoplectic onset, severe headache, nausea, vomiting, and focal neurologic deficits; exam shows hemiparesis, obtundation, sensory deficits, conjugate eye deviation contralateral to hemiparesis (toward hemiparesis if brain stem), rapidly developing coma in pontine or cerebellar hemorrhage, elevated blood pressure.

▶ Diagnosis

CT or MRI of head to assess extent of bleeding, LP may be bloody but nonspecific and may induce herniation.

▶ Disease Severity

Both pontine and cerebellar hemorrhages carry increased risk; cerebellar hemorrhage is usually treated surgically if large.

▶ Concept and Application

Hypertensive hemorrhages are due to aneurysmal dilatation (Charcot–Bouchard aneurysms) of small-caliber arteries as a result of lipohyalinosis. Amyloid deposition in older patients (amyloid angiopathy).

▶ Treatment Steps
1. Supportive therapy, management of intracranial hypertension, careful control of systemic hypertension.
2. Lobar and cerebellar hemorrhages may be amenable to surgical resection.

## D. Subarachnoid Hemorrhage

▶ H&P Keys

Acute onset of worst headache of patient's life, nausea, vomiting, variable loss of consciousness, may have had previous "warning" headaches; nuchal rigidity, obtundation; hemiparesis in middle cerebral territory; third cranial nerve palsy in posterior communicating artery distribution; leg weakness, confusion in anterior cerebral artery territory. Two thirds of ruptured aneurysms occur in anterior circulation.

▶ Diagnosis

CT of head positive in about 90% of cases; MRI may miss initial picture; LP shows elevated pressure, markedly bloody and xanthochromic, protein elevated, leukocytosis in 48 hours. Cerebral angiography is mandatory for definitive diagnosis; if initially negative (vasospasm) repeat in 6–12 weeks. Delay study if severe vasospasm present.

▶ Disease Severity

Outcome depends on mental status at time of ictus. Lethargic or obtunded patients have poorer outcome. Vasospasm and seizures add to morbidity. Disease associated with polycystic kidneys. Multiple aneurysms in many cases.

▶ Concept and Application

Hypertension, arteriosclerosis cause weakness of large-artery walls at bifurcations, leading to saccular dilatation. Rupture of this dilatation with associated arterial pressure results in symptoms. Reflex vasospasm causes oligemia and in severe cases, infarcts. Arteriovenous malformation can also rupture.

▶ Treatment Steps

1. Control of hypertension.
2. Reduction of Valsalva with stool softeners, quiet room.
3. Reduction of vasospasm with nimodipine.
4. Reduction of increased intracranial pressure with osmotic agents.
5. Hyperventilation and ventriculostomy if necessary.
6. Treatment of seizures with anticonvulsants.
7. Surgery when stable.

### E. Venous Thrombosis

▶ H&P Keys

History of sinus or ear infection, cyanotic heart disease, sickle cell anemia, or hypercoagulable state. Headache, papilledema, nausea, and vomiting; seizures with cortical vein involvement. Cranial nerves IX, X, XI involved in transverse sinus thrombosis; proptosis, periorbital ecchymosis and edema with cranial nerves II, IV, VI in cavernous sinus thrombosis; visual field defects, crural monoplegia in sagittal sinus thrombosis.

▶ Diagnosis

MRA (angiogram) and MRV (venogram) are preferred. Arteriography with venous phase will show thrombosis also; LP shows raised intracranial pressure and xanthochromia but may be contraindicated because of risk of herniation.

▶ Disease Severity

Because many thrombi are caused by septic infection, abscesses and meningitis may appear concurrently.

▶ Concept and Application

Thrombosis of venous drainage resulting from infection or inappropriate coagulation impedes venous flow, causing increased intracranial pressure, infarction of tissue.

▶ Treatment Steps
1. Antibiotics if septic, anticoagulants otherwise.
2. Supportive management.
3. Treatment of seizures.
4. Acutely, intravenous thrombolysis is highly successful and a lifesaving procedure.

## VI. TOXIC DISORDERS

### A. Heavy Metals

1. Lead

    ▶ H&P Keys

    In adults, exposure occurs from burning lead batteries, water ingestion (lead pipes), "moonshine" ingestion, gasoline fumes. Colic (usually precipitated by alcohol intoxication), anemia, and neuropathy presenting as wrist drop or predominantly motor polyneuropathy. In children, exposure occurs from ingestion of lead paint. Clinical presentations include anorexia, colic, ataxia, followed by drowsiness, stupor, seizures, and coma (most frequently in summer if ingestion continues).

    ▶ Diagnosis

    Basophilic stippling in RBCs, urine porphyrins elevated, increased blood levels of lead. Lead lines along metaphysis in children.

2. Mercury

    ▶ H&P Keys

    History of mercury exposure in thermometer manufacturing plants, mirrors, x-ray machines. Presents with tremor of arms, lips, tongue, and legs; ataxia; and chorea.

    ▶ Diagnosis

    Elevated mercury levels in blood.

3. Arsenic

    ▶ H&P Keys

    Usually suicidal (intentional ingestion) attempts with herbicides or rat poison. Headaches, drowsiness, confusion, and seizures if acute, associated with hemolysis, weakness, and myalgia if chronic.

    ▶ Diagnosis

    Transverse (Mees') white lines on the fingernails, scaly desquamation, and gastrointestinal (GI) symptoms. Elevated arsenic levels in hair and urine.

4. Manganese

    ▶ H&P Keys

    History of exposure in miners separating ore from manganese. Present with a parkinsonlike syndrome including marked drooling, tremors, rigidity, and retropulsive gait.

▶ Diagnosis

Elevated levels of manganese in blood.

▶ Disease Severity

Improvements in symptoms depend on timing of initiation of therapy in relation to onset. Manganese poisoning in children can be fatal or result in mental deficiencies.

▶ Concept and Application

Calcarine neuronal loss, cerebellar granule cell loss in mercury; diffuse punctate hemorrhages in arsenic; endothelial damage and swelling in lead poisoning; pallidal and striatal neuronal loss in manganese poisoning.

▶ Treatment Steps

1. Chelation with dimercaprol (BAL) for lead and arsenic poisoning.
2. *N*-Acetylpenicillamine for mercury poisoning.
3. L-Dopa for manganese poisoning.
4. Mannitol for edema and anticonvulsants for seizures for lead poisoning in children.

## B. Medications

### 1. Opioids

▶ H&P Keys

High incidence of addiction; inadvertent poisoning or suicidal attempts, results in varying degrees of obtundation followed by decreased ventilation, miosis, bradycardia, and hypothermia.

### 2. Barbiturates

▶ H&P Keys

High incidence of addiction; suicide attempts or accidental poisoning result in progressive unarousal, respiratory depression; pupillary response present and pulmonary edema.

### 3. Benzodiazepines

▶ H&P Keys

Similar to barbiturates.

### 4. Antipsychotic Drugs

▶ H&P Keys

Use of phenothiazines and butyrophenones, treatment of schizophrenia; side effects are parkinsonian syndrome, buccolingual involuntary movements (tardive dyskinesias), inability to sit still (akathisia), and a syndrome of severe rigidity, fever, and confusion (neuroleptic malignant syndrome), which can prove fatal in 20% of cases even when treated.

### 5. Cocaine

▶ H&P Keys

History of dependency; can be administered nasally, intravenously, or smoked; symptoms of intoxication include tremor, myoclonus, seizures, and psychosis. Stroke, seizures, and subarachnoid hemorrhages have been described.

## VII. NEOPLASMS

### A. Glioblastoma

▶ H&P Keys

Most common type of primary CNS tumor in adults (Fig. 10–5); history of hemiparesis or other focal neurologic signs, also seizures, confusion, obtundation, and late headache. No clear predisposing factors; most common cause of new-onset seizures in middle age. Exam correlates with complaints.

▶ Diagnosis

Contrast CT or MRI will show characteristic ring-enhancing lesion; rarely may be multicentric or across corpus callosum. Other studies are negative, including search for a metastatic origin. MR spectroscopy, PET, functional MRI, and cerebral blood flow techniques add to the current diagnostic arsenal. Biopsy shows typical pseudopallisading, hemorrhage, pleomorphism, and hypercellularity, and necrosis and endothelial hyperplasia.

▶ Disease Severity

Younger patients have better prognosis than older ones. Less than one fifth of all patients survive more than a year.

▶ Concept and Application

Likely arises from anaplasia of astrocytes. Secondary characteristics of the tumor lead to further tissue invasion and mass effect.

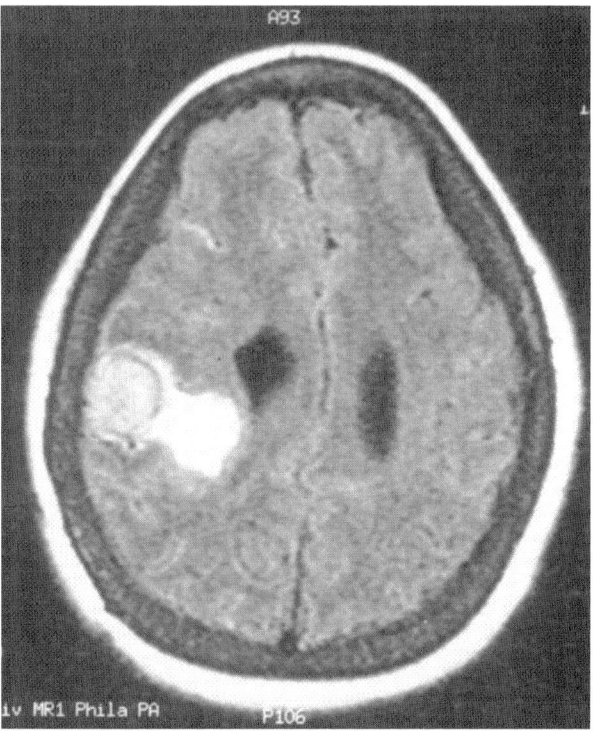

Figure 10–5. Fluid-attenuated inversion recovery MRI of right frontal glial tumor demonstrating vasogenic edema and midline shift.

▶ Treatment Steps
1. Surgery to debulk tumor.
2. Radiation accompanied by use of corticosteroids (vasogenic edema) and anticonvulsants is routine because of patients symptoms.
3. Chemotherapy with timazolamide or BCNU.
4. New radiothearapy techniques include radioactive implants, stereotactic radiosurgery, radiation with radiosensitizers, hyperthermia.
5. Monoclonal antibodies did not prove useful.
6. Genetic modification is the most promising future approach.

## B. Meningioma

▶ H&P Keys

Benign tumor, causes symptoms by compression or irritation. Convexity tumors present with hemiparesis, seizures, and headaches; parasagittal with bicrural asymmetric weakness and spasticity, with sphincter disorder. Can happen in spinal canal (mainly females) or on optic nerve. Exam relates to complaints and presentation.

▶ Diagnosis

CT of head will show a usually rounded dural lesion with mass effect; MRI may only show lesion clearly with contrast enhancement. It may calcify and show on plain roentgenograms.

▶ Disease Severity

Location of the tumor and potential for surgical resection determine outcome. Usually, tumor recurs if not completely resected.

▶ Concept and Application

Arise from arachnoid cells and may attain great size prior to development of symptoms. Usually cause exostosis rather than bone erosion. Some have progesterone, somatostatin, epidermal growth factor, and estrogen receptors and enlarge because of this. Psammoma bodies can be seen microscopically.

▶ Treatment Steps
1. Surgical resection when accessible, radiation otherwise if symptomatic.
2. Incidental tumors can be observed because of slow growth.
3. Corticosteroids for edema; anticonvulsants for seizures.

## C. Metastases

▶ H&P Keys

History of smoking, breast cancer, or other predisposing factors. Usually presents with focal neurologic signs, behavioral changes, headaches, or seizures. May be apoplectic if it bleeds.

▶ Diagnosis

MRI or CT scan shows single or multiple lesions with surrounding edema and enhancement. Physical examination including breast, gynecologic, and rectal exam; chest roentgenography; blood count may lead to diagnosis of primary. Biopsy of lesion if primary unknown will lead to separation from other etiologies.

▶ Disease Severity

Choriocarcinoma, melanoma, thyroid carcinoma, and hypernephroma may present with high incidence of bleeding. Solitary lesions have better prognosis and can be resected in some cases. Final outcome is relative to the primary disease itself.

▶ Concept and Application

Most commonly arises from lung, breast, or melanoma.

▶ Treatment Steps

Radiation, steroids, and anticonvulsants. Chemotherapy in appropriate cases.

## VIII. DEGENERATIVE DISEASES

### A. Alzheimer's Disease

▶ H&P Keys

Onset in late fifties or sixties; presents initially with deficit in retentive memory followed by dysnomia, spatial disorientation, personality changes, and gait disorder. The mental status examination shows findings related to these complaints. Seizures, paraparesis, and abulia can be seen in advanced cases.

▶ Diagnosis

CSF is normal, EEG is diffusely slow late in the disease, and the CT or MRI show atrophy; SPECT scan shows biparietal perfusion defects. PET scans and T2-weighted MRI imaging proven useful in diagnosis. Efforts are being made to develop a biologic marker.

▶ Disease Severity

Progressive dementia leads to both physical and mental dissolution and eventually death.

▶ Concept and Application

The etiology is unknown, but a relationship exists with chromosome 21 in familial cases, the same chromosome involved in Down syndrome. The latter condition has pathologic similarities to Alzheimer's disease. In familial autosomal dominat cases, mutation in presenilin 1 and 2 and amyloid precursor protein genes are found. E4 alelle inheritance of apolipoprotein E gene carries genetic risk.

▶ Treatment Steps
1. Treatment includes acetylcholine esterase inhibitors (tacrine, donepezil, rivastigmine, galantamine) with effect on cognition and global measures.
2. Vitamin E demonstrated slowing in progression of dementia severity.

3. Psychotic symptoms are controlled with newer atypical antipsychotics.
4. Depression is treated with SSRIs.

## B. Amyotrophic Lateral Sclerosis

### ▶ H&P Keys

Progressive weakness, usually asymmetrically, involving all voluntary muscles except extraocular ones. Prominent cramps, fasciculations, accompanied by "stiffness," dysarthria, and dysphagia. Exam shows mainly distal weakness with atrophy and fasciculation. Reflexes are exaggerated, tone is increased (spastic), toes are extensor. Combination of weak limb with atrophy and hyperreflexia is very suggestive.

### ▶ Diagnosis

Do MRI of cervical spine if exam shows atrophy and weakness of arms with hyperreflexia of legs to rule out cervical lesion. EMG shows denervation and reinnervation as does the muscle biopsy. CK is minimally elevated in some cases. Do lead blood levels, hexosaminidase A, serum protein electrophoresis to exclude conditions that will mimic it, particularly when upper motor neuron signs are absent or mild. Familial cases secondary to SOD1 gene mutations are diagnosed with genetic testing.

### ▶ Disease Severity

The disease is fatal; bulbar forms have a shorter course. Respiratory failure and malnutrition are causes of death.

### ▶ Concept and Application

Neuronal loss in the anterior horn and motor cortex. Etiology is unknown, but glutamate excitotoxicity and free radical injury are implicated. Familial cases are associated with mutation of calcium or zinc superoxide dismutase gene.

### ▶ Treatment Steps

Riluzole is the first FDA-approved drug for ALS treatment.

## C. Parkinson's Disease

### ▶ H&P Keys

Progressive tremor, slowness, festinating gait, stooped posture. Early on, symptoms may be nonspecific ("arm discomfort"). Exam shows a resting tremor of 4–6 Hz, difficulty with passive motion (rigidity) evenly through the full range, decreased expression, paucity of movements (bradykinesia), and difficulty with posture. When tremor is added to the rigidity, "cogwheeling" results. Dementia occurs in 30% of cases.

### ▶ Diagnosis

No routine diagnostic studies exist; have decreased basal ganglia dopamine activity on PET scan. Exclude medications, progressive supranuclear palsy, olivopontocerebellar degeneration.

▶ Disease Severity
The disease eventually leads to disability in spite of therapy. Swallowing can be markedly affected.

▶ Concept and Application
Neuronal loss of the substantia nigra and other pigmented nuclei. Reduced dopamine levels. Similarity to a syndrome caused by the designer drug MPTP has raised question of environmental factor.

▶ Treatment Steps
1. Replace dopamine with L-dopa; added carbidopa (Sinemet) reduces peripheral effects. This medication can cause variations in clinical state not associated with dosing (on-off phenomenon).
2. Dopamine receptor agonists are also helpful (bromocriptine, pergolide, pramipexole, ropinirole).
3. Anticholinergics improve tremor but can worsen dementia.
4. Selegiline, a selective monoamine oxidase (MAO)-B inhibitor, is used to slow down the disease progression.
5. Catechol-O-methyltransferase (COMT) inhibitors prolong L-dopa availability.

## D. Huntington's Disease

▶ H&P Keys
Progressive mental deterioration; becoming irritable, impulsive, exhibiting poor self-control. Hand and face chorea develops and eventually all muscles follow. The exam shows chorea, dementia, oculomotor disturbances.

▶ Diagnosis
The CT or MRI shows caudate head atrophy; genetic studies can define the patient at risk and the subject with overt disease.

▶ Disease Severity
The disease is transmitted as autosomal dominant with complete penetrance. It is also fatal. Childhood cases present with rigidity and seizures also. Mode of transmission leads to anticipation (subsequent generations show earlier and more severe signs).

▶ Concept and Application
Autosomal dominant inheritance; gene located on the short arm of chromosome 4; multiple erroneous repeats of nucleic acid triplets (CGA) results in defective Huntington's gene.

▶ Treatment Steps
1. No known treatment. Genetic counseling available for receptive individuals.
2. Because there is no cure, patients or individuals at risk may commit suicide.

## IX. TRAUMA

### A. Subdural Hematoma

▶ H&P Keys

History of head trauma with progressive change in mentation, focal neurologic signs, often loss of consciousness but not always, hemiparesis, large unreactive pupil with ophthalmoplegia if acute; seizures, headache, progressive change in mentation if chronic.

▶ Diagnosis

CT of head, if performed without contrast, may miss an isodense (chronic) subdural hematoma. MRI of head with contrast (gadolinium) is the study of choice. Both will show crescentic lesion with signal compatible with blood.

▶ Disease Severity

Progressive focal neurologic deficit, progressive obtundation, requires quick intervention. Mass effect and shift of intracranial contents in radiologic studies also are usually suggestive of increased severity.

▶ Concept and Application

Ruptured bridging superficial cortical veins are responsible for blood accumulation. Chronic subdural may have recent rebleeding. Mass effect and cortical irritation are responsible for symptoms.

▶ Treatment Steps
1. Subdural hematomas with rapidly or incapacitating symptoms are best treated with surgical evacuation of the clot.
2. Prudent observation or corticosteroids can be used for small, incidental, or symptom-free subdural hematomas.

### B. Epidural Hematoma

▶ H&P Keys

Severe head trauma accompanied by loss of consciousness, transient recovery of consciousness followed by progressive obtundation, posturing, shallow respirations, seizures, focal neurologic signs, coma.

▶ Diagnosis

CT of head or MRI will show concave blood clot, white on CT, bright on T1- and T2-weighted images on MRI. Skull roentgenograms will show fracture through area of middle meningeal artery or, less commonly, across venous sinus.

▶ Disease Severity

If untreated, the condition is lethal; timing is of the essence.

▶ Concept and Application

Tear of middle meningeal artery or venous sinus results in accumulation of blood at great pressure in a potential space.

▶ Treatment Steps
1. Emergent surgical evacuation.
2. Supportive.

## C. Contusion

▶ H&P Keys

History of moderate to severe head trauma (unconscious for more than 5 minutes); returns to alertness with confusion and mild mutism. Exam shows extensor plantar reflexes, mild hemiparesis, elevated blood pressure and heart rate.

▶ Diagnosis

CT or MRI may show focal parenchymal swelling (most commonly frontal or temporal tip) or delayed hemorrhage.

▶ Disease Severity

Degree of alertness at the time of evaluation, time unconscious, degree of retrograde amnesia determine severity of injury if otherwise uncomplicated. Temporal lobe herniation is main cause of morbidity and mortality.

▶ Concept and Application

Sustained head trauma results in neuronal swelling and axonal shearing, often maximal 24–48 hours after event.

▶ Treatment Steps

Control of intracranial pressure with hyperventilation, ventriculostomy; barbiturate coma may lessen neuronal injury. Delayed physical and cognitive deficits may occur and will require therapy.

## X. DEMYELINATION

### A. Multiple Sclerosis

▶ H&P Keys

History of arm, leg, hand, or foot numbness (50% of patients); visual loss (25%); diplopia; incoordination; weakness; bladder dysfunction. Exam shows sensory loss in spinal distribution, afferent pupillary deficit, ataxia, dysarthria, hyperreflexia, internuclear ophthalmoplegia.

▶ Diagnosis

MRI will show periventricular white matter demyelination or lesion in the spinal cord or optic nerve (Fig. 10–6). LP shows lymphocytic pleocytosis (< 100 cells/mL), increased protein (< 100 mg/mL), normal glucose, increased IgG intrathecal production, and oligoclonal bands. Large myelinated pathways can be assessed with evoked potentials (visual, auditory, somatosensory). The disease can be mimicked by syphilis, Sjögren's syndrome, systemic lupus erythematosus, sarcoidosis, and Lyme disease. The diagnosis remains clinical and depends on finding different lesions on separate occasions.

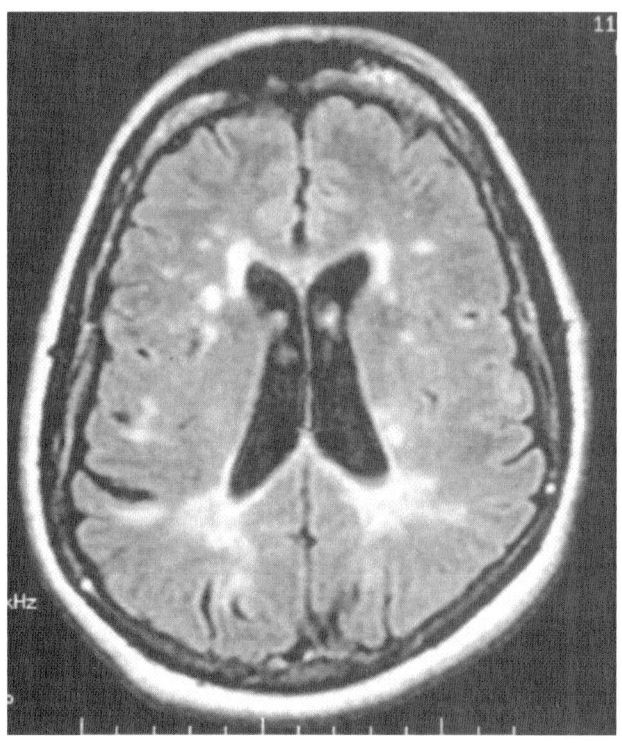

Figure 10-6. MRI of patient with multiple sclerosis demonstrating multiple white matter lesions with characteristic periventricular localization and perpendicular to ventricle orientation.

▶ Disease Severity

Pure spinal forms, chronic progressive, and early presentation are correlated with worst outcome. Elevation of body temperature (Uhthoff's phenomenon), stress, and infection can cause exacerbation.

▶ Concept and Application

The etiology of the disease is multifactorial, with environmental factors, increased incidence in temperate regions, immunogenetic factors such as certain HLA-Dw or DR antigens, followed by an aberrant immunologic response against CNS myelin.

▶ Treatment Steps
1. Acute attacks respond to IV corticosteroids.
2. Chronic prophylaxis can be obtained with interferon beta or glatinamer acetate.
3. The tremor responds to isoniazid, propranolol, clonazepam, or primidone; baclofen orally or intrathecally reduces spasticity.
4. Fatigue responds to amantadine, pemoline, or modafinil.
5. Gait disability, bladder disorders require appropriate care.

## XI. SPINE DISEASE

### A. Spinal Stenosis

1. Cervical

   ▶ H&P Keys

   Neck pain; gait difficulty; progressive leg and arm weakness; spasticity of weak limbs; hyperreflexia; Babinski's and Lhermitte's signs.

   ▶ Diagnosis

   CT or MRI of cervical spine confirms diagnosis, usually due to spondylitic "bars" or disc herniation; EMG and nerve conductions document root involvement; post myelography CT scan delineates questionable stenosis.

   ▶ Disease Severity

   Bowel and bladder disorder; progressive paresis; clonus; anterior-posterior diameter of spinal canal under 8 mm of circumference.

   ▶ Concept and Application

   Repeated trauma on flexion–extension; spinal vascular insufficiency.

   ▶ Treatment Steps
   1. Conservative therapy may be of some help (NSAIDs, therapy).
   2. Neurogenic pain responds to gabapentin or lamotrigine.
   3. Surgery may be necessary.

2. Lumbar

   ▶ H&P Keys

   Progressive pain and weakness in lower extremities on exertion; back pain; weakness of the legs.

   ▶ Diagnosis

   As in cervical area.

   ▶ Disease Severity

   As in cervical area.

   ▶ Concept and Application

   Vascular insufficiency.

   ▶ Treatment Steps
   1. In the cervical area, immobilization has been advocated.
   2. NSAIDs, epidural analgesic injections, or anticonvulsants help reduce pain.
   3. Surgery remains the most definitive method of treatment to decompress.

### B. Radiculopathy

▶ H&P Keys

Pain and weakness in the distribution of a root, shoulder pain, deltoid and biceps weakness, absent biceps reflex (C5); arm, forearm, and first-digit pain, brachioradialis and biceps weakness, absent brachioradialis reflex (C6); more commonly in cervical area. Hip, lateral thigh, anterior leg, and big-toe pain, foot and big-toe extensor weakness (L5); posterior leg and thigh, small-toe pain, absent ankle jerk, foot extension weakness (S1).

▶ Diagnosis

Cervical or lumbar roentgenogram if history includes trauma; MRI of appropriate level to assess intervertebral disk herniation; EMG and NCV in 3–4 weeks to assess distribution of radiculopathy.

▶ Disease Severity

Severe weakness correlates with prominent nerve involvement. Prolonged deficits will improve slowly or not at all.

▶ Concept and Application

Root compression leads to axonal injury.

▶ Treatment Steps

1. Mild and moderate deficits can be treated conservatively with physical therapy.
2. Surgery may be used if physical therapy does not improve symptoms over 6–12 weeks or for severe deficits (drop foot).

## XII. SLEEP DISORDERS

### A. Sleep Apnea

▶ H&P Keys

Obesity, short neck, large tongue, large tonsils in children, myxedema, acromegaly, myotonic dystrophy in obstructive type; poliomyelitis, syringobulbia, and brain stem infarct in central type; history of heavy snoring, daytime sleepiness, fatigue, early morning headache, impotence.

▶ Diagnosis

Thyroid studies to rule out hypothyroidism; polysomnogram to exclude other etiologies of daytime sleepiness and to assess apneas and differentiate between central or obstructive type; multiple sleep latencies to assess the degree of nocturnal disturbance.

▶ Disease Severity

Six or more apneas per hour; oxygen desaturation; nocturnal cardiac arrhythmias. Sleep apnea is associated with cerebrovascular accidents, heart attacks.

▶ Concept and Application

Upper airway laxity and collapse on inspiration; reduced nocturnal respiratory drive in central type.

▶ Treatment Steps
1. Weight reduction of as few as 5 lb may reduce symptoms.
2. Continuous positive airway pressure (CPAP) for obstructive type, repeat studies and adjust settings.
3. Protriptyline for central apnea.

## B. Narcolepsy

▶ H&P Keys

Present with excessive daytime sleepiness; multiple daytime naps; paralysis with strong emotions in 70% (cataplexy); sleep paralysis; hypnagogic hallucinations; normal examination.

▶ Diagnosis

Sleep study (polysomnogram) is normal and will exclude other pathologies; multiple sleep latencies show rapid eye movement (REM) sleep onset in at least 2 out of 4 to 5 recordings; same abnormality can be seen with use of drugs, drug withdrawal, or sleep deprivation; therefore needs good clinical correlation.

▶ Disease Severity

Most patients have narcolepsy and cataplexy by history; there could be milder cases; few have all symptoms.

▶ Concept and Application

The disease may be due to abnormalities in the orexin neurotransmitter system.

▶ Treatment Steps
1. Nondrug therapy consists of short naps, avoidance of heavy meals.
2. Drug therapy (often needed) consists of pemoline, and if unsuccessful, methylphenidate (Ritalin). Imipramine may be useful in controlling cataplexy. Modafinil, a newer drug is effective and with fewer side effects in the treatment of narcolepsy and excessive daytime sleepiness.

## XIII. DEVELOPMENTAL DISORDERS

### A. Tay-Sachs Disease

▶ H&P Keys

Mostly Jewish infants of Eastern European background; presents in early infancy with startle to noises, irritability, and subsequent developmental delay or regression of acquired milestones. Initial hypotonia is followed by spasticity, blindness, retinal cherry-red spot, and seizures. Death occurs in 3–4 years.

▶ Diagnosis

Exclude other cause of a similar syndrome, such as embryologic abnormalities or infections and other systemic diseases. The enzyme abnormality is the lack of hexosaminidase A, which can be measured in fibroblasts, WBCs, or serum. This enzymatic assay allows the recognition of the heterozygote asymptomatic carrier and permits genetic counseling.

▶ Disease Severity

Other variants of this disease are recognized, including one mimicking motor neuron disease in adults. The disease is invariably fatal.

▶ Concept and Application

Hexosaminidase A is needed for the cleavage of *N*-acetylgalactosamine, and its absence leads to ganglioside accumulation.

▶ Treatment Steps
1. No treatment is available.
2. Prevention depends on preconceptual identification of parents at risk and genetic counseling.

## DEFINITIONS

**aphasia** Language deficits of several types acquired after the acquisition of normal speech and reading skills. Often caused by a left hemispheric lesion. The type and degree of involvement of language depend on the localization of the injury.

**coma** Alteration of consciousness in which the subject appears asleep but is incapable of any response to external or internal stimuli. Degree may vary, and various vegetative functions may be absent or present, including breathing, pupillary response, corneal response, tendon reflexes, and reflex ocular movements. Coma can be reversible if caused by metabolic injuries (eg, hypothermia, drug intoxication).

**brain death** Medical and legal term that refers to complete absence of any brain activity with preserved cardiac or pulmonary function without reversible causative factor. Legally, the diagnosis allows the discontinuation of life-support measures, and its definition depends on finding no evidence of any neurologic function other than spinal reflexes. This includes absent corneal reflexes, reflex eye movements to caloric stimulation, pupillary responses, or significant response to pain. The absence of a respiratory drive is tested by oxygenating the patient through a cannula without mechanical assistance. Absent electroencephalogram (EEG) potentials larger than 2 µV, absent brain stem–evoked potentials, or lack of cerebral circulation on arteriography are supportive of but often not absolutely required for the diagnosis.

**dementia** Defined as a loss of various intellectual functions including memory (often the earliest), language, and abstract reasoning. In addition, behavioral and personality changes (such as paranoia) often accompany the intellectual dissolution.

**dyslexia** Reading or reading and spelling disability that is unexpected based on development and general aptitude. Often associated with attention deficit disorders in the child.

**syncope** Transitory loss of consciousness secondary to hypoperfusion of the brain. Often secondary to a vasovagal reflex (eg, during blood donation), can also be the presentation of cardiac arrhythmias, inability to sustain adequate blood pressure, etc. It is in the differential diagnosis of seizure but different from it because it is often preceded by prolonged warnings, is of short duration, is not accompanied by tongue biting or sphincter disorder, and consciousness is recovered quickly with supine position.

▶ on rounds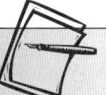

## NEUROLOGY

### Meningitis CSF Findings

- Aseptic: Pleocytosis, predominantly lymphocytic, mild protein elevation, normal glucose, negative bacterial cultures
- Bacterial: Pleocytosis up to 10,000, mainly neutrophils, low glucose, elevated protein, positive culture
- Fungal: Lymphocytic and monocytic pleocytosis, positive fungal culture in weeks
- TB: Lymphocytic pleocytosis, elevated protein, low glucose, positive acid-fast bacillus stain

### Degenerative Diseases

- Alzheimer's
  Onset late 50s or 60s
  Retentive memory deficit, personality changes, gait disorder
  Normal CSF, CT/MRI may show atrophy
  No treatment
- Amyotrophic lateral sclerosis
  Progressive asymmetric weakness of voluntary muscles
  Due to neuronal loss in the anterior horn and motor cortex
  No treatment
- Parkinson's disease
  Resting tremor 4–6 Hz, cogwheel rigidity, bradykinesia
  No diagnostic tests available
  Results from neuronal loss of the substantia nigra, reduced dopamine levels
  Treatment: L-dopa, carbidopa, anticholinergics, MAO-B inhibitors
- Huntington's disease
  Progressive mental deterioration, hand and face chorea, dementia
  CT or MRI positive for caudate head atrophy
  Transmitted as an autosomal dominant with complete penetrance, gene on the short arm of chromosome 4
  No treatment

## BIBLIOGRAPHY

Adams RD, Victor M, Ropper AH. *Principles of Neurology.* 6th ed. New York: McGraw-Hill Book Co; 1997.

Bradley WG, Daroff RB, Fenichel GM, Marsden CD. *Neurology in Clinical Practice.* 3rd ed. Boston: Butterworth Heinemann; 2000.

Bogousslavsky J, Fisher M. *Textbook of Neurology.* Boston: Butterworth Heinemann; 1998.

Haerer AF. *DeJong's The Neurologic Examination.* Philadelphia: Lippincott-Raven; 1992.

Goetz CG, Pappert EG. *Textbook of Clinical Neurology.* Philadelphia: WB Saunders Co.; 1999.

Joynt RJ, Griggs RC, eds. *Baker's Clinical Neurology.* Philadelphia: Lippincott Williams & Wilkins; 2001.

Mayo Clinic Department of Neurology. *Mayo Clinic Examinations in Neurology.* 7th ed. St. Louis: Mosby; 1998.

Samuels MA, ed. *Hospitalist Neurology.* Boston: Butterworth Heinemann; 1999.

# Male and Female Reproduction | 11

I. **UTERUS** / 341
   A. Malignant Neoplasm / 341
   B. Leiomyomata Uteri / 341
   C. Other Disorders / 343

II. **OVARY** / 344
   A. Malignant Neoplasm / 344
   B. Ovarian Cysts / 344

III. **CERVIX** / 345
   A. Malignant Neoplasm / 345
   B. Cervicitis and Sexually Transmitted Diseases / 345
   C. Cervical Dysplasia and Management of Abnormal Pap Smear / 347

IV. **VAGINA AND VULVA** / 348
   A. Malignant Neoplasms / 348
   B. Candidiasis of the Vulva and Vagina / 349
   C. Vaginitis and Vulvovaginitis / 350
   D. Pelvic Relaxation/Urinary Incontinence / 350

V. **MENSTRUAL DISORDERS** / 351
   A. Dysmenorrhea / 351
   B. Premenstrual Syndrome / 351
   C. Disorders of Menstruation / 352

VI. **MENOPAUSE** / 353
   A. Menopausal Symptoms / 353

VII. **BREAST** / 353
   A. Malignant Neoplasm / 353
   B. Fibroadenoma / 355
   C. Inflammatory Disease of the Breast / 355
   D. Fibrocystic Disease / 356

## VIII. OTHER PROBLEMS / 356
- A. Infertility, Male and Female / 356
- B. Pelvic Inflammatory Disease / 358

## IX. HEALTH MAINTENANCE / 359
- A. Gynecologic Examination and Screening / 359
- B. General Counseling for Contraception / 359
- C. Sterilization / 360
- D. Genetic Counseling / 360

**BIBLIOGRAPHY / 361**

## I. UTERUS

### A. Malignant Neoplasm

#### 1. Endometrial Cancer

▶ H&P Keys

Obesity, nulliparity, chronic anovulation, diabetes, hypertension, postmenopausal bleeding, median age 61, early menarche, late menopause, history of tamoxifen therapy, unopposed estrogen therapy.

▶ Diagnosis

Fractional dilatation and curettage, endometrial biopsy, hysteroscopy, transvaginal ultrasonography (thickened endometrial "stripe").

*Advanced Disease*—Chest roentgenogram, intravenous pyelogram (IVP), computerized tomographic (CT) scan, barium enema, cystoscopy.

▶ Disease Severity

International Federation of Gynecology and Obstetrics (FIGO).

FIGO Staging (1988)

*Stage I*—Endometrium, myometrium.

*Stage II*—Cervix.

*Stage III*—Serosal, adnexal involvement:
- Positive peritoneal cytology.
- Vaginal mets.
- Pelvic/periaortic nodes.

*Stage IV*—Bladder, bowel mucosa.
- Distant mets.

▶ Concept and Application

Relationship between estrogen production and endometrial proliferation; overgrowth of the endometrium in response to unopposed estrogen.

▶ Treatment Steps

*Early Disease*—Total abdominal hysterectomy and bilateral salpingo-oophorectomy (± lymph node sampling).

*Adjunctive Therapy*
1. External beam radiation.
2. Preoperative radiation.

*Recurrent Endometrial Carcinoma*
1. High-dose progestins, eg, medroxyprogesterone.
2. Chemotherapy, eg, adriamycin, platinum.

### B. Leiomyomata Uteri

▶ H&P Keys

Present in 20% of whites, 33% of blacks by 30 years of age; pain, abnormal uterine bleeding, pressure, infertility (recurrent pregnancy loss), uterine enlargement, urinary frequency, rectal pressure (Fig. 11–1).

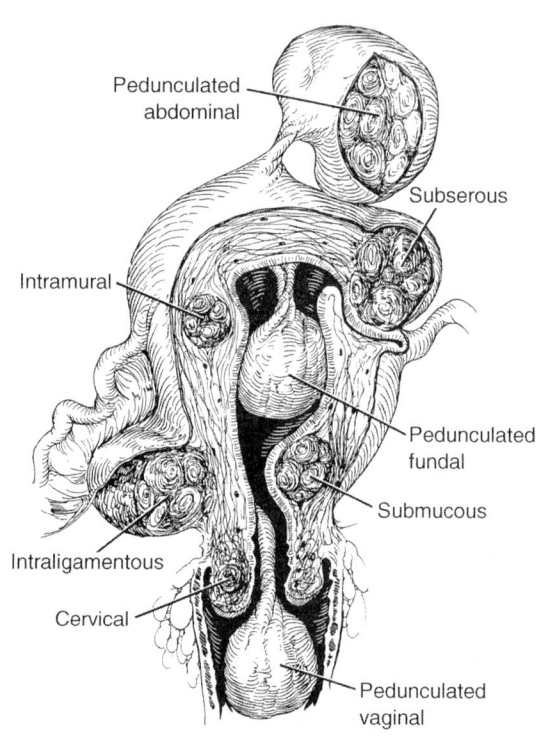

Figure 11–1. Common types of uterine fibroids. (Reproduced, with permission, from Pernoll ML, Benson RC (editors): *Current Obstetric & Gynecologic Diagnosis & Treatment,* 9th ed. Appleton & Lange, 2002.)

### ▶ Diagnosis
Complete blood count (CBC) with differential, pelvic ultrasound, and in extremely large tumors, an IVP will rule out urinary tract compression. (CT and magnetic resonance imaging [MRI] are not cost-effective.)

### ▶ Disease Severity
Severity of pain, anemia, urinary frequency or retention, hydronephrosis, uterine size beyond 12 weeks.

### ▶ Concept and Application
Localized proliferation of smooth muscle cells, estrogen-dependent, shrinkage after menopause. Arises from a single smooth muscle cell.

### ▶ Treatment Steps
1. *Observation:* pelvic examinations specifically bimanual exams, serial ultrasonograms, monitoring for continued enlargement and possible hydronephrosis.
2. *Medical:* Gonadotropin-releasing hormone (GnRh) agonists to induce a hypoestrogenic state, thus resulting in shrinkage.
3. *Surgical:* Myomectomy (via hysteroscopy, laparoscopy, or laparotomy), total abdominal hysterectomy as a last resort.

## C. Other Disorders

### 1. Endometriosis

▶ H&P Keys

Premenstrual dysmenorrhea, premenstrual spotting or staining, dyspareunia, infertility, chronic pelvic pain, retroverted uterus, uterosacral nodularity, nonmobile uterus.

▶ Diagnosis

History and physical examination, bimanual examination, pelvic ultrasonography (for presence of endometrioma), laparoscopy (gold standard of diagnosis; Fig. 11–2), biopsy if possible (histology shows endometrial glands and stroma). (CA 125 of questionable help and very nonspecific.)

▶ Disease Severity

American Fertility Society stages I to IV (minimal through severe), extent of pelvic pain, duration of infertility. Scored on a point system based on pelvic involvement.

▶ Concept and Application

Retrograde menstruation (most commonly accepted theory), hematogenous spread, lymphogenous spread, genetic and family predisposition, coelomic metaplasia, estrogen-dependent growth of endometriosis, resolves after menopause.

▶ Treatment Steps

Depends on age of patient, duration of infertility, severity of symptoms, extent of disease.

1. Expectant therapy.
2. Medical therapy consists of GnRH agonist (medical treatment of choice), progestogens, oral contraceptives, nonsteroidal anti-inflammatory drugs (NSAIDs).
3. Conservative surgery.
4. Radical surgery via laparoscopy, laparotomy.
5. Danazol not currently used because of androgenic side effects.

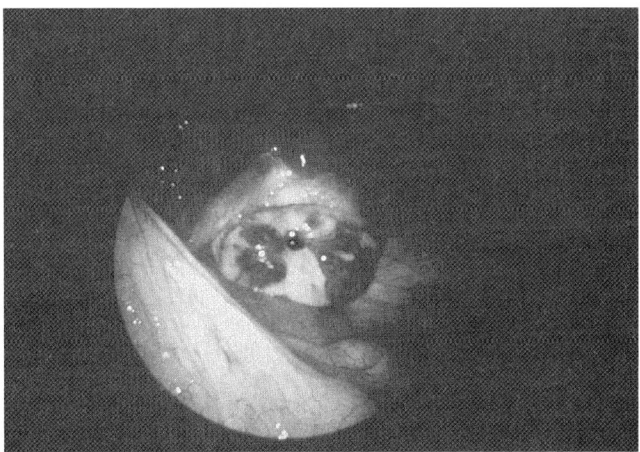

Figure 11–2. Implants of endometriosis are seen on the ovarian surface at the time of laparoscopy. These are "powder-burn" in appearance and characteristic of classical endometriosis.

## II. OVARY

### A. Malignant Neoplasm

#### 1. Ovarian Cancer

▶ H&P Keys

Fifth most common of all cancers in women, higest mortality rate because asymptomatic more than two thirds of the time. Affects 1 in 70 women in the United States. Ascites, abdominal distention, pelvic mass in advanced stages.

▶ Diagnosis

Usually diagnosis made when disease has reached stage III or IV. History and physical exam, pelvic ultrasonography, CA 125, CT scan, barium enema, chest roentgenogram, surgical staging.

▶ Disease Severity

*Surgical Staging*—Stage I limited to the ovaries; stage II pelvic extension; stage III intraperitoneal metastases outside the pelvis; stage IV distant metastases.

*Main Histologic Types*—Epithelial tumors (80%), sex-cord stromal tumors (3%), germ cell tumors (5%).

▶ Concept and Application

Spread to adjacent peritoneal surfaces; most common death result of bowel obstruction.
  BrCA1 gene associated with ovarian Ca ~5% of cases.
  Also associated with mutations in p53 tumor suppressor gene.

▶ Treatment Steps
1. Total abdominal hysterectomy, bilateral salpingo-oophorectomy, omentectomy.
2. Adjunctive chemotherapy.
3. Radiation therapy.
4. Second-look laparotomy or laparoscopy. Overall 5-year survival rate: 30%.

### B. Ovarian Cysts

▶ H&P Keys

Abdominal pain; anovulation, irregular bleeding, irregular periods, reproductive age group; usually unilateral, bimanual exam.

▶ Diagnosis

CBC and differential, pelvic ultrasonography (size, loculations, unilaterality versus bilaterality, calcifications), β-human chorionic gonadotropin (β-hCG) to rule out ectopic pregnancy.

▶ Disease Severity

Amount of pain, cyst size, presence of loculations, fluid in the peritoneal cavity (rare).

▶ Concept and Application

Most common is functional cyst related to anovulation. Follicular cyst continues to develop and enlarge without ovulation, thereby causing pain, possibly intraperitoneal rupture, and irregular menses. Eighty-five percent will resolve by 9 weeks.

▶ Treatment Steps
1. Observation, recheck at 3-week intervals.
2. Serial ultrasonograms.
3. Serial CBC with differential if suspicion of intraperitoneal bleeding.
4. Surgery if danger of torsion.
5. Possible laparotomy, ovarian cystectomy, or oophorectomy.

## III. CERVIX

### A. Malignant Neoplasm

▶ H&P Keys

STDs play the main role in the pathogenesis of cervical cancer, specifically human papillomavirus (HPV) infection. Multiple sexual partners, cigarette smoking, early intercourse, high-risk sexual behaviors, abnormal Pap smears, mean age 45 years, postcoital bleeding, abnormal discharge, occasional pelvic pain.

▶ Diagnosis

Pap smear, colposcopy, cone biopsy, endocervical curettage (ECC), LEEP (loop electrosurgical excision procedure), HPV serotyping, chest roentgenogram, IVP, barium enema, cystoscopy, proctosigmoidoscopy, MRI (optional).

▶ Disease Severity (FIGO Staging—1985)

*Stage I*—Confined to cervix.

*Stage II*—Upper vagina, not pelvic sidewall.

*Stage III*—Extending to pelvic sidewall.

*Stage IV*—Beyond pelvis: distant organs.

▶ Concept and Application

Associated with sexually transmitted diseases: HPV, herpes simplex virus type II, metaplasia of the cervical transformation zone (where squamous epithelium merges into columnar epithelium). Death in advanced cancer results from uremia secondary to ureteral obstruction.

▶ Treatment Steps
1. Total abdominal hysterectomy (cure rate 95%).
2. Stage IB–IIA: Radical hysterectomy or radiotherapy.
3. Recurrence of advanced stage: chemotherapy, radiotherapy.
4. Possible pelvic exenteration.

### B. Cervicitis and Sexually Transmitted Diseases

▶ H&P Keys

*Herpes*—Inguinal nodes, fever, multiple tender vesicles.

*Gonorrhea*—Discharge, fever, abdominal pain, asymptomatic.

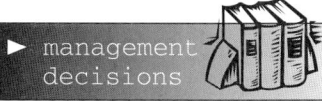

▶ management decisions

**BENIGN ADNEXAL MASSES**

**Ovarian Corpus Luteum Cyst**
Observation; serial ultrasonography; cyst usually resolves within 9 weeks, with or without oral contraceptive suppression. Rarely, surgical intervention is needed.

**Ovarian Hemorrhagic Corpus Luteum Cyst**
As above.

**Ovarian Follicular Cyst**
Observation; usually associated with anovulatory cycle; ultrasound for size; progestin to bring on menses; occasionally, oral contraceptives will help shrink cyst. Rarely, surgery is needed.

**Endometrioma**
Observation; analgesics, GnRH agonists to suppress growth of endometriosis, serial ultrasonography to check response to GnRH agonist. Surgery may be needed to drain cyst, remove cyst wall, or even perform oophorectomy.

**Pedunculated Fibroid**
Observation, serial ultrasonography; rarely need surgery if rapid growth in size, or pain from torsion or pressure.

**Ovarian Cyst with Torsion**
Stat admission to OR, to detorse ovary if no ischemia present; otherwise, emergency oophorectomy performed.

*Syphilis*—Chancre, fever, secondary skin rash, condyloma latum.

*Chlamydia*—Mucopurulent discharge. Asymptomatic or endocervicitis, inguinal lymphadenopathy.

*Chancroid*—Ulcerative disease: soft, painful ulcers.

*Human Papillomavirus (HPV)*—Multifocal fleshy warts may be papular, pedunculated, or flat.

*Lymphogranuloma Venereum (LGV)*—"Groove sign" (line between lymph nodes), buboes.

▶ Diagnosis

*Herpes*—Clinical examination; viral culture.

*Gonorrhea*—Gram negative intracellular diplococci seen on Gram stain. Culture on Thayer–Martin medium.

*Syphilis*—VDRL, fluorescent treponemal antibody (FTA), rapid plasma reagin (RPR).

*Chlamydia*—Culture; chlamydia antibody titers may indicate prior infection.

*Chancroid*—Biopsy, LGV, complement fixation.

▶ Disease Severity

*Herpes*—Primary lesions 2–3 weeks, recurrent lesions.

*Gonorrhea*—Severity of symptoms may progress to overt pelvic inflammatory disease with tubo-ovarian abscess formation; advanced stages: arthritis.

*Syphilis*—Primary, secondary, tertiary syphilis.

*Chlamydia*—Primary, secondary, tertiary stages may progress to overt pelvic inflammatory disease with tubo-ovarian abscess formation. Most common pathogen associated with pelvic inflammatory disease.

*Chancroid*—Severity of symptoms.

*HPV*—Severity of infection, HPV serotyping done to gauge malignant potential.

*HPV type 6,11*—Low-risk oncoviruses.

*HPV type 31,33,35,42*—Intermediate-risk oncoviruses.

*HPV type 16,18*—High-risk oncoviruses.

*LGV*—Severity of symptoms.

▶ Concept and Application

Transmitted sexually via oral, vaginal, and anal contact; also associated with specific microorganism; also with body fluid contact.

*Herpes*—Herpes simplex virus. Type I (more commonly oral) and II (more commonly genital).

*Gonorrhea*—*Neisseria gonorrhoeae*.

*Syphilis*—*Treponema pallidum*.

*Chlamydia*—Chlamydia trachomatis.

*Chancroid*—Haemophilus ducreyi.

*HPV*—Human papillomavirus.

*LGV*—Chlamydia trachomatis.

▶ Treatment Steps

*Herpes*—Acyclovir.

*Gonorrhea*
1. Ofloxacin and azithromycin (to cover chlamydia as well).
2. Ceftriaxone (most effective single dose treatment).
3. Cefoxitin.

*Syphilis*—Benzathine penicillin.

*Chlamydia*
1. Azithromycin.
2. Doxycycline.

*Chancroid*—Oral sulfonamides, tetracycline.

*HPV*—Chemical destructive techniques (podophyllin), cryotherapy, electrocautery, laser vaporization, 5-fluorouracil, interferon, bichloroacetic acid.

## C. Cervical Dysplasia and Management of Abnormal Pap Smear

▶ H&P Keys

Early age of coitus, sexual promiscuity, multiple sexual partners, cigarette smoking, high-risk male partner, abnormal Pap, HPV infection, cervical discharge, postcoital bleeding.

▶ Diagnosis

Pap smear, colposcopy, colposcopic biopsy, endocervical curettage (ECC), cone biopsy.

▶ Disease Severity

Based on Bethesda 2001 classification:

- Negative for squamous intraepithelial (SIL) lesion.
- ASCUS.
- ASCUS, cannot exclude high-grade SIL.
- Low-grade SIL (LSIL).
- High-grade SIL (HSIL).
- Squamous cell Ca.

▶ Concept and Application

Oncogenic agents such as sexually transmitted viruses help induce malignant transformation of the cervical transformation zone.

Histologic classification of abnormal Pap smears (see Fig. 11–3).

▶ Treatment Steps
1. CIN 1:
   - Observation with follow-up cytology.
   - Local ablation, eg, TCA, podophyllin, hysterectomy.

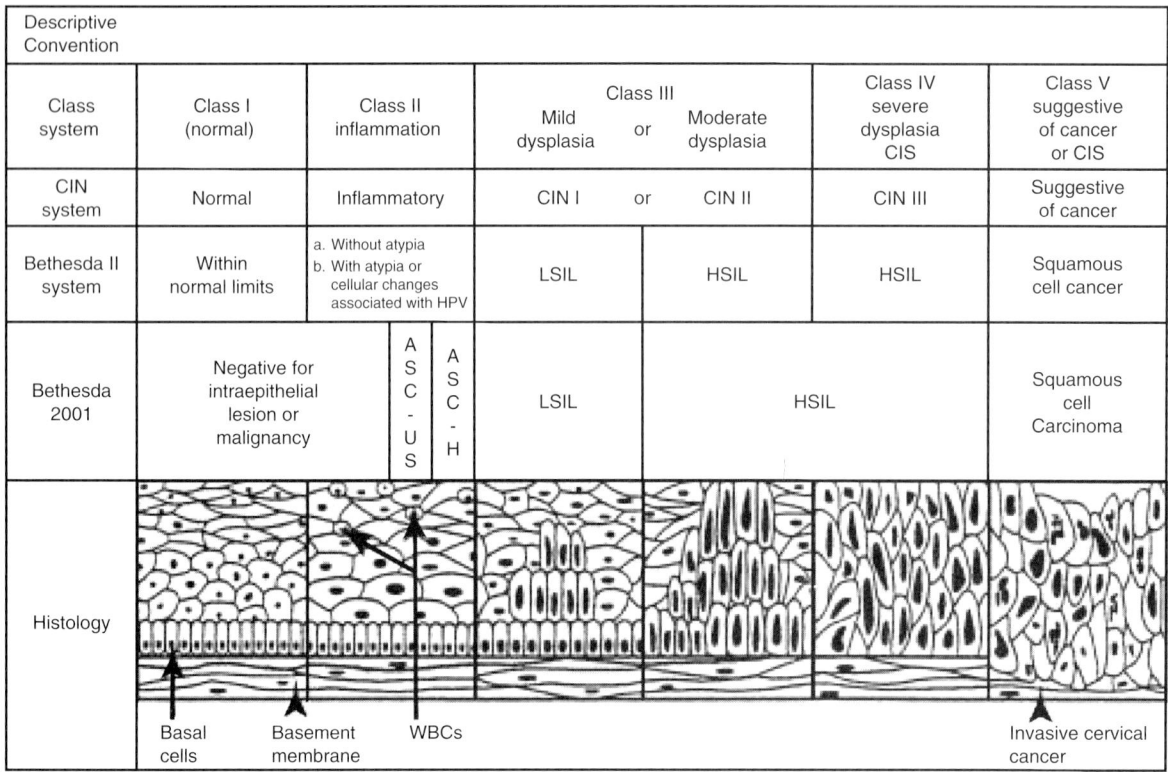

Figure 11–3. Comparison of Pap smear descriptive conventions. CIN = cervical intraepithelial neoplasia; CIS = carcinoma in situ; HPV = human papilloma virus; WBCs = white blood cells. ASC-US = atypical squamous cells of undetermined significance; ASC-H = atypical squamous cells, cannot exclude HSIL; LSIL = low grade squamous intraepithelial lesion; HSIL = high grade squamous intraepithelial lesion.

2. HSIL, CIN 2–3; CIS:
- Ablation or excision, eg, cryosurgery, electrocautery, LEEP, cone biopsy.
3. All patients with noninvasive lesions should have Pap smears every 4–6 months for about 2 years.

## IV. VAGINA AND VULVA

### A. Malignant Neoplasms

1. Vulvar Carcinoma

▶ H&P Keys

Chronic vulvar irritation or itching, labial lesion that does not heal, history of condyloma; age range 60–80 years.

▶ Diagnosis and Evaluation

Toluidine blue stain of vulva. Incisional or excisional biopsy, CXR, IVP, preoperative cystoscopy, and proctoscopy.

▶ Disease Severity

Staging based on T-N-M system (FIGO—1988). Clinical assessment of tumor size (T), node assessment (N), metastases (M).

▶ Concept and Application

Little known; may be associated with HPV 16 and 18 or other oncogenic serotypes.

▶ Treatment Steps
1. Wide local incision for microinvasive carcinoma.
2. Radical vulvectomy for stages I and II.
3. Adjunct radiation therapy or exenteration for advanced stages III and IV.

2. Vaginal Cancer

▶ H&P Keys

Vaginal discharge, urinary symptoms; very rare, may be associated with a history of diethylstilbestrol (DES) ingestion in mother (clear cell adenocarcinoma).

▶ Diagnosis

Pap smear, colposcopy, biopsy.

▶ Disease Severity

Staging: stage I limited to the vaginal mucosa, stage II to subvaginal tissue involvement, stage III to extension to pelvic sidewall, stage IV beyond true pelvis.

▶ Concept and Application

Ninety-five percent are squamous cell carcinoma: Most commonly in upper vagina, possibly of sexually transmitted disease origin.

▶ Treatment Steps
1. Depends on stage.
2. Radiation therapy, surgery, chemotherapy.
3. Overall 5-year survival rate 50%.

B. Candidiasis of the Vulva and Vagina

▶ H&P Keys

Thick whitish discharge, cottage cheesy, itching, non-malodorous, burning, swelling, dysuria. Obesity, frequent douching, diabetes, HIV disease, antibiotic usage, immunosuppressed patients.

▶ Diagnosis

Microscopic specimen examination including potassium hydroxide (KOH) and saline wet mount; hyphae on wet-mount exam; no odor.

▶ Disease Severity

Severity of symptoms.

▶ Concept and Application

*Candida albicans.*

▶ Treatment Steps
1. Clotrimazole, miconazole, terconazole.
2. Avoidance of perfumed soaps and douches.
3. Advise cotton underwear, avoid tight-fitting clothing.
4. Recurrence with severe yeast infections, oral agents possibly required.

## C. Vaginitis and Vulvovaginitis

▶ **H&P Keys**

*Trichomoniasis*—May be asymptomatic, greenish-gray, frothy, malodorous discharge, strawberry spots on cervix and vagina, vaginal pH between 5 and 6.

*Bacterial Vaginosis*—Watery malodorous discharge, pH 5.0–5.5.

▶ **Diagnosis**

*Trichomonas*—Saline wet mount and KOH prep show trichomonad organisms intermixed with clumps of white blood cells (WBCs).

*Bacterial Vaginosis*—"Clue" cells (squamous cells with coccobacilli bacteria obscuring the sharp borders and cytoplasm), fishy odor, positive "whiff" test, when mixed with KOH.

▶ **Disease Severity**

Severity of symptoms.

▶ **Concept and Application**

*Trichomonas*—*Trichomonas vaginalis*.

*Bacterial Vaginosis*—*Gardnerella vaginalis*.

▶ **Treatment Steps**

*Trichomonas*—Metronidazole (PO).

*Bacterial Vaginosis*—Metronidazole (PO or intravaginal).

## D. Pelvic Relaxation/Urinary Incontinence

▶ **H&P Keys**

Varies, based on structure or structures involved and the degree of prolapse, pressure, heaviness, urinary (stress) incontinence, frequency, hesitancy, incomplete voiding, recurrent infections, painful or incomplete defecation. Ten to fifteen percent of women suffer significant recurrent urinary loss.

▶ **Diagnosis**

*Cystourethrocele:* Q-tip test; evaluation of urinary function, urodynamic testing, anoscopy, sigmoidoscopy.

▶ **Disease Severity**

First degree, second degree, third degree; procidentia (uterus completely outside vagina).

▶ **Concept and Application**

Loss of uterine support, paravaginal tissue support, bladder wall and urethrovesicle angle support, and support overlying the distal rectum, associated with aging and multiple childbirth.

▶ **Treatment Steps**

1. Order of treatment depends on severity and etiology of prolapse and/or urinary incontinence.

2. Bladder training, biofeedback, anticholinergic drugs, β-sympathomimetic agonists, antidepressants, estrogen replacement therapy, Kegel exercises, pessaries, surgery: colporrhaphy, obliteration of the rectovaginal space (Moschowitz procedure), vaginal hysterectomy.

## V. MENSTRUAL DISORDERS

### A. Dysmenorrhea

▶ H&P Keys

Pelvic pain with menses with variable onset of pain compared to day 1 of flow; nausea, diarrhea, headache, ovulatory menstrual cycles.

▶ Diagnosis

Ovulatory menses, menstrual pain history.

▶ Disease Severity

Severity of symptoms, from mild to incapacitating.

▶ Concept and Application

Result of uterine contractions, caused by prostaglandins.

*Primary Dysmenorrhea*—No associated pelvic pathology.

*Secondary Dysmenorrhea*—Associated with pelvic pathology: endometriosis, fibroids, etc.

▶ Treatment Steps

*Primary Dysmenorrhea*
1. NSAIDs to inhibit prostaglandin synthetase and thereby decrease smooth muscle contractility.
2. Combination oral contraception to inhibit ovulation.
3. GnRH agonists in severe cases if suspicion of endemetriosis is present.
4. No relief, laparoscopy may be needed to rule out pelvic pathology (eg, secondary dysmenorrhea).

### B. Premenstrual Syndrome

▶ H&P Keys

Anxiety, breast tenderness, crying spells, depression, fatigue, irritability, weight gain around the luteal phase of the cycle; prior to the onset of menses, usually relieved with the onset of bleeding.

▶ Diagnosis

Basal body temperature charts; symptom-recording diaries; daily weight recordings.

▶ Disease Severity

Severity of symptoms. PMS is classified into 4 major groups by symptoms: Group A—anxiety group; group C—carbohydrate group; group H—edema group; group D—depression group.

▶ Concept and Application

Unknown, but progesterone deficiency is one of the more popular theories.

▶ Treatment Steps

There are no studies in evidence-based medicine with respect to any specific treatment to be effective. Treatments include exercise, vitamin $B_6$, progesterone, diuretics, oral contraceptives.

## C. Disorders of Menstruation

### 1. Amenorrhea

▶ H&P Keys

*Primary* amenorrhea is defined by no menses by age 16. *Secondary* is 3 months or longer of amenorrhea in a normally cycling individual. Possible sexual ambiguity or virilization; possible absence of secondary sex characteristics.

▶ Diagnosis

History and physical examination, β-hCG, prolactin, follicle-stimulating hormone (FSH), luteinizing hormone (LH), progesterone withdrawal test. If virilization, testosterone, dehydroepiandrosterone sulfate (DHEAS). *Primary:* Karyotype, FSH, estradiol.

▶ Disease Severity

Presence or absence of secondary sex characteristics; no breast development by age 14.

▶ Concept and Application

*Primary*—Müellerian agenesis, testicular feminization (androgen insensitivity), Turner's syndrome.

*Secondary*—Pregnancy, Asherman's syndrome (intrauterine synechiae), polycystic ovarian disease, congenital adrenal hyperplasia, hyperandrogenism, hypothyroidism, hyperprolactinemia.

*Hypothalamic*—Associated with weight loss, chronic anxiety, excessive exercise, eating disorder (anorexia nervosa), marijuana, tranquilizers, head injury, chronic medical illness, central nervous system (CNS) tumor, IV drug use (opium derivatives).

*Note*—In the absence of all the above, diagnosis is dysfunctional uterine bleeding.

▶ Treatment Steps

1. *Primary:* Obtain karyotype if < 30 years old. If abnormal karyotype, phenotypic female: estrogen replacement therapy for completion of secondary sex characteristics. Müllerian agenesis requires surgery.
2. *Secondary:* Requires cyclic menstrual function to prevent endometrial hyperplasia: cyclic combination oral contraceptive therapy or monthly progestin therapy.
3. *Hypothalamic:* Hormone replacement therapy to prevent osteoporosis and maintain normal physiologic status.
4. *Asherman's syndrome:* Amenorrhea not responsive to estrogen–progesterone cycle; hysteroscopic surgical intervention.

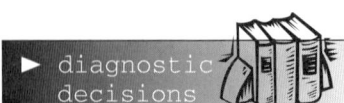

### SECONDARY AMENORRHEA

**Pregnancy**
Most common etiology of secondary amenorrhea in reproductive age women. Look for sexual activity with partner—unprotected intercourse. Usually 1 to 2 weeks beyond expected date of menses. Check pregnancy test.

**Menopause**
Most common etiology of secondary amenorrhea in older women. Average age of menopause is 51.4 years in the United States. Look for a history of hot flashes; vaginal dryness; abnormal menstrual bleeding patterns, followed by amenorrhea. If this occurs before age 40, it is called premature ovarian failure. Check FSH levels and estradiol levels.

**Hypothalamic Amenorrhea**
History of exercise; eating disorder (usually anorexia); decreased body fat; high-stress lifestyle; heroin or opiate usage. Measure patient's height, weight, and BMI; check bone density for osteoporosis. Obtain good dietary history.

**Polycystic Ovarian Disease (PCOD)**
History of obesity, hirsutism, and infertility. Usually familial as well; look for height, weight; ↑ BMI; hirsutism on face, chest, abdomen, male escutcheon; bilateral ovarian cystic enlargement; obtain LH, FSH, and check if positive withdrawal bleed to progestins.

## VI. MENOPAUSE

### A. Menopausal Symptoms

▶ H&P Keys

Changes in menstrual cycle regularity, decreased cycle interval, finally cessation of menses; mean age 51.4 years; atrophy of estrogen-dependent tissue (uterus, breasts, vagina), vasomotor symptoms (hot flashes), osteoporosis, urethral changes, increased frequency of cystitis, insomnia.

▶ Diagnosis

FSH; estradiol; if osteoporosis severe, DEXA bone densitometry. Menopause prior to age 40 means premature ovarian failure; if menopause prior to age 30, check karyotype.

▶ Disease Severity
1. Skin collagen content decreases.
2. Worsening serum lipid profile.
3. Vaginal dryness with atrophy.
4. Breast atrophy.
5. Osteopenia leading to osteoporosis and possibly stress fractures.
6. Atherosclerotic coronary vessel disease.
7. Senility, Alzheimer's disease.

▶ Concept and Application

Sequelae of decreased estrogen result of loss of all remaining follicles. Estrone is principle estrogen in menopause, produced from androgen precursor androstenedione.

▶ Treatment Steps
1. Estrogen replacement therapy (if no uterus).
2. If uterus present, must add progestin; however, recent studies on estrogen/progestin replacement seem to indicate that long-term hormones have a greater risk than benefit.
3. Increase calcium intake.
4. Increase exercise.
5. Decrease fat intake. Daily Ca requirements 1,500 mg/day. Bisphosphonates may be helpful as well as SERMs (selective estrogen receptor modulators).

## VII. BREAST

### A. Malignant Neoplasm

▶ H&P Keys

Family history the most important epidemiologic factor genetic evaluation for BrCa1 and BrCa2 genes; long history of unopposed estrogen exposure, nulliparity obesity, high fat intake, alcohol; first child born after age 30, early menarche, late menopause; discrete lump, retracted nipple, puckering of breast skin (peau d'orange), axillary lymphadenopathy, nipple bleeding or discharge (Table 11–1).

### ▶ Diagnosis
Mammography, physical examination, fine-needle aspiration, thermography (not as useful).

### ▶ Disease Severity
Stated by T (tumor size), N (regional lymph nodes), and M (distant metastases). Evaluations done for hormone receptors reflect tumor responsiveness to chemotherapy.

### ▶ Concept and Application
Unknown, possibly related to hormones; or high-fat diet; surgical menopause appears to be protective; complex combination of environmental and genetic influences.

Tumor is analyzed for the presence of estrogen receptors and/or progesterone receptors.

### ▶ Treatment Steps

*Surgery*
1. Mammography.
2. Biopsy/Fine-needle aspiration.
3. Lumpectomy.

### 11-1 RISK FACTORS FOR BREAST CANCER

| Factor | Relative Risk |
| --- | --- |
| Family history of breast cancer | |
|     First-degree relative (sister or mother) | 1.2–3.0 |
| Menstrual history | |
|     Menarche < 12 years of age | 1.3 |
|     < 40 menstrual years | 1.5–2.0 |
| Oral contraceptive use | No effect |
| Estrogen replacement < 10 years | No effect |
| Pregnancy | |
|     First delivery > 35 years of age | 2.0–3.0 |
|     Nulliparous | 3.0 |
| Other neoplasms | |
|     Contralateral breast cancer | 5.0 |
|     Carcinoma of uterus or ovary | 2.0 |
|     Carcinoma of major salivary gland | 4.0 |
| Other conditions | |
|     Atypical hyperplasia | 4.0–6.0 |
|     Previous biopsy | 1.9–2.1 |
|     North American (white or black) | 5.0 |
|     Age 60 vs. age 40 years | 2.0 |
|     Moderate alcohol use | 1.5–2.0 |
|     Radiation exposure (> 90 rads) | 4.0 |
|     Obesity | Suggested but unknown |
|     Large bowel cancer | Suggested but unknown |
|     Increased dietary fat | Suggested but unknown |

(Reproduced, with permission, from Gant NF, Cunningham FG. *Basic Gynecology and Obstetrics*. Norwalk, CT: Appleton & Lange, 1993.)

4. Simple mastectomy (if necessary).
5. Radical mastectomy (if necessary).

*Hormonal Therapy*—If positive hormone receptors, progestins.

## B. Fibroadenoma

This is a benign breast neoplasm.

▶ H&P Keys

Younger women, peak age 21–25, single breast mass, smooth, well-circumscribed, firm, mobile, and rubbery nodule. Intraductal papilloma most common cause of unilateral bloody nipple discharge.

▶ Diagnosis

Mammography, sonography, fine-needle aspiration, cytologic smear of discharge.

▶ Disease Severity

Severity of symptoms.

▶ Concept and Application

Unknown.

▶ Treatment Steps

1. Fine-needle aspiration to make diagnosis.
2. Subsequent observation.
3. Possible lumpectomy needed.

## C. Inflammatory Disease of the Breast

▶ H&P Keys

*Mastitis*—Usually in nursing women; pain, fever, erythema.

*Breast Abscess*—Fluctuant lesions, well localized, difficult to palpate.

*Superficial Thrombophlebitis*—Acute pain, redness, upper outer quadrant.

▶ Diagnosis

Diagnosed by history, CBC with differential, fever.

▶ Disease Severity

Elevation of WBCs, fever, severity of symptoms.

▶ Concept and Application

*Mastitis*—Penicillin-resistant *Staphylococcus aureus* from the infant's nose and throat; organism enters the breast through fissure or abrasion in nipple.

▶ Treatment Steps

1. *Mastitis:* dicloxacillin.
2. *Breast abscess:* incision and drainage and antibiotics.
3. *Superficial thrombophlebitis:* warm compresses, non-narcotic analgesics.

### D. Fibrocystic Disease

▶ H&P Keys

Cyclic bilateral pain (mastalgia) and breast engorgement, may radiate to shoulders or upper arms, diffuse bilateral nodularity, "lumpy-bumpy" pattern.

▶ Diagnosis

Mammography, physical examination, history.

▶ Disease Severity

According to symptoms.

▶ Concept and Application

May be hormone related; initially with proliferation of stroma, especially in the upper outer quadrant, followed by adenosis, leading to cyst formation, then marked proliferation of the ducts and alveolar cells.

▶ Treatment Steps

Regular breast exams.

1. Diet therapy.
2. Avoidance of caffeine and tobacco.
3. Occasionally medical therapy is helpful, eg, progestins.
4. Diuretics.
5. Danazol.
6. Bromocriptine.
7. Tamoxifen.

## VIII. OTHER PROBLEMS

### A. Infertility, Male and Female

▶ H&P Keys

*Primary Infertility*—Never having conceived, despite 12 months of having unprotected intercourse.

*Secondary Infertility*—Previous history of conception but currently unable to establish a subsequent pregnancy despite 12 months of unprotected intercourse.

▶ Diagnosis

Complete history and physical on both partners, semen analysis, postcoital test, hysterosalpingogram, progesterone level (midluteal phase), endometrial biopsy (Fig. 11–4).

▶ Disease Severity

Directly proportional to the duration of the infertility; worse prognosis with longer duration of infertility.

▶ Concept and Application

Forty-five percent male factor, 45% female factor; 10% unexplained.

One sixth of all U.S. couples are infertile.

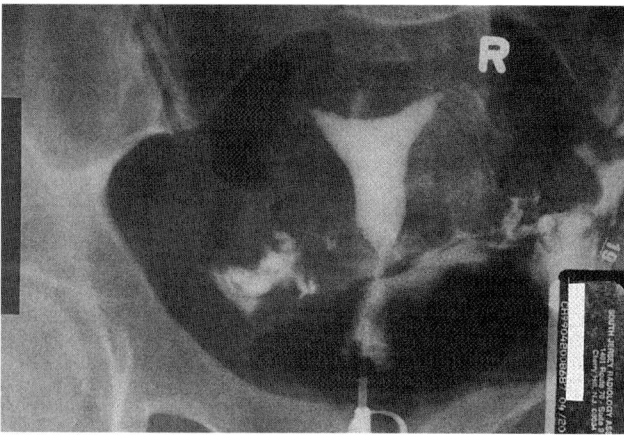

Figure 11–4. A normal hysterosalpingogram is shown in this photograph. The uterus takes on a classic "goblet" shape, and both tubes are patent. There is free dye throughout the peritoneal cavity.

*Male Factor*—Most commonly associated with varicocele (etiology of infertility uncertain). Other factors include infection, trauma, impotence, antisperm antibodies, etc.

*Female Factor*—Blocked tubes, ovulatory dysfunction, peritoneal factor (pelvic adhesive disease, endometriosis, etc).

▶ management decisions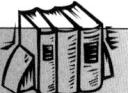

### INFERTILITY

#### Ovulatory dysfunction
One third of all infertility etiologies. Determine cause of oligo/anovulation. If abnormal thyroid function, replace thyroid hormone, then await resumption of menses. If elevated prolactin levels, determine etiology—use bromocriptine (dopamine agonist) to decrease prolactin, then await resumption of menses. If elevated androgen levels of adrenal origin, give glucocorticoid to inhibit adrenals, then add ovulation induction agent (eg, clomiphene, human menopausal gonadotropins). If elevated androgen levels of ovarian origin (eg, PCOD) ovulation induction agents. If hypothalamic amenorrhea, remove etiologic agent if possible (eg, dietary correction, ceasing drug usage, decreasing severe exercise, etc).

#### Tubal obstruction
One third of all infertility etiologies. Associated with poor prognosis if longstanding. Also risk of ectopic pregnancies. Surgery is first-line treatment; attempt to open tube(s) via laparoscopy/hysteroscopy or laparotomy. Overall success rate is 10%. Assisted reproductive technology (ART) if surgery not possible. IVF provides up to 20–25% success rate/cycle. Involves ovulation induction with potent injectable gonadotropins, oocyte retrieval, and embryo transfer.

#### Male Factor
Third main cause of overall infertility. Semen analysis shows most abnormalities, although sperm antibody testing, and postcoital testing very important. If low count, or antisperm antibody positive, then intrauterine insemination is suggested (with/without ovulatory induction drugs). If unsuccessful, ART with ICSI (intracytoplasmic sperm injection). Finally, donor semen is used in the most severe cases.

▶ Treatment Steps

*Ovulatory Dysfunction*—Ovulation-induction agents.

*Tubal Factor*
1. Surgery.
2. Assisted reproductive technology (ART):
   - In vitro fertilization (IVF).
   - Gamete intrafallopian transfer (GIFT).

*Cervical Mucus Factor*—Intrauterine insemination, bicarbonate douching.

*Peritoneal Factor*
1. Laparoscopy confirms diagnosis.
2. If endometriosis, ablation of peritoneal implants, lysis of adhesions, restoration of normal pelvic anatomy ± GnRH agonist.
3. If pelvic adhesions, as above ± antibiotic postop therapy.

*Male Factor*—Intrauterine insemination, ART, intracytoplasmic sperm injection, Donor sperm.

## B. Pelvic Inflammatory Disease

▶ H&P Keys

Pain, adnexal tenderness, fever, nausea and vomiting, dysuria, vaginal discharge, adnexal masses, peritoneal signs, cervical motion tenderness.

▶ Diagnosis

Cervical Gram stain (for gonorrhea), gram negative intracellular diplococci, laparoscopy, ultrasound, β-hCG, elevated WBC count, elevated sedimentation rate.

▶ Disease Severity

Depends on extent of signs and symptoms, multiple episodes of pelvic inflammatory disease (PID) may result in infertility, chronic pelvic pain, increased ectopic pregnancy rate. Tubo-ovarian abscess (TOA) formation may be in later stages.

▶ Concept and Application

Infection of the upper genital tract, usually polymicrobial consisting of *Chlamydia trachomatis*, *Neisseria gonorrhoeae*, endogenous aerobes (*Escherichia coli*, *Proteus*, etc), and endogenous anaerobes (*Bacteroides*, *Peptostreptococcus*), *Mycoplasma hominis*. *Chlamydia* is most common pathogen associated with PID.

▶ Treatment Steps

*Outpatient*
1. Aqueous procaine penicillin G, ampicillin with probenecid, doxycycline, ceftriaxone.
2. Recheck patient in 2–3 days for possible need to admit.

*Inpatient*
1. IV antibiotics. Doxycycline plus intravenous cefoxitin, clindamycin plus gentamicin, doxycycline plus metronidazole.
2. Bed rest in semi-Fowler position.
3. Pelvic rest, ie, vaginal precautions.

---

▶ diagnositc decisions

### CHRONIC PELVIC PAIN

**Endometriosis**
Chronic pelvic pain of more than 6 months duration; family history positive (mother, sister, daughter, etc.); dysmenorrhea several days to a week *before* onset of menses; premenstrual spotting or staining; dyspareunia (deep thrusting); afebrile, pain usually diffuse, bilateral; uterine retroversion, decreased mobility; abnormal vaginal discharge usually absent; rectovaginal nodularity; uterosacral implants; bilateral adnexal tenderness, normal WBC; check ultrasound for ovarian cysts.

**Chronic PID**
Chronic pelvic pain of more than 6 months duration; STI etiology; history of more than one chlamydial infection; fever, chills; mucopurulent cervical thick copious discharge; cervical motion tenderness; bilateral adnexal tenderness; peritoneal signs; elevated WBCs, elevated sed rate; check ultrasound for tubo-ovarian abscesses.

4. Pelvic ultrasound. If TOA present and unresponsive, then surgical drainage.
5. In severe cases patient may require surgery with colpotomy or actual laparotomy with total abdominal hysterectomy and bilateral salpingo-oophorectomy.

## IX. HEALTH MAINTENANCE

### A. Gynecologic Examination and Screening

▶ H&P Keys

*Menstrual History*—Age at menarche, cycle length, duration of flow; vaginal discharge; pelvic pain; sexual history; history of abnormal cervical cytology; obstetrical history (gravidity and parity), contraception usage.

*Review of Systems*—Gastrointestinal, urinary, endocrine, metabolic, cardiovascular, hematologic.

*Physical Examination*—Vital signs, breast exam (sitting and supine), thyroid exam, axillary lymph nodes, abdomen, hair distribution.

*Pelvic Examination*—External genitalia, speculum examination, cervical cytology, evaluation of vaginal contents.

*Bimanual Examination*—Cervix, uterus, adnexal masses.

*Rectal Examination*—Rectovaginal exam, uterosacral nodularity, guaiac test.

▶ Diagnosis

CBC with differential, gonorrhea culture (GC), chlamydia culture, Pap smear, lipid profile, rubella status (if interested in conception), RPR.

*Note*—General gynecologic exam should be done annually along with counseling about tobacco, alcohol, caffeine, exercise, and diet.

### B. General Counseling for Contraception

*Types*—Natural family planning; spermicides and barrier contraceptives (spermicide, condoms, diaphragms, sponges, cervical caps); intrauterine devices (IUDs) (Progesta-Sert, Paraguard); steroid oral contraceptives: contraceptive patch, vaginal ring, combination oral contraceptive, progestin-only contraceptives; injectable and implantable contraceptives (medroxyprogesterone acetate, Levonorgestrel implants (Norplant); postcoital contraception (emergency contraception), oral abortifacients (RU-486, methotrexate and misoprostol).

*Effectiveness (Given as Failure Rate)*—Oral contraceptives: < 1–2%; Norplant: < 1–3%; IUD: 2–4%; diaphragm with spermicide: 10–20%; condom: 5–15%.

*Surveillance of Prescribed Contraceptives*—Oral contraceptives: regular breast, thyroid, liver, and pelvic examinations, initial blood pressure check; IUD: string check 6 weeks after insertion.

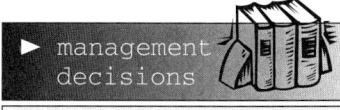
▶ management decisions

**FAMILY PLANNING**

**Teenage Girl**
The most important two issues here are to prevent pregnancy *and* to prevent transmission of STIs, especially in light of multiple partners. Condoms plus hormonal contraception would provide this coverage. Hormonal contraception consists of either oral contraceptives or long-acting injectable progestins (eg, Depo-Provera), contraceptive patch, or vaginal ring.

**Woman in Long-term Monogamous Relationship**
*Completed child-bearing:* Laparoscopic tubal sterilization or vasectomy is most highly recommended, if permanent contraception desired. Otherwise, long-acting progestins, or IUD.
*Not completed child-bearing:* Long-acting progestins, or oral contraceptives, or IUD.

**Woman over 35, Smoker, in Monogamous Relationship**
Condoms or long-acting injectable progestins, or IUD.

**Perimenopausal woman**
Ultra low-dose oral contraception assuming no contraindications to estrogen; long-acting progestins; tubal sterilization if permanent contraception desired.

### C. Sterilization

Most frequent method of controlling fertility in the United States.

*Male Sterilization*—Vasectomy failure rate 1%.

*Female Sterilization*—Postpartum failure rate 1 in 250; interval (between pregnancies) failure rate 1 in 500.

Counseling must include permanent nature of procedure, operative risk, failure rate. Despite careful counseling, approximately 1% of patients undergoing sterilization subsequently request reversal. Most common reason, new sexual partner.

### D. Genetic Counseling

Assessment of risk for developing disease and providing information to the patient regarding appropriate screening or diagnostic tests. Chromosome abnormalities account for 50–60% of first-trimester spontaneous abortions, 5% of stillbirths, and 2–3% of couples experiencing repeated pregnancy loss. Overall, 6% of live-born infants have a chromosomal abnormality.

▶ H&P Keys

Data forms, questionnaires, pedigree construction, and patient interviews, family medical history, parental exposure to harmful substances.

▶ Diagnosis

Karyotype, extensive family history, pedigree. If patient pregnant, chorionic villus sampling, amniocentesis.

*Indications for Prenatal Cytogenetic Analysis*—Advanced maternal age, previous child with chromosome abnormality, parental chromosome abnormality (balance translocation).

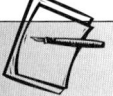

▶ on rounds

---

### VAGINITIS

#### Candidiasis
- Thick white discharge, itching, swelling, no odor
- Diagnosis by KOH preparation, saline wet mount
- Treatment—clotrimazole, miconazole, terconazole

#### Trichomoniasis
- Green-gray discharge, frothy, bad odor, strawberry spots on cervix
- Diagnosis by wet mount (trichomonads)
- Treatment—metronidazole

#### Bacterial Vaginosis
- Watery discharge, bad odor
- Diagnosis by "clue cells," fishy odor, "whiff" test
- Treatment—metronidazole—oral or vaginal

# BIBLIOGRAPHY

Beckman CRB, Ling FW, et al. *Obstetrics and Gynecology.* 4th edition. Baltimore: Lippincott Williams & Wilkins; 2002.

DeCherney AH, Pernoll ML. *Current Obstetric and Gynecologic Diagnosis and Treatment.* Norwalk, CT: Appleton & Lange; 2002.

Gant NF, Cunningham FG. *Basic Gynecology and Obstetrics.* Norwalk, CT: Appleton & Lange; 1993.

# Obstetrics 12

I. **UNCOMPLICATED PREGNANCY / 365**
   A. Health and Health Maintenance / 365
   B. Rh Immunoglobulin Prophylaxis / 365
   C. Prenatal Diagnosis / 366
   D. Teratology / 366
   E. Immediate Care of the Newborn / 367
   F. Postpartum Care of the Mother / 367
   G. Lactation / 368
   H. Normal Labor and Delivery / 368

II. **COMPLICATED PREGNANCY / 369**
   A. Adolescent Pregnancy / 369
   B. Ectopic Pregnancy / 370
   C. Spontaneous Abortion / 371
   D. Induced Abortion / 372
   E. Septic Abortion / 372
   F. Placenta Previa / 373
   G. Abruptio Placentae / 374
   H. Preeclampsia / 374
   I. Eclampsia / 375
   J. Premature Labor / 376
   K. Infections of the Genitourinary Tract / 376
   L. Hepatitis B Infection Complicating Pregnancy / 377
   M. Incompetent Cervix / 378
   N. Central Nervous System Malformation in the Fetus and Neural Tube Defect / 378
   O. Trisomy / 380
   P. Rh Incompatibility or Isoimmunization / 380
   Q. Multiple Gestation / 381
   R. Gestational Trophoblastic Disease / 382
   S. Maternal Mortality / 383
   T. Depression / 383

- U. Preterm Premature Rupture of Membranes / 384
- V. Hyperemesis Gravidarum / 384
- W. Abnormalities of Labor, Dystocia / 385
- X. Postpartum Hemorrhage / 386
- Y. Postpartum Sepsis / 386
- Z. Obstetric Forceps and Vacuum Extractor / 387
- AA. Diabetes, Gestational / 388
- BB. Diabetes, Overt / 389
- CC. Asthma / 389

**BIBLIOGRAPHY / 390**

## I. UNCOMPLICATED PREGNANCY

### A. Health and Health Maintenance

#### 1. Prenatal Care

▶ H&P Keys

Accurate dating! Presumptive signs of pregnancy: amenorrhea with nausea and breast tenderness and bluish vaginal mucosa. Probable: positive pregnancy test (β-human chorionic gonadotropin [β-hCG]), uterine change, and outlining of fetus. Diagnostic: fetal imaging (ultrasonography, etc), auscultation of the fetal heart.

▶ Diagnosis

Prenatal evaluation. Complete blood count (CBC), urine analysis (UA), urine culture and sensitivity (C&S), blood type and Rh factor, antibody screen, hepatitis B surface antigen, rubella titer, syphilis serology, Pap smear gonorrhea and chlamydia cultures at first visit. Maternal serum-alpha fetoprotein (MS-AFP) at 15 to 18 weeks and 50-g glucose screening at 24–28 weeks. Also consider HIV, hemoglobin electrophoresis screening for group B strep at approximately 36 weeks.

▶ Disease Severity

Surveillance for complications: preeclampsia, low birth weight, malnutrition, pre- and postterm delivery, anemia, and common infections, gestational diabetes, abnormal lab tests.

▶ Concept and Application

Prevention and early treatment of pregnancy complications.

▶ Treatment Steps

*Initial Care*—Accurate dating and diagnosis, education.

*Emergency Care*—Refer to specific problems.

*Continued Care*—Routine education, surveillance, and maintenance.

### B. Rh Immunoglobulin Prophylaxis

▶ H&P Keys

Rh-negative, Du-negative mother of an Rh-positive or unknown fetus.

▶ Diagnosis

Rh antibody screen to rule out preexisting sensitization.

▶ Disease Severity

Kleihauer-Betke test to determine quantity of fetal cells in the maternal circulation if large fetomaternal transfusion is suspected.

► Concept and Application

Rh immune globulin (RhIg) removes Rh-positive red blood cells (RBCs) prior to maternal sensitization. Three hundred micrograms neutralizes 15 mL of Rh-positive RBCs.

► Treatment Steps

*Initial Care*
1. Give at 28 weeks for prophylaxis.
2. Invasive fetal diagnostic procedures (amniocentesis, CVS) termination, or delivery at any gestation may result in fetomaternal transfusion.
3. Administer to all with indications within 72 hours of exposure.

*Emergency Care*—Same.

*Continued Care*—Same.

## C. Prenatal Diagnosis

► H&P Keys

Exposure to medications or teratogens, pedigree, accurate pregnancy dating, exam looking for expression of genotype.

► Diagnosis

Specific for condition evaluated: biochemical screening tests: MS-AFP, unconjugated estriol, and β-subunit hCG abnormal patterns are associated with neural tube defects and aneuploidy. Ultrasound screening: major structural anomalies, thickened nuchal fold, growth lag, and abnormal amniotic fluid volume.

► Disease Severity

Specific for condition evaluated.

► Concept and Application

Hundreds of biochemical, chromosomal, and genetic disorders can be diagnosed by condition-specific tests including: ultrasonography, identified structural change, karotyping, DNA analysis technologies, fetal tissue enzyme activity, and metabolic product accumulation in fetal cells obtained by chorionic villous sampling (CVS), amniocentesis, percutaneous umbilical blood sampling, or fetal biopsy.

► Treatment Steps
1. Specific for the condition evaluated.
2. Nondirective counseling is used.

## D. Teratology

► H&P Keys

Exposure of potential teratogens and gestational age of fetus. Examination of fetus is limited to high-resolution ultrasonography.

► Diagnosis

Specific for the condition evaluated.

---

► diagnostic decisions

### PRENATAL DIAGNOSIS

**Chorionic Villus Sampling (CVS)**
Provides direct DNA analysis of fetus by sampling chorionic tissue. Evaluation can be done between 10 and 14 weeks.

**Amniocentesis**
Provides direct DNA analysis of fetus by sampling the somatic cells of the fetus. Evaluation is done after 15 to 16 weeks.

**Triple Screen**
Provides indirect biochemical analysis of alpha fetal protein, estriol, and β-hcg as markers for fetal abnormalities specifically open neural tube defects and chromosomal abnormalities. Evaluation is done between 15 and 18 weeks.

**Ultrasound**
Provides a visual image of the fetus at any gestational age.

▶ Disease Severity
Specific for the condition evaluated.

▶ Concept and Application
Three percent of all pregnancies have a major congenital anomaly, and another 3% will have a minor one. There are very **few known teratogens:** viruses (rubella), parasites (toxoplasmosis), bacteria (syphilis), heavy metals (mercury), cancer chemotherapeutics (folic acid antagonists), antiepileptics, maternal conditions (phenylketonuria [PKU]), anticoagulants (warfarin), antibiotics (tetracycline), as well as ethanol and radiation.

▶ Treatment Steps
1. Specific to the exposure and evaluation.

### E. Immediate Care of the Newborn

▶ H&P Keys
Prenatal history, labor history. Assess the dry baby for neonatal depression, anomalies, respirations, heart rate, and meconium while under the warmer.

▶ Diagnosis
Heel stick blood sugar if mother is diabetic or if there are signs that the baby is hypoglycemic.

▶ Disease Severity
Apnea, heart rate < 100, central cyanosis.

▶ Concept and Application
Resuscitation based on Apgar score alone results in a 45-second delay. A chilled baby requires more oxygen.

▶ Treatment Steps

*Initial Care*
1. Stimulation or resuscitation as needed.
2. Intubate and aspirate if meconium stained; dry and stimulate.
3. Apneic or heart rate < 100: bag and mask; < 60: closed chest cardiac massage.

### F. Postpartum Care of the Mother

▶ H&P Keys
Childbirth in the preceding 6 weeks. Lochia changes from red to brown to serous over first 2 weeks. Episiotomy heals rapidly. Uterus is in pelvis at 2 weeks and normal size at 6 weeks.

▶ Diagnosis
Pap smear at postpartum visit if no recent pap smear.

▶ Disease Severity
Infection: endomyometritis (mixed aerobic and anaerobic flora), mastitis (*Staphylococcus aureus*), breast abscess. Depression: > 50% will have a week of "the blues," 10% will be depressed, and 0.05% suicidal. See section on postpartum hemorrhage and lactation.

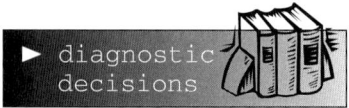

## COMPLICATIONS OF LACTATION

**Breast Engorgement**
Diffuse distension, firmness and nodularity of the breast secondary to normal edema and lymphatic engorgement as a result of the milk coming in. It is sometimes associated with tenderness and a transient fever. Treatment depends upon whether the mother is breast-feeding or bottle-feeding.

**Galactocele**
Blocked milk duct with collection of milk behind it. It is an isolated lump which may be mildly tender. Treatment includes warm compresses, massage, and breast-feeding.

**Mastitis**
Infection in the breast which presents with pain, erythema, fever, malaise. It usually presents in one segment of the breast. *Staph aureus* is the most common organism. Treatment includes antibiotics along with hot compresses and continuation of breast-feeding.

▶ Concept and Application
Fifty percent of nonlactating women ovulate between 28 and 90 days postpartum. Cardiac output normalizes in several hours. Glomerular filtration rate (GFR) is down to normal in a few weeks.

▶ Treatment Steps

*Initial Care*
1. Evaluation, support and problem specific therapy.
2. Rh immune globulin if indicated.

*Emergency Care*—Problem-specific.

### G. Lactation

▶ H&P Keys
Absence of pain, erythema, localized induration, abscess, nipple fissures or cracks. Prefeeding engorgement and discomfort is common in the first couple weeks. Limit medications to those necessary and not contraindicated.

▶ Diagnosis
None.

▶ Disease Severity
Same as history and physical examination.

▶ Concept and Application
Human breast milk best nutrition and immunologic stimulation for the baby. Prolactin is essential. Suckling stimulates the neurohypophysis to release oxytocin, which contracts the breast's myoepithelial cells, allowing milk "let-down." Less than 1% of most medications is found in breast milk. Nipple fissures and cracks allow ingress of bacteria, causing cellulitis to abscess.

▶ Treatment Steps

*Initial Care*—Encourage relaxation and hydration to facilitate breast-feeding.

*Emergency Care*
1. Treat mastitis with antibiotics effective against *S. aureus*, and continue breast-feeding.
2. Abscess may require surgical drainage.

### H. Normal Labor and Delivery

▶ H&P Keys
Progressive uterine contractions associated with cervical change; progressively intense, about every 3 minutes and lasting 60 seconds.

▶ Diagnosis
Normal latent phase lasts a maximum of 20 hours in the nulligravida and 14 hours in the multipara. Normal active phase dilatation is at least 1.2 cm/hr in the nulligravida and 1.5 cm/hr in the multipara (Fig. 12–1).

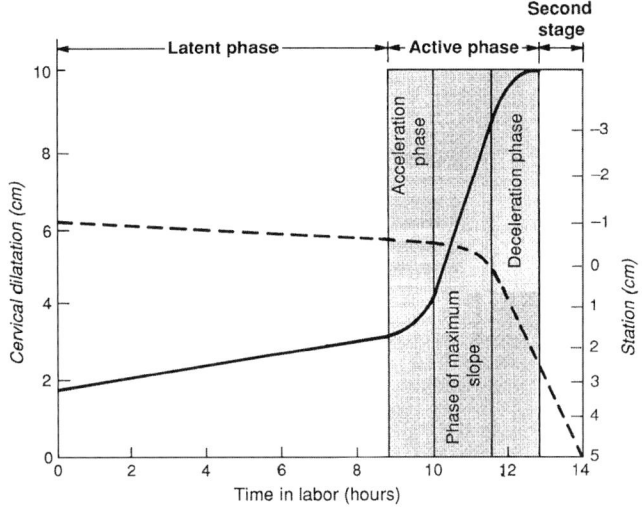

Figure 12–1. Stages of labor. (Reproduced, with permission, from Cohen W, Friedman EA (editors): *Management of Labor*. 2nd ed. University Park Press, 1988.)

Reassuring fetal heart tracing, normal rate between 120 and 160 beats per minute with adaquate variability and tolerance of the stress of the contractions.

▶ Disease Severity

Failure of acceptable progress.

▶ Concept and Application

Increased prostaglandins cause an increased number of myometrial gap junctions that allow cells to communicate and rhythmically depolarize in labor.

▶ Treatment Steps

*Initial Care*—Make diagnosis by serial examinations and initiate management.

*Continued Care*
1. When cephalopelvic disproportion is diagnosed, a cesarean section is used for delivery.
2. Hypotonic dysfunction is treated with oxytocin augmentation.

## II. COMPLICATED PREGNANCY

### A. Adolescent Pregnancy

▶ H&P Keys

Nineteen years old and younger, sexually transmitted disease surveillance, nutritional deficiency, substance abuse, sexual abuse.

▶ Diagnosis
Same for pregnancy; assist with social support network.

▶ Disease Severity
Disease-specific.

▶ Concept and Application
Seventeen percent have *Chlamydia trachomatis,* and 3% *Neisseria gonorrhoeae* per year; increased need for calcium (1,600 mg/day) and calories (2,700 cal/day); 89% of 10th graders have alcohol exposure, and 8% have cocaine, up to 38% have had nonvoluntary sexual activity.

▶ Management
Routine prenatal care with a special emphasis in support services and screening and intervention for problems.

## B. Ectopic Pregnancy

▶ H&P Keys
Early pregnancy symptoms and signs, amenorrhea, abnormal vaginal bleeding, and abdominal pain, colicky and lateralizing to the affected side. Shoulder pain, rectal pain, syncope, and peritoneal signs are associated with intraperitoneal bleeding. Passage of the decidual cast is confused with spontaneous abortion (SAB).

▶ Diagnosis
Quantitative β-subunit (BSU) of hCG rising less than 66% every 48 hours, serum progesterone less than 5 ng/mL, and inability to identify an intrauterine pregnancy by transabdominal ultrasonography when the β-hCG > 5,000 mIU/mL or by transvaginal ultrasonography if the β-hCG is > 2,000. Culdocentesis to identify hemoperitoneum if ultrasonography is not available. Blood type and Rh.

▶ Disease Severity
Transvaginal sonography and serial measurement of the β-hCG diagnose many unruptured ectopics.

▶ Concept and Application
Ectopic pregnancy is implantation outside of the uterine cavity; 78% are ampullary. Incidence of ectopic pregnancy has increased to 1 in 66 pregnancies. Risk factors include salpingitis, tubal surgery (including prior ectopic pregnancy), infertility treatments, and advanced age. RhIg if Rh negative.

▶ Treatment Steps

*Initial Care*
1. **Early diagnosis.**
2. Protocols are available for the nonsurgical management (methotrexate) of the small, unruptured ectopic pregnancy.
3. More commonly, conservative laparoscopic surgery, removing only the products of conception through a slit in the

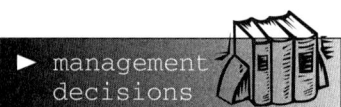

### TREATMENTS FOR ECTOPIC PREGNANCY

**Methotrexate**
Medical treatment for ectopic pregnancy, which meets specific criteria. The treatment is given intramuscularly and under strict supervision.

**Salpingectomy**
Surgical treatment where the fallopian tube is removed.

**Salpingostomy**
Removal of the ectopic pregnancy from the tube by making an incision in the antimesenteric side of the fallopian tube. After the tissue is removed, the incision in the tube is left open.

**Salpingotomy**
Removal of the ectopic pregnancy as above except the incision in the fallopian tube is then sutured closed.

tube (slit salpingostomy), or removal of a limited portion of the tube is performed—partial salpingectomy (segmental resection).

*Emergency Care*—Salpingectomy for hemoperitoneum with a large ruptured ectopic pregnancy.

## C. Spontaneous Abortion

▶ H&P Keys

Spontaneous fetus loss at or before 20 weeks from first day of last menstrual period or 500 g. Vaginal bleeding, rupture of membranes, cervical dilatation, passage of tissue.

▶ Diagnosis

β-hCG, transabdominal and transvaginal ultrasonography, progesterone, blood type, and Rh factor.

▶ Disease Severity

*Threatened Abortion*—Bleeding in the first 20 weeks of an intrauterine pregnancy. This occurs in 20–25% of women and approximately half of these go on to abort the pregnancy.

*Inevitable Abortion*—Cervix is dilated, or membranes are ruptured.

*Incomplete Abortion*—Some tissue is retained.

*Complete Abortion*—All tissue is passed.

*Missed Abortion*—Retention of nonviable pregnancy in the uterus for 4–8 weeks after the demise.

▶ Concept and Application

Fifty to 75% of conceptions end in spontaneous abortion. Most of these are unrecognized. Fifteen to 20% of recognized pregnancies are lost in the first and early second trimester. At least 50% of SABs are caused by genetic factors, including nondisjunction and translocation. Endocrine problems, principally luteal-phase deficiency, are present in 25%. Second-trimester losses are more often related to maternal diseases and uterine structural anomalies.

▶ Treatment Steps

*Initial Care*
1. Threatened abortion is usually managed by observation and prevention of the introduction of infection. There is no evidence to support that bed rest will prevent early spontaneous abortion.
2. Incomplete abortion is treated by uterine evacuation.
3. RhIg for the Rh-negative woman.

*Emergency Care*—Same as initial care.

*Continued Care*
1. Emotional support for the patient and family.
2. Prepregnancy evaluation if recurrent (three or more).

### D. Induced Abortion

▶ H&P Keys

Termination of an otherwise viable pregnancy for medical or personal reasons. A legal termination is consistent with statutory authority. An illegal or criminal one is not.

▶ Diagnosis

Same as initial pregnancy evaluation.

▶ Disease Severity

Advanced gestational age.

▶ Concept and Application

Compliance with the patient's wishes. Procedures are safest when performed in the first trimester. They can be done either surgically or medically using a combination of methotrexate followed by prostaglandins. In experienced hands, second-trimester surgical terminations are safer and less traumatic than medical terminations.

▶ Treatment Steps

*Initial*—Same as routine early pregnancy care, RhIg.

*Emergency Care*
1. Patients having a criminal abortion are at increased risk for serious complications including sepsis, abscess, and structural damage.
2. Intravenous hydration, broad-spectrum antibiotics, expeditious uterine evacuation, and evaluation for associated injury are indicated.

### E. Septic Abortion

▶ H&P Keys

Same as SAB, except for symptoms of infection, fever, foul-smelling discharge, and pain. Possible history of illegal abortion.

▶ Diagnosis

Same as SAB.

▶ Disease Severity

Same as SAB except for associated infection, septic shock, renal failure.

▶ Concept and Application

Same as SAB except for possibility of perforation and associated organ injury.

▶ Treatment Steps
1. Same as SAB, plus inspection of injury and administration of broad-spectrum antibiotics prior to or during procedure pending culture results.

## F. Placenta Previa

▶ H&P Keys

Frequent incidental ultrasonographic finding in early pregnancy. Patients present with painless vaginal bleeding in the third trimester. Most first bleedings are limited as long as digital examination does not occur.

▶ Diagnosis

Transabdominal and transvaginal ultrasonography is used in most cases (Fig. 12–2).

▶ Disease Severity

Degree of placenta previa present and the amount of bleeding.

▶ Concept and Application

Implantation of the placenta in the lower uterine segment covering the entire cervix (complete or central), partially covering the internal os (partial), or encroaching on the internal os (marginal). It is related to poor uterine vascularization (high multiparity, cesarean section) or large placental mass (multiple gestation or hydrops). Poor mechanical hemostasis causes heavy intra- and postpartum bleeding. Five percent of second trimester pregnancies are found to have a placenta previa, 90% of these resolve by term. A patient with a previous cesarean section and placenta previa has a 25% risk of placenta accreta.

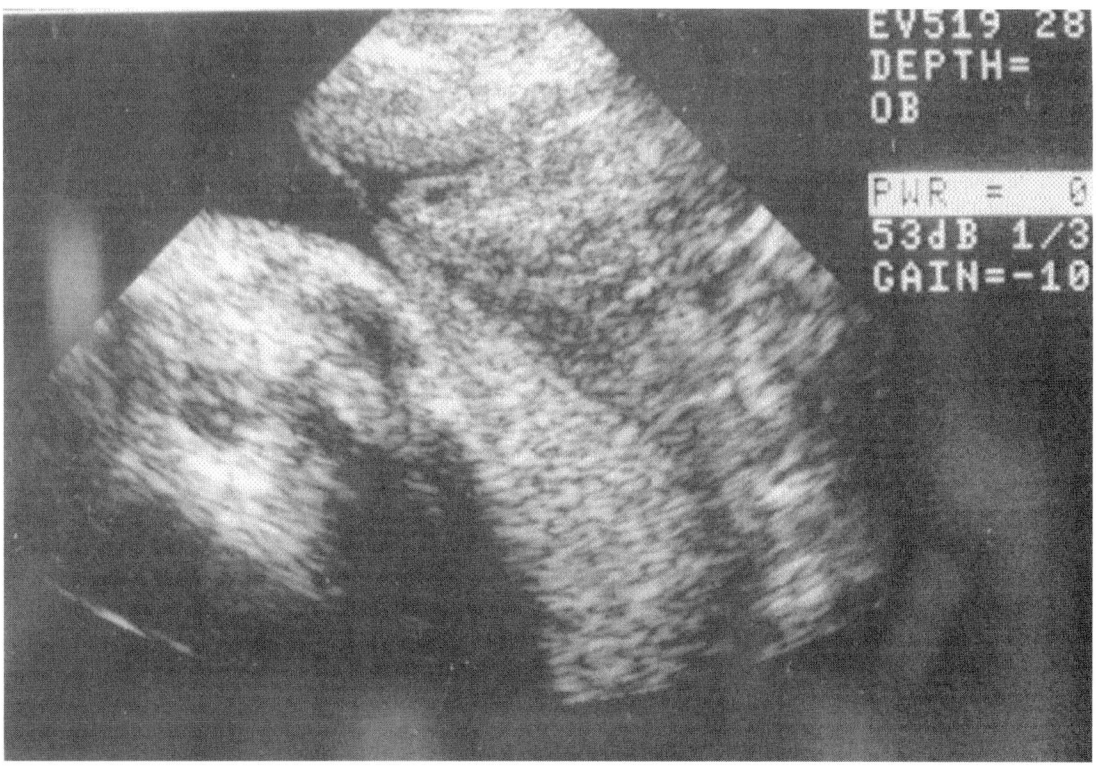

Figure 12–2. Placenta previa.

▶ Treatment Steps

*Initial Care*
1. Asymptomatic patient education, and coital restriction in the third trimester.
2. Serial ultrasonograms for fetal growth and placental location.

*Emergency Care*—A patient who has bleeding is hospitalized for hemodynamic stabilization and fetal assessment.

*Continued Care*
1. Delivery is usually by cesarean section after 36 weeks with documented fetal maturity or uncorrectable fetal compromise.
2. Patients with marginal placenta previa may attempt a vaginal delivery.

### G. Abruptio Placentae

▶ H&P Keys

Painful contractions, tender uterus, and vaginal bleeding. Fetal monitoring may suggest cause for alarm.

▶ Diagnosis

Clinical diagnosis, CBC, platelet count, fibrin split products, fibrinogen and prothrombin time (PT) and partial thromboplastin time (PTT) for disseminated intravascular coagulation (DIC). Ultrasonography is of limited value.

▶ Disease Severity

Shock out of proportion to the observed blood loss, especially if concealed hemorrhage. Fetal demise possible if > 50% abruption.

▶ Concept and Application

Bleeding into the decidua basalis. Couvelaire uterus is caused by blood extravasating into the myometrium (ecchymosis). Abruptio may be caused by hypertension, cocaine, smoking, uterine decompression, and trauma.

▶ Treatment Steps

*Initial and Emergency Care*
1. Hemodynamic stabilization, observation for complications, and delivery of the mature fetus.
2. Vaginal delivery is attempted if the patient is stable hemodynamically and the fetal monitoring is reassuring.
3. Immature fetus may be expectantly managed in mild abruptions.

### H. Preeclampsia

▶ H&P Keys

Hypertension (140/90 mm Hg) and proteinuria (< 300 mg/24 h) and edema after 20 weeks. Signs and symptoms of HELLP syndrome (**H**emolysis, **E**levated **L**iver functions, **L**ow **P**latelets).

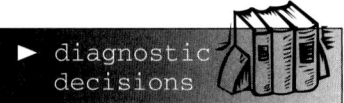

### THIRD TRIMESTER BLEEDING

**Placenta Previa**
Look for painless bleeding with the placenta located low in the uterus in the area of the cervix.

**Placental Abruption**
Look for bleeding associated with pain and contractions. Look carefully for fetal compromise.

**Bloody Show**
Painless bleeding often mixed with mucus. Bleeding is usually minimal and is often accompanied with early labor.

▶ Diagnosis

Careful blood pressure (BP) measurement, 24-hour urine for protein and creatinine clearance, CBC with platelets, and uric acid. Aspartate aminotransferase (AST, formerly SGOT), bilirubin, and lactate dehydrogenase (LDH) may be elevated. Fetal growth and well-being assessment.

▶ Disease Severity

Mild preeclampsia is without symptoms and signs of severe preeclampsia. Severe preeclampsia if BP > 160/110 mm Hg, > 5 g of proteinuria in 24 hours, visual disturbances, headache, pulmonary edema, cyanosis, epigastric pain, right upper quadrant pain, liver dysfunction, oliguria, thrombocytopenia, intrauterine growth restriction, or oligohydramnios.

▶ Concept and Application

Diffuse multiorgan vasospastic disease starting months before diagnosis, characterized by decreased sensitivity to angiotensin II and increased thromboxane: prostacyclin ratio. Delivery is the only specific therapy.

▶ Treatment Steps

*Initial Care*—Gestational age, fetal, and maternal assessment.

*Term*—Delivery.

*Preterm*
1. Weighing the risks and benefits of expectant management for the baby and the mother.
2. Bed rest is the mainstay of expectant care.

*Emergency Care*
1. Magnesium sulfate (4- to 6-g load and 2 g/hr) is used for seizure prophylaxis.
2. Monitoring blood pressure, respiration, reflexes, and urinary output.
3. Diastolic blood pressures over 110 mm Hg are treated with antihypertensive medications like hydralazine (5-mg boluses).

## I. Eclampsia

▶ H&P Keys

Preeclampsia with tonic–clonic seizures of no other etiology.

▶ Diagnosis

Same as preeclampsia.

▶ Disease Severity

Same as preeclampsia.

▶ Concept and Application

Same as preeclampsia.

▶ Treatment Steps

*Initial and Emergency Care*
1. Same as preeclampsia.
2. Treatment of seizures with magnesium sulfate.
3. Delivery when mother is stable.

### J. Premature Labor

▶ H&P Keys

Uterine contractions with cervical change prior to 37 weeks. Symptoms: cramps, backache, pressure, and uterine contractions.

▶ Diagnosis

Monitor for contractions, rule out rupture of membranes, check for cervical change, culture vagina for group B streptococcus, evaluate for urinary tract infection or other processes which might be causing the contractions, confirm dating if indicated.

▶ Disease Severity

No tocolysis if: rupture of membranes, advanced cervical dilatation (5+ cm), fetal distress, fetal anomalies, mature fetus, in utero infection, and conditions made worse by tocolysis.

▶ Concept and Application

Preterm labor associated with: premature rupture of membranes (PROM), incompetent cervix, infection, uterine overdistention, abnormal placentation, dehydration, and idiopathic causes. Prostaglandin activation is a common final pathway. β-Sympathomimetics (ritodrine and terbutaline), magnesium sulfate, prostaglandin synthetase inhibitors (indomethacin), and calcium channel blockers (nifedipine) have been used to treat preterm labor (PTL). All tocolytics can be associated with serious complications. Steroid treatment to help with fetal lung maturity is also recommended.

▶ Treatment Steps

*Emergency Care*
1. Monitoring, hydration, and evaluation of the patient; administration of tocolytic (SQ terbutaline 0.25 mg 3–6 doses every 20–30 min or incremental increases from IV 0.050 mg/min or IV $MgSO_4$ 6-g load and 2–3 g/hr) and monitoring for complications (pulmonary edema, etc).
2. Penicillin for group B streptococcus prophylaxis.
3. Betamethasone IM 12 mg every 12 hours for two doses to hasten pulmonary maturity and decrease hemorrhagic disorders and necrotizing enterocolitis.

*Continued Care*—Outpatient on oral β-sympathomimetics.

### K. Infections of the Genitourinary Tract

▶ H&P Keys

Infection in the urinary tract are the most common type of infection in the pregnant female. Asymptomatic bacteriuria [> 100,000 colony-forming units per milliliter (CFU)] progresses to cystitis about 25% of the time and to pyelonephritis in 1% to 3% of gravidas. Increased nocturia, urgency, frequency, dysuria are common symptoms. Pyelonephritis is associated with a significantly elevated temperature, flank pain, costovertebral angle (CVA) tenderness.

▶ Diagnosis

Urinalysis positive for leukocyte esterase, nitrate, white blood cells (WBCs), RBCs. 10,000 CFU/mL is significant in the symptomatic patient.

▶ Disease Severity

Pyelonephritis: evaluate for intrauterine infection, sepsis in 2% of patients, rarely associated with septic shock and adult respiratory distress syndrome (ARDS).

▶ Concept and Application

Urinary stasis (decreased tone, mechanical ureteral or bladder compression) and glucosuria facilitate bacterial (*Escherichia coli*) overgrowth; 8% have asymptomatic bacturia.

▶ Treatment Steps

*Initial Care*

*Lower Tract*—Antibiotic therapy by local sensitivities (usually 7–10 days of ampicillin or nitrofurantoin).

*Pyelonephritis*—IV, then oral therapy. Monitoring for preterm labor.

*Continued Care*—Reculturing monthly. If recurrent infection, prophylactic antibiotics.

## L. Hepatitis B Infection Complicating Pregnancy

▶ H&P Keys

Malaise, jaundice 15–50 days following exposure to infected blood or body secretions; high-risk groups (patients and partners) include IV drug users, multiple sexual partners, and health care workers.

▶ Diagnosis

Bilirubin, AST (SGOT), alaninine aminotransferase (ALT, formerly SGPT), hepatitis B surface antigen (HBsAg), antibody to hepatitis B core antigen (HBcAb), antibody to hepatitis Be antigen (HBeAb), and hepatitis Be antigen (HBeAg).

▶ Disease Severity

Fewer than 10% develop chronic infection. Hepatic failure, coma, and death. Vertical transmission is highest (80%) in HBeAg-positive.

▶ Concept and Application

Major cause of jaundice in pregnancy, 80% HBV; 10% HAV; and 10% HCV, HDV, and HEV. Well-nourished patients usually tolerate the disease.

▶ Treatment Steps

*Initial Care*
1. Uninfected at-risk pregnant patient may be vaccinated.
2. Supportive and serial liver function evaluation.

*Emergency Care*—Treatment of newborn with hepatitis B immune globulin and hepatitis B vaccine.

## M. Incompetent Cervix

▶ H&P Keys

Painless preterm (second trimester) effacement and dilatation of the cervix. Patient complains of several days of vaginal or pelvic pressure, watery-to-pink vaginal discharge, or backache prior to rupture of the membranes. There is no history consistent with uterine contractions. The process usually recurs in multiple pregnancies if there is no intervention. Although there is no specific known causes risk factors include trauma to the cervix including surgery and DES exposure.

▶ Diagnosis

Internal os dilated > 1 cm or painless passage of a #8 Hegar dilator. The appearance of cervical funneling on ultrasound. No documentation of uterine contractions. History of similar occurrences in previous pregnancies.

▶ Disease Severity

Associated with deep lacerations or conizations and cervical amputations.

▶ Concept and Application

Cervix is not able to maintain closure pressure against the expanding gestation.

▶ Treatment Steps

*Initial Care*—Prophylactic transvaginal cerclage at 12–16 weeks.

*Emergency Care*—An emergency cerclage may be placed after PTL is ruled out.

*Continued Care*—Physical and coital activities may be restricted.

## N. Central Nervous System Malformation in the Fetus and Neural Tube Defect

▶ H&P Keys

Ninety percent of NTDs occur in pregnancies in which there is no identifiable increased risk and are due to multifactorial inheritance. There is a 10-fold increased risk in a subsequent pregnancy. Preconceptional poor glycemic control increases risk in diabetics. Presents in the United States as an incidental ultrasonographic finding and during the evaluation of an elevated MS-AFP.

▶ Diagnosis

Elevated MS-AFP, amniotic fluid (AF)-AFP, elevated AF acetylcholinesterase. Directed scan (Fig. 12–3).

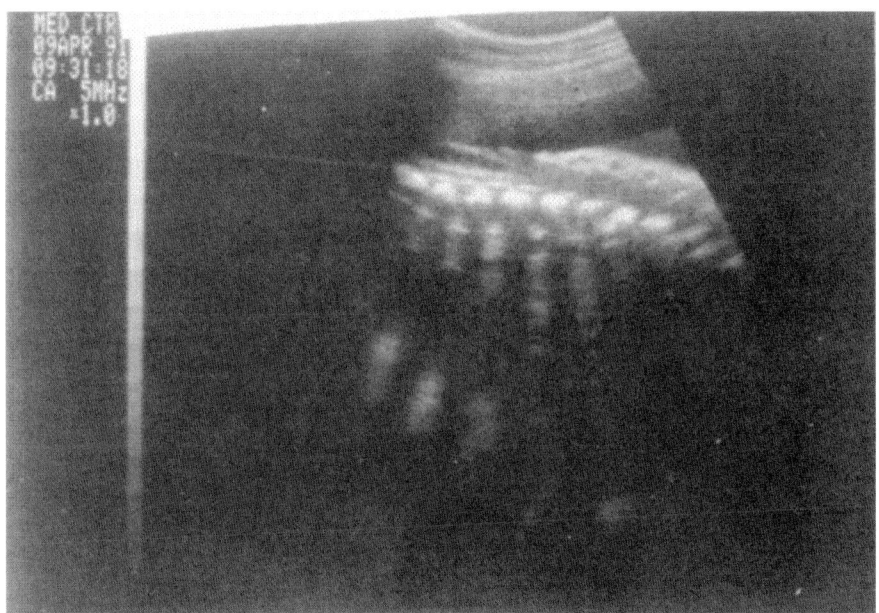

A

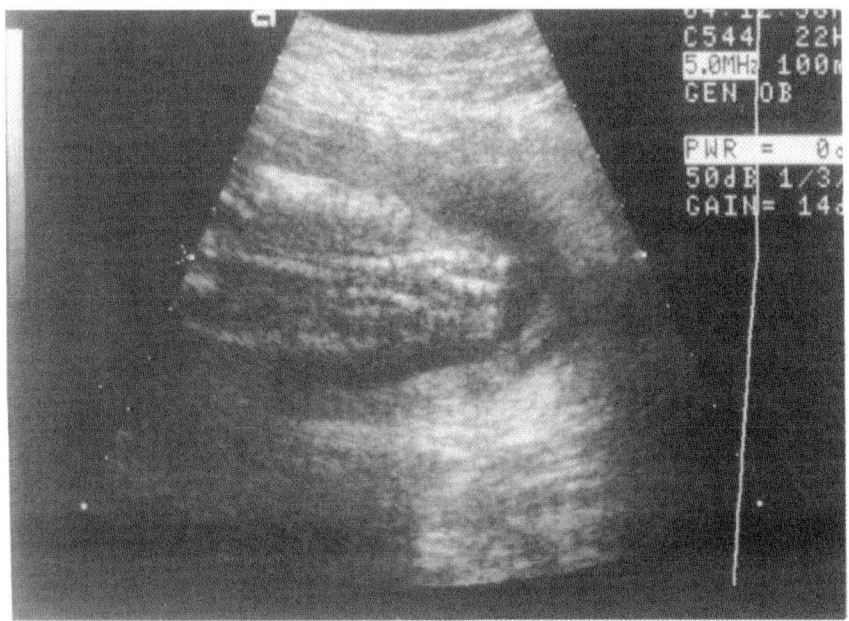

B

Figure 12–3. CNS malformation.

▶ Disease Severity

Anencephaly (failure of development of the forebrain) occurs in 50% of neural tube defects (NTDs). Spina bifida may occur at any level.

▶ Concept and Application

Failure of closure of at least a portion of the neural tube prior to the 28th day postconception. Prepregnancy folic acid decreases the risk.

▶ Treatment Steps

*Initial Care*—Diagnosis, nondirective genetic counseling and option counseling.

*Emergency Care*—Delivery by cesarean section is recommended for fetuses with isolated neural tube defects.

*Continued Care*—If pregnancy is maintained, monitoring for hydrocephalus.

## O. Trisomy

▶ H&P Keys

Advanced maternal age, previous history, balanced translocation, low MS-AFP. Trisomy 21 is most common accounting for 1 in 800 live births.

▶ Diagnosis

Fetal sampling via CVS, amniocentesis, or percutaneous umbilical blood sample (PUBS) is definitive.

▶ Disease Severity

Babies with a mosaicism may not fully express the typical phenotype.

▶ Concept and Application

Aneuploidy results from nondisjunction in the first meiotic division or from an unbalanced translocation. Trisomy 21 is most common, followed by trisomy 18 and trisomy 13.

▶ Treatment Steps

*Initial Care*—Nondirective counseling, support of the patient's decision within the legal and ethical framework.

## P. Rh Incompatibility or Isoimmunization

▶ H&P Keys

Inadequate or no RhIg after Rh-positive RBC exposure in Rh-negative woman; Kell-negative recipient of Kell-positive transfusion.

▶ Diagnosis

Serial maternal antibody titering; amniocentesis or PUBS once greater than the critical titer.

▶ Disease Severity

Delta OD450 (a measure of bilirubin in amniotic fluid) in zone III is associated with imminent fetal death from erythroblastosis fetalis. PUBS is used for both diagnosis (hemoglobin and hematocrit and antigen determination) and treatment (transfusion).

▶ Concept and Application

Maternal hemolytic IgG antibody formation to fetal red cell antigens (Rh, Kell, Duffy, Kidd, etc), extramedullary hematopoiesis in the fetal liver, decreased oncotic protein production and edema, anasarca (erythroblastosis fetalis). Rh-negative woman has a 15% risk of sensitization in the first exposed Rh-positive, ABO-compatible pregnancy if not treated with Rhogam.

▶ Treatment Steps

*Initial Care*
1. Serial measurement of the indirect Coombs' and antibody titering.
2. Amniocentesis or PUBS (diagnostic and therapeutic) is performed once critical titer is reached.

*Emergency Care*—PUBS or delivery.

*Continued Care*—Serial studies and therapy are determined by previous results.

## Q. Multiple Gestation

▶ H&P Keys

High index of suspicion when size greater than dates, multiple heart beats positive family history, ovulation induction; 1 of 80 black women, 1 of 100 white women.

▶ Diagnosis

Ultrasonogram, elevated MS-AFP. See Figure 12–4.

▶ Disease Severity

Serial ultrasonographic evaluation for growth and polyhydramnios.

▶ Concept and Application

Seventy percent of twins are dizygotic where two eggs are fertilized by two sperm. This type of twinning is affected by race, heredity, age and parity as well as infertility treatments.

Thirty percent are monozygotic—one egg fertilized by one sperm; 70% of monozygotic are monochorionic diamniotic (division days 3–8).

Risks: 15% perinatal mortality, preterm labor, discordant growth or intrauterine growth retardation, malformations, preeclampsia, anemia, abruption, polyhydramnios, malpresentation.

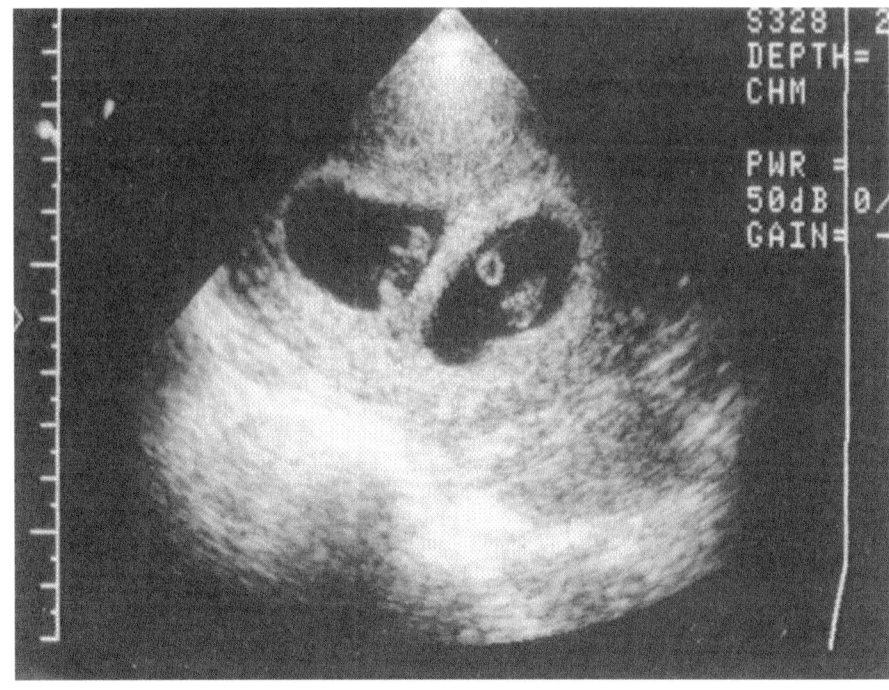

Figure 12-4. Multiple gestation.

▶ Treatment Steps

*Initial Care*—Increased calories and iron, preterm labor education, a management program of maternal and fetal surveillance.

*Emergency Care*—Treatment of specific complications.

*Continued Care*—Following through on the management plan.

### R. Gestational Trophoblastic Disease

▶ H&P Keys

Size–date discrepancy (usually greater size than norm); hyperemesis gravidarum; preeclampsia before 20 weeks; hyperthyroidism, and bleeding especially in the first trimester.

▶ Diagnosis

β-hCG, ultrasonography, and histology.

▶ Disease Severity

Malignant gestational trophoblastic disease (GTD) with a poor prognosis has pretreatment β-hCG > 40, 000 mIU/mL, more than 4 months' duration, brain or liver metastases, failed chemotherapy, or antecedent term pregnancy. Complete moles increase risk of serious complications.

▶ Concept and Application

Incidence is 1 in 1,000 pregnancies. Complete moles are paternal in origin (46,XX > 46,XY) and are histologically distinct (absence of fetus and blood vessels, diffuse villous edema, and variable trophoblastic proliferation). Partial moles may coexist with a normal pregnancy and are 69,XXX or XXY.

▶ Treatment Steps

*Initial Care*
1. After diagnosis, chest roentgenogram and labs.
2. Suction curettage.

*Continued Care*
1. Serial β-hCG every 1–2 weeks until normal, then every month for the remainder of a year.
2. Serial pelvic exams.
3. Contraception.

## S. Maternal Mortality

▶ H&P Keys

Maternal mortality is defined as the death of a woman from any pregnancy related problem during pregnancy or within 42 days of termination of pregnancy.

▶ Diagnosis

Self-evident.

▶ Disease Severity

Self-evident.

▶ Concept and Application

Causes: embolism (24%), hypertensive disease (20%), hemorrhage (16%), and infection (10%) are the most common. Rates have been declining since the mid-1970s.

▶ Management

Initial care: prevention.

## T. Depression

▶ H&P Keys

Mean age 40 years; disturbance of mood, intense anguish, and loss of a sense of control; predisposing factors include: victim of abuse, childhood loss of a parent, genetic predisposition, deprivation, and lifestyle stress.

▶ Diagnosis

High index of suspicion: a high score on the Beck Depression Inventory.

▶ Disease Severity

Suicide threats and attempts.

▶ Concept and Application

Most common psychiatric disorder in women.

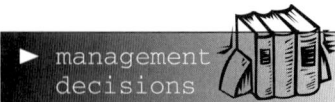

### management decisions

**EVALUATION OF RUPTURE OF MEMBRANES**

**Pooling**
Speculum exam reveals large amount of fluid in the vagina. False-positive results can come from recent intercourse.

**Nitrazine**
Amniotic fluid turns nitrazine paper blue. False-positive results can result from urine, semen, cervical mucus, blood contamination, antiseptic solution, or vaginitis. False-negative results can be from minimal leakage or exam remote from the time of rupture of membranes.

**Ferning**
The deposition of salt crystals on a glass slide when the amniotic fluid dries. False-positive can result from cervical mucus. False-negative can result from contamination with blood or urine or antiseptic solution or very early gestational age.

▶ Treatment Steps

*Initial Care*
1. Mild to moderate depression is treated with psychotherapy.
2. Severe, chronic, recurrent depression is treated with antidepressants and psychotherapy.

*Emergency*—Hospitalization and psychotherapy for suicidal ideation.

## U. Preterm Premature Rupture of Membranes

▶ H&P Keys

Leakage of amniotic fluid (AF) from vagina prior to term.

▶ Diagnosis

Demonstration of ferning and nitrazinepositive fluid. Culture the cervix for gonorrhea, group B Streptococcus, and *Chlamydia trachomatis*. Quantitative AF volume. Vaginal pool specimen for maturity studies.

▶ Disease Severity

Chorioamnionitis or fetal distress.

▶ Concept and Application

Rupture allows bacteria access to the fetus. If < 24 weeks, risks of pulmonary hypoplasia, contractures, and limb anomalies increase.

▶ Treatment Steps

*Initial Care*—Observation for symptoms and signs of infection (uterine tenderness or irritability, fever, maternal or fetal tachycardia, leukocytosis, purulent fluid) labor and fetal well being.

*Emergency Care*—Delivery if mature lungs or fetal or maternal indications.

*Continued Care*—Initial care plus periodic fetal assessment.

## V. Hyperemesis Gravidarum

▶ H&P Keys

Intractable nausea and vomiting associated with significant weight loss, dehydration, electrolyte imbalance, or ketonemia. This occurs predominately prior to 16 weeks of gestation.

▶ Diagnosis

Rule out other causes: gastroesophageal reflux, pancreatitis, hepatobiliary disease, and other gastrointestinal disorders.

▶ Disease Severity

Protracted negative protein balance and ketonemia adversely affect fetal growth.

▶ Concept and Application

Etiology unknown.

▶ Treatment Steps

Frequent small, bland meals with liquids at separate intervals, antiemetics.

*Emergency Care*
1. Intravenous hydration.
2. Hyperalimentation is used rarely.

## W. Abnormalities of Labor, Dystocia

▶ H&P Keys

Patient in labor with abnormal progress based on graphic analysis (see Table 12–1).

▶ Diagnosis

Graphic analysis of labor, assessment of pelvis and fetal attitude, position, and presentation.

▶ Disease Severity

Prolonged latent phase: no progress from latent to active phase (nulligravidas > 20 hours, multiparas > 40 hours. Protracted active phase dilatation: nulligravidas 1.2 cm/hr, multiparas 1.5 cm/hr. Arrest of dilatation: no change in 2 hours. Arrest of descent: no descent in 1 hour.

▶ Concept and Application

Reason for over one quarter of all cesarean sections. Uterine contractions may be ineffective when associated with mechanical factors.

### 12-1 ABNORMAL LABOR PATTERNS, DIAGNOSTIC CRITERIA, AND METHODS OF TREATMENT

| Labor Pattern | Diagnostic Criterion | | Preferred Treatment | Exceptional Treatment |
| --- | --- | --- | --- | --- |
| | Nulliparas | Multiparas | | |
| **Prolongation disorder** | | | | |
| Prolonged latent phase | > 20 h | > 14 h | Therapeutic rest | Oxytocin or cesarean deliveries for urgent problems |
| | | | Expectant and supportive | Cesarean delivery for CPD[2] |
| **Protraction disorders** | | | | |
| Protracted active phase dilatation | < 1.2 cm/h | < 1.5 cm/h | | |
| Protracted descent | < 1.0 cm/h | < 2 cm/h | | |
| **Arrest disorders** | | | | |
| Prolonged deceleration rate | > 3 h | > 1 h | Without CPD: oxytocin | Rest if exhausted |
| Secondary arrest of dilatation | > 2 h | > 2 h | With CPD: cesarean delivery | Cesarean delivery |
| Arrest of descent | > 1 h | > 1 h | | |
| Failure of descent | No descent in deceleration phase or second stage of labor | | | |

*Source:* Cohen W, Friedman EA (editors): *Management of Labor.* University Park Press, 1983.

▶ Treatment Steps

*Initial and Continuing Care*
1. Prolonged latent phase, therapeutic rest or augmentation.
2. Protracted dilatation, augmentation if no disproportion.
3. Arrest of dilatation, same.
4. Arrest of descent, same or obstetric forceps if indicated.
5. Labor is augmented by IV pitocin. The pitocin is titrated to achieve three contractions in 10 minutes of adequate intensity.

## X. Postpartum Hemorrhage

▶ H&P Keys

*Uterine Atony*—Predisposing factors: prolonged labor, precipitous labor, infection, uterine overdistention, multiparity, fibroids, oxytocin augmentation, and magnesium sulfate.

*Genital Tract Laceration*—Predisposing factors: instrumented vaginal delivery, precipitous delivery, macrosomic infant, previous genital tract laceration, and in utero manipulation.

*Retained Placental Fragments*—From incomplete removal of normal placenta, retained accessory lobe, or partial placenta accreta.

▶ Diagnosis

Vital signs, CBC, blood product availability, and search for the source of the bleeding.

▶ Disease Severity

Normal blood loss: singleton, vaginal, 500 mL; twin, vaginal, 1,000 mL; cesarean section, 1,000 mL. Normal parturient can lose 900 mL without any symptoms; 1,500 mL is associated with tachycardia, narrowed pulse pressure, positive blanch test; 2,000 mL is associated with hypotension; 2,400 mL is associated with profound hypotension and vasoconstriction.

▶ Concept and Application

Uterine blood flow is 500–600 mL/min. Interference with the normal mechanisms of hemostasis may result in significant blood loss.

▶ Treatment Steps

*Emergency Care*
1. Uterine massage, oxytocin, methylergonine maleate (Methergine) or 15-methylprostaglandin $f_2\alpha$.
2. Transfusion if hemodynamically unstable.
3. Determination of etiology of the hemorrhage; definitive treatment.
4. Hysterectomy is last resort.

## Y. Postpartum Sepsis

▶ H&P Keys

Predisposing factors: cesarean section, prolonged rupture of membranes, chorioamnionitis, prolonged labor, multiple pelvic exams, internal monitors, obesity, and anemia. Febrile morbidity: temperature of > 100.4°F on two occasions at least 6 hours apart 24 hours postpartum.

▶ Diagnosis

Endomyometritis presents with uterine tenderness and fever; cultures are not reliable. Wound infection presents with fever, pain, tenderness, erythema, and swelling; wound cultures are helpful. Pyelonephritis, pneumonia, and atelectasis should be ruled out.

▶ Disease Severity

Evaluate for septic pelvic thrombophlebitis, which presents as persistent fever and tachycardia after presumed effective antibiotic treatment; responds to the addition of heparin.

▶ Concept and Application

Uncontrolled sepsis results in physiologic instability, organ failure, and death.

▶ Treatment Steps

*Initial Care*—Endomyometritis: broad-spectrum antibiotics until afebrile for 24–48 hours and patient is asymptomatic.

*Wound Infection*
1. Probe for fascial integrity.
2. Drainage, wound care, and broad-spectrum antibiotics until resolved.

*Emergency Care*—Same.

## Z. Obstetric Forceps and Vacuum Extractor

▶ H&P Keys

Adequate anesthesia, empty bladder (if not outlet), full cervical dilatation, known fetal attitude, position, and station.

▶ Diagnosis

Clinical assessment of fetal size and pelvis.

▶ Disease Severity

Mid: Station engaged but > +2. Low: Station is at least at +2 but not on the pelvic floor, and rotations of > 45 degrees. Outlet: Fetal head is at or on the perineum and the rotation is < 45 degrees.

▶ Concept and Application

Shortening of the second stage for a variety of fetal and maternal reasons.

▶ Treatment Steps

After prerequisites are met, apply instruments, check application, and apply traction with contractions. Inspect genital tract for injury after delivery. If unsuccessful proceed to cesarean section.

### 12-2 PRISCILLA WHITE CLASSIFICATION

| Class | Age at Onset | | Duration | Vascular Disease | Therapy |
|---|---|---|---|---|---|
| A | Any | | Any | None | Diet |
| B | Over 20 | OR | Under 10 | None | Insulin |
| C | 10–19 | OR | 10–19 | None | Insulin |
| D | Before 10 | OR | Over 20 | Benign Retinopathy | Insulin |
| F | Any | | Any | Nephropathy | Insulin |
| R | Any | | Any Retinopathy | Proliferative | Insulin |
| H | Any | | Any | Heart disease | Insulin |

## AA. Diabetes, Gestational

▶ **H&P Keys**

Universal screening or screen if risk factors are present (prior history, obesity, macrosomia, hydramnios, family history, excessive weight gain).

▶ **Diagnosis**

If 50-g glucola screen > 140 mg/dL, then proceed to 3-hour oral glucose tolerance test (GTT); abnormal if any 2 values exceed fasting blood sugar (FBS) > 105, > 190 at 1 hour, > 165 at 2 hours, or > 145 at 3 hours.

▶ **Disease Severity**

Start on diet of 30–35 kcal/kg of ideal body weight (IBW). If FBS is > 105 or 2-hour postprandial levels are > 120, evaluate for insulin. Fifteen percent of patients progress to insulin. Monitor for preeclampsia, bacterial infection, macrosomia, and hydramnios. See Table 12–2.

▶ **Concept and Application**

Pregnancy is diabetogenic. Prevalence 2%. Human placental lactogen (hPL) induces peripheral insulin resistance.

▶ **Treatment Steps**

*Initial*—Initiate diet, monitor BS, culture urine monthly, fetal well-being.

*Continued Care*
1. As in initial management, normalize blood sugar in labor.
2. Test for diabetes at 6 weeks postpartum.

## BB. Diabetes, Overt

▶ Diagnosis

Hemoglobin A1c, home glucose monitoring, ultrasound, 24-hour urine for protein and creatinine clearance, blood pressure, MS-AFP.

▶ Disease Severity

Elevated hemoglobin A1c increases risk of congenital anomalies (neural tube defect [NTD] and heart), maternal and fetal risks increase with duration of disease, presence of small-vessel disease (retinopathy, nephropathy, and intrauterine growth retardation [IUGR]). Increased incidence of preeclampsia.

▶ Concept and Application

Impaired insulin secretion and insulin resistance. Prone to ketoacidosis at lower blood sugar levels.

▶ Treatment Steps

1. Education, diet, exercise, normalization of blood sugar (FBS between 70 and 105, 2-hour postprandial < 120).
2. Monitor for complications.
3. Tight control of blood sugar in labor.

## CC. Asthma

▶ H&P Keys

Acute dyspnea, wheezing, cough. One third become better, one-third stay the same, one-third experience a worsening of the condition in pregnancy. Patients usually tolerate labor well.

▶ Diagnosis

Peak flow monitoring.

▶ Disease Severity

Accessory muscle usage, respiratory rate, pulse oximetry, arterial blood gases (ABGs).

▶ Concept and Application

Bronchospasm in response to allergens, antigens or irritants, infection.

▶ Treatment Steps

*Acute*
1. β-Agonist inhalers, parenteral glucocorticoids.
2. Evaluation of fetal well-being.

*Continued Care*
1. β-Agonist, inhaled glucocorticoids, cromolyn.
2. Peak flow monitoring.

▶ on rounds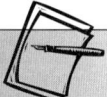

### PROBLEMS IN OBSTETRICS

#### Preeclampsia
- Hypertension and proteinuria or edema after 20 weeks.
- Diagnosis by blood pressure measurement, 24-hour urine for protein.
- Treatment includes bed rest (if preterm) and delivery (if term). Magnesium sulfate to prevent seizures.

#### Eclampsia
- Preeclampsia with tonic-clonic seizures.
- Diagnosis as in preeclampsia.
- Treatment includes stabilization of the mother and then delivery of the fetus.

#### Abruptio Placenta
- Vaginal bleeding, tender uterus, shock.
- Clinical diagnosis, ultrasound no help.
- Treatment includes hemodynamic stabilization and delivery (with mature fetus).

#### Placenta Previa
- Painless third-trimester vaginal bleeding, often at night.
- Diagnosis by ultrasound.
- Treatment for asymptomatic cases:
  Education
  Hematinics
  Serial ultrasounds
  Coital restriction in third trimester
- Urgent cases: hemodynamic stabilization.

## BIBLIOGRAPHY

Cunningham FG. *Williams Obstetrics.* 21st ed. Stamford, CT: Appleton & Lange; 2001.

DeChemey AH, Pernoll ML, eds. *Current Obstetric and Gynecologic Diagnosis and Treatment.* 9th ed. Norwalk, CT: Appleton & Lange; 2002.

Gabbe SG. *Obstetrics: Normal and Problem Pregnancies.* 4th ed. New York: Churchill Livingstone; 2002.

Martin DH. Sexually transmitted diseases. *The Med Clin North Am.* Philadelphia: WB Saunders Co; 1990.

Niswander KR. *Manual of Obstetrics, Diagnosis and Therapy.* 5th ed. Boston: Little, Brown & Co; 1996.

Sweet RL. *Infectious Disease of the Female Genital Tract.* 4th ed. Baltimore: Williams & Wilkins; 2002.

# Ophthalmology 13

I. CONJUNCTIVITIS / 393

II. DISORDERS OF THE EYELIDS / 396
    A. Blepharitis / 396
    B. Stye / 397
    C. Chalazion / 397
    D. Entropion / 398
    E. Ectropion / 398
    F. Epicanthus / 398
    G. Blepharoptosis / 399

III. DISORDERS OF THE LACRIMAL SYSTEM / 400
    A. Undersecretion / 400
    B. Acute Dacryocystitis / 400

IV. DISORDERS OF THE OPTIC NERVE / 401
    A. Elevation of the Disc / 401
    B. Pallor of the Disc, Optic Atrophy / 404

V. DISORDERS OF THE VISUAL PATHWAYS / 404
    A. Monocular Defects (Central Scotomas) / 404
    B. Bitemporal Defects / 405
    C. Homonymous Defects / 406

VI. AMBLYOPIA / 406

VII. STRABISMUS / 407

VIII. DIABETES WITH OPHTHALMOLOGIC MANIFESTATIONS / 409

IX. DISORDERS OF THE CORNEA / 410
    A. Corneal Ulcers / 410
    B. Herpes Simplex Keratitis / 411

C. Ophthalmic Herpes Zoster / 412
   D. Dry Eye (Keratoconjunctivitis Sicca) / 413
   E. Interstitial Keratitis / 413

X. **DISORDERS OF THE LENS / 414**
   A. Glaucoma / 414
   B. Cataract / 417

**BIBLIOGRAPHY / 418**

## I. CONJUNCTIVITIS

Hyperemia of conjunctival blood vessels. Types: allergic, bacterial, viral; common, often not serious.

### ▶ H&P Keys

Red eye, usually without blurred vision, pain, or colored halos. Exudation is more severe in bacterial, moderate in viral, and least in allergic (watery). Itching is pronounced in allergic. Ciliary flush is absent. Conjunctival injection is prominent in bacterial, moderate in viral, and least in allergic. Corneal disturbance may be present in viral, absent in bacterial and allergic. Pupil, anterior chamber depth, and intraocular pressure are normal. Preauricular lymph node may be present in viral but absent in bacterial and allergic (Tables 13–1, 13–2).

### ▶ Diagnosis

Correct diagnosis for cause of red eye determines effectiveness of treatment and reduces complications. Aside from conjunctivitis, other causes of red eye must be ruled out. Differentiate from acute glaucoma, acute iridocyclitis, and keratitis corneal lesions (Tables 13–3, 13–4, 13–5).

Most cases are managed without laboratory studies. Smear of exudates. Conjunctival scrapings for culture and sensitivities studies.
1. Allergic conjunctivitis: eosinophils.
2. Bacterial conjunctivitis: polymorphonuclear cells and bacteria.
3. Viral conjunctivitis: lymphocytes.

### ▶ Disease Severity

Assess vision, pupils, amount of pain, and sensitivity to light. Rule out red eye caused by acute glaucoma, corneal lesions, or iridocyclitis.

*Allergic Conjunctivitis*—Itching, watery discharge, chemosis, history of allergies, edematous lids, and no preauricular nodes.

*Bacterial Conjunctivitis*—Severe purulent discharge; may have subconjunctival hemorrhage. Red eye subconjunctival hemorrhage. Gram stain for causative bacteria.

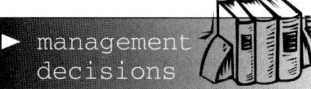

### ▶ management decisions

#### RED, INFLAMED EYE

**Acute Conjunctivitis**
Extremely common, minimal change in vision, minimal discomfort, diffuse conjunctival injection/hyperemia, tearing (purulent—bacterial, watery—viral), itchy—allergic.

**Corneal Ulcer**
Pain, photophobia, decreased vision, watery tearing, ciliary injection, contact lens use (especially soft lenses worn while sleeping).

**Acute Iridocyclitis**
Pain, photophobia, decreased vision, watery discharge, small pupil sometimes, ciliary injection, history of recent trauma (blunt or corneal abrasion) or autoimmune diseases.

**Acute Angle-closure Glaucoma**
Severe pain, nausea/vomiting, elderly, markedly decreased vision (Halo around light), mid-size dilated nonreacting pupil, diffuse conjunctival hyperemia, cloudy/opaque cornea.

### 13-1 SYMPTOMS OF CONJUNCTIVITIS

| Symptoms | Bacterial | Viral | Allergic |
|---|---|---|---|
| Exudation | +++ | ++ | + |
| Itching | 0 | 0 | ++ |
| Blurred vision | 0 | 0 | 0 |
| Colored halos | 0 | 0 | 0 |
| Pain | 0 | 0 | 0 |
| Photophobia | 0 | 0 | 0 |

+++, severe; ++, moderate; +, present; 0, absent.

## 13-2 SIGNS OF CONJUNCTIVITIS

| Signs | Bacterial | Viral | Allergic |
| --- | --- | --- | --- |
| Conjunctival injection | +++ | ++ | + |
| Discharge | +++ | ++ | + |
| Preauricular lymph node | 0 | + | 0 |
| Corneal opacification | 0 | 0/+ | 0 |
| Corneal epithelial disruption | 0 | 0/+ | 0 |
| Ciliary flush | 0 | 0 | 0 |
| Pupil | N | N | N |
| Anterior chamber depth | N | N | N |
| Intraocular pressure | N | N | N |

N, normal; +, present; 0, absent.

*Viral Conjunctivitis*—History of recent upper respiratory tract infection or contact with someone 7–10 days prior with a red eye. Usually gets worse the first few days after onset and may last for 2–3 weeks. Watery or mucous discharge, red and edematous eyelids. Eyelid sticking, worse in the morning. May have subconjunctival hemorrhages and corneal irritations. Palpable preauricular lymph nodes suggests viral cause.

▶ Concept and Application

Viral conjunctivitis associates with systemic problems, upper respiratory infection and fever, pharyngoconjunctival fever, adenovirus type 3 or type 7. Allergic conjunctivitis associates with seasonal rhinitis of hay fever, erythema multiforme, serious systemic disorders with ocular involvement, Stevens–Johnson syndrome, allergic reaction to medication (Table 13–5).

▶ Treatment Steps
(See Table 13–6.)

*Allergic Conjunctivitis*
1. Detection and removal of source of irritants.
2. Cold compress for comfort during waking hours.

## 13-3 SYMPTOMS OF RED EYE

| Symptoms | Acute Conjunctivitis | Acute Iritis | Acute Glaucoma | Corneal Lesions |
| --- | --- | --- | --- | --- |
| Exudation | +/+++ | 0 | 0 | 0/+++ |
| Itching | 0/++ | 0 | 0 | 0 |
| Blurred vision | 0 | +/++ | +++ | +++ |
| Colored halos | 0 | 0 | ++ | 0 |
| Pain | 0 | ++ | ++/+++ | ++ |
| Photophobia | 0 | +++ | + | +++ |

+++, severe; ++, moderate; +, present; 0, absent.

### 13-4 SIGNS OF RED EYE

| Signs | Acute Conjunctivitis | Acute Iritis | Acute Glaucoma | Corneal Lesions |
|---|---|---|---|---|
| Conjunctival injection | +/+++ | ++ | ++ | ++ |
| Discharge | +/+++ | 0 | 0 | 0/+ |
| Preauricular lymph node | 0/+ | 0 | 0 | 0 |
| Corneal opacification | 0/+ | 0 | +++ | 0/+++ |
| Corneal epithelial disruption | 0/+ | 0 | 0 | +/+++ |
| Ciliary flush | 0 | ++ | + | +++ |
| Pupil | N | Mid-dilated irregular | Small/irregular | N/small |
| Anterior chamber depth | N | N | Shallow | N |
| Intraocular pressure | N | Low | High | N |

+, present; ++, moderate; +++, severe; N, normal; 0, absent.

3. Vasoconstrictor/antihistamine or mild topical steroids to the affected eyes. Improvement should be noted immediately or within 2–3 days.
4. Persistent irritation requires consultation and further investigation.

*Bacterial Conjunctivitis*

1. Appropriate topical antibiotic drops during the waking hours of the day and ointment at night.
2. Washing away exudates and warm soaks of eyes for comfort.
3. Avoidance of topical steroids.

*Viral Conjunctivitis*

1. Usually subsides after its natural course. It is very contagious about 5 days after onset. Patients with red and weeping eyes should avoid spreading to other people.
2. Isolation from group gatherings.
3. Artificial tears and cold compresses as often as needed for comfort.
4. Frequent hand washing.

### 13-5 ASSOCIATED SYSTEMIC DISEASES IN CONJUNCTIVITIS

| Systemic Diseases | Bacterial Conjunctivitis | Viral Conjunctivitis | Allergic Conjunctivitis |
|---|---|---|---|
| Pharyngoconjunctival fever (adenovirus type 3, type 7) | 0 | + | 0 |
| Seasonal rhinitis of hay fever | 0 | 0 | + |
| Erythema multiforme (Stevens–Johnson syndrome) | 0 | 0 | + |

+, present; 0, absent.

## 13-6 MANAGEMENT OF CONJUNCTIVITIS

| | Bacterial Conjunctivitis | Viral Conjunctivitis | Allergic Conjuctivitis |
|---|---|---|---|
| Topical antibiotics | Sulfa, tobramycin polymixin B, erythromycin | 0 | 0 |
| Topical mastcell stabilizers, NSAIDs | 0 | 0 | +++ |
| Antihistamines (oral) | 0 | 0 | ± |
| Isolation precaution | 0 | ++ | 0 |
| Remove irritants | + | ++ | +++ |

+, of some benefit; ++, moderate benefit; +++, treatment of choice; ±, may or may not help; 0, no benefit.

## II. DISORDERS OF THE EYELIDS

### A. Blepharitis

Chronic bilateral inflammation of the lid margins.

▶ H&P Keys

Itching, irritation, burning of lid margins, red rims, scales of lashes, ulcerated areas along lid margins.

▶ Diagnosis

Lid margin ulceration or no ulceration, scales oily or dry.

▶ Disease Severity

Check scalp, brows, ears for seborrhea. Smear and stain of scraping from lid margins. Stain cornea. Evaluate for ulceration.

▶ Concept and Application

*Seborrheic Blepharitis*—Associated with seborrhea of scalp, brows, ears. Nonulcerative lid margin, scales oily, *Pityrosporum ovale* present.

*Staphylococcal Blepharitis*—*Staphylococcus aureus* or *Staphylococcus epidermidis*, coagulase-negative, ulcerative lid margin, hordeola, chalazia, epithelial keratitis lower one third of cornea, marginal infiltrates, recurrent conjunctivitis.

▶ Treatment Steps

*Seborrheic Blepharitis*—Soap-and-water shampoo of scalp. Removal of scales from lid margins with baby shampoo.

*Staphylococcal Blepharitis*
1. Daily antibiotic ointment against staphylococcus.
2. Long-term low-dose systemic antibiotic therapy.

## B. Stye

External hordeolum (glands of Zeis or Moll, hair follicles).

### ▶ H&P Keys
Recent onset; localized red, swollen tender area of the lid, frequently preceded by diffuse edema of the lid.

### ▶ Diagnosis
Red, swollen gland with pore opening can be seen at the lid margin. Tender area can be identified with a cotton tip.

### ▶ Disease Severity
Pain is related to the amount of swelling. Pus tends to point to the skin surface of the lid margin.

### ▶ Concept and Application
Common staphylococcal infection of Zeis's or Moll's glands of the lids. A small abscess sometimes is formed.

### ▶ Treatment Steps
1. Warm compresses over affected lids 10 minutes three times a day after application of antibiotic ointment.
2. Incision and drainage of pus when needed.

## C. Chalazion

Internal hordeolum (meibomian gland).

### ▶ H&P Keys
Persistent nontender lump palpable or visible along the margin of upper or lower eyelid. Inflammation and swelling develop over a period of days and can remain for months.

### ▶ Diagnosis
When the lid is everted, the nodules usually point toward the conjunctival side and can be detected as reddened, elevated areas. Absence of acute inflammation is seen in fully developed chalazion.

### ▶ Disease Severity
1. Evaluate for malignancy if recurrent at same site.
2. Assess visual disturbance caused by the lump on the lids.
3. Perform biopsy if recurrent.

### ▶ Concept and Application
A granulomatous inflammation of the meibomian gland. Seldom subsides spontaneously. Langhans' giant cells, yellowish, fatty content. Large chalazion pressing on the eyeball, can cause astigmatism. Recurrence at same site after excision suggests malignant disease.

### ▶ Treatment Steps
1. Warm compresses.
2. Topical antibiotics.
3. Local steroid injection.
4. Excision if large and disturbs vision.
5. Biopsy if recurrent.

### D. Entropion
Turning inward of the lid margin, usually affects the lower lid.

▶ **H&P Keys**
Tearing, irritation of the cornea. Eyelashes turn inward, touching cornea.

▶ **Diagnosis**
Check the lid margin, position of the eyelashes, and the integrity of the cornea. Early detection of corneal ulcer.

▶ **Disease Severity**
Entropion can cause trichiasis, the turning inward of the lashes so that they rub on the cornea. Irritation of the cornea can predispose to corneal ulcer.

▶ **Concept and Application**
*Senile* type caused by degeneration of fascial attachments in the lower lid. *Cicatricial* type caused by scarring of the palpebral conjunctiva and the tarsus. Common in trachoma, Stevens–Johnson syndrome, chemical burns, and trauma.

▶ **Treatment Steps**
1. Temporary taping to evert lid.
2. Corrective surgery.

### E. Ectropion
Turning outward of lower lid.

▶ **H&P Keys**
Tearing, irritation. Sagging and eversion of lid margin.

▶ **Diagnosis**
Test closure of lids and integrity of cornea.

▶ **Disease Severity**
Exposure keratitis. Fluorescein stain for corneal integrity.

▶ **Concept and Application**
Bilateral. Older persons. Relaxation of orbicularis oculi. Present in aging and seventh cranial nerve palsy.

▶ **Treatment Steps**
1. Protection of cornea.
2. Lubrication with artificial tears or ointment.
3. Surgical correction of deformed lid.

### F. Epicanthus
Wide nasal folds.

▶ **H&P Keys**
Vertical folds of skin over medial canthi; in Asians and most children of all races.

▶ Diagnosis

Corneal light reflex test is normal. So-called esotropia, or turning in of the eye, appears present on side gaze.

▶ Disease Severity

Prominent epicanthal folds in children becomes less obvious as child grows older.

▶ Concept and Application

The large skin fold covers the nasal sclera and causes pseudo-esotropia. Frequent concern as strabismus. A common cause for referral.

▶ Treatment Steps

Explanation and understanding. No treatment needed.

## G. Blepharoptosis

Droopy eyelids.

▶ H&P Keys

May be noted at birth; congenital or acquired. Drooping of upper lids when both eyes are open. Unilateral or bilateral. Constant or intermittent.

▶ Diagnosis

Determine amount of movement of upper lid and severity in blocking of vision. Assess cosmesis and skin position.

▶ Disease Severity

Degree of upper lid movement and occlusion of pupillary axis for vision. Concern with visual development in children. May cause amblyopia.

▶ Concept and Application

*Congenital*—Developmental failure of levator muscle of the lid, anomalies of superior rectus muscle, complete external ophthalmoplegia. Dominant transmission.

*Acquired*

*Mechanical Factors*—Edema of lids, swelling, tumor, fat.

*Myogenic Causes*—Muscular dystrophy, myasthenia gravis.

*Neurogenic (Paralytic)*—Weakness of cranial nerve III.

▶ Treatment Steps
1. Conservative: no cosmetic or visual acuity disturbance.
2. Myasthenia gravis: neostigmine.
3. Special spectacle frames.
4. Surgery for improvement of vision or cosmesis: frontalis sling for no action of levator, to lift upper lid; levator strengthening for partial weakness of levator.

## III. DISORDERS OF THE LACRIMAL SYSTEM

### A. Undersecretion
Dry-eye syndrome, Sjögren's disease.

#### 1. Dry-eye Syndrome (Keratoconjunctivitis Sicca)

▶ H&P Keys

Dry, irritative conjunctiva. Dry, sore mouth. Foreign-body sensation, scratchy and sandy feeling of the eyes. Itchy, burning, photosensitivity, excessive mucus, redness, pain, dry lids. Grossly, normal-looking eyes.

▶ Diagnosis

Dry undersecretion is confirmed by Schirmer's test with strip of blotting paper (4 mm × 30 mm). The strip is inserted onto the lower lid margin so that the strip protrudes forward from the eye. The rate of lacrimation is measured. By the end of 5 minutes the strip should be moistened for at least 15 mm in a normal response. In Sjögren's disease, the moistening rarely extends beyond 5 mm along the strip, suggesting inadequate tear production.

▶ Disease Severity

Undersecretion of tears. Evaluation studies for corneal epithelium and conjunctival defects with vital stain such as rose bengal (1%). The affected areas will be colored bright red. Collagen-vascular diseases, conjunctival scarring, drugs and vitamin A deficiency should be investigated, if not yet diagnosed.

▶ Concept and Application

Dryness of eye may have many causes. Hyposecretion, excessive evaporation, mucin deficiency are predisposing factors.

Sjögren's disease is a general glandular atrophy. It affects the lacrimal and salivary glands and associates with rheumatic diathesis. Postmenopausal women. Dryness affects conjunctiva, cornea, mouth, trachea.

▶ Treatment Steps
1. Search for cause.
2. Artificial tears, methylcellulose are used frequently.

### B. Acute Dacryocystitis

▶ H&P Keys

Infection of lacrimal sac. Common acute or chronic. Infants or in patients over 40. Tearing and discharge. Swelling lump, redness, pain, tenderness over tear sac area. May have fever.

▶ Diagnosis

Persistent tearing. Purulent material can be expressed from tear sac. Nasolacrimal duct is blocked. Staining of conjunctival smear to identify infectious organisms.

▶ **Disease Severity**

Tearing in mild cases. Purulent discharge in moderate to severe blockage of nasolacrimal ducts.

▶ **Concept and Application**

Blockage of nasolacrimal duct is the cause of infection. May be developmental.

▶ **Treatment Steps**

In children, forceful massage of the tear sac is tried initially. Irrigation and probings of nasolacrimal duct are usually effective in adults.

*Acute*
1. Warm compresses.
2. Appropriate antibiotics.
3. Incision and drainage if necessary.

*Chronic*—Surgical removal of obstruction of nasolacrimal duct (dacrocystorhinostomy).

## IV. DISORDERS OF THE OPTIC NERVE

### A. Elevation of the Disc

#### 1. Congenital Anomalous Disc Elevation

Blurred optic disc since birth, caused by developmental anomaly.

▶ **H&P Keys**

No symptoms, blurred disc margin, elevated disc substance, obliterated cup, no edema, no hemorrhage.

▶ **Diagnosis**

Dilated ophthalmoscopy; document with optic disc photography, pseudopapilledema; visual field, intravenous fluorescein angiography (Tables 13–7, 13–8).

**13-7 SYMPTOMS OF BLURRED OPTIC NERVE HEAD**

| Symptoms | Papilledema | Papillitis | Pseudopapilledema |
|---|---|---|---|
| Etiology | Acute swelling of optic disc<br>• Increased intracranial pressure<br>• Brain tumor<br>• Hypertension<br>• Pseudotumor cerebri | Acute blurred disc margin<br>• Ischemia<br>• Inflammation<br>• Multiple sclerosis | Blurred disc<br>• Congenital, developmental anomalies<br>• Hyperopia |
| Acute loss of vision | + | +++ (Severe) | 0 |
| Headaches | +++ | 0/+ | 0 |
| Retrobulbar pain on eye movement | 0 | +/+++ | 0 |

+, present; ++, moderate; +++, severe; 0, absent.

## 13-8 SIGNS OF BLURRED OPTIC NERVE HEAD

| Signs | Papilledema | Papillitis | Pseudopapilledema |
|---|---|---|---|
| Hyperemia of disc | +++ | +++ | 0 |
| Hemorrhages | +++ | + | 0 |
| Tortuosity of veins, capillaries | +++ | ++ | + |
| Disc margin blurred, | +++ | +++ | +++ |
| elevated | +++ | 0/+ | ++ |
| One eye affected | Rare | +++ | ++ |
| Both eyes affected | +++ | Rare | Rare |
| Afferent pupillary defect | 0 | +++ | 0/+ |
| Visual field defect | 0/+ | +++ | 0/+ |

+, present; ++, moderate; +++, severe; 0, absent.

▶ **Disease Severity**
Benign, nonprogressive; rule out true papilledema.

▶ **Concept and Application**
Hyperopia, glial tissue, persistent hyaloid remnants, drusen of the disc.

▶ **Treatment Steps**
Detection and follow-up through serial examinations to monitor possible progression.

2. **Papilledema**
Swelling of optic disc caused by increased intracranial pressure (Fig. 13–1).

▶ **H&P Keys**
Symptoms of brain tumor, hyperemia of optic disc, tortuosity of veins and capillaries, blurring and elevation of disc margin, hemorrhages on and surrounding nerve head.

▶ **Diagnosis**
Studies for brain lesions, computed tomographic (CT) scan, magnetic resonance imaging (MRI), magnetic resonance angiography (MRA), intravenous fluorescein angiography.

▶ **Disease Severity**
Brain tumor, pseudotumor cerebri, severe systemic hypertension.

▶ **Concept and Application**
Swelling of optic disc secondary to increased intracranial pressure, brain tumor 50%.

▶ **Treatment Steps**
Detection and referral for evaluation by neurologists or neurosurgeons.

3. **Papillitis**
Anterior optic neuritis. Inflammatory edema of the optic nerve head visible by ophthalmoscope.

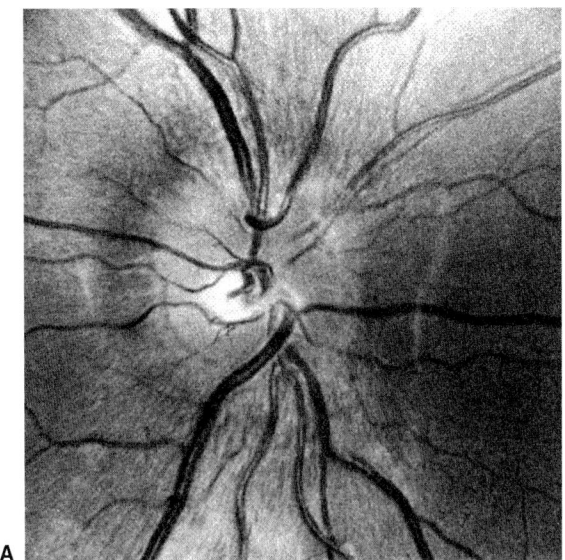

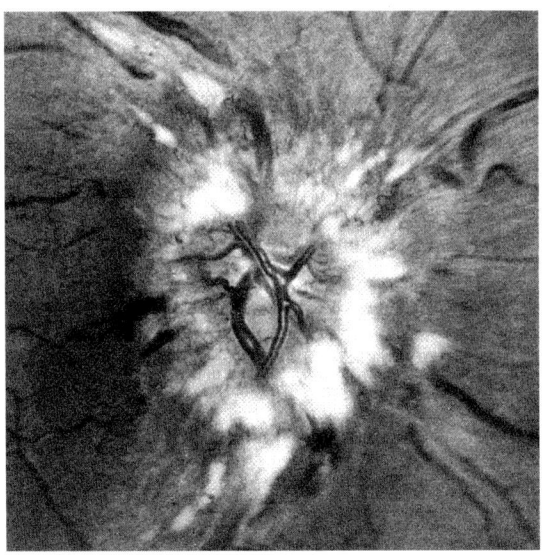

Figure 13–1. (A) Mild papilledema with blurred disc margins superiorly and inferiorly. (B) Acute papilledema with cotton-wool spots and hemorrhages. (Reproduced, with permission, from Vaughan DG (editor): *General Ophthalmology,* 15th ed. Stamford, CT: Appleton & Lange, 1999).

► H&P Keys

Sudden loss of central vision, usually in one eye. Pain behind the eyeball on movement of the affected eye. Reduced vision. Swinging light test for relative afferent pupillary defect.

► Diagnosis

Ophthalmoscopy. Visual field test for central scotoma. CT of orbits and chiasm, MRI, and MRA of the brain.

▶ Disease Severity
Search for multiple sclerosis, Lyme disease, and neurosyphilis. Rule out compressive lesions of optic nerve and chiasm.

▶ Concept and Application
Inflammation of optic nerve. Idiopathic. Associated with multiple sclerosis, Lyme disease, and neurosyphilis. Prognosis for return vision after single attack is good. Spontaneous resolution can follow in weeks to months.

▶ Treatment Steps
1. IV corticosteroid versus no treatment for acute phase.
2. Oral prednisone treatment is contraindicated in the treatment of idiopathic optic neuritis.

### B. Pallor of the Disc, Optic Atrophy
Optic nerve degeneration.

▶ H&P Keys
Decreased vision, visual field loss, relative afferent pupillary defect, fixed dilated pupil, pale optic disc.

▶ Diagnosis
Vision, pupillary reaction to light, swinging light test, ophthalmoscopy; compare both discs for asymmetry of color, cupping, fine-vessels pattern.

▶ Disease Severity
Intraocular pressure for glaucoma, orbital mass compression of nerve. Intravenous fluorescein angiography of disc.

▶ Concept and Application
History of diseases that damage nerve fiber layer of retina, optic nerve, optic chiasm, optic tracts. Common causes: optic neuritis, long-standing papilledema, compression of the nerve by a mass, meningioma, ischemic optic neuropathy, glaucoma.

▶ Treatment Steps
Detection and referral for investigation and treatment.

## V. DISORDERS OF THE VISUAL PATHWAYS

### A. Monocular Defects (Central Scotomas)
Anterior to chiasm.

▶ H&P Keys
Loss of central vision in one eye. Reduction of visual acuity (Fig. 13–2).

▶ Diagnosis
Visual acuity testing. Pupillary reaction to light. Swinging light test for relative afferent pupillary defect. Ophthalmoscopy. Visual field testing. Red-color appreciation. Amsler grid.

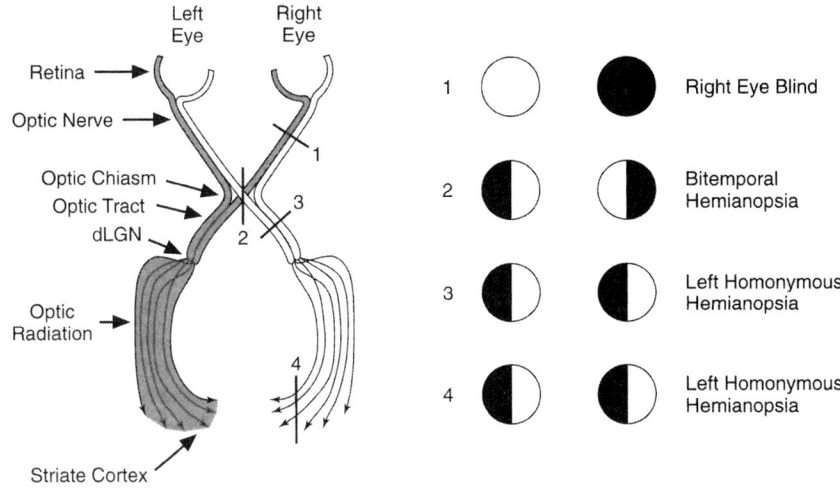

Figure 13-2. Visual pathways with associated field defects. (Reproduced, with permission, from Schwartz SH, *Visual Perception*, 2nd ed. New York: McGraw-Hill; 1999).

▶ Disease Severity

Ophthalmoscopy for macular and optic nerve diseases. Rule out retinal detachments, vascular occlusions, such as central retinal artery occlusion, branch retinal artery occlusion, central retinal vein occlusion. Intravenous fluorescein angiography.

▶ Concept and Application

Prechiasmal lesions mean monocular loss of vision. Optic nerve lesions. Scotoma is a blind or partially defective area in the visual field. Central scotoma means central vision is affected. Optic neuritis. Ischemic optic neuropathy. Multiple sclerosis.

▶ Treatment Steps

Detection and referral.

## B. Bitemporal Defects

At the chiasm.

▶ H&P Keys

Visual field defect affects both eyes, bitemporal hemianopsia, side vision defect of both eyes (see Fig. 13–2). Confrontation testing with red object.

▶ Diagnosis

Vision. Visual fields testing. CT scan, MRI/MRA.

▶ Disease Severity

CT scan. Check out enlarged sella turcica for pituitary tumor.

▶ Concept and Application

Bitemporal visual field defects means chiasmal lesions; suspect pituitary tumor.

▶ Treatment Steps

Detection and referral.

### C. Homonymous Defects
Posterior to chiasm.

▶ **H&P Keys**
Loss of visual fields of both eyes on the same side (see Fig. 13–2). Visual field defects on the right or left side. Confrontation testing with red object.

▶ **Diagnosis**
Visual field testing. Intracranial studies. CT scan. MRI.

▶ **Disease Severity**
Check out neurologic symptoms and signs for brain tumor and cerebral vascular lesions, stroke.

▶ **Concept and Application**
Defects indicate lesions behind the chiasm. Lesions affect optic tract opposite the defects, extending to occipital cortex. The more posterior the lesion, the more similar in shape, size, and severity the damage in the two eyes. Check out tumor, cerebral vascular diseases.

▶ **Treatment Steps**
Detection and referral.

## VI. AMBLYOPIA
Defective vision, uncorrectable by glasses, in an otherwise normal eye.

▶ **H&P Keys**
Eye fixation pattern, vision test, ophthalmoscopy.

▶ **Diagnosis**
Refraction, check out anisometropia.

▶ **Disease Severity**
Check out visual loss caused by organic diseases, congenital cataracts, retinoblastoma.

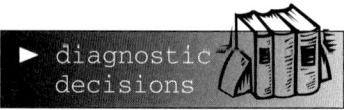

**THREE COMMON CAUSES OF VISION LOSS**

**Amblyopia**
Child, positive family history, decreased vision in one eye uncorrectable with glasses, no organic disease, strabismus in 50% (exotropia—eye turns out, esotropia—eye turns in).

**Diabetic Retinopathy**
Frequency increases with duration of disease, vision may be normal, decreased vision is often a late sign, hypertension, exacerbated with puberty and pregnancy.

**Glaucoma (Open-angle)**
Positive family history, advanced age (especially 80+ years), diabetes, hypertension, normal vision, constricted peripheral vision, thinning of optic disc rim/asymmetrical opic nerve rims, increased intraocular pressure (> 21 mm Hg).

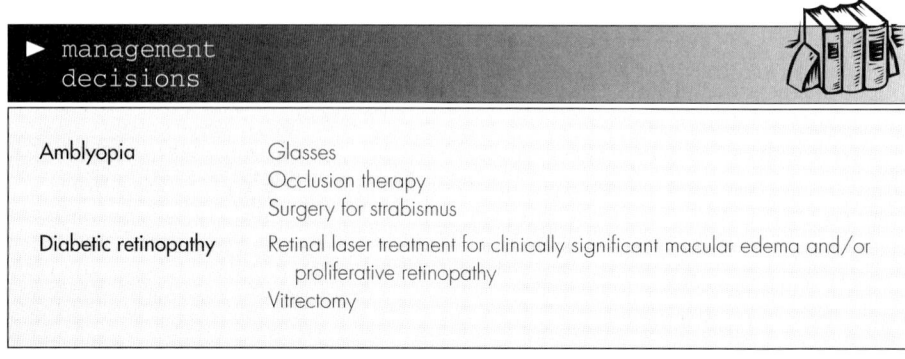

| management decisions | |
|---|---|
| Amblyopia | Glasses |
| | Occlusion therapy |
| | Surgery for strabismus |
| Diabetic retinopathy | Retinal laser treatment for clinically significant macular edema and/or proliferative retinopathy |
| | Vitrectomy |

### 13-9 PROGRESSION OF DIABETIC RETINOPATHY

Nonproliferative retinopathy
    Microaneurysms
    Hemorrhages (dot and blot, flame)
    Hard exudates
    Retinal edema
Preproliferative retinopathy
    Retinal nerve fiber layer infarcts (cotton-wool patches)
    Venous dilation, loops, and beading (irregularities of the vein caliber)
    Telangiectasias (intraretinal microvascular abnormalities)
Proliferative diabetic retinopathy
    Neovascularization of the retina, optic disc, or vitreous
    Preretinal and vitreous hemorrhages
    Fibrous proliferation
    Tractional retinal detachment

▶ Concept and Application

Preventable blindness. Strabismus in 50% of patients with amblyopia. Amblyopia secondary to strabismus. Organic visual loss causes strabismus. Predisposing factors: strabismic amblyopia, refractive amblyopia, form-deprivation and occlusion amblyopia.

▶ Treatment Steps

Early detection. Early treatment before age 5 (Table 13–9).

## VII. STRABISMUS

Misalignment of two eyes so that both eyes cannot be directed toward the object of fixation (Fig. 13–3).

▶ H&P Keys

Family history, head trauma, systemic disease, neurologic disorder.

▶ Diagnosis

General inspection, corneal light reflex, cover test, dilated ophthalmoscopy.

▶ Disease Severity

Check for intraocular lesions, cataract, retinoblastoma, other retinal abnormalities. Examine for neurologic disorder.

▶ Concept and Application

Early detection (Tables 13–10, 13–11). Delayed diagnosis affects vision, eye, and systemic problems.

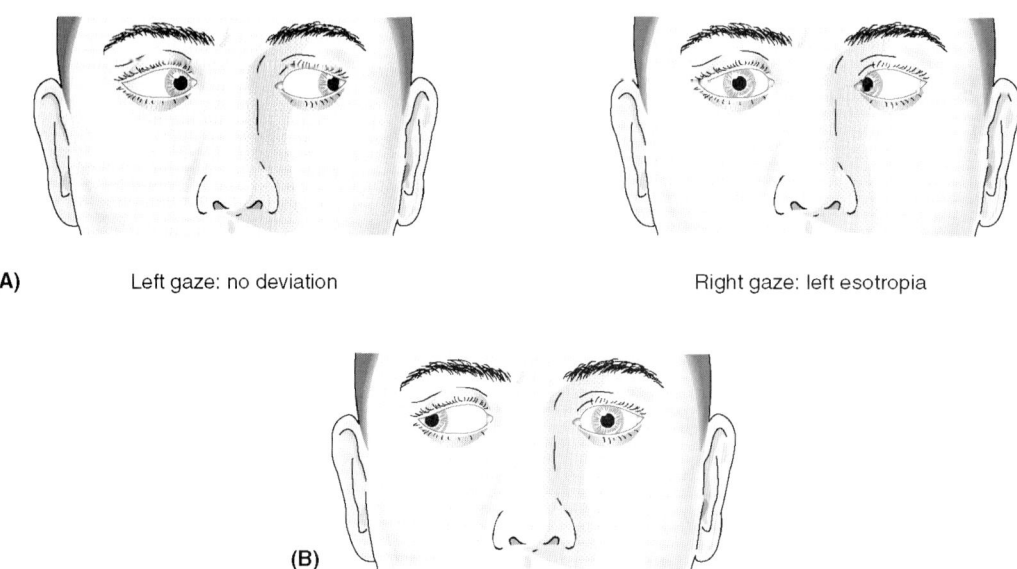

Figure 13-3. (A) Right esotropia. (B) Right exotropia. (Reproduced, with permission, from Vaughan DG (editor): *General Ophthalmology,* 15th ed. Stamford, CT: Appleton & Lange, 1999).

▶ Treatment Steps
1. Detection early to allow diagnosis and treatment.
2. Search for serious organic conditions that cause strabismus.

## 13-10 CLASSIFICATION OF STRABISMUS

|  | Comitant (Nonparalytic) Strabismus | Noncomitant (Paralytic) Strabismus |
|---|---|---|
| Onset | Childhood (under 6 y) | Later in life |
| Angle of misalignment *varies* with direction of gaze | 0 | + |
| Extraocular muscles palsy | 0 | + |
| Associated neurologic disease* | 0 | + |

*Blowout fracture; palsy of cranial nerve III; orbital diseases; thyroid.
+, present; 0, absent.

### 13-11 TYPES OF IMBALANCE OF THE TWO EYES

|  | Tropia (Visible Turning) | Phoria (Tendency to Turn) |
|---|---|---|
| **Horizontal** | | |
| Inward turning | Esotropia | Esophoria |
| Outward turning | Exotropia | Exophoria |
| **Vertical** | | |
| Upward turning | Hypertropia | Hyperphoria |
| Downward turning | Hypotropia | Hypophoria |

## VIII. DIABETES WITH OPHTHALMOLOGIC MANIFESTATIONS

### ▶ H&P Keys

Decreased vision often a late symptom that may not be evident until ocular damage is severe. The longer a patient is diabetic, the more likely the retinopathy and visual loss. Age of onset, type of diabetes, history of hypertension, and presence of obesity are relevant to disease severity and management. Changes in refraction of lens, decreased or abnormal pupillary responses, extraocular muscle palsy, cataract, iris neovascularization, optic neuropathy, or retinopathy. Diabetic retinopathy progresses in severity from nonproliferative or background retinopathy to preproliferative and proliferative changes (see Table 13–11).

### ▶ Diagnosis

Direct ophthalmoscopy detects most ophthalmic clinical manifestations of diabetes, including retinopathy, optic neuropathy, blockage of the red reflex by cataract (Fig. 13–4). Indirect oph-

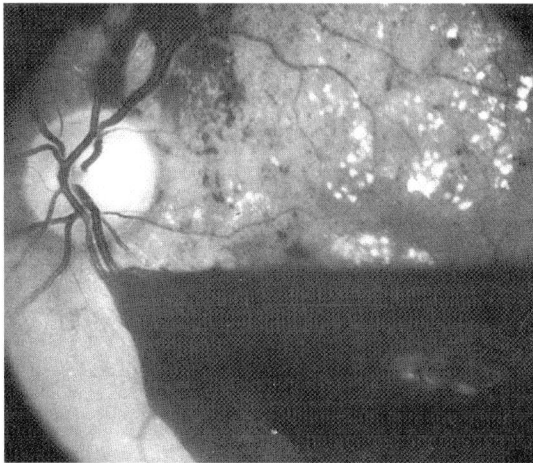

Figure 13–4. Proliferative diabetic retinopathy with preretinal hemorrhage obscuring the inferior macula. Macular exudate, microaneurysms, and intraretinal hemorrhages are also present. (Reproduced, with permission, from Vaughan DG (editor): *General Ophthalmology*, 15th ed. Stamford, CT: Appleton & Lange, 1999).

thalmoscopy: wider, stereoscopic view of retina. Biomicroscopy with a slit lamp: useful in evaluating for diabetic changes in anterior segment including cataracts and iris neovascularization. Pupillary dilation for easier, more thorough examination of retina and lens. Ultrasonography for internal structure (eg, tractional retinal detachment), when blood, debris, or membranes impede direct visualization of retina.

### ▶ Disease Severity
Biomicroscopy with a contact lens system provides stereoscopic, detailed view of structures of retina; especially valuable in diagnosis of macular edema. Fluorescein angiography to assess extent of disease, such as leakage from abnormal vessels in suspected neovascularization, and in guiding laser photocoagulation treatment of clinically evident macular edema by revealing characteristic lesions and pathologic processes of retinopathy, eg, microaneurysms, capillary leakage, and nonperfusion areas. Images of retina.

### ▶ Concept and Application
Cellular edema, pericyte destruction, endothelial damage and dysfunction from increased intracellular sorbitol and hypoxia lead to capillary hyperpermeability. Abnormal retinal vascular permeability leads to macular edema, which threatens vision and may be an indication for laser therapy. Increased hemoglobin $A_{1c}$ oxygen affinity impairs oxygen release, resulting in retinal hypoxia. Basement membrane thickening and increased platelet and red blood cell aggregability predispose to regions of microvascular occlusions, retinal hypoxia, and release of vasogenic factors with subsequent neovascularization of the retina, optic nerve, or iris. Widespread panretinal laser photocoagulation reduces release of vasogenic stimuli and therefore neovascularization.

### ▶ Treatment Steps
1. Tight medical control with long-term near-normalization of blood sugar level slows the progression of diabetic retinopathy. Aggressive control of blood pressure to 130/80 or better.
2. Laser photocoagulation for diabetic retinopathy with clinically significant macular edema and high-risk proliferative retinopathy.
3. Vitrectomy may be indicated for severe vitreous or preretinal hemorrhages, or tractional retinal detachment.

## IX. DISORDERS OF THE CORNEA
See Table 13–12.

### A. Corneal Ulcers

#### ▶ H&P Keys
Pain, photophobia, blepharospasm, lacrimation, discharge, and decreased vision often present. The lesion begins as a dull, grayish, circumscribed superficial infiltration of the cornea that subse-

## 13-12 DISEASES OF THE GLOBE

A. Cornea
  1. Ulcers
  2. Herpes simplex keratitis
  3. Ophthalmic herpes zoster
  4. Dry eye (keratoconjunctivitis sicca)
  5. Interstitial keratitis
B. Sclera
  1. Scleritis
C. Uvea
  1. Uveitis
    a. Anterior
    b. Posterior
D. Retina
  1. Retinal detachment
  2. Vascular occlusions
    a. Arteriolar
    b. Venous
  3. Hypertensive retinopathy
  4. Retinitis pigmentosa
  5. Age-related macular degeneration
E. Penetrating injuries

quently ulcerates. Conjunctival and limbal injection is usual and blood vessels may grow in from the limbus in long-standing cases (pannus). Pus may appear in the anterior chamber (hypopyon). Corneal perforation with iris prolapse may occur.

▶ Diagnosis

The ulcer stains green with fluorescein. Bacterial and fungal cultures from corneal scrapings should be obtained prior to starting antibiotic treatment.

▶ Disease Severity

Slit-lamp biomicroscopy may be used to determine the extent of corneal thinning and infiltration and the presence of hypopyon.

▶ Concept and Application

Bacterial or fungal infection following trauma, corneal foreign body, contact lens wear, or previous corneal disease. Assume bacterial until proven otherwise.

▶ Treatment Steps

1. Cycloplegia (scopalamine), broad-spectrum or fortified topical antibiotics, subconjunctival antibiotics.
2. Eye shield if corneal thinning.
3. Pain medication (acetaminophen).
4. Avoid steroids.

## B. Herpes Simplex Keratitis

▶ H&P Keys

Red eye, foreign-body sensation, photophobia, tearing, decreased vision, skin vesicles. Decreased corneal sensation. Dendritic corneal branching lesion. Possible recent topical steroids, systemic steroids, or immune deficiency state.

▶ Diagnosis

Edge of herpetic lesions are heaped up with swollen epithelial cells, which stain with rose bengal, whereas the central ulceration stains with fluorescein. Corneal or skin lesion scraping for multinucleated giant cells and intranuclear inclusion bodies. Viral culture.

▶ Disease Severity

Slit-lamp examination with intraocular pressure measurement. Concomitant corneal infiltrates, iritis, hypopyon, or glaucoma may occur. Bacterial superinfection must be ruled out.

▶ Concept and Application

Self-limited primary ocular herpes keratoconjunctivitis, regional lymphadenitis, vesicular blepharitis, or skin involvement. Herpes virus establishes presence in trigeminal ganglion, allowing chronic recurrent disease.

▶ Treatment Steps

1. Skin vesicles (antibiotic ointment); eyelid margin involvement, conjunctivitis, corneal epithelial disease (topical trifluorothymidine or vidarabine).
2. Consider mechanical debridement of infected corneal epithelium.
3. Topical steroids contraindicated for corneal epithelial involvement.

### C. Ophthalmic Herpes Zoster

▶ H&P Keys

Acute vesicular skin rash of fifth cranial nerve dermatome. Fever, malaise, blurred vision, eye pain, red eye. Conjunctivitis, corneal involvement (eg, pseudodendrites), uveitis, optic neuritis, retinitis, glaucoma. Postherpetic neuralgia may occur late. Involvement of tip of nose by vesicles (Hutchinson's sign) associated with corneal involvement. Immunocompromised or risk factors for AIDS?

▶ Diagnosis

Clinical diagnosis based on pattern of skin rash. Pseudodendrites stain poorly with fluorescein. Regional lymphadenopathy with associated pain occurs in primary disease.

▶ Disease Severity

Slit-lamp examination with intraocular pressure measurement. Dilated optic nerve and retinal examination. Immunodeficiency workup if less than 40 years old or immunodeficiency suspected.

▶ Concept and Application

Primary herpes zoster: acute infection of dorsal root ganglion by chickenpox virus. Secondary eruption following ganglion involvement may be associated with immune compromise from neoplastic, inflammatory, or infectious processes.

▶ Treatment Steps
1. Systemic acyclovir if started in first 5–7 days of skin rash.
2. Antibiotic ointment to skin lesions.
3. Consider systemic steroids and cimetidine in nonimmunocompromised, nondiabetic patients over age 60 to reduce postherpetic neuralgia.

## D. Dry Eye (Keratoconjunctivitis Sicca)

▶ H&P Keys

Initial reduction of tear production leads to burning and irritation. Corneal epithelium develops scattered cellular loss called superficial keratitis; may be associated with photophobia or blepharospasm. Keratinization of the ocular surface occurs in advanced stages, often with loss of normal conjunctival fornices. Corneal ulceration, vascularization, and scarring may lead to severe visual disability. Dry eye may be an isolated phenomenon or associated with systemic diseases such as rheumatoid arthritis or lupus erythematosus (Sjögren's syndrome).

▶ Diagnosis

Reduced tear meniscus at lid margin. Fluorescein or rose bengal stains reveal superficial keratitis with scattered staining of corneal surface and premature tear drying over the corneal surface.

▶ Disease Severity

Tear production may be measured by the use of strips of blotting paper with (boneline tear production) or without topical anesthesia (reflex and baseline tear production) (Schirmer test). Baseline and reflex.

▶ Concept and Application

Dryness of the eye may be associated with hypofunction of the lacrimal glands (eg, Sjögren's syndrome, familial dysautonomia, sarcoidosis, atropine), excessive evaporation of tears (eg, exposure keratopathy, dry climate, deficient blinking), mucin deficiency (eg, Stevens–Johnson syndrome, chemical burns, ocular pemphigoid, avitaminosis A).

▶ Treatment Steps
1. Frequent use of artificial tears and ointments.
2. Occlusion of the nasolacrimal punctum to reduce tear drainage.
3. Partial tarsorrhaphy to reduce tear evaporation may be tried in more severe cases.

## E. Interstitial Keratitis

▶ H&P Keys

Acute: pain, tearing, photophobia, red eye. Corneal stromal blood vessels, corneal edema, anterior uveitis. Old disease: deep corneal scarring and haze, corneal stromal thinning, and ghost vessels. Associated with maternal venereal disease, saddle nose, frontal bossing, Hutchinson's teeth, chorioretinitis, optic atrophy (congenital syphilis); hearing deficit, tinnitus, vertigo, polyarteritis nodosa (Cogan's syndrome); hypopigmented or anesthetic skin lesions, loss of temporal eyebrow or eyelashes, thickened corneal nerves, iris nodules (leprosy); tuberculosis.

▶ Diagnosis

Slit-lamp and dilated fundus examination. Rapid plasma reagin (RPR), fluorescent treponemal antibody absorption (FTA-ABS), purified protein derivative (tuberculin) (PPD) tests with anergy panel, chest roentgenogram, sedimentation rate.

▶ Disease Severity

Slit-lamp examination for corneal edema, scarring or thinning, or uveitis.

▶ Concept and Application

Chronic nonulcerative infiltration of the deep layers of the cornea with uveal inflammation.

▶ Treatment Steps

1. Acute corneal involvement: topical cycloplegia, topical steroids, treatment of underlying disease.
2. Corneal transplant surgery for central corneal scarring with impaired vision.

## X. DISORDERS OF THE LENS

### A. Glaucoma

▶ H&P Keys

*Primary Open-angle Glaucoma*—Usually asymptomatic in the early stages. Risk factors include advanced age, African ancestry, immediate family members with glaucoma, myopia (nearsightedness), diabetes mellitus, hypertension. The optic nerve may show an increased ratio of the physiologic cupping diameter to disc diameter, pallor, displacement of retinal vessels to the rim, and asymmetry compared to the contralateral eye.

*Acute Angle-closure Glaucoma*—Presents with severe ocular pain, blurred vision, halos around lights, headache, nausea, and vomiting. Examination shows red eye, mid-dilated sometimes oval pupil, cloudy cornea, marked elevation of intraocular pressure, shallow anterior chamber, and closed angle by gonioscopy. Highly farsighted patients are at greater risk. An attack may be precipitated by dim light, emotional stress, or dilating drops.

*Congenital Glaucoma*—Presents with light sensitivity, corneal cloudiness, and excessive tearing. Chronically, there may be slow development and learning disabilities.

*Secondary Glaucomas*—May occur with chronic exposure to steroids (topical generally), ocular trauma, retinal vein occlusion, intraocular inflammation, intraocular tumor, diabetes mellitus, and carotid vascular disease.

► Diagnosis

Intraocular pressure measurement may be performed with Schiotz' (indentation) or applanation tonometry. Individuals may present with normal intraocular pressures and have glaucoma. A patient who has elevated intraocular pressure but shows no sign of optic nerve damage or visual field loss is generally considered to be a glaucoma suspect. Visual field defects start insidiously. They are characterized by arcuate-shaped scotomas or a silent contraction of the peripheral field, sparing the central vision until late in the disease process.

► Disease Severity

The severity of disease is based on the clinical appearance of the optic nerve and on the visual field. Response to treatment is evaluated with regard to relationship of lowering of intraocular pressure to stability of changes in the optic nerve appearance and visual field (Fig. 13–5).

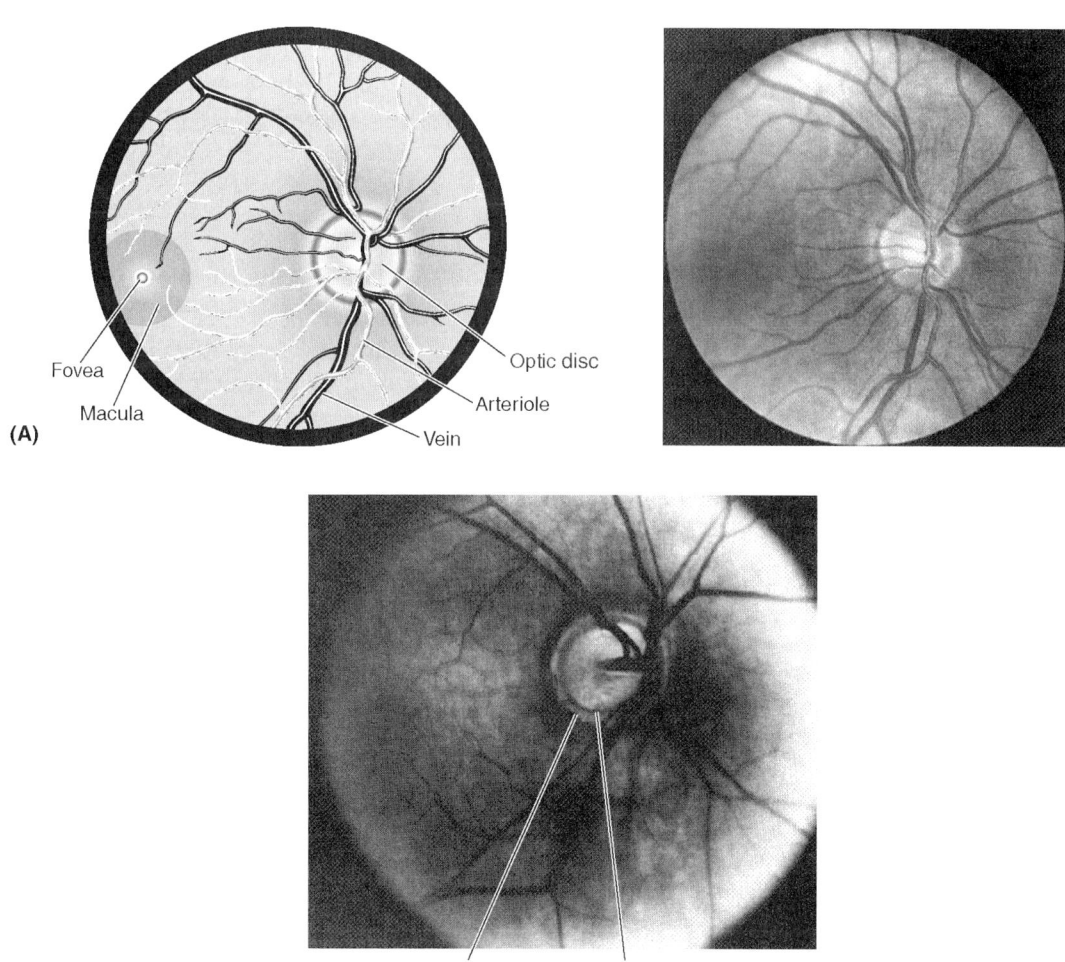

Figure 13–5. **(A)** Normal optic disc. (Photo by Diane Beeston.) **(B)** Glaucomatous optic disc. (Reproduced, with permission, from Vaughan DG (editor): *General Ophthalmology*, 15th ed. Stamford, CT: Appleton & Lange, 1999).

▶ Concept and Application

Glaucoma is in general a condition in which the intraocular pressure is too elevated for the health of the optic nerve, resulting in damage and visual field loss. This is generally due to increased resistance to aqueous outflow. In primary open-angle glaucoma, there appears to be an increased resistance to aqueous outflow through the trabecular meshwork. In primary angle-closure glaucoma, the peripheral iris closes off the angle structures, preventing aqueous outflow. Neovascularization, pigmentary or inflammatory debris, traumatic damage, or cellular changes from chronic steroid exposure all increase resistance to aqueous outflow. Both the medical and surgical treatment of glaucoma is based on the reduction of intraocular pressure by promoting aqueous outflow or reducing aqueous production.

▶ Treatment Steps

*Open-Angle Glaucoma*

1. β-Adrenergic antagonists (eg, timolol), topical carbonic anhydrase inhibitors (eg, dorzolamide, brinzolamide), and adrenergic agonists (eg, epinephrine) decrease aqueous production.
    α-Adrenergic agonists (eg, brimonidine, clonidine, apraclonidine), prostaglandin analogs (eg, latanoprost; travaprost), and miotics (eg, pilocarpine) reduce outflow resistance.
2. Laser trabecular burns promote aqueous outflow.
3. Surgical filtration procedures promote aqueous outflow.

*Angle-Closure Glaucoma*

1. Acutely treat with topical β-blockers, topical pilocarpine, oral carbonic anhydrase inhibitors, and osmotic agents such as oral glycerin or intravenous mannitol.
2. A laser or surgical peripheral iridectomy must be performed for definitive treatment of the anatomic problem.

▶ management decisions

### GLAUCOMA

| | |
|---|---|
| Open-angle | β-Adrenergic antagonists, α-adrenergic agonists, prostaglandin analogs, topical carbonic anhydrase inhibitors, miotics, adrenergic agonists. |
| | Laser trabecular burns. |
| | Surgical filtration procedures. |
| Closed-angle | Topical β-blockers pilocarpine, carbonic anhydrase inhibitors. Oral carbonic anhydrase inhibitors, osmotics (glycerin), IV mannitol. |
| | Laser peripheral iridotomy—for definitive treatment. |

## B. Cataract

▶ H&P Keys

A cataract is a lens opacity. Complaints of painless blurred vision, glare, increasing nearsightedness, or monocular double vision. History of previous eye conditions, injury, or surgery or of concurrent diseases may suggest cause of cataract. Assessment of visual acuity with optical correction by means of Snellen letter chart or a number chart, or picture charts or ability to fixate on and follow or reach for a moving object for young children or adults with severe mental disability. Preferential viewing techniques may estimate visual acuity in infants. The lens is best examined for cataracts with a dilated pupil. The simplest way is with a handheld direct ophthalmoscope showing dark lenticular opacities blocking the normal red reflex of the retina. The slit-lamp biomicroscope is routinely used to detect the location and density of any opacity within the lens.

▶ Diagnosis

Potential visual acuity that might be expected with removal of the cataract may be estimated by the use of a potential acuity meter (PAM) or a laser interferometer. Both instruments are based on the ability of a patient to resolve letters or lines projected onto the retina.

When significant lens opacification prevents direct retinal examination, B-scan ultrasonography may be used to detect severe abnormalities of the retina, such as retinal detachment or tumors.

▶ Disease Severity

The clinical degree of cataract formation, assuming that no other eye disease is present, is judged primarily by the visual acuity. With direct ophthalmoscopy of the posterior pole through the cataract, the ocular fundus becomes increasingly more difficult to visualize as the lens opacity becomes denser. Slit-lamp biomicroscopy allows judgment of lens clarity and location of the cataract. Glare testing and contrast sensitivity testing are new methods for quantitatively estimating the functional impact a cataract has on vision.

▶ Concept and Application

A cataract is an opacity or loss of transparency within the lens. Cataracts may be classified by their age of onset, location, and etiology (Table 13–13). The most common indication for cataract surgery is the patient's desire for improved visual function. Medical indications for cataract surgery include phacolytic glaucoma, phacomorphic glaucoma, phacotoxic uveitis, and dense cataracts that obscure the view of the fundus and interfere with the diagnosis and management of other ocular diseases such as diabetic retinopathy or glaucoma. In children, cataract extraction is performed early to prevent otherwise irreversible visual impairment from amblyopia, the loss of visual maturation from visual sensory deprivation.

## 13-13 CLASSIFICATION OF CATARACTS

A. Age-related
   1. Nuclear sclerotic
   2. Posterior subcapsular
   3. Cortical
   4. Mature
   5. Morgagnian and hypermature
B. Congenital
C. Juvenile
   1. Inborn errors of metabolism
   2. Chromosomal abnormalities
D. Secondary
   1. Traumatic or physical damage
   2. Associated with intraocular disease
      a. Chronic or recurrent uveitis
      b. Retinitis pigmentosa
      c. Retinal detachment or tumors
   3. Associated with systemic disease (eg, hypoparathyroidism, Down syndrome, diabetes mellitus)
   4. Toxic
      a. Steriods
      b. Miotic agents
      c. Intraocular metals: copper or iron

▶ Treatment Steps

No current medical treatment conclusively delays, prevents, or reverses the development of cataracts in adults.

1. Pupillary dilation, increased ambient illumination, or improved spectacle correction may be temporarily helpful until cataract progression causes additional symptoms.
2. Surgical removal of the cataract with or without artificial lens implantation is the definitive treatment.

## BIBLIOGRAPHY

Foundation of the American Academy of Ophthalmology. *Ophthalmology Monographs*. Italy: 1999.

Kanski, JS, *Clinical Opthalmology: A Systematic Approach*. 5th ed. Butterworth-Heinemann Medical, 2003.

Spalton DJ, Hitchings RA, Hunter PA. *Atlas of Clinical Ophthalmology*. 2nd ed. London: Wolfe Publishing; 1994.

Vaughan D. *General Ophthalmology*. 15th ed. Stamford, CT: Appleton & Lange; 1999.

# Pediatrics 14

**I. NEUROLOGY / 421**
- A. Febrile Seizures / 421
- B. Infantile Botulism / 421
- C. Neural Tube Defects / 422
- D. Malformations / 423

**II. RHEUMATOLOGY / 425**
- A. Henoch–Schönlein Purpura / 425
- B. Kawasaki Disease / 425

**III. GENITOURINARY SYSTEM / 426**
- A. Hypospadias / 426
- B. Posterior Urethral Valves / 426
- C. Prune-belly Syndrome (Eagle–Barrett Syndrome) / 427
- D. Vesicoureteral Reflux / 427
- E. Infantile Polycystic Disease / 428
- F. Multicystic Kidney Disease / 428
- G. Undescended Testis / 428
- H. Bladder Extrophy / 429

**IV. NEONATOLOGY / 429**
- A. Transient Tachypnea of the Newborn (TTN) / 429
- B. Respiratory Distress Syndrome / 430
- C. Meconium Aspiration / 431
- D. Rh Incompatibility / 431
- E. Neonatal Hyperbilirubinemia / 432
- F. Developmental Dysplasia of the Hip / 433

**V. INFECTIOUS DISEASES / 434**
- A. Bronchiolitis / 434
- B. Otitis Media / 343
- C. Epiglottitis (Supraglottitis) / 435

D. Laryngotracheitis (Croup) / 435
E. Varicella (Chickenpox) / 436
F. Pharyngitis / 436
G. Bacterial Meningitis / 437
H. Congenital Infections (STORCH) / 437
I. Hemolytic Uremic Syndrome / 440

VI. GASTROENTEROLOGY / 440
A. Cleft Lip or Palate / 440
B. Tracheoesophageal Fistula (TEF) / 441
C. Pyloric Stenosis / 441
D. Malrotation of the Small Intestine / 441
E. Intussusception / 442
F. Necrotizing Enterocolitis (NEC) / 443
G. Colonic Aganglionosis (Hirschsprung Disease) / 443

VII. GENETICS / 444
A. Down Syndrome (Trisomy 21) / 444
B. Trisomy 18 / 445
C. Trisomy 13 / 445
D. Gonadal Dysgenesis 45,XO (Turner Syndrome) / 445
E. Fragile X Syndrome / 446

VIII. PULMONOLOGY / 446
A. Congenital Laryngeal Stridor (Laryngomalacia) / 446
B. Congenital Lobar Emphysema / 446
C. Cystic Adenomatoid Malformation / 447
D. Pulmonary Sequestration / 447

IX. SKIN CONDITIONS / 448
A. Acne / 448
B. Fungal Infections / 448

X. DISORDERS OF MUSCULOSKELETAL SYSTEM / 448
A. Scoliosis / 448
B. Kyphosis / 449
C. Slipped Capital Femoral Epiphysis / 449
D. Osgood-Schlatter Disease / 449
E. Osteochondritis Dissecans / 449
F. Chondromalacia Patellae / 450

**BIBLIOGRAPHY / 450**

## I. NEUROLOGY

### A. Febrile Seizures

▶ H&P Keys

Occurs in children 6 months to 6 years of age. Signs and symptoms include generalized, tonic, atonic, tonic–clonic, or focal seizures and fever. Risk factors include positive family history developmental delay, day care, prematurity, perinatal maternal smoking.

▶ Diagnosis

Diagnosis of exclusion. Studies based on history and physical exam. Evaluate for source of infection or metabolic imbalance. May include lumbar puncture, blood and urine cultures, electrolytes, glucose, calcium, and complete blood count (CBC) based on clinical presentation.

▶ Disease Severity

*Simple Febrile Seizure*—Generalized seizure lasting < 15 minutes, occurring once in a 24-hour period.

*Complex Febrile Seizure*—A focal seizure or a generalized seizure lasting more than 15 minutes, or more than one seizure in a 24-hour period.

▶ Concept and Application

Genetic factors play a role, ie, an increased incidence if a first-degree relative has had a febrile seizure. Thirty percent recurrence after first seizure. Unclear etiology.

▶ Treatment Steps

1. ABC (airway, breathing, circulation).
2. Lorazepam (Ativan) or diazepam (Valium) for prolonged seizures.
3. Antipyretics.
4. Prophylactic anticonvulsants are controversial.

### B. Infantile Botulism

▶ H&P Keys

An acute neurologic disease caused by the toxin of *Clostridium botulinum*. *C. botulinum* spores can be found in soil, dust, lakes, and contaminated food products, including honey. Signs and symptoms include weakness, poor feeding, weak cry, constipation, respiratory failure, symmetric descending flaccid paralysis, loss of a gag reflex, and ptosis.

▶ Diagnosis

Stool culture for *C. botulinum* and toxin. Electrophysiologic studies.

▶ Disease Severity

Neurologic changes. Pulmonary function tests. Arterial blood gases (ABG).

▶ Concept and Application

Botulinum toxin irreversibly binds to the neuromuscular junctions and inhibits exocytosis of acetylcholine, which results in flaccid paralysis.

▶ Treatment Steps
1. Supportive care.
2. Antitoxin (neutralizes circulating toxin before it binds to nerve endings). Must be given expediently.
3. No antibiotics. Aminoglycosides contraindicated.

## C. Neural Tube Defects

▶ H&P Keys

Failure of neural tube to close in utero (normally closes by day 26). Signs and symptoms depend on the region of spinal cord involved and the extent of the lesion. Clues to diagnosis are a tuft of hair, dimple, or birthmark over the spine.

▶ Diagnosis

Prenatal ultrasonography. Maternal α-fetoprotein (AFP). Clinical exam. Magnetic resonance imaging (MRI) and CT scanning.

▶ Disease Severity

Asymptomatic or disturbances of bowel, bladder, motor function. Degrees of severity include: spina bifida occulta (incomplete closure of the posterior lumbosacral spinal cord) (see Fig. 14–1), meningocele (herniation of the meninges through the spinal

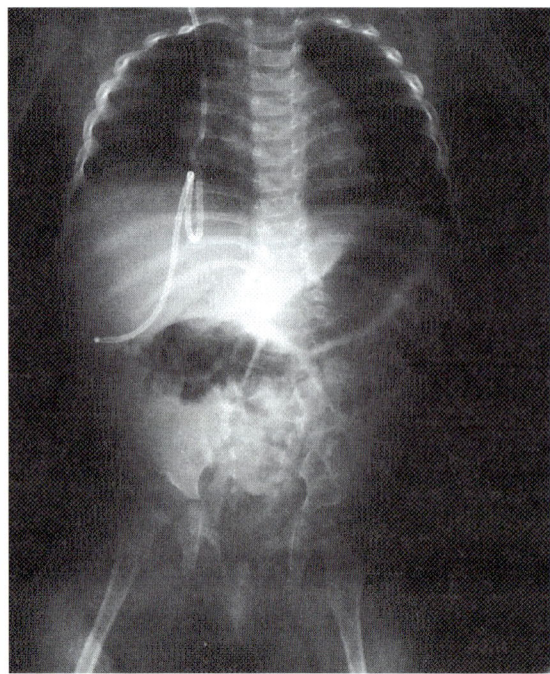

Figure 14–1. Spina bifida. Radiographic study of an 11-month-old with a lumbothoracic myelomeningocele who had undergone a surgical repair as a neonate. A right ventriculoperitoneal shunt was placed for the associated hydrocephalus.

canal defect without neural tissue), encephalocele (herniation of the meninges and brain substance through a skull defect), myelomeningocele (severe spinal dysraphism with herniation of the meninges and spinal cord), anencephaly (congenital absence of the cerebral hemisphere and cranial vault). More than 75% of myelomeningoceles are associated with hydrocephalus (usually related to an Arnold–Chiari malformation). Majority have normal intelligence.

▶ Concept and Application
Multifactorial. Maternal folate supplementation during pregnancy has decreased its frequency.

▶ Treatment Steps
Multidisciplinary approach.

### D. Malformations

1. Hydrocephalus

    ▶ H&P Keys
    A congenital or acquired condition resulting from impaired circulation, absorption or overproduction of cerebrospinal fluid (CSF). Can cause increased intracranial pressure. Signs and symptoms include headaches, vomiting, nausea, irritability, lethargy, third and sixth cranial nerve palsies, papilledema, bulging anterior fontanelle, rapid increase in head circumference, setting-sun sign, long-tract signs, vital sign changes.

    ▶ Diagnosis
    Clinical exam. Computed tomographic (CT) scan. Avoid lumbar punctures (risk of herniation).

    ▶ Disease Severity
    Evidence of herniation: Cushing's triad (bradycardia, hypertension, and irregular breathing), vomiting, change of mental status.

    ▶ Concept and Application

    *Communicating*—Results from either an obstruction of CSF flow from outside the ventricular system or an overproduction of CSF. Etiologies include intraventricular hemorrhages (premature infants), postinfectious state, tumors, hemorrhagic trauma.

    *Noncommunicating*—Results from obstruction of CSF flow within the ventricular system. Etiologies include aqueductal stenosis, Chiari malformation (low cerebellar tonsils), and Dandy–Walker malformation of the fourth ventricle.

    ▶ Treatment Steps
    Placement of a ventriculoperitoneal (VP) shunt if needed.

2. Congenital Glaucoma

    ▶ H&P Keys
    Incidence of about 1 in 100,000 births; 30% are unilateral. Signs and symptoms include photophobia, tearing, blepharospasm, and clouding or enlargement of the cornea.

▶ Diagnosis
Intraocular pressure measurements. Clinical exam.

▶ Disease Severity
Blindness if not treated promptly.

▶ Concept and Application
Maldevelopment of the trabecular meshwork of the eye resulting in increased intraocular pressure as a result of decreased aqueous humor outflow. Autosomal recessive. Associated with conditions such as congenital rubella, neurofibromatosis, Sturge–Weber syndrome (facial port-wine stain, seizures, central nervous system [CNS] calcifications), chromosomal abnormalities, and retinopathy of prematurity.

▶ Treatment Steps
Surgery.

3. Congenital Cataracts

▶ H&P Keys
Unilateral or bilateral opacification of the lens. Signs and symptoms include decreased visual attentiveness, light sensitivity, decreased vision, and opacification of the lens.

▶ Diagnosis
Ophthalmologic exam. Ocular ultrasonography. Rule out associated systemic conditions.

▶ Disease Severity
Varies by the degree of opacification. Blindness. Amblyopia.

▶ Concept and Application
Often idiopathic but may have an autosomal dominant inheritance pattern. May occur as part of a systemic disease including intrauterine infections (rubella, cytomegalovirus [CMV]), metabolic diseases (galactosemia), syndromes (Marfan, Alport), or be associated with chromosomal disorders (trisomies).

▶ Treatment Steps
1. Surgical removal of lens.
2. Evaluate for associated underlying problems.

4. Congenital Deafness

▶ H&P Keys
Conductive (abnormal sound transmission to the middle ear) or sensorineural (poorly functioning auditory nerve) hearing disorders. Signs and symptoms include delay in language skills, poor attentiveness.

▶ Diagnosis
Clinical suspicion (especially by caretaker). Brain stem auditory evoked response potentials (BAER). Audiology assessment.

▶ Disease Severity
Depends on etiology.

▶ Concept and Application
Genetic (dominant, recessive, or X-linked). Ototoxic drugs. Congenital infection (CMV, rubella). Prematurity (low birth weight). Associated with many syndromes (Pierre Robin, Treacher–Collins, Crouzon, Waardenburg [white forelock] and Alport [nephritis]).

▶ Treatment Steps
1. Early amplification.
2. Surgical implants.
3. Sign language.
4. Social support.

## II. RHEUMATOLOGY

### A. Henoch-Schöenlein Purpura

▶ H&P Keys
Small-vessel vasculitis occurring in children ages 1–7 years. Male-to-female ratio 2:1. Signs and symptoms include abdominal pain, rash, vomiting, hematemesis, and joint pain. Purpura, most commonly found on the buttocks and lower extremities, is the first sign in > 50% of cases. Patients may also have fever, gastrointestinal (GI) bleeding, intussusception (3%), and hematuria.

▶ Diagnosis
No pathognomonic laboratory tests. Normal platelet count and coagulation studies. Mild increase in white blood cell (WBC) count and erythrocyte sedimentation rate (ESR). Elevation of serum IgA and IgM in 50% of cases. Skin lesions show leukocytoclastic vasculitis.

▶ Disease Severity
Morbidity and mortality related to the extent of GI or kidney involvement. May lead to GI hemorrhage, intussusception, or end-stage renal disease.

▶ Concept and Application
Leukocytoclastic vasculitis often involving the synovium, GI tract, or renal glomerulus. An immune complex disease (IgA-involved).

▶ Treatment Steps
1. Supportive care.
2. Corticosteroids (if GI hemorrhage).
3. Anti-inflammatory agents if needed for arthritis.
4. Urinalysis to evaluate for hematuria.

### B. Kawasaki Disease

▶ H&P Keys
Fever of ≥ 5 days associated with at least four of the following: bilateral conjunctival injection, nonsuppurative cervical lymphadenopathy, rash, mucous membrane changes (strawberry tongue, erythema of the lips or oropharynx), extremity changes (edema, erythema).

▶ Diagnosis
Clinical presentation. Findings may include an elevated WBC count with a left-shift, elevated ESR and C-reactive protein (CRP), pyuria, uveitis, hydrops of the gallbladder, thrombocytosis (second week of illness), desquamation of the hands and feet.

▶ Concept and Application
Etiology unknown.

▶ Disease Severity
Aneurysms of the coronary arteries and other large arteries. Electrocardiographic (ECG) changes.

▶ Treatment Steps
1. Intravenous gamma globulin.
2. Aspirin.
3. Cardiac evaluation (ECG, ECHO).

## III. GENITOURINARY SYSTEM

### A. Hypospadias

▶ H&P Keys
Urethral meatus located proximal to its normal position at the tip of the glans (any point along the course of the anterior urethra from the perineum to the tip of the glans). Abnormal urinary stream.

▶ Diagnosis
Clinical presentation.

▶ Disease Severity
Dependent on the location.

▶ Concept and Application
Failure of the urethral folds to fuse completely over the urethral groove.

▶ Treatment Steps
Surgical correction. Avoid circumcision (foreskin used in repair).

### B. Posterior Urethral Valves

▶ H&P Keys
Most common cause of anatomic bladder outlet obstruction in male children. Signs and symptoms include a poor urinary stream, dribbling, absence of voiding, abdominal distention, vomiting, and failure to thrive.

▶ Diagnosis
Voiding cystourethrogram.

▶ Disease Severity
Chronic renal failure. Hydronephrosis.

▶ Concept and Application
Mucosal folds obstruct the posterior urethra.

▶ Treatment Steps
Early surgical repair.

## C. Prune-belly Syndrome (Eagle-Barrett Syndrome)

▶ H&P Keys
Male infant with deficiency of the abdominal wall musculature, urinary tract abnormalities, and bilateral intra-abdominal testes. Associated with cardiopulmonary, GI, and orthopedic malformations. Signs and symptoms include marked laxity of the abdomen with bulging of the flanks.

▶ Diagnosis
Clinical presentation. Urologic evaluation. Renal ultrasonography (dilated urinary tract).

▶ Disease Severity
Urinary tract infection. End-stage renal disease.

▶ Concept and Application
Etiology unknown.

▶ Treatment Steps
1. Monitoring for urinary tract infections and signs of renal failure.
2. Correction of electrolyte imbalances.
3. Vitamin D supplementation (prevent hypocalcemia and renal osteodystrophy).

## D. Vesicoureteral Reflux

▶ H&P Keys
Often asymptomatic. May develop features of urinary tract infection (fever, vomiting, flank pain, dysuria, frequency, urgency, irritability).

▶ Diagnosis
Voiding cystourethrogram.

▶ Disease Severity
Renal scarring. Pyelonephritis.

▶ Concept and Application
Abnormal backflow of urine from the bladder into the ureters or kidneys. Increased incidence of reflux in siblings.

▶ Treatment Steps

Management depends on grade of reflux and the amount of renal scarring.

1. Medical management includes treatment of the urinary tract infection and prophylactic antibiotics.
2. Surgical correction of the anatomic defect if severe reflux or scarring.

### E. Infantile Polycystic Disease

▶ H&P Keys

Signs and symptoms include enlarged palpable kidneys, oliguria, and respiratory insufficiency in the neonate. Older infants may present with hepatosplenomegaly, flank masses, renal tubular acidosis, and hypertension.

▶ Diagnosis

Renal ultrasonography.

▶ Disease Severity

Renal insufficiency. Hypertension. Portal hypertension. Hepatic fibrosis. Variable cortical atrophy.

▶ Concept and Application

Bilateral renal cystic disease. Autosomal recessive inheritance.

▶ Treatment Steps

1. Treatment of hypertension.
2. Management of chronic renal failure.
3. Management of portal hypertension.

### F. Multicystic Kidney Disease

▶ H&P Keys

A unilateral, dysplastic, nonfunctioning kidney. Usually an asymptomatic abdominal mass.

▶ Diagnosis

Renal ultrasonography.

▶ Treatment Steps

1. Evaluation of renal function.
2. Monitoring.
3. Kidney not routinely removed.

### G. Undescended Testis

▶ H&P Keys

Nonpalpable testis.

▶ Diagnosis

Clinical exam. Ultrasonography (location of testis).

▶ Disease Severity

More prone to testicular torsion, malignant degeneration, and impaired fertility.

▶ Concept and Application
Result of mechanical hindrance, abnormal epididymal development, or endocrine dysfunction during fetal development.

▶ Treatment Steps
1. Surgical orchiopexy before 2 years of age.
2. Consider hormonal therapy.

## H. Bladder Extrophy

▶ H&P Keys
Externalization of the bladder and epispadias.

▶ Diagnosis
Clinical presentation.

▶ Disease Severity
Repair depends on the capacity of the bladder.

▶ Concept and Application
Failure of the abdominal wall to close inferior to the umbilicus with separation of the pubis symphysis. This anomaly leads to evulsion and protuberance of the posterior bladder wall.

▶ Treatment Steps
Surgery.

## IV. NEONATOLOGY

### A. Transient Tachypnea of the Newborn (TTN)

▶ H&P Keys
Mild self-limited respiratory disorder seen more frequently in infants born by cesarean section. Signs and symptoms include increased respiratory rate, mild cyanosis, and retractions.

▶ Diagnosis
Chest roentgenogram (CXR) shows prominent vascular markings with fluid in the fissures. Diagnosis of exclusion.

▶ Disease Severity
Respiratory rate. Cyanosis. ABG. Pulse oximetry.

▶ Concept and Application
Delayed resorption of fetal lung fluid.

▶ Treatment Steps
1. ABCs.
2. Supportive care.

## B. Respiratory Distress Syndrome

▶ H&P Keys

Incidence inversely proportional to the newborn's gestational age and birth weight. Signs and symptoms include respiratory distress (tachypnea, grunting, nasal flaring, retractions) soon after delivery.

▶ Diagnosis

CXR shows a fine reticular granularity of the lung fields and air bronchograms (Fig. 14–2). Must differentiate from other causes of respiratory distress in newborns (sepsis, heart disease, CNS disorders, lung anomalies).

▶ Disease Severity

ABG. Pulse oximetry. Hemoglobin. Metabolic disturbances. Cardiovascular compromise. Long-term complications include bronchopulmonary dysplasia (BPD), cor pulmonale, retinopathy of prematurity, poor growth, and persistent patent ductus arteriosus.

▶ Concept and Application

Secondary to lung immaturity (surfactant deficiency), incomplete structural lung development, and highly compliant chest wall. Results in atelectasis, hyaline membrane formation, and pulmonary edema.

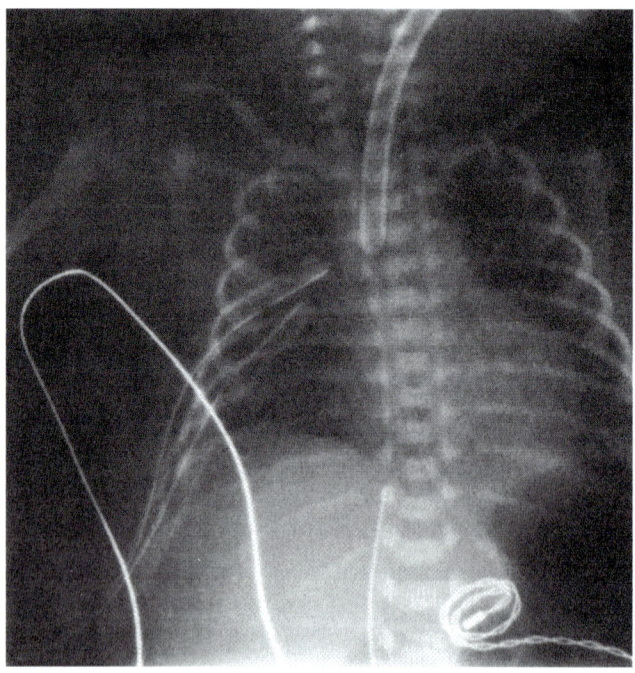

Figure 14–2. Respiratory distress syndrome. Radiographic study of a 2-week-old infant who was prematurely born at 23-week gestation. This neonate requires ventilator support for his persistent respiratory distress. The lung fields show a fine reticular granularity and air bronchograms. Two chest tubes noted in right lung field.

▶ Treatment Steps
1. Prevention of prematurity.
2. Maternal steroid administration 48–72 hours prior to delivery to stimulate fetal surfactant production.
3. Neonatal surfactant via endotracheal tube at delivery for premature infants (surfactant serves to reduce surface tension of the alveoli).
4. Supportive care (correction of hypoxia, acidosis, and hypercapnia).

## C. Meconium Aspiration

▶ H&P Keys

Presence of meconium in the amniotic fluid and the newborn's trachea. Signs and symptoms include retractions, increased respiratory rate, cyanosis, and hypoxia.

▶ Diagnosis

Clinical presentation. CXR.

▶ Disease Severity

Severe respiratory distress with increased respiratory rate, retractions, and hypoxia requiring ventilatory support. Pneumothorax. Pulmonary hypertension.

▶ Concept and Application

Aspiration of meconium-contaminated amniotic fluid leading to airway obstruction and poor gas exchange.

▶ Treatment Steps
1. Suctioning the infant on the perineum.
2. Direct visualization and suctioning of the trachea in distressed infants.
3. ABCs.
4. Chest physiotherapy.
5. Supplemental oxygen.
6. Mechanical ventilation if needed.

## D. Rh Incompatibility

▶ H&P Keys

Infant of a gravida 2 Rh-negative mother. Signs and symptoms include pallor, respiratory distress, cardiomegaly, edema.

▶ Diagnosis

Rh type, ABO group, Coombs' test (positive), hemoglobin, blood smear (hemolysis), reticulocyte count (increased), and bilirubin (increased).

▶ Disease Severity

Hydrops fetalis. Severe anemia leading to heart failure, ascites, pleural and pericardial effusions. Thrombocytopenia. Organomegaly. Elevated bilirubin leading to kernicterus (staining of the basal ganglia).

▶ Concept and Application

Sensitization and antibody formation in an Rh-negative mother exposed to Rh-positive fetal blood (contains D antigen). This antibody crosses the placenta causing hemolytic disease in the fetus. Rarely occurs during the first pregnancy.

▶ Treatment Steps

1. Supportive therapy, including volume expansion, red blood cell (RBC) transfusion, and ventilatory support if needed.
2. Exchange transfusion in extreme cases.
3. Prevention in Rh-negative mothers with the administration of $Rh_o(D)$ immune globulin (RhoGAM).

### E. Neonatal Hyperbilirubinemia

▶ H&P Keys

Signs and symptoms depend on the etiology. Ascertain a maternal history (blood type, race, illnesses during pregnancy, drug usage, family history of anemia), and an infant history (birth weight, onset of jaundice, stooling pattern, trauma, feeding pattern [breast-feeding], emesis).

▶ Diagnosis

Total and direct bilirubin (normal total levels rise to a mean of 6.5 ± 2.5 mg/dL in a full-term formula-fed infant). Hemoglobin, smear, reticulocyte count, maternal and infant blood type, direct Coombs' (evidence of hemolysis), albumin level. Urine Clinitest. Culture if sepsis is suspected.

▶ Disease Severity

Elevated bilirubin in the first 24 hours of life is pathologic. Kernicterus (bilirubin staining and necrosis of neurons in the basal ganglion) especially with hemolytic disease.

▶ Concept and Application

Physiologic jaundice is found in 60% of newborns with maximum values reached in the second to fourth day (6 to 8 mg/dL) as a result of inefficient bilirubin conjugation and excretion. Jaundice due to breast feeding reaches a maximum level of 7.3 ± 3.9 mg/dL. The etiology is unknown. Elevated levels of bilirubin also occur with increased turnover of RBCs from hemolysis (ABO or Rh incompatibility), significant bruising, cephalhematomas, structural or metabolic abnormalities of RBCs, or hereditary defects of bilirubin conjugation (Crigler–Najjar syndrome, Gilbert disease).

▶ Treatment Steps

1. Evaluation and treatment for underlying pathologic etiologies.
2. Encouragement of fluid intake.
3. Phototherapy with pathologically elevated bilirubin levels.
4. Exchange transfusion in severe cases.

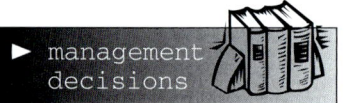

### ▶ management decisions

**Febrile Seizures**
ABC (airway, breathing, circulation); lorazepam (Ativan) or diazepam (Valium) for prolonged seizures; prophylactic anticonvulsants are controversial.

**Kawasaki Disease**
Intravenous gamma globulin; aspirin; cardiac evaluation (electrocardiogram, echocardiogram).

**Neonatal Hyperbilirubinemia**
Evaluation and treatment for underlying etiology; encouragement of fluid intake; phototherapy with pathologically elevated bilirubin levels; exchange transfusion in severe cases.

## F. Developmental Dysplasia of the Hip

▶ H&P Keys

A higher incidence with breech deliveries, first-born children, females, and oligohydramnios. Left hip more commonly involved. Twenty percent have a positive family history. Signs and symptoms include Barlow sign (posterosuperior movement of the femur over the limbus with adduction and posteriorly directed pressure), Ortolani sign (relocation of the hip with abduction, causing a dull clunk) (see Fig. 14–3), asymmetric leg lengths, and asymmetric thigh creases. A limitation of abduction is seen in older infants.

▶ Diagnosis

Clinical exam. Hip ultrasonogram. Radiography.

▶ Disease Severity

Three degrees of hip dysplasia in order of increasing severity: subluxable, dislocatable, dislocated. Can lead to avascular necrosis and decreased range of motion.

▶ Concept and Application

Multifactorial (mechanical, hormonal, and hereditary).

▶ Treatment Steps

1. Goal is to restore contact between the femoral head and the acetabulum.
2. Management depends on the degree of hip dysplasia and the age at diagnosis. Harness. Closed reduction (traction). Open reduction.

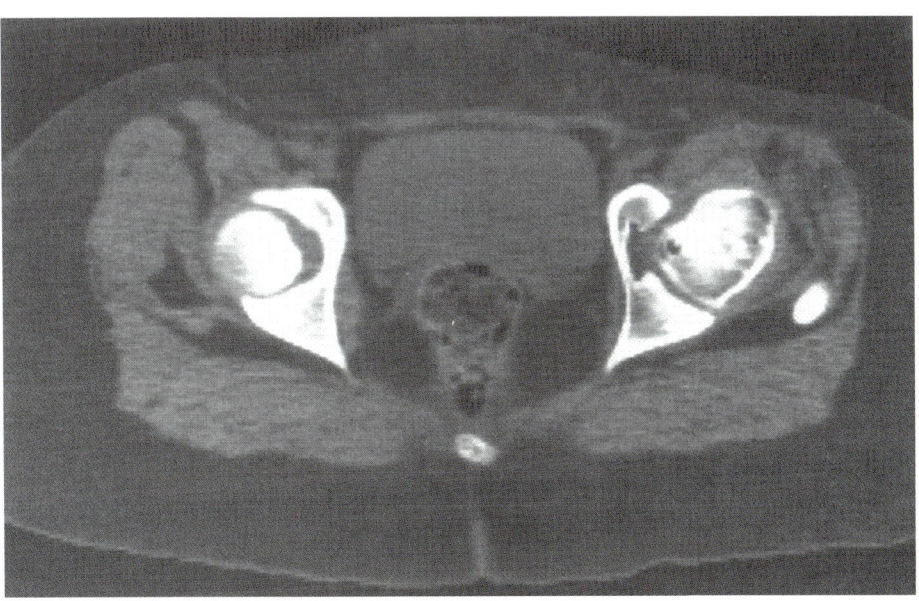

Figure 14–3. Developmental dysplasia of the hip (DDH). A hip ultrasound of a 3-week-old infant with a positive Ortolani sign (relocation of the hip with abduction) of the left hip. Dysplasia of the left acetabulum and head of the femur is visualized on sonography.

## V. INFECTIOUS DISEASES

### A. Bronchiolitis

▶ H&P Keys

Common (60% of infants). Winter-to-spring months. Peak age under 24 months. Signs and symptoms include cough, rhinorrhea, with or without low-grade fever, scattered wheezing with or without rales, labored breathing.

▶ Diagnosis

Clinical features (age, season, physical). Evaluation of nasopharyngeal secretions (viral culture, enzyme-linked immunosorbent assay, or immunofluorescence). CXR has nonspecific changes (hyperinflation, atelectasis, with or without interstitial infiltrates).

▶ Disease Severity

General appearance, mental status changes, labored breathing (tachypnea, nasal flaring, retractions, accessory muscle use), cyanosis, pulse oximetry, ABG if severe distress. Higher morbidity and mortality if infant has underlying pulmonary or cardiac disease, immunodeficiency disease, underlying chronic disease, history of prematurity, or is under 6 weeks old.

▶ Concept and Application

Viral infection (primary cause is respiratory syncytial virus) of lower respiratory tract. Transmission by direct contact. Respiratory mucosal injury, inflammation or edema, mucous production.

▶ Treatment Steps
1. Prevention by hand washing.
2. Supportive care including oxygen if hypoxic.
3. Aerosolized $\beta_2$-adrenergic agent trial.
4. Use of ribavirin and steroids controversial.

### B. Otitis Media

▶ H&P Keys

Peak age under 24 months. Winter season. Signs and symptoms include pain, fever, hearing loss, cough, and congestion as well as hyperemia, dullness, decreased mobility, retraction or bulging (loss of landmarks) of tympanic membrane. Asymptomatic in 50% of cases.

▶ Diagnosis

Pneumatic otoscopy. Tympanometry. Audiometry.

▶ Disease Severity

Overall appearance. Degree of discomfort or hearing loss. Response to therapy. Higher morbidity if young age (< 6 months), environmental setting (passive smoking, day care), genetic factors (familial, trisomy 21, Native American), immunodeficiency, congenital anomalies (cleft palate, choanal atresia).

▶ Concept and Application

Bacterial infection (usually *Streptococcus pneumoniae*, nontypable *Haemophilus influenzae*, *Moraxella catarrhalis*) of middle ear. Viral copathogens (40%). Often results from a dysfunctional eustachian tube.

▶ Treatment Steps
1. First-line antibiotics include aminopenicillins. [Amoxil]
2. Consider coverage for pneumococcal resistant organisms in high risk groups (eg, day care, age < 2 years, recent antibiotic use).
3. Consider prophylactic antibiotics if recurrent episodes (≥ 3 bouts in 6 months, ≥ 4 in 12 months) although concern of resistant organisms.
4. Consider myringotomy tubes if persistent effusion with hearing loss, failure of prophylaxis, or high-risk groups (eg, trisomy 21, cleft palate, known sensorineural hearing loss).

## C. Epiglottitis (Supraglottitis)

▶ H&P Keys

Ages 2–7 years if unvaccinated. Winter months. Signs and symptoms include acute hyperpyrexia (39°C), hoarseness, drooling, dysphagia, anxious or toxic appearance, stridor, and respiratory distress. Rare in vaccinated children.

▶ Diagnosis

Clinical presentation (high index of suspicion!). Lateral neck radiograph (thumb-shaped epiglottis, ballooning of hypopharynx) only if presentation not classical. Cultures of epiglottis and blood after airway secured.

▶ Disease Severity

Overall appearance. Mental status changes. Respiratory distress (tachypnea, inspiratory stridor, retractions, cyanosis). Hypoxia and hypercapnia.

▶ Concept and Application

Edema or cellulitis of epiglottis resulting in glottic narrowing. Primarily *Haemophilus influenzae* type b (> 90%).

▶ Treatment Steps
1. Prevention is key.
2. Early suspicion.
3. ABCs.
4. Minimal disturbance to child.
5. Direct visualization and culture of epiglottis in operating room followed by intubation.
6. Emergent cricothyrotomy if complete airway obstruction.

## D. Laryngotracheitis (Croup)

▶ H&P Keys

Ages 6–36 months. Nocturnal. Severity of disease peaks at 3–5 days. Signs and symptoms include barklike cough, hoarseness, upper respiratory symptoms, inspiratory stridor.

▶ Diagnosis

Clinical presentation. Steeple sign (subglottic swelling) on CXR.

▶ Disease Severity

Overall appearance. Mental status changes. Respiratory distress. Hypoxia and hypercapnia.

▶ Concept and Application

Mucosal edema and swelling of subglottis and trachea leading to hypoxia and atelectasis. Primarily caused by parainfluenza virus.

▶ Treatment Steps

1. Supportive (especially airway).
2. Minimal disturbance.
3. Mist.
4. Oxygen if hypoxemia.
5. Racemic epinephrine or dexamethasone if severe respiratory distress.

### E. Varicella (Chickenpox)

▶ H&P Keys

Intubation period of 14–15 days. Winter or spring months. Contagious period is 4–5 days prior to exanthem and until rash scabs. Signs and symptoms include fever, malaise, vesicles with erythematous base ("teardrop on rose petal") beginning on hairline or trunk and spreading to extremities.

▶ Diagnosis

Characteristic rash. Fluorescein monoclonal antibody.

▶ Disease Severity

Worse course if under 1 year of age, teenager or adult, or visceral involvement (lungs, CNS, liver, joints, heart, kidneys).

▶ Concept and Application

Human herpes varicella-zoster virus. Respiratory (direct contact) transmission. Cutaneous tissue involvement after primary or secondary viremia. Life-long immunity after infection.

▶ Treatment Steps

1. Prevention is key (varicella vaccine).
2. Antipruritic drug.
3. Antimicrobial therapy if secondary infection (usually group A streptococcus).
4. Acyclovir if child is immunocompromised, older, or severely involved.

### F. Pharyngitis

▶ H&P Keys

Signs and symptoms include fever, sore throat, hoarseness, cough, abdominal pain, tonsillar erythema or enlargement or exudate, petechiae of palate, anterior cervical adenopathy, "sandpaper" rash. Concomitant nasal symptoms suggest viral etiology.

▶ Diagnosis
Throat culture. Rapid streptococcus antigen test.

▶ Disease Severity
Clinical discomfort. Suppurative complications (cervical adenitis, otitis media, septicemia). Nonsuppurative complications (rheumatic fever, nephritis).

▶ Concept and Application
Cellulitis of pharynx and tonsils. Organisms include group A β-hemolytic streptococci, adenovirus, influenza virus, Epstein–Barr virus.

▶ Treatment Steps
1. Self-limiting if viral etiology.
2. Penicillin (erythromycin if penicillin allergy) for 10 days if group A β-hemolytic streptococci.

### G. Bacterial Meningitis

▶ H&P Keys
Signs and symptoms include fever, lethargy, irritability, neck stiffness or pain, headache, altered consciousness, nuchal rigidity, Kernig's sign, Brudzinski's sign.

▶ Diagnosis
Bacterial culture of CSF is gold standard. CSF cytology and biochemical parameters. Bacterial antigen test if child currently on antibiotics.

▶ Disease Severity
Mental status change. Focal or persistent neurologic deficit. Syndrome of inappropriate secretion of antidiuretic hormone (SIADH). Neonatal infection. Focal or late-onset seizures. Long-term sequelae include learning disability, hearing impairment, seizure disorders.

▶ Concept and Application
Primarily hematogenous spread to CSF. *S. pneumoniae* and *Neisseria meningitidis,* are usual pathogens in childhood (group B streptococcus, *Escherichia coli,* or other gram-negative enteric bacilli, *Listeria monocytogenes* in neonates).

▶ Treatment Steps
1. Age-specific antibiotics pending cultures. Respiratory isolation.
2. Identification and treatment of associated complications if necessary.
3. Prevention (vaccine, treatment of carrier state).
4. Consider dexamethasone in infants > 6 weeks.

### H. Congenital Infections (STORCH)

#### 1. Congenital Syphilis

▶ H&P Keys
Characteristic features include skin rash (palms and soles), hepatosplenomegaly, snuffles (blood-tinged nasal discharge), Par-

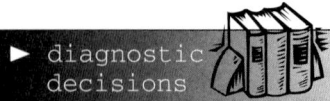

### diagnostic decisions

#### CONGENITAL INFECTIONS (STORCH)

**Syphilis**
*Treponena pallidum*; snuffles, palm and sole rash, anemia, hepatosplenomegaly, periostitis, peg teeth, saddle nose; prescription penicillin.

**Toxoplasmosis**
*Toxoplasma gondii*; oocysts from cat litter and meat; hydrocephalus, chorioretinitis, scattered CNS calcifications; prescription pyrimethamine.

**Other**
HIV, hepatitis B, varicella.

**Rubella**
Blueberry muffin lesions, hepatosplenomegaly, anemia, cardiac lesions, deafness, cataracts.

**Cytomegalovirus**
Most common congenital infection; usually asymptomatic; hepatosplenomegaly, jaundice, deafness, microcephaly, perventricular CNS calcifications.

**Herpes Simplex**
Usually acquired at birth; seizures (temporal lobe); encephalitis, vesicles, overwhelming sepsis, hepatitis; prescription acyclovir.

---

rot's pseudoparalysis (periostitis), saber shins, Hutchinson (peg) teeth, thrombocytopenia, anemia, jaundice, saddle nose, hepatitis.

▶ **Diagnosis**
Serology (rapid plasma reagin [RPR], fluorescent treponemal antibody absorption [FTA-ABS]), darkfield examination (organism).

▶ **Concept and Application**
Spirochete (*Treponema pallidum*).

▶ **Treatment Steps**
1. Prevention.
2. Prenatal screening.
3. Penicillin for all infected mothers and infants with positive serology without documented adequate treatment.

### 2. Congenital Toxoplasmosis

▶ **H&P Keys**
Characteristic features include chorioretinitis, scattered CNS calcifications, hydrocephalus, developmental delay.

▶ **Diagnosis**
Serology (organism isolation).

▶ **Concept and Application**
Intracellular protozoan parasite (*Toxoplasma gondii*).

▶ **Treatment Steps**
1. Prevention (avoid cat litter and undercooked meat).
2. Multidisciplinary approach.
3. Pyrimethamine and/or sulfadiazine have variable effectiveness.

### 3. Human Immunodeficiency Virus (HIV)

▶ **H&P Keys**
One third of infants of HIV-positive mothers will develop AIDS. Presentation variable (eg, frequent infections, developmental or growth delay, lymphadenopathy, persistent thrush).

▶ **Diagnosis**
1. Polymerase chain reaction (PCR) useful in diagnosis and viral load detection.
2. Serology.

▶ **Concept and Application**
Human retrovirus that infects tissue cells (including helper T cells).

▶ **Treatment Steps**
Azidothymidine (AZT). Antimicrobial therapy for infections. Poor prognosis.

1. Prevention is key.
2. Treatment of infected pregnant women has decreased the incidence of vertical transmission.

3. Antiretroviral drugs and immunomodulators.
4. Vaccines are under investigation.

4. Congenital Rubella Infection (German Measles)

▶ H&P Keys

Characteristic features include intrauterine growth retardation (IUGR), congenital cardiac defects, cataracts, deafness, thrombocytopenia, "blueberry muffin" skin lesions, hepatosplenomegaly.

▶ Diagnosis

Serology (organism isolation).

▶ Concept and Application

Multiorgan damage by the virus.

▶ Treatment Steps

1. Prevention is key (rubella vaccine).
2. Prenatal screening.
3. Multidisciplinary approach.

5. Congenital Cytomegalovirus Infection (CMV)

▶ H&P Keys

Majority of cases are asymptomatic. Characteristic features include jaundice, hepatosplenomegaly, microcephaly, chorioretinitis, deafness, periventricular CNS calcification, IUGR.

▶ Diagnosis

Organism isolation (serology).

▶ Concept and Application

Herpes virus. Multiorgan involvement. Transmission with primary or recurrent maternal infection.

▶ Treatment Steps

1. Prevention by handwashing.
2. Multidisciplinary approach.
3. Antiviral treatment controversial.

6. Herpes Simplex Virus

▶ H&P Keys

Incidence of HSV: 1 in 5,000 deliveries. Characteristic features include vesicular skin rash, chorioretinitis, meningoencephalitis, seizures, microcephaly.

▶ Diagnosis

Organism isolation (Tzanck test, immunofluorescent studies).

▶ Concept and Application

HSV-2 (70%). Transmission more likely during primary maternal infection.

▶ Treatment Steps

1. Antiviral (acyclovir) therapy.
2. Supportive care.

## I. Hemolytic Uremic Syndrome

▶ H&P Keys

Children usually between 2 months and 8 years of age. Triad of uremia, thrombocytopenia, and microangiopathic hemolytic anemia. Signs and symptoms include preceding illness (diarrhea or upper respiratory infection [URI]), irritability, bloody diarrhea, poor urinary output, pallor, petechiae, edema, hypertension.

▶ Diagnosis

CBC with platelets and smear (RBC morphology). Coombs' test (negative). Electrolytes.

▶ Disease Severity

Seizures, stroke, coma, cardiac failure, metabolic imbalance (metabolic acidosis).

▶ Concept and Application

No one causative factor (viral, bacterial, drugs). Peripheral destruction of platelets. RBC hemolysis secondary to mechanical destruction by fibrin strands in small renal vessels.

▶ Treatment Steps
1. Supportive care.
2. Correction of fluid and electrolyte imbalance.
3. Correction of hypertension.
4. Dialysis and RBC transfusion if needed.

## VI. GASTROENTEROLOGY

### A. Cleft Lip or Palate

▶ H&P Keys

Common (1/1,000 live births). Family history.

▶ Diagnosis

Clinical.

▶ Disease Severity

Feeding problems. Frequent ear infections. Speech problems. Associated with many anomalies.

▶ Concept and Application

Failure of primary (lip) and secondary (cleft) palate closure. Multifactorial inheritance (3–5% recurrence with an affected parent or sibling; 10% if two affected parents or siblings).

▶ Treatment Steps
1. Multidisciplinary approach.
2. Surgical repair.

## B. Tracheoesophageal Fistula (TEF)

▶ H&P Keys

Signs and symptoms of TEF include excessive oral secretions, coughing or choking on foods, tachypnea, wheezing, rales.

▶ Diagnosis

Inability to pass nasal catheter to stomach. Surgical exploration. Barium studies rarely needed.

▶ Disease Severity

Respiratory distress. Signs and symptoms of aspiration pneumonia.

▶ Concept and Application

Failure of trachea and esophagus to separate during embryogenesis. Proximal esophageal atresia with a tracheal-to-distal esophageal fistula is most common type (85%).

▶ Treatment Steps
1. Surgery.

## C. Pyloric Stenosis

▶ H&P Keys

Average age 3–4 weeks of life. First-born males. Signs and symptoms include progressive nonbilious projectile emesis, peristaltic abdominal waves in epigastrium, palpable right upper quadrant mass ("olive").

▶ Diagnosis

Clinical. Sonogram or upper GI (UGI) series ("tram-track" sign) if necessary. Hypochloremic hypokalemic metabolic alkalosis.

▶ Disease Severity

Cachexia. Profound dehydration. Severe metabolic imbalance.

▶ Concept and Application

Mechanical gastric outlet obstruction results from congenitally hypertrophied pyloric muscle.

▶ Treatment Steps
1. Correction of fluid and electrolyte abnormality.
2. Surgical repair (pyloromyotomy).

## D. Malrotation of the Small Intestine

▶ H&P Keys

Bilious projectile emesis. Abdominal distention.

▶ Diagnosis

Clinical. Barium study.

▶ Disease Severity

Melena (secondary to intestinal ischemia). Sepsis. Signs and symptoms of peritonitis or perforation.

► Concept and Application
Mechanical obstruction from either poor fixation of cecum to abdominal wall (midgut volvulus or twisting) or extrinsic bands.

► Treatment Steps
Surgery (15–20% mortality rate).

### E. Intussusception

► H&P Keys
Most common cause of intestinal obstruction ages 3–12 months. Signs and symptoms include intermittent colicky pain, bilious emesis, mental status changes, palpable "sausage-shaped" abdominal mass, "currant jelly" stools (Fig 14–4).

► Diagnosis
Clinical. Barium enema.

► Disease Severity
Severe metabolic acidosis. Evidence of intestinal ischemia or infarction. Severe dehydration.

► Concept and Application
Invagination or telescoping of proximal bowel into more distal bowel. Lymphatic and venous compromise. Primarily ileocolic region. Leadpoint lesion (eg, polyp, lymphoma) in older children.

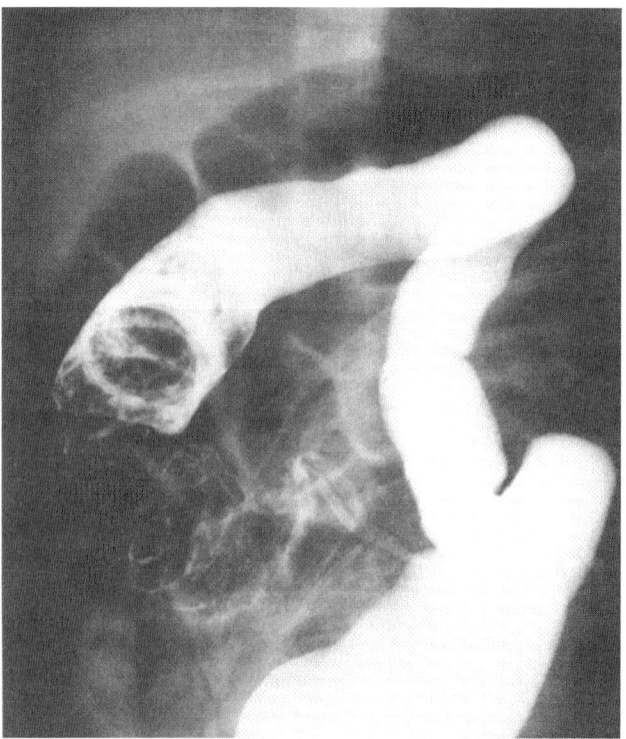

Figure 14–4. Intussusception. Barium enema of a 4-month-infant with intermittent colicky pain, pallor, poor tone, and a palpable "sausage-shaped" abdominal mass. The contrast material did not descend into the ileocecal region. The diagnosis was confirmed during an explorative laparoscopy.

▶ Treatment Steps
1. Barium enema reduction.
2. Antibiotics if peritoneal signs.
3. Occasionally surgical reduction.

### F. Necrotizing Enterocolitis (NEC)

▶ H&P Keys

Characteristic features of NEC include prematurity (75%), poor feeding or regurgitation, emesis, hematochezia, temperature instability, gastric retention, abdominal distention with decreased bowel sounds.

▶ Diagnosis

Clinical. Blood or reducing substances in stool. Thrombocytopenia. Prolonged prothrombin time (PT) and partial thromboplastin time (PTT). Pneumatosis intestinalis, bowel wall edema, biliary air, or free air in peritoneum on abdominal radiograph.

▶ Disease Severity

Evidence of sepsis, hemorrhage, disseminated intravascular coagulation (DIC), shock, severe metabolic acidosis, mental status changes.

▶ Concept and Application

Unknown. Presentation consistent with bowel ischemia or infarction.

▶ Treatment Steps
1. Bowel rest.
2. Fluid resuscitation.
3. Parenteral nutrition.
4. Broad-spectrum antibiotics.
5. Surgery if failure of medical management or if complications.

### G. Colonic Aganglionosis (Hirschsprung Disease)

▶ H&P Keys

Absence of meconium stools in first week of life. Signs and symptoms include emesis, abdominal distention, minimal stool in rectal vault.

▶ Diagnosis

Clinical. Rectal biopsy. Barium study in older children (Fig. 14–5).

▶ Disease Severity

Presentation can simulate sepsis or NEC.

▶ Concept and Application

Absence of colonic ganglia resulting in persistent colonic contraction.

▶ Treatment Steps

Surgery.

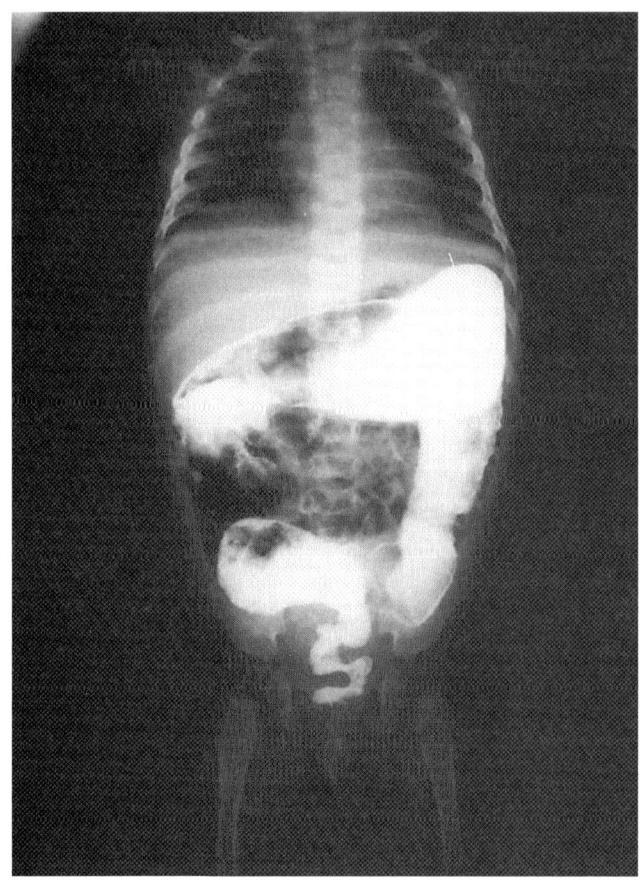

Figure 14–5. Hirschsprung's disease. Barium enema of a 4-day-old infant with abdominal distention, green emesis, a tight rectum, and an explosive liquid stool following the rectal examination. The lumen of the rectum is contracted with proximal colonic dilatation, suggesting congenital aganglionosis. The diagnosis was confirmed with a rectal biopsy.

## VII. GENETICS

### A. Down Syndrome (Trisomy 21)

▶ H&P Keys

Characteristic features include epicanthal folds, upslanting palpebral fissures, transverse palmar (simian) creases, cardiac anomalies (40%) including septal defects, atlantoaxial instability (12%), duodenal atresia (4–7%), short stature, leukemia (1%), thyroid disease, sterility in males, early Alzheimer's disease, shortened lifespan (Fig. 14–6).

▶ Diagnosis

Clinical. Chromosome analysis (classical trisomy [95%], translocation [4%], mosaic [1%]). Prenatal screening (amniocentesis, chorionic villus sampling) in high-risk groups (advanced maternal age).

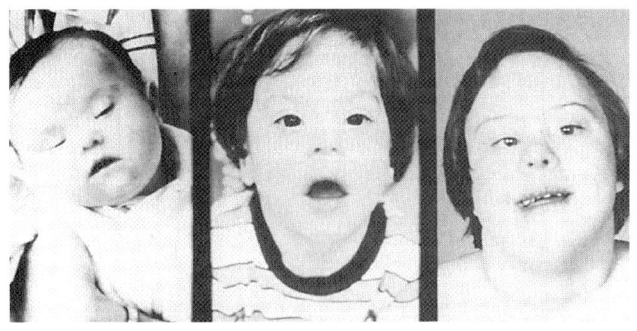

Figure 14–6. Typical phenotype in Down syndrome.

▶ Treatment Steps
1. Supportive care.
2. Cardiac evaluation.
3. Correction of anomalies.
4. Genetic counseling.
5. Special education.

## B. Trisomy 18

▶ H&P Keys
Characteristic features include IUGR, micrognathia, clenched hands with overlapping fingers, congenital heart disease (ventricular septal defect [VSD], patent ductus arteriosus [PDA]), mental retardation.

▶ Diagnosis
Clinical. Chromosome analysis.

▶ Treatment Steps
Same as for trisomy 21.

## C. Trisomy 13

▶ H&P Keys
Characteristic features include cleft lip or palate (60–80%), microcephaly, urinary tract malformations, CNS and ocular malformations, aplasia cutis congenita, polydactyly.

▶ Diagnosis
Clinical. Chromosome analysis.

▶ Treatment Steps
Same as for trisomy 21.

## D. Gonadal Dysgenesis 45,XO (Turner Syndrome)

▶ H&P Keys
Characteristic features include transient lymphedema of feet and hands at birth (80–90%), short stature, short webbed neck, short fourth metacarpal bone, cardiac defects (coarctation of aorta), re-

---

▶ diagnostic decisions

### CHROMOSOMAL ABNORMALITIES

**Trisomy 21**
Down syndrome; 1/700 births; mental retardation, cardiac (AV canal), duodenal atresia, simian creases, epicanthal folds.

**Trisomy 13**
Poor prognosis; 1/10,000 births; cleft lip/palate, CNS malformations (holoprosencephaly), renal and ocular malformations.

**Trisomy 18**
Poor prognosis; 1/5,000 births; IUGR, clenched hands, rocker-bottom feet, cardiac (VSD, PDA).

**5P**
Cri-du-chat; cat-like cry, mental retardation, microcephaly.

**45,XO**
Turner syndrome; 1/2,000 newborn girls; short webbed neck, horseshoe kidney, coarctation of aorta, primary amenorrhea.

**47,XXY**
Klinefelter syndrome; 1/1,000 boys, seminiferous tubule dysgenesis, hypogonadism, tall stature, gynecomastia, infertility.

nal anomalies (horseshoe kidney), lack of secondary sex characteristics with primary amenorrhea. Normal intelligence. Most spontaneously abort in early pregnancy.

▶ Diagnosis

Clinical. Chromosome analysis.

▶ Treatment Steps
1. Evaluation for and correction of anomalies.
2. Psychosocial counseling.
3. Estrogen replacement at puberty.
4. Consider growth hormone therapy.

### E. Fragile X Syndrome

▶ H&P Keys

Characteristic features include mental retardation (MR), hyperactivity, seizures, prominent ears, long face, macro-orchidism. Common cause of MR in males (1/1,000).

▶ Diagnosis

Chromosome analysis with fragile X studies.

▶ Treatment Steps
1. Genetic counseling.
2. Supportive.

## VIII. PULMONOLOGY

### A. Congenital Laryngeal Stridor (Laryngomalacia)

▶ H&P Keys

Signs and symptoms include noisy "crowing" respirations (positional) and stridor.

▶ Diagnosis

Clinical. Fluoroscopy or direct visualization.

▶ Disease Severity

Respiratory distress (tachypnea, retractions, poor air movement).

▶ Concept and Application

Delayed maturation of newborn larynx, resulting in increased flexibility.

▶ Treatment Steps

Positioning (self-limited).

### B. Congenital Lobar Emphysema

▶ H&P Keys

Most common congenital lung lesion. Respiratory distress in early infancy.

▶ Diagnosis
Chest radiograph (radiolucent lobe, mediastinal shift). Mimics pneumothorax.

▶ Disease Severity
Severe respiratory distress or cyanosis.

▶ Concept and Application
In utero bronchial obstruction with normal alveolar histology. Usually unilateral.

▶ Treatment Steps
Surgical resection.

### C. Cystic Adenomatoid Malformation

▶ H&P Keys
Respiratory distress in infancy.

▶ Diagnosis
Chest radiograph (mediastinal shift, multiple cystic areas). Mimics diaphragmatic hernia.

▶ Concept and Application
Early embryonic insult with cysts and little normal lung tissue.

▶ Treatment Steps
Surgical resection. Significant mortality and morbidity.

### D. Pulmonary Sequestration

▶ H&P Keys
Fever, hemoptysis, and respiratory symptoms if intralobar. Respiratory symptoms, heart failure, or no symptoms if extralobar. Dullness to percussion. Heart murmur.

▶ Diagnosis
CXR (mass). Further investigation includes bronchoscopy, sonogram, and aortogram.

▶ Concept and Application
Segments of nonfunctioning embryonic lung tissue that are nourished by anomalous systemic circulation. Intralobar type occurs within normal visceral pleura. Extralobar type has separate visceral pleural covering.

▶ Treatment Steps
Surgical resection.

## IX. SKIN CONDITIONS

### A. Acne

▶ Description
Increased sebum production in follicles. *Propionibacterium acnes* bacteria uses sebum to attract a white blood cell response, leading to local inflammatory reaction.

▶ Diagnoses
Comedo-hyperkeratosis of follicular epithelium. Whiteheads are closed comedones; blackheads are open comedones containing melanin.
   Cystic acne evolves from nodules to erythematous papules (pimples) to pus filled papules (pustules).

▶ Treatment
Goal is to reduce sebum production and decrease bacterial activity. Comedolytic and antikeratolytic agents include topical retinoic acid and benzoyl peroxide. Antibacterial agents consist of topical or systemic antibiotics.

### B. Fungal Infections

▶ Description
The second most common skin infection in adolescents. Common organisms include *Microsporum, Trichophyton, Epidermophyton,* and *Pitryrosporon*. Can infect the body (tinea corporis), the groin (tinea cruris), the feet (tinea pedis), or the head (tinea corporis).

▶ Diagnoses
Clinical appearance. Can also examine scraped specimen under a microscope or obtaining fungal cultures.

▶ Treatment
Topical antifungals for weeks of therapy. Tinea capitis requries the use of systemic antifungal.

## X. DISORDERS OF MUSCULOSKELETAL SYSTEM

### A. Scoliosis

▶ Description
A lateral curvature of the spine involving the thoracic and/or lumbar vertebrae.

▶ Diagnosis
Clinical evaluation of patient's back in an erect and a bent-at-the-hips position. Radiographs can quantitate any curvature > 10 degrees.

▶ Treatment

Depends on severity of curvature. Follow curves < 15–20 degrees closely at interval health maintenance visits. If curvature is > 20 degrees, the patient should be referred to an orthopedic surgeon for additional therapy, which may include bracing or surgical intervention.

## B. Kyphosis

▶ Description

An excessive roundback of the thoracic spine.

▶ Diagnosis

Physical examination. Radiography may be used to differentiate a postural and structural defect.

▶ Treatment

Improvement of posture, back exercises, braces.

## C. Slipped Capital Femoral Epiphysis

▶ Description

Posterior-medial displacement of femoral head. Occurs most frequently in males and is associated with obesity.

▶ Diagnosis

History significant for pain in hip or knee region. Radiograph of the hip shows femoral head displacement.

▶ Treatment

Surgical intervention required.

## D. Osgood–Schlatter Disease

▶ Description

Stress changes at the tibial tuberosity. Most commonly seen in adolescent males during growth spurt.

▶ Diagnosis

Clinical. Point tenderness at tibial tuberosity with occasional associated swelling.

▶ Treatment

Supportive.

## E. Osteochondritis Dissecans

▶ Description

Separation of bone from cartilage in the medial or lateral femoral condyle. Typically occurring in males and most cases unilateral. Associated with recurrent, diffuse knee pain.

▶ Diagnosis

Radiography reveals separation of bone.

▶ Treatment

Casting for mild cases; most require surgical repair.

### F. Chondromalacia Patellae

▶ Description

Patellar cartilage destruction resulting from instability of the patella. Most common cause of knee pain in women, worse with increased activity.

▶ Diagnosis

Clinical with evidence of patellar displacement with knee extention.

▶ Treatment

Supportive including rest, pain control, and improvement of muscle tone.

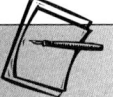

▶ on rounds

**PEDIATRIC INFECTIONS**

**Croup**
- Ages 6–36 months, also termed *laryngotracheitis*.
- Bark-like cough, hoarseness, inspiratory stridor, CXR positive Steeple sign (subglottic swelling).
- Worse at night.
- Supportive treatment, mist, $O_2$.

**Epiglottitis**
- Ages 2–7.
- Fever, drooling, dysphagia, stridor, may have abnormal lateral neck roentgenogram, possible toxic appearance, anxious.
- Winter most often.
- Support airway, visualization in OR followed by intubation.

**Bronchiolitis**
- Peak age under 2.
- Cough, wheezing, labored breathing, nonspecific CXR.
- Winter to spring occurrence.
- Supportive treatment.

## BIBLIOGRAPHY

Avery GB. *Neonatology: Pathophysiology and Management of the Newborn*. 5th ed. Philadelphia: Lippincott Williams & Wilkins; 1999.

Behrman RE, Kliegman RM, Jenson HB. *Nelson Textbook of Pediatrics*. 16th ed. Philadelphia: WB Saunders Co; 2000.

Burg FD, Ingelfinger JR, Polin RA, Gershon AA. *Gellis & Kagan's Current Pediatric Therapy*. 17th ed. Philadelphia: WB Saunders Co; 2002.

McMillan JA, DeAngelis CD, Feigin RD, Warshaw JB. *Oski's Pediatrics Principles & Practice*. 3rd ed. Philadelphia: Lippincott Williams & Wilkins; 1999.

# Psychiatry 15

I. **PSYCHOSES** / 453
- A. Schizophrenia / 453
- B. Affective Psychoses: Mania and Psychotic Depression / 454
- C. Delusional Disorder / 456
- D. Other Psychoses / 456
- E. Psychoses Originating in Childhood / 458

II. **MOOD DISORDERS** / 459
- A. Major (Unipolar) Depression / 459
- B. Dysthymia / 460
- C. Bipolar Disorders / 461
- D. Cyclothymia / 462

II. **ANXIETY DISORDERS** / 462
- A. Panic Disorder / 462
- B. Generalized Anxiety Disorder / 464
- C. Obsessive–Compulsive Disorder / 464
- D. Posttraumatic Stress Disorder (PTSD) / 465
- E. Acute Stress Disorder / 466
- F. Phobias / 466

IV. **ADJUSTMENT DISORDERS** / 467

V. **PERSONALITY DISORDERS (AXIS II)** / 468
- A. Odd, Eccentric / 468
- B. Dramatic, Emotional / 468
- C. Anxious, Fearful, Inhibited / 468

VI. **SOMATOFORM DISORDERS** / 469
- A. Somatization Disorder / 469
- B. Pain Disorder / 470
- C. Conversion Disorder / 471

      D. Hypochondriasis / 471
      E. Body Dysmorphic Disorder / 472
      F. Related Disorders / 472

**VII. ATTENTION DEFICIT/HYPERACTIVITY DISORDER (ADHD) / 472**

**VIII. CONDUCT DISORDER / 473**

**IX. EATING DISORDERS / 474**
      A. Anorexia Nervosa / 474
      B. Bulimia Nervosa / 475

**X. SUBSTANCE-RELATED DISORDERS / 477**
      A. Overview / 477
      B. Alcohol Dependence / 478
      C. Other Alcohol Syndromes / 479
      D. Drug Dependence / 480

**XI. SEXUAL DYSFUNCTIONS / 484**

**XII. DELIRIUM / 485**

**XIII. ABUSE SYNDROMES / 486**
      A. Child Physical and Sexual Abuse / 486
      B. Adult Domestic Violence / 487
      C. Elder Abuse / 488

**XIV. BEREAVEMENT / 488**
      A. Uncomplicated Bereavement / 488
      B. Sudden Infant Death Syndrome / 489

**BIBLIOGRAPHY / 489**

# I. PSYCHOSES

## A. Schizophrenia

### ▶ H&P Keys

*History*—Family history; onset most often late teens through twenties, often triggered by stressful situation; increased in lower socioeconomic groups; may have premorbid schizotypal features; symptom duration at least 6 months.

*Physical and Mental Status Exam*—Hallucinations, delusions, disorganized speech, bizarre behavior (positive symptoms); agitated, constricted, and/or inappropriate affect, social withdrawal, poor self-care, anhedonia, poverty of speech, lack of motivation, attentional impairment (negative symptoms); may have soft neurologic signs, motoric abnormalities.

### ▶ Diagnosis

No pathognomonic signs or lab studies; rule out general medical etiology (eg, substance abuse, temporal lobe epilepsy, delirium, medications, central nervous system [CNS] infections, trauma, tumors, endocrine and metabolic disorders); psychotic affective, schizophreniform, schizoaffective, delusional, personality disorders; obtain complete history, physical and neurologic exams, routine labs (including complete blood count, electrolytes, renal and liver function tests), thyroid function tests (TFTs), serology, human immunodeficiency virus (HIV), toxicology, $B_{12}$, folate; electroencephalogram (EEG), brain imaging indicated with first episode, unusual presentation (eg, older age, rapid onset of new symptoms, visual or olfactory hallucinations, clouded sensorium, catatonia, focal neurologic signs).

### ▶ Disease Severity

Worse prognosis with poor premorbid social history, early onset, insidious onset, lack of insight, nonparanoid subtype, absence of mood symptoms, neurologic abnormalities, male gender, negative symptoms, brain imaging abnormalities. Course is variable. Early treatment of psychosis improves prognosis. Exacerbations associated with medication noncompliance (50% in first year), high levels of criticism and hostility in families ("expressed emotion"). Increased risk for medical illness, incarceration, violence, substance use, victimization, poverty, suicide (10–15%).

### ▶ Concept and Application

Dopamine hypothesis: Schizophrenia associated with altered dopaminergic activity in the mesolimbic and mesocortical tracts. Antipsychotic efficacy of "typical" neuroleptics is a function of dopamine receptor blockade. Newer "atypical" neuroleptics also affect serotonin and other receptors. Negative symptoms associated with enlargement of cerebral ventricles and cortical atrophy. Functional neuroimaging demonstrates hypofrontality. Twin and adoption studies support both (polygenic) genetic and environmental contributions.

---

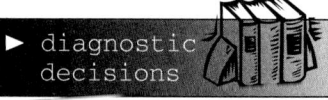

▶ diagnostic decisions

**PSYCHOSIS**

**Mood Disorders**
Bipolar, unipolar, schizoaffective—40%.

**Drug-induced States**
Withdrawal delirium, intoxication—25%.

**Schizophrenia**
Spectrum disorders—5–10%.

**Neurologic Disease**
Epilepsy, head trauma, CVA, dementia (especially subcortical), basal ganglia disease, delirium, masses, infection, others—20–25%.

Modified from Taylor, MA, *The Fundamentals of Clinical Neuropsychiatry*, New York: Oxford University Press, 1999, p. 264.

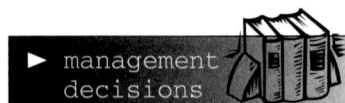

### management decisions

**ACUTE PSYCHOSIS**

**Maintain Safety, Manage Agitation/Arousal**
Calming environment and staff behavior. "Show of force" if necessary. Benzodiazepine, eg, lorazepam 2 mg PO or IM and/or neuroleptic, eg, haloperidol 5 mg PO or IM given q 30–60 min until patient is calm. Seclusion, restraint only if necessary after previous interventions.

**Identify Serious Medical Problems**
History, vital signs, physical exam. Review all medications (prescribed, over-the-counter, borrowed). Drug and alcohol screen, CBC, chemistries, LFTs, TFTs, brain imaging for first or atypical presentations, abnormal neuro exam.

**Assessment and Tentative Diagnosis**
Further treatment dictated by diagnostic category.

▶ Treatment Steps

*Acute*

1. Hospitalization for stabilization, protection of self and others (may require involuntary commitment).
2. Benzodiazepines and antipsychotics for acute agitation.
3. Rule out general medical, substance-induced etiologies.
4. Antipsychotic medication: "atypicals" (olanzapine, risperidone, quetiapine) may have fewer side effects and treat negative symptoms better than older antipsychotics. Require 4–6 weeks for full effect. Clozapine indicated for refractory symptoms (weekly complete blood count [CBC] to rule out agranulocylosis).

*Continued Care*

1. Continuation of antipsychotics (oral or long-acting intramuscular) reduces relapse rate.
2. Assess for development of side effects, eg, tardive dyskinesia (5% incidence per year with older antipsychotics); anticholinergic effects, sexual dysfunction, weight gain, sedation, hypotension, extrapyramidal symptoms.
3. Addition of lithium, anticonvulsants may benefit some.
4. Psychosocial treatments, including patient and family education, social skills training, residential and day treatment, vocational rehabilitation, supportive psychotherapy, contribute independently to outcome.

B. **Affective Psychoses: Mania and Psychotic Depression**

▶ H&P Keys

*History*—Personal and family history of affective disorder; clinical features of mood disorders that have been present preceding psychosis; illness course generally episodic rather than continuous; alcohol and drug abuse common.

*Physical and Mental Status Exam*—Mania: hyperactivity, rapid and pressured speech, flight of ideas, elated or irritable affect with lability, decreased need for sleep, distractibility, impulsivity, poor judgment. Forty percent have psychotic symptoms, eg, grandiose or paranoid delusions. Depression: psychomotor retardation or agitation, slowed and impoverished speech, signs of weight loss, poor self-care, guilty ruminations, somatic delusions, derogatory hallucinations, suicidal preoccupation. Either mania or depression may present with catatonia.

▶ Diagnosis

No pathognomonic signs or studies; rule out general medical etiologies (thyroid and adrenal dysfunction, medications, [eg, sympathomimetics, L-dopa, steroids, antidepressants], Parkinson's disease, head injury, multiple sclerosis, dementing illnesses, pancreatic and other malignancies, epilepsy, lupus, CNS tumors, cerebrovascular accidents [CVAs], viral illnesses); psychiatric disorders including personality disorders, substance intoxication or abuse (eg, stimulants, anabolic steroids).

## ▶ differential diagnosis

### PSYCHOTIC MANIA OR DEPRESSION VERSUS SCHIZOPHRENIA

| Psychotic mania or depression | Schizophrenia |
|---|---|
| Premorbid adjustment good | Premorbid adjustment poor in ≥ 50% |
| Family history of affective disorder | Family history affective disorder less likely |
| Personality and functioning usually preserved between episodes | Chronic, often deteriorating course |
| Prior mood episodes | No prior mood episodes |
| Mood disturbance always present and begins before onset of psychosis | Psychosis usually precedes any mood symptoms |
| Psychotic features usually reflect underlying mood disturbance (eg, somatic delusions in depression, grandiose delusions in mania) | Psychotic features often bizarre, persecutory, nihilistic |

### ▶ Disease Severity

*Mania*—Severe hyperactivity can lead to exhaustion, dehydration, cardiac death; impaired judgment, irritability, grandiosity, assaultiveness may result in danger to self and others; assess progression of symptoms, support system.

*Depression*—Increased suicide risk (15% overall) with presence of delusions; previous attempt; plan and means (especially firearm); male; concurrent substance abuse; social isolation; recent loss; family history; poor health; unemployment. Assess self-care ability, potential life-threatening medical problem.

*Both*—Mood-incongruent psychotic features predict poorer prognosis. Mixed and rapid cycling disorders difficult to treat with high suicide risk.

### ▶ Concept and Application
See Section II.

### ▶ Treatment Steps

*Acute*
1. Hospitalization for protection of self and others, treatment (may need involuntary commitment).
2. Rule out general medical, substance-induced etiologies.
3. For mania: may require restraint IV/IM benzodiazepines and antipsychotics; may use loading doses of lithium or valproate; use IM antipsychotic only if necessary for control of agitation. Electroconvulsive therapy (ECT) for toxic mania, rapid control, pregnancy.
4. For psychotic depression: ECT most effective and rapid; antidepressant (AD) combined with antipsychotic also effective; poor response to AD used alone.

*Continued Care*—See Section II.

## C. Delusional Disorder

▶ H&P Keys

Primary, often sole, manifestation is fixed, nonbizarre, systematized delusion; common types are erotomanic (one is loved by a famous other), grandiose, jealous, persecutory (most common), somatic. Age of onset and psychosocial functioning variable.

▶ Diagnosis

No pathognomonic signs or studies; rule out general medical disorders (early dementias, CNS tumor, endocrine and metabolic disorders, stimulant abuse, basal ganglia trauma); schizophrenia associated with bizarre delusions, prominent hallucinations, thought disorder, deteriorating course, younger onset; paranoid personality disorder has no true delusions.

▶ Disease Severity

Course is variable; worsens with stress.

▶ Concept and Application

Etiology unknown. Predisposed by immigration, deafness, severe stress, visuospatial deficits.

▶ Treatment Steps

*Acute*
1. Hospitalize for inability to control suicidal or homicidal impulses; extreme impairment, including danger associated with delusions.
2. General medical workup.
3. Supportive and psychoeducational therapies with attention to building trust.

*Continued Care*
1. Low-dose antipsychotic for delusions may help.
2. Antidepressants for depression.

## D. Other Psychoses

### 1. Schizoaffective Disorder

▶ H&P Keys

Concurrent symptoms of schizophrenia and depression or mania, with at least 2 weeks of psychotic symptoms alone.

▶ Disease Severity

Poorer prognosis with depressive subtype, family history of schizophrenia, insidious onset, poor premorbid history, predominance of psychotic symptoms. Somewhat better prognosis than for schizophrenia.

▶ Concept and Application

Mood syndrome defines subtype (manic versus depressive); depressive subtype thought to be related to schizophrenia; manic or "bipolar" subtype to bipolar disorder.

▶ Treatment Steps
1. Hospitalization as in other psychoses.
2. Rule out general medical etiology.

   *Bipolar Type*—Lithium and/or other mood stabilizer, eg, valproic acid (VPA), carbamazepine (CBZ) with antipsychotic if necessary; antipsychotic may be discontinued or reduced after stabilization; ECT if necessary. $Li^{++}$, VPA, CBZ maintenance; atypical neuroleptics also used.

   *Depressive Type*—Neuroleptic with or without antidepressant; ECT, $Li^{++}$, anticonvulsants also used.

2. Schizophreniform Disorder

   ▶ H&P Keys
   History, signs, symptoms, and differential as in schizophrenia but duration < **6 months.**

   ▶ Disease Severity
   Good prognosis associated with acute onset, confusion and disorientation, full affect, good premorbid functioning.

   ▶ Treatment Steps
   1. Hospitalize as needed.
   2. Neuroleptics for at least 6 months.

3. Brief Psychotic Disorder

   ▶ H&P Keys
   Acute onset psychosis with emotional turmoil and confusion often following obvious stressor, duration < 1 month, full return to premorbid functioning. Young adult. Predisposed by personality disorder, posttraumatic stress disorder [PTSD]. Rule out schizophreniform and mood disorders, general medical etiology, factitious disorder, malingering, substance induced.

   ▶ Disease Severity
   Prognostic factors as in schizophreniform disorder. Suicide risk.

   ▶ Treatment Steps
   1. Hospitalization as needed.
   2. Antipsychotic or antianxiety agent.
   3. Psychotherapy when stabilized.

4. Shared Psychotic Disorder

   ▶ H&P Keys
   Patient's delusion (usually persecutory) develops in context of submissive, dependent, isolated relationship with person with established delusion. Suicide or homicide pacts.

   ▶ Treatment Steps
   1. Hospitalize as necessary.
   2. Separate the people involved.
   3. Antipsychotic medication as indicated.

5. **Psychotic Disorder Not Otherwise Specified**

   ▶ **H&P Keys**
   Psychotic symptoms that do not meet criteria for other disorders or when enough information is unavailable. Includes postpartum psychoses, culture-bound syndromes. Former occurs 2–3 weeks postpartum, usually primipara, carries risk of infanticide or suicide.

   ▶ **Treatment Steps**
   1. Ensure safety.
   2. Symptomatic treatment.

E. **Psychoses Originating in Childhood**

   1. **Autistic Disorder**

      ▶ **H&P Keys**
      A type of pervasive developmental disorder (PDD) with severe impairments in reciprocal social interaction, verbal and nonverbal communication, imaginative activity, repertoire of interests; frequent self-stimulating, stereotyped behaviors, rigid routines; no prominent hallucinations or delusions, no relationship to psychotic disorders. Onset by age 3, boys > girls; associated mental retardation (70%) with uneven cognitive profile; seizure disorder (25%); multiple neurologic syndromes and biological abnormalities. Genetic predisposition; specific biologic etiology unknown. Other PDDs: Asperger's (no language delay), Rett's, childhood disintegrative disorder (normal development followed by degenerative course).

      ▶ **Diagnosis**
      Neurologic exam, screening for hearing and vision, EEG, CT or MRI, heavy metals, serum ceruloplasmin, phenylketonuria (PKU), karyotype, IQ testing.

      ▶ **Disease Severity**
      Better prognosis with higher IQ, language, and social skills. May be associated with neurologic or genetic medical disorders.

      ▶ **Treatment Steps**
      1. Evaluate as above.
      2. Structured classroom training behavioral modification, family support.
      3. Haloperidol, risperidone for hyperactivity, stereotypies, irritability. Selective serotonin reuptake inhibitors (SSRIs) may help with social interaction, compulsive behaviors.

   2. **Childhood Schizophrenia**
      Diagnosed using adult criteria; extremely rare; average onset age 7, boys ≥ girls; family history of psychosis, possible neonatal CNS injury; rule out autistic disorder, mood disorder, brain tumor or trauma, toxicity caused by heavy metals or poisoning, seizures, nutritional deficiencies. Monitor use of high-potency neuroleptics; family support; special schooling.

3. **Psychotic Mood Disorders**

In adolescence may be misdiagnosed as schizophrenia. Bipolar disorder and major depression diagnosed with same criteria used for adults; children may show irritability, somatic complaints, behavioral disturbance. Good premorbid functioning, normal IQ, prominent manic symptoms, family history of mood disorder predict bipolar diagnosis in children and adolescents, as does acute onset, psychomotor retardation, hypersomnia, psychosis, and bipolar family history in first-episode depression. Lithium or anticonvulsants with careful monitoring, supportive psychotherapy, family education.

## II. MOOD DISORDERS

### A. Major (Unipolar) Depression

▶ **H&P Keys**

Two weeks of sustained depressed mood or loss of interest and pleasure (anhedonia), and at least four of the following: weight and appetite change, insomnia or hypersomnia, fatigue, psychomotor agitation or retardation, low self-esteem or guilt, trouble concentrating, recurrent thoughts of death or suicide. Associated with social withdrawal, loss of libido, abnormal menses, constipation, diurnal mood variation, impoverished speech, somatic preoccupation (cardiac, gastrointestinal [GI], genitourinary [GU], back pain, headache), indecisiveness, obsessive rumination, tearfulness, anxiety. "Masked depression" presents with (often vague) physical complaints. Children and adolescents may have irritability, behavioral problems, somatic complaints, failure to gain weight. Elderly may present with cognitive complaints (pseudodementia). Twenty-five percent identify precipitating event, often loss. Personal and family history. Females > males; > 50% recurrence rate; pattern may be seasonal. Predisposed to by chronic medical or psychiatric illness, substance abuse.

▶ **Diagnosis**

Clinical diagnosis. Lab tests based on neuroendocrine dysfunction (dexamethasone suppression test, thyrotropin-releasing hormone [TRH] stimulation test, sleep EEG) not specific or sensitive enough to use clinically. Rule out mood disorder caused by substance use, medications, or illness; dysthymia (chronic, less severe); personality disorder (lifelong pattern of mood instability; may be comorbid); dementia (less likely history of affective disorder; deficits stable; patient may try to hide deficits, rather than complain about them; insidious onset); bipolar depression (history of mania); bereavement (self-limiting, lacks morbid preoccupation with worthlessness, suicidal ideation, psychomotor retardation, marked functional impairment). Diagnosis may be difficult in medically ill because of overlapping symptoms.

▶ **Disease Severity**

Same as for affective psychoses; untreated episodes last > 6 months; 60% recover, 30% partially recover, 5–10% develop

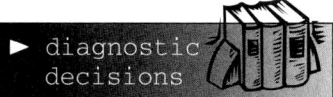

▶ diagnostic decisions

**MAJOR DEPRESSION**

Sustained, distinct depressed mood for 2 weeks plus at least 4 of the following
(SIG E CAPS):
**S**leep (increased or decreased)
**I**nterest (loss of interest or pleasure)
**G**uilt (worthlessness)
**E**nergy (decreased)
**C**oncentration (decreased)
**A**ppetite (increased or decreased)
**P**sychomotor change (retardation or agitation)
**S**uicidality (active or passive)

chronic course. Worse prognosis with late-life onset, concurrent personality, anxiety, substance abuse, chronic medical problems, dysthymic disorder, psychosocial stress. Aggressive treatment reduces suicide risk (15%) and improves comorbid medical disorders. Each recurrence increases risk of further recurrence.

▶ Concept and Application

Dysregulation of neurotransmitters and neuroendocrine system, especially in HPA axis; decreased serotonergic activity associated with suicide. Late-onset may have subcortical cerebrovascular disease. Antidepressants increase available monoamines at nerve terminals, alter receptor sensitivity and density. Genetic component. Twenty-five percent identify precipitant, often loss. Higher incidence and earlier age of onset in younger age groups (cohort effect) supports psychosocial contribution. Psychiatric or medical illness, substance abuse, and early parental loss predispose.

▶ Treatment Steps

*Acute*—See Section I.B. for psychotic depression (20%).
1. Hospitalization if suicide risk or incapacity warrants.
2. Rule out general medical, medication, substance induced etiology.
3. Moderate to severe symptoms indication for somatic therapy. Antidepressants (ADs) successful in 65–75% after 4–6 weeks treatment; good response predicted by vegetative signs, previous response, severe symptoms, acute onset.
4. Serotonin reuptake inhibitors (SRIs) have fewer side effects, less toxicity, less suicide risk than older classes of ADs, tricyclic antidepressants (TCAs) or monoamine oxidase inhibitors (MAOIs). Other newer ADs include bupropion, venlafaxine, mirtazapine. AD, lithium, or triiodothyronine ($T_3$) augmentation for nonresponders. Antipsychotic plus AD needed for psychotic depression. ECT for psychotic depression drug nonresponders (70–80% respond), previous good response, rapid response, pregnancy, cardiac disease.
5. Psychotherapy alone may be effective for mild major depression; psychotherapy plus antidepressants more effective than either treatment alone.
6. Seasonal pattern may respond to phototherapy.
7. Diagnose and treat comorbid psychopathology.

*Continued Care*
1. First episode, continuation of antidepressants for 6–12 months; recurrent depression indication for long-term maintenance; observe for weight gain, jitteriness, insomnia, sexual dysfunction, dry mouth. Lithium prophylaxis also effective.
2. Psychotherapy.

**B. Dysthymia**

Chronic depression of at least 2 years' duration with at least two of the following: appetite disturbance, sleep disturbance, fatigue, low self-esteem, difficulty concentrating, hopelessness; no history of major depression within first 2 years or of manic episode. May be secondary to other psychiatric or general medical illness, chronic stress. Insidious onset childhood through early adulthood; women > men; family history of depression. Rule out major depression, personality disorder (may coexist), chronic illnesses, such as uncontrolled diabetes, hypothyroidism, chronic fatigue syndrome. 10%/year develop "double depression" (major depression superimposed on dysthymia), worsens prognosis of both. Treat with antidepressants, psychotherapy, possibly exercise.

## C. Bipolar Disorders

### ▶ H&P Keys

(See Section I.B. above.) One or more manic episodes (distinct period of elated or irritable mood with at least three of the following: grandiosity, decreased need for sleep, talkativeness, racing thoughts, distractibility, hyperactivity or increased goal-directed activity, impulsivity [eg, excessive spending, gambling, promiscuity]; causing marked impairment or hospitalization) usually accompanied by one or more major depressive episodes. Bipolar depressions may have hypersomnia, severe lethargy. Manic episode may be precipitated by psychosocial stressor, sleep deprivation. Subtypes include:

*Type I*—History of full-blown mania and major depression.

*Type II*—History of hypomania (less severe manic symptoms and impairment) and major depression.

*Rapid Cycling*—Four or more mood episodes per year (10%).

*Mixed*—Full symptoms of both mania and depression intermixed or rapidly alternating. Often psychotic. High suicide risk.

### ▶ Diagnosis

Same as for affective psychoses. Rapid cycling may be associated with thyroid abnormalities, CNS insult. If onset > age 40, likely general medical etiology.

### ▶ Disease Severity

Suicide risk of 10–15%. Worse prognosis with substance abuse, early onset, mixed features, rapid cycling, psychosis. Women have more rapid cycling and more depressive episodes. Adolescents at high risk of relapse. Women at risk for postpartum episodes. Cycling increases with age.

### ▶ Concept and Application

Strong genetic component, likely of several different mechanisms. Various data consistent with heterogeneous dysregulations of biogenic amine systems. One theory implicates kindling (sensitization due to repeated subthreshhold stimulation of neuron generating action potential) in limbic system.

### ▶ Treatment Steps

*Acute Mania*—(See Section I.B.)
1. Hospitalize if necessary.
2. Rule out medical, substance-induced causes, eg, hyper- or hypothyroidism, CNS disorders (head injury, seizures, MS),

substance intoxication or withdrawal, medications (eg, steroids, antidepressants, stimulants, sympathomimetics).
3. Mood stabilizers: $Li^{++}$ serum levels 1.0–1.5. Family history of affective disorder or $Li^{++}$ responsiveness, euphoric mania predict good response; for rapid cycling or dysphoric mania, valproic acid or carbamazepine (obtain serum levels), may be added or substituted. Bipolar depression may respond to $Li^{++}$ or anticonvulsants alone or may need additional antidepressant or ECT. Observe for precipitation of mania.

*Continued Care*

1. More than 80% recurrence without prophylaxis, warranted after second episode or first in adolescents, high genetic loading, or sudden onset with suicidal or highly disruptive symptoms. Lithium levels 0.8–1.0; observe for nausea, diarrhea, weight gain, polyuria, tremor, cognitive dysfunction; avoid dietary $Na^{++}$ fluctuations; monitor thyroid, renal function. Anticonvulsants for lithium nonresponders, substance abusers, rapid cycling, and mixed forms. Obtain CBC, LFTs, pregnancy test, follow serum levels. Antipsychotics, benzodiazepines may be useful in acute mania. Antidepressants may precipitate rapid cycling or mania but may be indicated for bipolar depression unresponsive to mood stabilizers alone.
2. Psychotherapy may increase adaptation, compliance, long-term stability.
3. Family support, education.
4. Stress reduction.

### D. Cyclothymia

Chronic fluctuating mood disturbance of at least 2 years' duration with symptoms of hypomania and depression insufficient to be diagnosed as major depression or bipolar disorder. Onset adolescence, early adulthood. Family history of affective disorder. Rule out personality disorder, substance abuse. May respond to lithium or anticonvulsants, psychotherapy.

## III. ANXIETY DISORDERS

### A. Panic Disorder

▶ H&P Keys

*History*—Recurrent, initially unexpected, sudden episodes of intense fear or discomfort accompanied by autonomic hyperarousal, depersonalization, fears of dying or going crazy; often associated with agoraphobia, fear of situations in which escape is difficult or help unavailable, such as outside the home alone, in a crowd, traveling, on a bridge; may be housebound. Attacks cause anticipatory anxiety, concern about implications, and/or change in behavior (eg, phobic avoidance). Increased history of separation anxiety disorder, family history of panic disorder, other anxiety disorders. Onset mid-

20s, women > men. Nonpsychiatric physicians usually consulted first for symptoms.

*Physical and Mental Status Exam*—Trembling, systolic hypertension, sweating, hyperventilation, flushing, tachycardia, palpitations, dilated pupils, piloerection, cold hands; complaints of chest pain, dyspnea, difficulty swallowing, dizziness, nausea, choking, paresthesias, fear of dying, losing control, going crazy, impending doom. Mitral valve prolapse present in 20–50% of cases.

▶ Diagnosis

Rule out general medical etiology (suspect if onset after 35): cardiac insufficiency, arrhythmias, hypoxia, hyperthyroidism, hyperparathyroidism, hypoglycemia, asthma, COPD, seizure disorders, pheochromocytoma, vestibular disease, caffeinism, hypoglycemia, carcinoid syndrome, autoimmune disorders, Parkinson's disease, postconcussion syndrome, MS, sedative or alcohol withdrawal, stimulants. Situationally bound (cued) panic attacks occur with phobias, obsessive–compulsive disorder, PTSD. Depression often accompanied by anxiety symptoms; look at course, predominant symptoms.

▶ Disease Severity

Chronic, intermittent course, with disability caused by phobic avoidance, substance use, depression (> 50%), associated with lack of prompt diagnosis, treatment. Excess risk of irritable bowel syndrome, peptic ulcer disease, hypertension, mitral valve prolapse, cardiovascular mortality, suicide attempts.

▶ Concept and Application

Genetic contribution. Biologic models include disturbances in locus coeruleus (norepinephrine), serotonergic (5-HT) and γ-aminobutyric acid (GABA) neurotransmission. Benzodiazepines facilitate GABA transmission, and antidepressants downregulate CNS β-adrenergic receptors. Substances that induce panic include carbon dioxide, lactate, isoproterenol. Onset often associated with stressful event.

▶ Treatment Steps

*Acute*
1. Emergency management of panic attack via reassurance, benzodiazepine.
2. Rule out acute medical event, eg, myocardial infarction (MI), pulmonary embolism (PE), substance withdrawal, CNS insult, hypoglycemia, electrolyte abnormalities.
3. Prompt psychiatric referral; avoidance of interminable medical workups.

*Continued Care*
1. Antidepressants first line; start with low doses and increase slowly; high-potency benzodiazepines also effective but may be difficult to discontinue. Mood stabilizing anticonvulsants also used. Buspirone often ineffective. Taper should be attempted in 6–12 months; 70% eventually relapse.

2. Cognitive-behavioral therapies effective for agoraphobia and in preventing relapses in many.
3. Supportive, educational approaches correcting misconceptions.
4. Eliminate caffeine.
5. Diagnose and treat comorbid disorders.

### B. Generalized Anxiety Disorder

▶ H&P Keys

More than 6 months of unrealistic, persistent anxiety and worry unrelated to another psychiatric disorder. Associated with ≥ 3 of following: restlessness, fatigability, difficulty concentrating, irritability, muscle tension, sleep disturbance. Other somatic complaints common.

▶ Diagnosis

Differential is same as for panic disorder.

▶ Disease Severity

Often seek treatment from cardiologists, etc; 25% develop panic disorder. Comorbid depression common.

▶ Concept and Application

Heterogeneous illness; possible genetic component.

▶ Treatment Steps
1. Cognitive–behavioral therapy effective for milder cases.
2. Medications for more severe, chronic disorder; many require prolonged or intermittent treatment. Antidepressants effective, especially with comorbid depression. Buspirone as effective as benzodiazepines without causing sedation, psychomotor impairment, risk of tolerance, abuse potential, rebound; delayed onset of action, headache, nausea, dizziness. Benzodiazepines give immediate relief; abuse rare without substance abuse history.

### C. Obsessive-Compulsive Disorder (OCD)

▶ H&P Keys

Recurrent intrusive thoughts, impulses, images (obsessions) and perseverative ritualistic behaviors (compulsions), that produce anxiety if resisted. In most cases, experienced as senseless product of own mind (as versus delusion). Typical obsessions involve contamination, sin, aggression, loss of control, order, doubt; common compulsions are washing, checking, counting. Onset childhood through early adulthood (men have earlier onset); 25% have obsessions only. Comorbid depression (> 50%), other anxiety disorders, Tourette's syndrome (5–7%), alcoholism, anorexia nervosa. Dermatologic problems due to excessive washing.

▶ Diagnosis

Clinical diagnosis; obsessive–compulsive symptoms in depression, schizophrenia, accompanied by other symptoms of those disorders and respond to specific treatments. "Compulsive" behaviors such as eating, shopping, gambling give pleasure, whereas true compulsions reduce anxiety. Obsessive–compulsive personality lacks true obsessions/compulsions and related anxiety.

▶ **Disease Severity**

Chronic intermittent course; worse prognosis with coexisting schizotypal personality, early onset, severe depression, noncompliance with treatment.

▶ **Concept and Application**

Genetic contribution, also linked to Tourette syndrome. Positron emission tomographic (PET) scans show hypermetabolism in prefrontal cortex and caudate nuclei. Psychobiologic probes suggest abnormality in serotonin system; treated with SSRIs. Autoimmunity to streptococcus linked to some childhood cases.

▶ **Treatment Steps**

1. Rule out temporal lobe epilepsy, postencephalitic states, Tourette syndrome, MS, basal ganglia lesions, post concussion syndrome, Sydenham's chorea.
2. Serotonergic antidepressants (SSRIs, clomipramine); may need higher doses and 4–12 weeks for effect. Observe for nausea, agitation, insomnia (SSRIs); weight gain, sedation, anticholinergic effects (clomipramine); sexual dysfunction (both). Rapid relapse common.
3. Behavioral therapy based on exposure, response prevention; good long-term response in ritualizers. Combined treatment most effective.
4. Support, education.
5. Diagnose and treat comorbid disorders.

## D. Posttraumatic Stress Disorder (PTSD)

▶ **H&P Keys**

Exposure to markedly stressful event causing terror and helplessness, eg, combat, rape, sexual abuse, torture, natural disaster. Symptoms from three categories: reexperiencing (eg, intrusive recollections, nightmares, play in children); emotional numbing (eg, avoidance, amnesia, restricted affect); autonomic arousal (eg, insomnia, irritability). Onset may be delayed, with initial presentation one of shock, confusion, detachment. Comorbid depression, anxiety, dissociation, substance abuse, personality problems, poor impulse control, suicide attempts.

▶ **Diagnosis**

Toxicology, head injury workup as indicated. Chronic PTSD may present with a variety of somatic and psychiatric symptoms; obtain trauma history routinely. PTSD symptoms following, eg, divorce, bereavement diagnosed as adjustment disorder.

▶ **Disease Severity**

Worse prognosis in children and the elderly; with preexisting psychopathology or brain injury, more severe, repetitive stressor; stressor of human design; insidious onset; poor social support; physical injury. Symptoms often persistent, worsen during periods of stress.

▶ Concept and Application

Traumatic memories may be processed differently from nontraumatic ones, making them more difficult to access and integrate in psychotherapy.

▶ Treatment Steps

*Acute*

1. Hospitalize for suicide, violence risk.
2. Rape victims require careful documentation (including photos), thorough physical exam, speculum exam with vaginal smear; fingernail scrapings; pregnancy prevention; rule out sexually transmitted disease (STD); plan for immediate safety; legal advice.
3. Ongoing cognitive behavioral and exposure therapies shown to help. Early intervention important for "working through" the trauma; ventilation, immediate support, validation, encouraging assumption of control, behavioral approaches based on desensitization, group therapy all of value.
4. Mild sedation, eg, with benzodiazepine, as indicated. Treat comorbid disorders. SSRIs helpful.

*Continued Care*

1. Individual, cognitive-behavioral and supportive therapies, peer group therapy, family education for chronic symptoms.
2. Antidepresants (SSRIs).
3. Treatment of concurrent disorders.

### E. Acute Stress Disorder

▶ H&P Keys

Symptoms of dissociation (eg, numbing, detachment, derealization, depersonalization) experienced during/following extreme trauma, followed by reexperiencing, avoidance, and arousal symptoms as in PTSD. Diagnosis predicts development of PTSD. Psychotherapy aims at reducing dissociation and acknowledging trauma. If symptoms still present after 4 weeks, diagnose PTSD.

▶ Treatment Steps
1. Psychotherapy.
2. Mild sedation as indicated.

### F. Phobias

1. Social Phobia

▶ H&P Keys

Fear of scrutiny of others; may be specific (eg, eating in public, public speaking) or more generalized. Situations avoided or endured with anxiety. Onset in adolescence, chronic course, may develop depression, substance abuse.

▶ Treatment Steps
1. Cognitive–behavioral therapy.
2. Breathing retraining.
3. ADs (SSRIs, MAOIs) for generalized symptoms; high-potency benzodiazepines also used.
4. β-Blockers used for performance anxiety.

2. Specific Phobia

▶ H&P Keys

Irrational, excessive fear and avoidance of object or situation (other than of panic or social situation), eg, snakes, heights, blood.

▶ Treatment Steps

Behavioral and cognitive therapies (systematic desensitization).

## IV. ADJUSTMENT DISORDERS

▶ H&P Keys

Pathologic, excessive emotional and behavioral responses to recognizable psychosocial stressor resulting in impaired functioning. Stressors within range of normal experience (eg, school problems, marital discord, job loss, illness). Onset within 3 months, persists no longer than 6 months after termination of stressor. Classified by major symptom: depression, anxiety, mixed emotional features, conduct disturbance, mixed disturbance of conduct and emotions. Adolescents frequently have behavioral symptoms; adults have mood, anxiety symptoms.

▶ Diagnosis

PTSD preceded by stressors outside range of normal experience. If one instance in a typical pattern of overreaction, diagnose personality disorder. Rule out substance intoxication, abuse. Not diagnosed with uncomplicated bereavement or if patient meets criteria for any specific Axis I or II mental disorder.

▶ Disease Severity

Greater vulnerability with history of childhood parental loss, serious medical illness. Most recover fully, but 20% of adults and 40% of adolescents have mental disorder at 5-year follow-up. Increased risk of suicide, medical noncompliance.

▶ Concept and Application

Vulnerability to stress may be a function of underlying constitution, developmental experiences, temperament, personality structure, as well as severity of stressor.

▶ Treatment Steps

1. Evaluate suicide risk, risk of medical noncompliance, substance abuse.
2. Psychotherapy to help patient clarify concerns, resources, options, develop plan of action.
3. Stress reduction may include social support, exercise, relaxation, cognitive reframing techniques, attention to health habits, peer group support.
4. Antianxiety/antidepressant medication as indicated for short-term symptom relief.

## V. PERSONALITY DISORDERS (AXIS II)

▶ H&P Keys

Persistent, inflexible, maladaptive patterns of thinking, feeling, and behaving causing dysfunction, subjective distress; frequent interpersonal problems, fragility under stress, depression; traits often egosyntonic. Onset late adolescence. Ten disorders (three clusters) in the *Diagnostic and Statistical Manual of Mental Disorders* (DSM):

### A. Odd, Eccentric
1. **Paranoid:** suspicious, hypervigilant; ascribes malicious intent, hidden meanings to others; hypersensitivity to criticism; nonpsychotic.
2. **Schizoid:** isolated, indifferent to social relationships, restricted affective expression.
3. **Schizotypal:** minor thought disorder (eg, ideas of reference, magical thinking), peculiar behavior, constricted affect, social anxiety.

### B. Dramatic, Emotional
1. **Antisocial (ASP):** pattern of exploitative, socially irresponsible, destructive, impulsive behavior with no remorse; comorbid substance abuse; conduct disorder in childhood.
2. **Borderline:** problems with intense, unstable relationships, affect regulation, impulse control, identity; suicide gestures common.
3. **Histrionic:** self-absorbed, seductive, with shallow, labile affect, excess need for praise, reassurance.
4. **Narcissistic:** grandiose, exploitative, entitled, rageful if humiliated, lacks empathy.

### C. Anxious, Fearful, Inhibited
1. **Avoidant:** fearful of rejection, timid, inhibited but desirous of relationships (as versus schizoid); comorbid anxiety disorders.
2. **Dependent:** submissive, passive, clingy; lets others make important decisions; easily hurt; preoccupied with abandonment; predisposed by chronic illness.
3. **Obsessive–Compulsive:** preoccupied with rules; rigid, perfectionistic, ambivalent, stingy, controlling, restricted affect; persistent, task-oriented.

▶ Diagnosis

Onset late teens to early twenties. Acute personality changes in adulthood due to Axis I or general medical disorders (eg, substance intoxication, abuse; CNS trauma, tumor, disease, eg, multiple sclerosis, lupus; mood disorders; psychosis; psychic trauma; temporal lobe epilepsy); diagnose coexistent Axis I mood, anxiety, psychotic, substance use, eating, somatization disorders. Personality disorders must have long-term, persistent pattern; may need to defer diagnosis in presence of Axis I pathology.

▶ Disease Severity

Hospitalize for protection of self and others (suicide risk significant in borderlines, antisocials, schizotypals, particularly in presence of substance use); psychotic decompensation (borderline, schizotypal, schizoid, paranoid); severe Axis I pathology.

▶ Concept and Application

Personality disorders result from interaction of constitution, temperament, developmental experiences, environment; genetic contribution in antisocial, schizotypal, paranoid; childhood sexual or physical abuse in many borderlines, avoidants, antisocials; nonspecific neurologic abnormalities; decreased CNS serotonin functioning associated with impulsivity, aggression; schizotypals genetically and biologically related to schizophrenia.

▶ Treatment Steps

1. Evaluate suicidal or aggressive risk; hospitalize if necessary.
2. Diagnose and treat comorbid Axis I disorders.
3. Psychotherapy: cognitive–behavioral, interpersonal/psychodynamic, family, group modalities all used depending on specific disorder and patient. May require long term treatment.
4. Medication for predominant symptoms. Schizotypals may respond to low-dose antipsychotics; SSRIs, mood stabilizers, low-dose antipsychotics used for borderline personality disorders. Antianxiety, antidepressant medications used for anxious, fearful, inhibited disorders.

## VI. SOMATOFORM DISORDERS

### A. Somatization Disorder

▶ H&P Keys

Recurrent, multiple, unfeigned somatic complaints not fully explained by physical disorder, for which medical attention has been sought. Onset before age 30; half have onset before age 15, often with menstrual difficulties; rare in men. Frequent complaints, presented vaguely and dramatically, involve chronic pain in different systems; GI symptoms, eg, irritable bowel, vomiting; cardiopulmonary symptoms, eg, unexplained dyspnea, dizziness; pseudoneurologic symptoms, eg, paralysis, blindness; reproductive tract, sexual problems. High medical utilizers, treated by multiple doctors, extensive, costly evaluations; may have polysurgeries, eg, early hysterectomy. Childhood sexual abuse predisposes; at risk for concurrent spousal abuse. Common comorbid disorders: alcohol, analgesic, sedative abuse; depression (80–90%); anxiety (25–45%); personality disorders.

▶ Diagnosis

Rule out disorders that present with vague, multiple, confusing complaints, eg, multiple sclerosis, porphyria, lupus, hyperparathyroidism; physical symptoms of panic disorder occur only during attacks; conversion disorder involves only pseudoneurologic symptoms; in factitious disorder, person consciously controls production of symptoms.

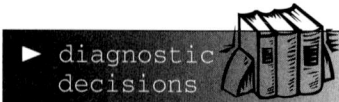

### diagnostic decisions

**SOMATOFORM AND RELATED DISORDERS**

**Somatoform Disorders**
Symptoms are not intentionally produced.
Symptoms not fully explained by medical condition.
Symptoms linked to psychological factors.
  a. Somatization disorder: multiple somatic complaints
  b. Conversion disorder: neurologic symptoms
  c. Pain disorder
  d. Hypochondriasis: fear of specific disease
  e. Body dysmorphic disorder: preoccupation with defect in appearance

**Factitious Disorder**
Intentional production of symptoms for unconscious psychological reasons (the sick role).

**Malingering**
Intentional production of symptoms for recognizable gain

**Psychological Factors Affecting a Medical Condition**
Known medical condition develops/is exacerbated by psychological factors.

▶ **Disease Severity**
Chronic course; suicide associated with substance abuse.

▶ **Concept and Application**
Family and adoption studies confirm that both genetic and environmental factors contribute; familial association with substance abuse and antisocial personality in males. Psychologically interpreted as expression of psychological pain, elicits care, secondary gain.

▶ **Treatment Steps**
1. Rule out general medical etiology.
2. Regularly scheduled visits with primary care physician.
3. Tests, consultations only with evidence of illness.
4. Treat depression, anxiety with antidepressants.
5. Avoid opiates, benzodiazepines.
6. Psychiatric referral if possible.

### B. Pain Disorder

▶ **H&P Keys**
Persistent preoccupation with pain without adequate physical findings or pathophysiologic mechanism to account for intensity or disabling psychosocial sequelae. Onset usually at age 30–50 years, women > men; high utilizers of medical care, surgery; complaints may be vague, diffuse; frequent analgesic, substance abuse; comorbid depression, anxiety, insomnia; inactivity, invalidism, isolation. Resistant to psychologic interpretation.

▶ **Diagnosis**
Dramatic presentation of pain (due to cultural or personality traits) lacks related impairment; lacks plethora of symptoms of somatization disorder; psychogenic disorders with known pathophysiologic mechanisms, eg, tension headache, diagnosed as psychologic factors affecting physical condition; in malingering, symptoms intentionally produced in pursuit of obvious goal. Rule out reflex sympathetic dystrophy (RSD).

▶ **Disease Severity**
Addiction to prescription drugs may require hospital detoxification. Evaluate psychosocial impairment. Suicide associated with severe depression.

▶ **Concept and Application**
Subjective pain experience has cognitive, affective, behavioral components, which may be modified through cognitive–behavioral interventions; serotonergic, adrenergic, endorphin systems involved in pain may be modulated with antidepressants, analgesics.

▶ **Treatment Steps**
1. Rule out RSD, other medical etiologies.
2. Team approach with "gatekeeper."
3. Cognitive behavioral and supportive therapies. (Behavioral evaluation, relaxation, contingency management.)

4. Nonsteroidal antiinflammatory agents, antidepressants for pain.
5. Family therapy, education.
6. Vocational rehab.

## C. Conversion Disorder

### ▶ H&P Keys

Involuntary psychogenic loss or alteration of functioning suggesting a physical disorder, not limited to pain or sexual disturbance. Temporal relationship between psychologically painful stressor and onset of symptoms. Classic cases involve pseudoneurologic symptoms, eg, blindness, paralysis, mutism, pseudoseizures, difficulty swallowing because of lump in throat (globus hystericus). Antecedent physical disorder (eg, seizure disorder), exposure to persons with physical disorders, preexisting gross brain pathology predispose. More common in women, rural, lower socioeconomic strata. Comorbid somatization, depressive, panic, substance, personality, dissociative disorders.

### ▶ Diagnosis

Diagnosis of exclusion, requiring careful neurologic exam and testing, psychiatric consultation. May have inconsistency of symptoms with known neuroanatomy and physiology, eg, glove distribution of anesthesia. Up to 30% subsequently develop neurologic or other illness that explains symptom, eg, multiple sclerosis, lupus, especially with onset > 35.

### ▶ Disease Severity

Improvement or complete resolution associated with abrupt onset, clear precipitant, absence of general medical or psychiatric illness; recurrence predicts chronicity.

### ▶ Treatment Steps

1. Rule out neurologic, medical disorders (eg, lupus, MS, HIV encephalopathy).
2. Reassurance, suggestion, attention to any stressful precipitant.
3. Diagnose and treat underlying psychopathology.
4. Hypnosis or amobarbital interview may be helpful.

## D. Hypochondriasis

### ▶ H&P Keys

Preoccupation with fear of having serious disease despite medical reassurance to the contrary, not of delusional intensity, duration at least 6 months. Selective attention to and misinterpretation of somatic signs and symptoms. Onset age 20–40. History of doctor shopping, resistance to psychiatric referral. Comorbid depression, anxiety, dependence, hostility. Associated with past experience of illness in self or family member.

### ▶ Diagnosis

Rule out subtle medical illness; psychotic disorder with somatic (fixed) delusions; in somatization disorder, patients preoccupied with symptoms rather than specific illness; symptoms must not be due to panic attacks or part of OCD.

▶ Disease Severity
Usually chronic, with functional impairment.

▶ Treatment Steps
1. As for somatization disorder; avoid repeated costly medical workups.

### E. Body Dysmorphic Disorder
Excessive preoccupation with imagined or slight defect in appearance, causing marked distress or impairment (not including anorexia nervosa). Generally not of delusional intensity. Onset adolescence, chronic course. May seek repeated cosmetic surgery. Comorbid depression, delusional disorder, social phobia, OCD. Evaluate social impairment, suicide potential. Psychotherapy, SSRI.

### F. Related Disorders

1. **Psychological Factors Affecting Physical Condition (Psychosomatic Disorders)**
A psychologic factor is believed to have contributed significantly to the development or exacerbation of physical symptom or illness, evidenced by temporal relationship with psychologically meaningful stressor; commonly, headaches, peptic ulcer disease, asthma, skin diseases, vomiting, obesity, low-back pain, ulcerative colitis, arrhythmias, others. Physical condition noted on Axis III. Stress management, psychotherapy may increase adjustment, reduce medical costs.

2. **Factitious Disorders**
Intentional (but often compulsive) production of or feigning of physical or psychological symptoms, presumably for psychologic reasons unknown to the patient, eg, unsatisfied dependency needs met in achieving "sick role." Includes reporting or intentionally producing false symptoms, eg, injection of contaminated substance, surreptitious use of medications, thermometer manipulation, self-induced bruises. Early adult onset; chronic, severe impairment; comorbid severe personality disorders, substance abuse; may have medical occupation, history of illness. Psychiatric consultation, confrontation may be helpful.

3. **Malingering**
Intentional production of physical or psychological symptoms for obvious recognizable external incentive, eg, to avoid military service, financial reward, evading prison, obtaining drugs. Discrepancy with objective findings, vague, uncooperative. Comorbid antisocial personality, substance abuse.

## VII. ATTENTION DEFICIT/HYPERACTIVITY DISORDER (ADHD)

▶ H&P Keys
At least 6 months of age-inappropriate degree of inattentiveness, hyperactivity, and impulsivity; manifested by difficulty following

instructions, organizing and completing tasks; easy distractibility; restlessness and fidgetiness; interrupting and talking out of turn; inability to sustain play activity; accident-proneness. Onset before age 7, boys > girls. Associated with academic underachievement, low self-esteem, mood lability, low frustration tolerance, temper outbursts, academic skills disorders, soft neurologic signs, clumsiness. Older children may develop comorbid conduct disorder, oppositional defiant disorder. Predisposed by CNS abnormalities, eg, fetal alcohol syndrome, Tourette's disorder, chaotic environments, possibly by child abuse. Family history.

▶ Diagnosis

Clinical diagnosis, may be assisted by careful neurologic exam, neuropsychologic testing, teachers' and parents' reports using Conner's scale; obtain EEG, TFTs, lead level, hearing assessment. Diagnose specific learning disabilities; rule out pervasive developmental disorders, tic disorders, mood disorder, seizure disorder, mental retardation, pathologic environment. Comorbid chronic otitis media.

▶ Disease Severity

Poorer outcomes associated with more severe symptoms, coexisting conduct disorder, low IQ, mental disorder in parents; many have continued symptoms in adulthood; 25% develop antisocial personality disorder; higher rates of substance abuse, arrests, suicide attempts, accidents, comorbid psychiatric problems. Children at higher risk for abuse.

▶ Concept and Application

Familial aggregation, also with mood, substance abuse, and personality disorders. Decreased frontal cerebral blood flow on positron emission tomography (PET) scan. Possible congenital and acquired CNS insults. Catecholamine or dopamine abnormalities; medications increase CNS dopamine and norepinephrine availability.

▶ Treatment Steps
1. Medical and psychiatric assessment as outlined previously.
2. Behavioral and environmental management by family, school.
3. Psychostimulant medication, eg, methylphenidate (10–60 mg/d) or dextroamphetamine (5–40 mg/d). May inhibit growth. Observe also for headache irritability, insomnia, abdominal pain, dysphoria, tics. TCAs, bupropion, clonidine also used.
4. Individual, family therapy as indicated.

## VIII. CONDUCT DISORDER

▶ H&P Keys

Age-inappropriate, persistent violation of societal norms and rights of others, manifested by aggression to people and animals, property destruction, deceitfulness and theft, and serious rule violations. May lack empathy, remorse; poor frustration tolerance, irritability, recklessness, low academic achievement. Onset late childhood to early adolescence.

▶ Diagnosis

Rule out response to immediate social context, eg, runaway episodes due to abuse, "adaptive delinquency." Obtain history from multiple sources.

▶ Disease Severity

Early onset, attentional problems, low intelligence, fire setting, family deviance, and large size predict worse prognosis. One third to one half develop ASP as adults; high mortality rates.

▶ Concept and Application

Genetic, neurodevelopmental, and environmental risk factors, including parental rejection/neglect; harsh and inconsistent discipline and abuse; parental ASP, substance abuse, other psychiatric disorder; poverty; evidence of genetic transmission; neurologic abnormalities, including attention deficits, seizures, perinatal insults, head injuries. Biological markers suggest autonomic underarousal, possibly associated with decreased anxiety or stimulus seeking, mediators of antisocial behavior.

▶ Treatment Steps

1. Evaluate suicide and violence potential.
2. Containment may involve hospitalization, parents, schools, legal system, residential placement, peers.
3. Aggression may respond to SSRI, mood stabilizer, clonidine, neuroleptic.
4. Individual, group, family therapies, behavioral management.
5. Evaluate and treat comorbid ADHD, LD, mood, anxiety, substance use disorders.

## IX. EATING DISORDERS

### A. Anorexia Nervosa

▶ H&P Keys

Refusal to maintain minimal normal body weight (< 85%), intense fear of gaining weight, distorted body image, 3 months amenorrhea; associated features include obligate exercise, peculiar food behaviors, bulimic symptoms (see below), emaciation, hypothermia, hypotension, lanugo hair, bradycardia, edema, hair loss, hyposexuality, compulsive behaviors. No loss of appetite. Onset adolescence, 95% women, premorbid history perfectionism, inflexibility and need for control, anxiety, possibly sexual abuse, mid- to upper socioeconomic strata, may be precipitated by stress, dieting. Comorbid depression, personality, OCD.

▶ Diagnosis

Rule out weight loss due to major depression, AIDS, cancer, GI disorders, substance abuse (lacks other criteria); in depression, appetite is diminished whereas anorexics have normal appetite;

in schizophrenia, bizarre eating patterns related to psychosis; in bulimia, weight does not fall below 85%; underweight persons without anorexia recognize their low weight. May have: leukopenia, anemia, electrolyte abnormalities, signs of dehydration, decreased TFTs, prepubertal hormone levels, sinus bradycardia.

▶ Disease Severity

Thirty percent have chronic course, 5–18% mortality. Poorer outcome associated with longer duration of illness, older age at onset, prior psychiatric hospitalizations, poor premorbid adjustment, comorbid personality disorder. May result in cardiovascular problems, impaired renal function, anemia, osteoporosis.

▶ Concept and Application

Genetic component; psychologically interpreted as resistance to social or sexual demands of adolescence; cultural preoccupation with extreme slimness rare in nonindustrialized societies. Biologic theories focus on hypothalamic disturbance, supported by amenorrhea preceding weight loss; reduced CNS, serotonin, and norepinephrine activity.

▶ Treatment Steps

*Acute*
1. Hospitalize for starvation, dehydration, electrolyte imbalance, hypotension, hypothermia, suicide risk.
2. Monitor and treat metabolic imbalances.
3. Strict enforcement of treatment contract for weight goal with daily weights, nutritional supplements, intake-output, supervised feeding (nasogastric tube as needed), reinforcement, nutrition education.
4. Treat comorbid depression with antidepressants (avoid bupropion because of seizure risk).

*Continued Care*
1. Residential, partial hospital treatment may prevent relapse.
2. Cognitive–behavioral, individual, family therapies with goal of weight maintenance, normalization of eating behaviors.

## B. Bulimia Nervosa

▶ H&P Keys

Recurrent binge eating (two episodes per week for 3 months) with lack of control over eating; self-induced vomiting (70–95%), use of laxatives or diuretics, strict dieting, vigorous exercise to prevent weight gain; overconcern with body weight, which is usually normal. Purging and nonpurging types. Onset in late adolescence and early adulthood, often during strict dieting; 95% women; mid- to upper socioeconomic strata. Complications include dental erosion and caries, parotid enlargement, calloused fingers, electrolyte abnormalities (50%), dehydration, weakness, lethargy, GI problems, cardiac arrhythmias; rarely, esophageal tears, gastric rupture, pancreatitis, sudden death. Comorbid anorexia, depression, personality disorders, stealing, substance abuse common.

> diagnostic decisions

### SIGNS AND SYMPTOMS OF SUBSTANCE INTOXICATION AND WITHDRAWAL

| Substance Category | Intoxication | Withdrawal |
|---|---|---|
| *CNS depressants:* alcohol, sedatives, hypnotics, anxiolytics | Disinhibition, slurred speech, drowsiness, ataxia, confusion, blackouts **Overdose:** respiratory depression, coma, death; barbiturates have low therapeutic index | Autonomic hyperactivity, anxiety, malaise, headache, nausea, vomiting, fever, mydriasis, seizures, delusions, hallucinations, delirium, death, can be life-threatening |
| *CNS stimulants:* amphetamine, cocaine, other sympathomimetics | Euphoria, alertness, increased energy, loquaciousness, anorexia, insomnia, mydriasis, autonomic hyperactivity **Overdose:** agitation, aggression, fever, chills, arrhythmias, seizures, sudden cardiac death, cerebrovascular accident; paranoid psychosis, hallucinosis, delirium | Fatigue, insomnia or hypersomnia, anxiety, dysphoria, vivid dreams, agitation, drug craving; not life threatening (unless suicidal) |
| *Opioids* | Euphoria, analgesia, drowsiness, hypoactivity, miosis, anorexia, constipation, pruritus, nausea, vomiting, ataxia **Overdose:** hypotension, bradycardia, CNS and respiratory depression, pulmonary edema, seizures, coma | Flulike syndrome: myalgias, rhinorrhea, nausea, vomiting, diarrhea, tearing, dilated pupils, restlessness, yawning, sweating, piloerection, insomnia, anxiety, tachycardia, hypertension, craving |

### ▶ Diagnosis
Rule out seizure disorder, CNS tumor, Klüver–Bucy and Kleine–Levin syndromes; obtain ECG, electrolytes, amylase, LFTs.

### ▶ Disease Severity
Chronic intermittent disorder with range of impairment.

### ▶ Concept and Application
Genetic component; decreased CNS serotonin, norepinephrine activity; increased family history of mood disorders, obesity, substance abuse.

### ▶ Treatment Steps
1. Hospitalization for severe electrolyte abnormalities, suicide risk.

2. SSRIs reduce binging. Avoid bupropion.
3. Cognitive–behavioral, individual, group, and family therapies.
4. Nutritional counseling, monitor weight.

## X. SUBSTANCE-RELATED DISORDERS

### A. Overview

#### Definitions

*Abuse*—Recurrent maladaptive pattern of use during 12-month period despite physical hazard or legal, social, or occupational problems.

*Dependence*—Psychological (craving) or physical (withdrawal syndrome, tolerance); loss of control over use; preoccupation with obtaining and using substance; continued use despite adverse social, occupational, or health consequences. Frequent denial, minimization.

*Intoxication*—Maladaptive behavior associated with recent ingestion.

*Withdrawal*—Substance-specific syndrome following decreased use or cessation of regular use.

*Tolerance*—Increasing amount of drug needed to produce intoxication.

#### ▶ H&P Keys

Decrement in work or school performance; absenteeism; fights; family problems; injuries or accidents; acute personality change; driving under the influence, theft, prostitution; related medical and mental disorders (see below); frequent psychiatric comorbidity, particularly mood, anxiety, personality, schizophrenic, attention deficit disorders, chronic pain; may be self-medicating or symptoms may be caused by substance; defer diagnosis until patient clean ≥ 6 weeks. Needle tracks with IV use. Occurs in all ages, races, social classes.

#### ▶ Diagnosis

History (may need to obtain from other sources) and associated physical signs. Drug testing usually done on urine; blood used for alcohol; saliva, sweat, breath, hair also used. Preliminary assays (immunologic) sensitive but less specific than confirmatory tests (chromotography or spectrometry).

#### ▶ Disease Severity

Worse prognosis with long-term use; psychiatric comorbidity; unsupportive milieu; lack of employment, job skills; younger age of onset; may be suicidal, assaultive; dangerous withdrawal syndromes associated with alcohol, sedatives, dangerous overdoses with alcohol, narcotics, stimulants, phencyclidine. High blood level without signs of intoxication indicates tolerance. Intravenous drug use may lead to HIV infection, subacute bacterial endocarditis (SBE), hepatitis, thrombophlebitis, pneumonia, cellulitis; snorting cocaine, heroin may lead to nasal perforation, rhinitis, bleeding; inhaling or smoking marijuana, crack, inhalants may lead to bronchitis, asthma. Relapses are common.

▶ Concept and Application

Genetic component to alcohol dependence and possibly others; all abused substances acutely enhance brain reward mechanisms; use reinforced by relief of withdrawal symptoms; environmental learning important.

▶ Treatment Steps

*Acute*

1. Intoxication: observation and medical treatment for overdose, multiple substance ingestion; protection from injury.
2. Withdrawal: symptomatic treatment; may need to detoxify (especially sedatives, alcohol, opioids) under medical supervision.
3. (For specific strategies, see below.) Diagnosis and treatment of concurrent nonpsychiatric medical problems.

*Continued Care*

1. Often need to confront denial.
2. Initiate and maintain abstinence (or substitution pharmacotherapy, eg, methadone), through inpatient, residential, partial and outpatient rehabilitation programs.
3. Individual, cognitive-behavioral and group therapies; family therapy; self-help groups, eg, Alcoholics Anonymous (AA).
4. Pharmacologic treatments, eg, methadone maintenance, disulfiram (Antabuse), naloxone.
5. Diagnosis and treatment of comorbid psychiatric problems.

## B. Alcohol Dependence

▶ H&P Keys

Early: injuries, accidents, gastritis, diarrhea, headaches, insomnia, absenteeism, blackouts, irritability. Later: nutritional deficiencies, hepatitis, cirrhosis, GI bleeding, pancreatitis, heart disease, hypertension, palmar erythema, acne rosacea, gynecomastia, testicular atrophy, peripheral neuropathy, GI cancers, cardiomyopathy, fetal alcohol syndrome (craniofacial abnormalities, mental retardation, behavior problems, congenital malformations), depression, anxiety, insomnia, neuropsychiatric disorders (below). Onset late teens to 30s, men > women, family history. Associated abuse of other substances. Rule out underlying bipolar, anxiety, attention deficit, antisocial disorders. Diagnosis for 20–40% of homeless persons.

▶ Diagnosis

Clinical diagnosis; screen with CAGE (attempts to *C*ut down; *A*nnoyance with criticism of drinking; *G*uilt; morning *E*ye-opener; two positives suggest problem drinking, and three positives give 95% certain diagnosis). Blood level of > 150 mg/dL without intoxication evidence of tolerance. May have increased GGT, mean corpuscular volume (MCV), AST, ALT, uric acid, alkaline phosphatase, vertebral or rib fractures, abnormal liver, hepatic disease stigmata, hypertension, peripheral neuropathy on exam.

### ▶ Disease Severity
One quarter to one third have early onset; male, antisocial, family history, poor prognosis, responds best to structured milieu treatments; two thirds to three quarters have later, gradual onset, equal sex distribution, better prognosis; women have later onset but more virulent course, family and personal history mood disorder; complications include motor vehicle accidents, job loss, assaults, suicide, falls (rule out subdural hematoma), fires, poisonings, drownings.

### ▶ Concept and Application
Multiple causes: genetic factors, cultural patterns, learning all important: High heritability in males; nondrinking sons of alcoholics have altered evoked potentials, possibly greater tolerance; certain groups, eg, Asians, have protective unpleasant responses caused by aldehyde dehydrogenase isoenzyme.

### ▶ Treatment Steps

*Acute*
1. Treatment of withdrawal, detoxification as below.
2. Diagnose and treat acute comorbid medical and psychiatric problems.

*Continued Care*
1. Confrontation of denial.
2. Inpatient or outpatient rehabilitation programs include group, individual, family, 12-step AA, educational components.
3. Disulfiram (Antabuse), naltrexone, SSRIs used to promote abstinence in some.
4. Anxiety, depression lasting more than 2–4 weeks past detoxification may require specific treatment.

## C. Other Alcohol Syndromes

### 1. Intoxication
Disinhibition, mood lability, irritability, impaired judgment; incoordination, slurred speech, ataxia, nystagmus, flushing; may progress to blackouts, coma, death. Complicated by head injuries, motor vehicle accidents, delirium, aggressive acts, suicide. Approximate blood alcohol levels for nontolerant person:

100–150 mg/dL: incoordination, irritability (legal intoxication)
150–250 mg/dL: slurred speech, ataxia > 250 mg/dL: unconsciousness
Blood alcohol level > 150 mg/dL without intoxication evidence of dependence.
Treat supportively; evaluate for subdural, infection, other substances.

### 2. Alcohol Withdrawal Syndromes

*Alcohol Withdrawal*—Tremulousness, nausea, vomiting, autonomic hyperactivity, malaise, headache, insomnia, irritability, agitation, transient perceptual disturbance, grand mal seizures (< 3%), lasting up to 5–7 days postcessation.

***Alcohol Withdrawal Delirium (Delirium Tremens)***—History of recent (2–3 days) cessation or reduction of heavy use in medically compromised patients with 5- to 15-year history of dependence; result of unmasking of downregulation of inhibitory GABA receptors; delirium (see below), autonomic hyperactivity, vivid auditory, visual and tactile hallucinations, paranoid delusions, agitation, tremor, fever, seizures occurring before delirium ("rum fits"). Diagnose and treat underlying pneumonia, GI bleed, hepatic failure, subdural hematoma, electrolyte imbalance, dehydration: obtain CBC, chemistries, vitamin $B_{12}$, folate, LFTs, UA, tox screen, chest roentgenogram, ECG; possible blood cultures, lumbar puncture (LP), CT of head, EEG; frequent vital signs, observation. Thiamine 100 mg (give *before* IV glucose), folate 1.0 mg, multivitamin, benzodiazepine, eg, chlordiazepoxide (or oxazepam with hepatic dysfunction) adjusted to control symptoms and tapered 20–25% daily; phenytoin may be used with history withdrawal seizures. Decrease stimulation, use seclusion, restraint as necessary.

***Alcohol Hallucinosis***—Vivid, persistent auditory or visual hallucinations without delirium within 48 hours of cessation or reduction; rarely become chronic. Treat with benzodiazepines, IV fluids, nutrition. Neuroleptic treatment if chronic.

3. **Alcoholic Encephalopathy (Wernicke's Encephalopathy)**

Abrupt onset of nystagmus, ophthalmoplegia, ataxia, confusion resulting from thiamine deficiency associated with alcoholism; early treatment with thiamine may prevent Korsakoff's syndrome. Give thiamine before giving IV glucose. Diagnose concurrent infection, hepatic failure.

4. **Alcohol-Induced Persisting Amnestic Disorder (Korsakoff's Syndrome)**

Severe, persistent retrograde and anterograde amnesia, confabulation, apathy, polyneuritis resulting from thiamine deficiency, following episode of Wernicke's encephalopathy.

5. **Alcohol-Induced Persisting Dementia**

Dementia following prolonged, heavy ingestion; distinguished from alcohol amnestic disorder by presence of cognitive deficits other than memory; exclude other causes of dementia.

D. **Drug Dependence**

1. **Stimulants (Amphetamines, Cocaine, "Diet Pills," Others)**

Highly addictive; ingested, injected, snorted, purified to free-base form and smoked (crack). *Intoxication* produces euphoria, alertness, increased energy, anxiety or panic, talkativeness, psychomotor agitation, impaired judgment, sexual arousal, anorexia, insomnia, pupillary dilatation, hypertension, tachycardia; may progress to hyperpyrexia; nausea and vomiting; visual or tactile hallucinations ("cocaine bugs"); paranoid ideation; seizures, CVA, MI, sudden cardiac death. Treat symptomatically, eg, severe agitation with benzodiazepine, tachyarrhythmia with antiarrhythmic; acidify urine. Assess for suicidality. *Delirium* lasting 1–6 hours with olfactory or tactile hallucinations, may lead to seizures, death. Chronic use and *dependence* associated with tolerance to euphoric effects; severe social, financial, health losses including STD risk through IV use, prostitution, poor judgment; weight loss; depression, irritability, sexual dysfunction, memory impairment, paranoia, persecutory delusions (*delusional disorder*). *Withdrawal* (crash) may be self-treated with sedatives, eg, alcohol, marijuana; associated with insomnia or hypersomnia, hunger, fatigue, dysphoria, agitation, anxiety, suicidal ideations, craving. Not physically dangerous; assess suicide risk, treat supportively, refer for drug treatment. Treat depression persisting > 2 weeks after withdrawal.

2. **Opioid Dependence (Heroin, Methadone, Meperidine, Codeine, Pentazocine, Others)**

   More common in urban settings, males, blacks, health care professionals, chronic pain patients. Opium smoked; heroin snorted, injected intravenously or subcutaneously ("skin popping"); speedball is heroin plus stimulant; pharmaceutic opioids ingested. *Dependence* associated with tolerance, compulsive use, weight loss, hyposexuality, amenorrhea, multiple medical problems (eg, HIV infection, SBE, cellulitis), criminal involvement, suicide, accidents. *Intoxication* produces euphoria, analgesia, hypoactivity, anorexia, drowsiness, constipation, nausea, vomiting, slurred speech, hypotension, bradycardia, pupillary constriction; CNS and respiratory depression, pulmonary edema, seizures, coma, death in overdose. Treat with IV naloxone, 0.8 mg, double dose q 15 min × 2 if no response; continue IV administration up to 3 days, support vital functions; diagnose polysubstance overdose. Assess for suicidality. *Withdrawal* severely uncomfortable but not a medical emergency; flulike syndrome of rhinorrhea, myalgias, nausea, vomiting, diarrhea, lacrimation, dilated pupils, restlessness, yawning, sweating, insomnia, piloerection, anxiety, craving, tachycardia, hypertension; methadone 15–25 mg q12h until symptoms suppressed, with gradual taper according to symptoms over 10–14 days; or buprenorphine withdrawal; symptomatic treatment with clonidine, antiemetics, analgesics also used; naltrexone used after detoxification to assist abstinence in highly motivated patient; progress to methadone maintenance or abstinence; pentazocine detoxified with pentazocine. Comorbid psychiatric disorder (ASP, depression, PTSD) in 80%.

3. **Sedative-Hypnotic Dependence (Benzodiazepines, Barbiturates, Methaqualone, Others)**

   Young, polydrug abusers (frequently combined with alcohol, opioids, stimulants) or middle-aged women, who become iatrogenically dependent. *Dependence* produces tolerance to euphoriant and sedative effects, fatigue, psychomotor impairment, amnesia, depression, headaches, GI disturbances; *intoxication* associated with slurred speech, drowsiness, incoordination, ataxia, impaired attention and memory, disinhibition. Flumetrazepam ("roofies") associated with date rape. Barbiturates have low therapeutic index, frequently used in suicide; *overdose* causes respiratory depression, coma; gastric lavage, charcoal, monitor closely, maintain airway and blood pressure. Benzodiazepines have high therapeutic index but may be lethal in combination with other CNS sedatives. Flumazenil (benzo antagonist) does not reverse respiratory inhibition. Mild *withdrawal* syndrome of anxiety, insomnia, headache, anorexia, dizziness common. Severe withdrawal syndrome is a medical emergency, associated with nausea, vomiting, malaise, autonomic hyperactivity, anxiety, photophobia, tremor, hyperreflexia, hyperthermia, insomnia, delirium, seizures, death; short-acting drugs cause most severe syndrome. Pentobarbital challenge tests determines substitute phenobarbital or long-acting benzodiazepine dose to begin gradual withdrawal. Give pentobarbital 200 mg PO, then 100 mg q 2 h (max 500 mg) until intoxication observed; substitute phenobarbital, 30 mg/each 100 mg pentobarbital; taper ≈ 10%/day, adjusting for signs of intoxication, withdrawal.

### 4. Cannabinoids (THC, Marijuana, Hashish, Bhang, Ganja)

Intoxication may produce euphoria or dysphoria, heightened sensation, time distortion, increased humorousness, impaired judgment, dry mouth, increased appetite, pupillary dilation, conjunctival injection, suspiciousness, anxiety, tachycardia, depersonalization, incoordination; rarely hallucinations, mild persecutory delusions; pupils are normal sized. Treatment rarely needed. Very high doses may produce prolonged (up to 6 weeks) psychosis, mild delirium, panic. Chronic use may lead to apathetic, amotivational syndrome, memory impairment, depression, anxiety, respiratory and reproductive problems; no characteristic withdrawal syndrome. Often used or mixed with other substances. Urine toxicology remains positive up to 4 weeks after cessation of heavy use.

### 5. Hallucinogens (LSD, Mescaline, DMT, Psilocybin, MDMA, Others)

Eaten, sucked from paper, smoked; intoxication produces wakeful hallucinosis, sympathomimetic effects (pupillary dilatation, tachycardia, diaphoresis), perceptual changes, emotional intensity and lability; may be associated with anxiety, depression, paranoia, panic reactions with belief that disturbed perceptions are real ("bad trips"); treat with reassurance, ensure safe environment; benzodiazepines, antipsychotics for severe symptoms. Prolonged psychosis may develop in vulnerable patients; posthallucinogen perception disorder ("flashbacks") distressing persistent reexperiencing of hallucinations with intact reality testing. Low-dose benzodiazepine acutely, antipsychotic if persistent.

### 6. Phencyclidine (PCP, Angel Dust)

Hallucinogen, smoked with marijuana, eaten, injected, snorted; euphorigenic, commonly causes unpredictable, paranoid, agitated, assaultive behavior; accompanied by dysarthria, diaphoresis, vertical and horizontal nystagmus, hypertension, tachycardia, analgesia (may result in injury). May develop muscle rigidity, ataxia, hyperacusis, hyperreflexia, myoclonic jerks, catatonia, seizures, respiratory depression, coma, renal failure, chest pain, palpitations. Pupils normal sized. Elevated CPK, myoglobinuria, ALT, BUN, creatinine. Chronic users may develop psychosis, mood disorder, delirium, long-term neuropsychologic damage. Ensure safety in nonstimulating environment; may need physical restraint; acidify urine to increase drug clearance, treat severe hypertension; may use benzodiazepines, antipsychotic symptomatically; evaluate for medical problems, other substance intoxication.

7. **Inhalants (Volatile Glues, Solvents, Gasoline, Cleaners, Nitrates, Others)**

   Frequently abused by male adolescents; causes light-headedness, euphoria, disinhibition, dizziness, intensification of orgasm, belligerence, impaired judgment, perceptual disturbances, delusions, ataxia, confusion, disorientation, slurred speech, hyporeflexia, nystagmus, poor judgment, accidents; can progress to delirium, coma; chronic use can result in weight loss, fatigue, breating problems, facial rash, halitosis, dementia, liver and kidney damage, bone marrow suppression, peripheral neuropathies, immunosuppression. Treat supportively. Substance abuse education, medical and psychiatric evaluation.

8. **Anabolic Steroid Abuse**

   Adolescents, athletes; ingested or intramuscular injection; chronic use associated with depression, mania, psychosis, acne, hepatic damage, infection from needle sharing, CVAs, testicular atrophy, and feminization in males, masculinization in females.

9. **Caffeine Dependence (Coffee, Tea, Cola, Chocolate, Over-the-counter Stimulants, Cold Preps)**

   Restlessness, insomnia, diuresis, anxiety, excitement, GI disturbance, flushing with intake > 250 mg/d (two cups brewed coffee); cardiac arrhythmia, muscle twitching, agitation, inexhaustibility with intake > 1 g. Withdrawal symptoms: headache, fatigue lasting 4–5 days.

10. **Nicotine Dependence (Tobacco Smoking, Chewing)**

    Strongly conditioned with rapid development of dependence; assessed by number of cigarettes smoked per day, use of morning cigarette; dependence causes pulmonary, cardiac, peripheral vascular, neoplastic diseases. Withdrawal associated with craving, irritability, headache, anxiety, difficulty concentrating, restlessness, bradycardia, increased appetite, weight gain, GI distress, increased cough, insomnia, impaired performance. Obtain commitment to stop on specific date. Counseling, self-help literature, smoking cessation groups, behavioral interventions, nicotine gum or patch for moderate to severe addiction (continued smoking with nicotine treatment can cause cardiac death); bupropion also effective, may be used in combination with nicotine replacement. Highly comorbid with other psychiatric, substance use disorders; depression may develop upon withdrawal.

## XI. SEXUAL DYSFUNCTIONS

▶ H&P Keys

Includes disorders of all phases of the sexual response cycle causing distress, interpersonal difficulty: *hypoactive sexual desire disorder* (deficient or absent sexual fantasies or desire); *sexual aversion disorder* (revulsion to and avoidance of sexual contact); *female sexual arousal disorder* (inability to attain or maintain adequate sexual excitement and lubrication); *male erectile disorder* (inability to attain or maintain adequate erection); *female and male orgasmic disorders* (persistent or recurrent delay or absence of orgasm following sexual excitement); *premature ejaculation* (persistent ejaculation with minimal stimulation before or shortly after penetration); *dyspareunia* (persistent genital pain with intercourse); and *vaginismus* (involuntary spasm of vaginal musculature during intercourse) classified as sexual pain disorders. All disorders may be lifelong or acquired, generalized or situational, due to psychological or combined with general medical or substance induced factors.

▶ Diagnosis

Rule out dysfunction due to another psychiatric disturbance (eg, depression, PTSD), substance dependence, diabetes, vascular disease, neurologic disease, including MS and trauma, endocrine disorders, hepatic or other systemic disease, surgical procedures; medications, commonly including antihypertensives, anticholinergics, antihistamines, antidepressants, antipsychotics, steroids. Spontaneous erections, morning erections, erections with masturbation rule out organic etiology of impotence. Complete gynecologic or urologic exam, measurement of nocturnal penile tumescence, pudendal nerve latency, penile blood pressure, serum glucose, LFTs, TFTs, prolactin, luteinizing hormone (LH), FSH as indicated.

▶ Disease Severity

Primary and chronic disorders more difficult to treat. Patient may have history of sexual victimization.

▶ Concept and Application

Illnesses, substance abuse, or medications that interfere with normal endocrine, neural, and vascular systems may produce sexual dysfunction. Psychological etiologies include ignorance and misinformation; unconscious guilt, anger and anxiety; conditioned responses; performance anxiety or fear of rejection; and lack of communication between partners. Major physical and psychological stresses may inhibit sexual functioning.

▶ Treatment Steps

1. Rule out medical or substance-related etiology.
2. Cognitive therapy, specific behavioral therapies, marital therapy, education (eg, importance of clitoral stimulation for orgasm in women). Behavioral therapies (eg, sensate focus for erectile dysfunction, squeeze technique for premature ejaculation, directed masturbation for anorgasmia) desensitize patient and decrease performance anxiety.

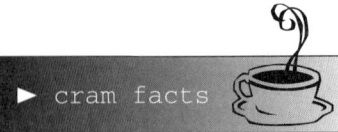

### SAFE SEX GUIDELINES

**Safe Sex Practices**
- Masturbation
- Dry kissing
- Hugging, massage
- Use of unshared vibrators, sex toys

**Low-risk Sex Practices**
- Wet kissing without mouth sores
- Mutual masturbation
- Intercourse (vaginal or anal) with condom
- Oral sex with use of barrier
- Skin contact with semen, urine with no skin sores or breaks

**Unsafe Sex Practices**
- Intercourse (vaginal or anal) without condom
- Oral sex without barrier
- Blood contact
- Sharing needles
- Sharing sex instruments
- Semen, urine, feces in mouth, vagina

3. Somatic treatments include alprostadil injections or sildenafil for impotence (contraindicated with use of nitrates, heart disease), SSRIs for premature ejaculation.

## XII. DELIRIUM

### ► H&P Keys

Syndrome of global cognitive impairment with reduced attention; disorganized thought with rambling or incoherent speech; reduced and fluctuating level of consciousness (clear, drowsy, stupor, coma); sensory (commonly visual) misperceptions, such as illusions, hallucinations; disorientation; disturbed sleep–wake cycle; psychomotor and memory disturbances; rapid onset, fluctuating course, brief duration ending in recovery, dementia, death. May have emotional disturbance (agitated or withdrawn); fearfulness; abnormal movements, eg, asterixis; autonomic hyperactivity. Increased susceptibility in children, elderly, prior brain damage (eg, dementia, AIDS). Prevalence 10–15% medical and surgical patients, 30% intensive care unit patients.

### ► Diagnosis

History, physical, lab studies to diagnose underlying problem. Common etiologies include systemic infection; metabolic disorders (hypoxia, hypoglycemia, thyroid disease, electrolyte imbalances, hepatic or renal disease, thiamine deficiency); postoperative states; seizures and postictal states; head injury; substance intoxication, withdrawal syndromes; anticholinergic, sedative, or other medications; toxins; autoimmune disorders; hypertensive encephalopathy; brain neoplasms; focal lesions (right parietal, inferomedial occipital). Symptoms differ from psychotic psychiatric disorder with random fluctuation; problems with attention, orientation, memory; lack of prior history. Clear sensorium in dementia (but may have comorbid dementia). In delirium, EEG shows background alpha wave slowing or low-voltage fast theta wave activity.

### ► Disease Severity

Delirium is a medical emergency, requiring rapid assessment and treatment.

### ► diagnostic decisions

#### DELIRIUM VERSUS DEMENTIA

| Delirium | Dementia |
| --- | --- |
| Rapid onset | Insidious onset |
| Fluctuating, clouded consciousness | Clear sensorium until late in course |
| Often reversible | Most irreversible and progressive |
| Perceptual disturbances, sleep–wake cycle abnormalities, incoherent speech common | These symptoms uncommon until late in course |

▶ Concept and Application

Final common pathway for acute brain insult. Dysfunction of brainstem reticular activating system.

▶ Treatment Steps

1. Diagnose and treat underlying disorder (history, physical exam, electrolytes, blood urea nitrogen [BUN], creatinine, CBC, LFTs, UA, erythrocyte sedimentation rate [ESR], toxicologies, HIV, blood cultures, ECG, EEG, CT or MRI of head, LP as indicated.
2. Monitor vital signs, cognitive status (eg, Mini-Mental State Exam).
3. Treat alcohol, sedative withdrawals as above; severe anticholinergic delirium treated with physostigmine.
4. Discontinue all unnecessary medications and avoid anticholinergic and sedative hypnotics.
5. Hydration, nutrition.
6. Reassurance; sensory environment should be individually optimized, eg, night light, soft music, relative or sitter in room, restraint, protection from injury as necessary.
7. Low-dose, high-potency antipsychotic, eg, haloperidol, for agitation.

## XIII. ABUSE SYNDROMES

### A. Child Physical and Sexual Abuse

▶ H&P Keys

Risk factors include parental history of child abuse, current substance abuse, depression, impulsivity; premature, hyperactive, emotionally disturbed, physically ill, or otherwise difficult child; stepchild; current toilet training; impairment, unavailability, abuse of mother; familial isolation, stress, poverty, conflict; child's running away. History of injury inconsistent with physical findings or developmental level; inconsistent stories; multiple injuries of different ages; delay in seeking care. Suspect when see linear or geometric marks; old scars; spiral, humerus, or rib fractures; geometric or symmetric lower body burns; ruptured viscera; facial and head trauma; retinal hemorrhages; may see genital or anal trauma or lesions; stomach or rectal pain; urinary tract infections with sexual abuse. Signs of disturbed attachment (eg, lack of physical contact or concern by parent, lack of separation anxiety by child, hypercritical attitude toward child). Delayed development, disturbed play, inappropriate sexual behavior may be present.

▶ Diagnosis

Rule out unintentional trauma, bleeding diathesis, dermatologic conditions, vitamin deficiencies, osteogenesis imperfecta, self-inflicted injuries; thorough physical exam; skeletal series, serologies, bleeding screening battery, CBC, creatine kinase (CK) as indicated.

▶ **Disease Severity**

Deaths usually occur only after numerous episodes; psychiatric sequelae (including PTSD, depression, substance abuse, personality disorders, dissociative identity disorder, sexual dysfunction, somatic complaints, repetition of abuse, suicidal or self-destructive behavior) worse with early-age onset, chronicity, severe abuse, use of force, multiple perpetrators, abuse by parental figure, lack of support.

▶ **Concept and Application**

Child may dissociate during abuse episode, resulting in later development of dissociative symptoms. Guilt, shame, rage, low self-esteem, self-destructive behavior, developmental delays, anxiety, withdrawal, antisocial behavior common.

▶ **Treatment Steps**

*Acute*
1. Interview of child alone; expert may be necessary to elicit abuse history; separate interviews of parents if possible.
2. Document findings, including pictures.
3. All states mandate reporting of suspected abuse (physical, emotional, sexual, severe neglect).
4. Ensure safety of child.

*Continued Care*
1. Treatment of child for physical, emotional sequelae; individual, group psychotherapy usually indicated.
2. Treatment for abusers ranges from support (emotional support, social services, education, Parent's Anonymous groups, hotlines, etc.) through mandated therapy, removal of parent abuser or child, legal prosecution.

**B. Adult Domestic Violence**

▶ **H&P Keys**

Risk factors include pregnancy, younger age, social isolation, child abuse in home; histories of child abuse, substance abuse, criminality in abuser; abused women not shown to have specific predisposing personality traits. History may be incompatible with injury. Trauma repetitive in most; no diagnostic injury pattern; head, face, neck, breast, abdomen frequent injury sites. PTSD symptoms, low self-esteem, somatic complaints, depression, anxiety, substance abuse, suicide attempts.

▶ **Diagnosis**

Battering present in 20% of women seeking medical care; 22–35% of women presenting to emergency departments; 23% of prenatal patients; 25% of women who attempt suicide; 45–58% of mothers of abused children. Routine inquiry in privacy makes diagnosis.

▶ **Disease Severity**

Increased risk of severe abuse when abused partner decides to leave; respect victim's judgment regarding her safety. Inquire about presence of firearms. High risk of marital rape.

▶ Concept and Application

Barriers to leaving abusive relationship include shock and denial, self-blame, feelings of helplessness, presence of children, financial dependency, lack of job skills, fear of retaliation.

▶ Treatment Steps
1. Interview victim alone.
2. Treat and document injuries.
3. Evaluate suicide/homicide potential.
4. Ensure confidentiality and safety of victim, children—risk of severe abuse increases when abused partner decides to leave.
5. Assess resources, continued risk (threats, extent of prior injury, presence of weapons, stalking, substance abuse).
6. Referrals for social, legal, medical, psychiatric resources.

### C. Elder Abuse

Abuser generally relative/caretaker; victim may fear disclosure due to dependency; family system with frustration, financial, or health stress, substance abuse, history of violence; previous injuries, physical deterioration: bruising, head injury, burns, decubiti, contractures, dehydration, lacerations, diarrhea, impaction, malnutrition, urine burns, signs of neglect, sexual assault, PTSD symptoms. Interview privately; social service for assessment of living situation; mandatory reporting in most states.

## XIV. BEREAVEMENT

### A. Uncomplicated Bereavement

Normal reaction to death of loved one or other significant loss; acute grief characterized by intense emotional distress, somatic symptoms, dissociation, preoccupation with deceased, anger, loss of habitual patterns of conduct; mourning can include full depressive syndrome with depressed mood, sleep disturbance, anorexia, guilt, crying, difficulty concentrating, loss of interest, fatigue, anxiety most common; duration varies, symptoms generally remit spontaneously, anniversary reactions common. Higher risk

▶ diagnostic decisions

#### DEPRESSION VERSUS BEREAVEMENT

| Depression | Bereavement |
| --- | --- |
| Mood pervasive, unremitting | Mood fluctuates |
| Pervasive low self-esteem, worthlessness | Self-reproach regarding deceased |
| May be suicidal | Usually not suicidal |
| May have sustained psychotic symptoms | May transiently hear voice or see image of deceased |
| Does not improve without treatment; average episode 6–9 months | Symptoms improve with time; severe symptoms usually gone by 2–6 months |
| Social withdrawal | Often welcomes social support |

of general medical and psychiatric illness and mortality during mourning. Signs of pathologic grief include marked psychomotor retardation, morbid preoccupation with worthlessness and hopelessness, prolonged functional impairment, persistent suicidal preoccupation; prolonged denial; absence of grief. Encouragement of expression of feelings, reminiscences; referral to community supports; medication generally contraindicated, but autonomous depressive disorder should be treated.

### B. Sudden Infant Death Syndrome

Sudden, unexpected, unexplained death of infant < 1 year old. African Americans and Native Americans have 2–3 times risk. Risk factors include sleeping prone, exposure to cigarette smoke, lack of prenatal care, prematurity. Associated with abnormalities in the arcuate nucleus.

Intense, severe grief reactions frequent in parents, including guilt, anger, hostility, somatic symptoms; delayed mourning; overactivity; social isolation; psychosis; agitated depression. Associated with decline in physical health, marital difficulties, behavioral disturbance in siblings, migration. Contact with dead infant; autopsy may help; education may reduce guilt and blame; parent support groups; involvement of siblings; extended social support; counseling regarding future pregnancy recommended.

## BIBLIOGRAPHY

American Psychiatric Association. *Diagnostic and Statistical Manual of Mental Disorders*. 4th ed. Text Revision. Washington, DC: American Psychiatric Association; 2000.

Fauman MA. *Study Guide to DSM IV*. Washington, DC: American Psychiatric Press, Inc.; 1994.

Kaplan HI, Sadock BJ. *Synopsis of Psychiatry*. 9th ed. Baltimore: Williams & Wilkins; 2002.

Rosher R. *Principles and Practice of Forensic Psychiatry*. 2nd ed. Edward Arnold, 2003.

Taylor MA. *The Fundamentals of Clinical Neuropsychiatry*. New York: Oxford University Press; 1999.

# Pulmonary Medicine 16

**I. INFECTIOUS DISORDERS / 493**
  A. Croup / 493
  B. Acute Epiglottitis / 493
  C. Acute Bronchitis / 494
  D. Acute Bronchiolitis / 494
  E. Pertussis / 494
  F. Bacterial Bronchopneumonia / 495
  G. Atypical Pneumonias / 497
  H. Pulmonary Tuberculosis / 499
  I. Fungal Pneumonias / 500

**II. OBSTRUCTIVE PULMONARY DISEASES / 503**
  A. Pulmonary Function Tests / 503
  B. Asthma / 503
  C. Chronic Obstructive Pulmonary Diseases / 505

**III. RESTRICTIVE PULMONARY DISEASES / 508**
  A. Idiopathic / 508
  B. Pneumoconiosis / 509

**IV. PLEURAL DISEASES / 512**
  A. Pleural Effusion / 512
  B. Pleurisy (Pleuritis) / 513
  C. Pneumothorax / 513

**V. DISEASES OF PULMONARY CIRCULATION / 514**
  A. Cardiogenic Pulmonary Edema (Congestive Heart Failure) / 514
  B. Adult Respiratory Distress Syndrome / 514
  C. Newborn Respiratory Distress Syndrome (Hyaline Membrane Disease) / 515
  D. Pulmonary Embolism / 515
  E. Pulmonary Vasculitis / 517
  F. Vasculitis: Goodpasture's Syndrome / 517
  G. Cor Pulmonale / 518

## VI. PULMONARY NEOPLASTIC DISEASES / 518
   A. Bronchogenic Carcinoma / 518
   B. Carcinoid Tumors / 519
   C. Metastatic Malignant Tumors / 520

## VII. ILL-DEFINED SYMPTOM COMPLEX / 520
   A. Cough / 520
   B. Dyspnea / 521
   C. Chest Pain / 521
   D. Hemoptysis / 522
   E. Wheezing and Stridor / 522
   F. Solitary Pulmonary Nodule (Coin Lesion) / 523
   G. Sleep Apnea Syndrome / 523

**BIBLIOGRAPHY / 525**

## I. INFECTIOUS DISORDERS

### A. Croup

▶ H&P Keys

Children under 6 years old following upper respiratory illness. Barking cough, inspiratory stridor, dyspnea, hoarseness, usually worse at night.

▶ Diagnosis

X-ray or MRI of upper airway (glottic and subglottic swelling). Diagnosis usually clinical.

▶ Disease Severity

Respiratory rate, pulse oximetry, accessory muscle use, stridor, intercostal muscle retractions.

▶ Concept and Application

Glottic and subglottic edema leading to upper airway obstruction. Multiple viral etiologies, including respiratory syncytial virus, influenza A and B, adenovirus, and rhinovirus.

▶ Treatment Steps
1. Humidification of inspired air.
2. Correction of hypoxemia.
3. Aerosol racemic epinephrine, systemic corticosteroids.
4. Intubation if severe (rarely needed).

### B. Acute Epiglottitis

▶ H&P Keys

Children < 7 years of age most common. High fever, stridor, dyspnea, hoarseness, dry cough, drooling, dysphagia, systemic toxicity, cherry-red epiglottis.

▶ Diagnosis

Lateral neck roentgenogram (soft-tissue shadow of enlarged epiglottis), blood culture, throat culture (but see below).

▶ Disease Severity

Roentgenographic findings, pulse oximetry, clinical distress, accessory muscle use, intercostal retractions.

▶ Concept and Application

Edema of epiglottis obstructing upper airway. Etiologic agent usually *Haemophilus influenzae* type b.

▶ Treatment Steps
1. Antibiotics active against *H. influenzae* (cefuroxime, ampicillin plus clavulinic acid, others).
2. Endotracheal intubation or tracheostomy in severe cases.

*Note:* Airway examination and throat culture may provoke laryngospasm and cardiopulmonary arrest!

## C. Acute Bronchitis

▶ **H&P Keys**

Severe, prolonged productive cough, fever, dyspnea.

▶ **Diagnosis**

History and physical, sputum culture, chest roentgenogram to rule out bronchopneumonia.

▶ **Disease Severity**

Respiratory rate, temperature.

▶ **Concept and Application**

Infection and inflammation of large airways. Usually viral (influenza, adenovirus). May be bacterial (*Mycoplasma pneumoniae, Bordetella pertussis, H. influenza, Streptococcus pneumoniae*).

▶ **Treatment Steps**

1. Symptomatic decongestants, cough suppressants.
2. If viral: consider zanamivir, oseltamivir, or rimantadine if influenza is suspected and symptoms < 48 hours.
3. If bacterial: broad-spectrum oral antibiotic (eg, macrolide, tetracycline derivative, broad-spectrum quinolone, others).

## D. Acute Bronchiolitis

▶ **H&P Keys**

Children under 2 years old following upper respiratory infection; tachypnea, inspiratory and expiratory wheezing, intercostal and suprasternal retractions, nasal flaring, hyperresonant chest, wheezing, inspiratory rales.

▶ **Diagnosis**

Chest roentgenogram: hyperinflated lungs, peribronchial thickening; may have concurrent bronchopneumonia. Normal white blood cell (WBC) count. Inspiratory "click."

▶ **Disease Severity**

Respiratory rate, intercostal retractions, pulse oximetry.

▶ **Concept and Application**

Acute inflammation of small airways causing hyperinflation, obstruction, and atelectasis. Majority associated with respiratory syncytial virus.

▶ **Treatment Steps**

Oxygen, hydration, aerosol ribavirin for respiratory syncytial virus.

## E. Pertussis

▶ **H&P Keys**

Usually occurs in infants under 2 years old.

*Catarrhal Stage*—Lasts 1–2 weeks. Presents similarly to viral illness: low-grade fever, injected conjunctiva.

*Paroxysmal Stage*—Lasts 2–4 weeks. Severe, paroxysmal, short coughs with inspiratory "whoop." Thick, tenacious secretions, usually afebrile.

▶ Diagnosis

Nasopharyngeal culture (requires special medium), elevated WBC count (mostly lymphocytes); increased polymorphonuclear neutrophils (PMNs) suggest bacterial superinfection.

▶ Disease Severity

WBC count. Presence of bacterial superinfection.

▶ Concept and Application

Infection of tracheobronchial tree with *Bordetella pertussis*. In severe cases, mucopurulent exudate obstructs small airways.

▶ Treatment Steps

1. Macrolide antibiotic in catarrhal stage (does not help in paroxysmal stage).
2. Supportive care.
3. Antibiotics for treatment of superinfection if present.

## F. Bacterial Bronchopneumonia

### 1. Pneumococcal Pneumonia

▶ H&P Keys

Acute onset of rigors, fever, productive cough of "rusty" sputum, tachypnea, respiratory distress, pleuritic chest pain, bronchial breath sounds. Dullness to percussion may indicate accompanying effusion or empyema.

▶ Diagnosis

Chest roentgenogram (lobar infiltrate), sputum Gram stain, sputum culture, blood culture, WBC.

▶ Disease Severity

Pulse oximetry, arterial blood gases (ABG), tachypnea, chest roentgenogram. Multilobed involvement, low WBC count, positive blood culture, and older age associated with worse prognosis.

▶ Concept and Application

Infection caused by *Streptococcus pneumoniae*. Most common cause of community-acquired pneumonia. Can cause otitis, meningitis, pleural effusion, empyema. Elderly, infants, asplenic, and immunocompromised patients at highest risk.

▶ Treatment Steps

1. Begin antibiotic immediately (penicillin G, erythromycin, broad-spectrum quinolone). Use vancomycin or quinolone if penicillin resistance is present or suspected.
2. Chest tube drainage if empyema present. Pneumococcal vaccine for high-risk individuals after acute episode resolves. Oxygen if hypoxic.

2. Staphylococcal Pneumonia

   ▶ H&P Keys

   Fever, dyspnea, cough with purulent sputum.

   ▶ Diagnosis

   Chest roentgenogram (multifocal infiltrates, abscess, pneumatocele, effusions), sputum Gram stain, sputum culture, blood culture, elevated WBC.

   ▶ Disease Severity

   Pulse oximetry, ABG, tachypnea, chest roentgenogram. Metastatic infection (central nervous system [CNS], bone, endocarditis, sepsis).

   ▶ Concept and Application

   Pulmonary infection caused by *Staphylococcus aureus*. Seen after influenza infection, chronic obstructive pulmonary disease (COPD), hematogenous spread from staph endocarditis (especially in intravenous drug abusers with right heart endocarditis), nosocomial infection.

   ▶ Treatment Steps

   1. *Begin antibiotic immediately* (β-lactamase–resistant penicillin; if resistant: vancomycin, quinupristin/dalfopristin, or linezolid).
   2. Oxygen if hypoxic.

3. *Haemophilus influenzae* Pneumonia

   ▶ H&P Keys

   Young children, chronic lung disease, alcoholics. Fever, cough, dyspnea, purulent sputum. May present with subacute presentation over several weeks.

   ▶ Diagnosis

   Sputum Gram stain, sputum and blood culture, chest roentgenogram (multilobar patchy infiltrates).

   ▶ Disease Severity

   Pulse oximetry, ABG, respiratory rate, chest roentgenogram. Empyema is rare.

   ▶ Concept and Application

   Pulmonary infection caused by *Haemophilus influenzae*.

   ▶ Treatment Steps

   Begin antibiotic immediately (broad spectrum quinolone if over 18 years of age, cefuroxime, ampicillin/clavulinic acid, chloramphenicol, others).

4. Gram-Negative Bacillary Pneumonias

   ▶ H&P Keys

   Usually nosocomial, fever, chills, dyspnea, cough productive of purulent and sometimes bloody sputum.

▶ Diagnosis

Sputum Gram stain, sputum and blood cultures, chest roentgenogram (lobar or multilobar, cavitary infiltrates), elevated WBC.

▶ Disease Severity

Pulse oximetry, ABG, respiratory rate, chest roentgenogram (multilobed involvement and cavitation). High mortality.

▶ Concept and Application

Aspiration of gram-negative bacilli from colonized oropharynx. *Klebsiella pneumoniae, Acinetobacter* and *Pseudomonas* species, Enterobacteriacae genera; common in immunocompromised and mechanically ventilated patients. *Klebsiella* common in alcoholics.

▶ Treatment Steps

1. Third-generation cephalosporin or semisynthetic penicillin (ticarcillin, piperacillin) plus either an aminoglycoside or a broad-spectrum quinolone.
2. Check antibiotic sensitivities (resistant strains common).
3. Oxygen if hypoxic.
4. May require intensive care unit monitoring.

### G. Atypical Pneumonias

#### 1. Legionnaire's Disease

▶ H&P Keys

Lethargy, headache, fever, rigors, anorexia, myalgias, nonproductive cough, nausea, vomiting, and diarrhea. Rales and rhonchi, abdominal tenderness, relative bradycardia.

▶ Diagnosis

Chest roentgenogram (lobar, nodular, or patchy subsegmental), low sodium and phosphate, elevated WBC. Sputum culture (requires special media), serologic titers, urinary antigen.

▶ Disease Severity

Symptoms, respiratory rate, pulse oximetry, ABG, chest roentgenogram.

▶ Concept and Application

Infection with *Legionella* species; transmitted through contaminated water system (not person to person). More common in immunocompromised, chronic disease, dialysis, alcoholics.

▶ Treatment Steps

1. Begin antibiotic immediately (macrolide, tetracycline, or quinolone).
2. Add rifampin in severe cases.
3. Oxygen if hypoxic.

#### 2. *Mycoplasma pneumoniae* Infection

▶ H&P Keys

Fever, chills, persistent nonproductive cough, headache, sore throat. Common in young adults.

▶ Diagnosis

Gram stain (many WBCs without predominant organism), chest roentgenogram (interstitial or diffuse alveolar infiltrates), cold agglutinins, serum complement fixation titers.

▶ Disease Severity

Usually does not require hospitalization.

▶ Concept and Application

Extrapulmonary manifestations common, including bullous myringitis, pharyngitis, meningitis, and erythema multiforme, Stevens–Johnson syndrome.

▶ Treatment Steps

Macrolide antibiotic, quinolone, or tetracycline.

3. *Pneumocystis carinii* Pneumonia

▶ H&P Keys

Opportunistic infection most commonly related to HIV or other immunodeficiency states. Subacute onset fever, dyspnea, nonproductive cough, tachypnea, tachycardia, diffuse rales.

▶ Diagnosis

Induced sputum cytology, bronchoscopic lavage or biopsy, elevated lactic dehydrogenase (LDH), HIV test, CD4 count, chest roentgenogram (diffuse interstitial or alveolar infiltrates, may be atypical or even clear).

▶ Disease Severity

Pulse oximetry, ABG, respiratory rate, and clinical appearance.

▶ Concept and Application

Molecular genetic data suggest organism is fungal.

▶ Treatment Steps

1. Trimethoprim and sulfamethoxazole (TMP-SMZ) or pentamidine.
2. Oxygen and systemic corticosteroids if hypoxic.
3. Prevent in susceptible patients with TMP-SMZ, dapsone, or aerosolized pentamadine. Aerosol less effective; risk of upper lobe disease.

4. Influenza Pneumonia

▶ H&P Keys

Abrupt onset fever, chills, headache, myalgias, and malaise. Nonproductive or productive cough, tachypnea and dyspnea follow.

▶ Diagnosis

Sputum Gram's stain (many WBCs without organisms); chest roentgenogram (bilateral diffuse midlung and lower-lung infiltrates), viral cultures of nose and throat, acute and convalescent serum titers.

▶ Disease Severity

Respiratory rate, clinical appearance.

▶ Concept and Application

Viral pneumonia caused by influenza A.

▶ Treatment Steps

1. Zanamivir, oseltamivir, or rimantadine if administered within 48 hours of onset, otherwise symptomatic treatment.
2. Prophylactic influenza vaccine for high- and moderate-risk groups.
3. Consider post-exposure prophylaxis of high-risk patients with zanamivir, oseltamivir, rimantadine, or amantadine.

## H. Pulmonary Tuberculosis

▶ H&P Keys

Fever, malaise, weight loss, dyspnea, night sweats; productive cough with hemoptysis, rales in area of involvement; amphoric breath sounds may indicate cavity.

▶ Diagnosis

Chest roentgenogram (upper-lobe cavitary disease if reactivation, lower-lobe infiltrates in primary infection, upper-lobe scarring may indicate prior inactive infection). Sputum culture, acid-fast smear; bronchoscopy if unable to get diagnosis on sputum studies. Purified protein derivative (tuberculin) (PPD) skin test.

▶ Disease Severity

Chest roentgenogram. Extrapulmonary involvement (lymphatic, pleural, peritoneal, genitourinary, miliary, bone and joint, meningeal) may be more problematic. Drug-resistant strains more difficult to treat.

▶ Concept and Application

Inhalation of *Mycobacterium tuberculosis* leads to primary lower-lobe infection. Localized inflammatory response usually halts infection. Reactivation disease occurs in upper lobes of lung or other areas of high oxygen content.

▶ Treatment Steps

*Prophylaxis*—Isoniazid for 6–12 months in appropriate patients with inactive infection (Table 16–1).

*Treatment*
1. Isoniazid and rifampin for 6 months, with pyrazinamide plus either ethambutol or streptomycin for first 2 months. In cities with frequent drug resistance, therapy may be started with five or six drugs. Drug-resistant strains require longer treatment with additional antibiotics.
2. Directly observed therapy highly recommended.

## 16-1 INTERPRETATION OF TUBERCULIN SKIN TESTING

1. A reaction of > 5 mm is classified as positive in the following groups of patients:
   - HIV positive
   - Recent close contact
   - Fibrotic changes on CXR c/w old TB
   - Immune suppressed (equivalent of ≥ 15 mg/d prednisone ≥ 1 mo)
2. A reaction of > 10 mm is classified as positive in persons who have other risk factors for tuberculosis or are in high-prevalence situations. These include:
   - Injection drug users
   - Diabetes mellitus
   - High risk job or environment exposure
   - Hematologic, head, neck malignancies
   - Chronic renal failure
   - Weight > 10% below ideal body weight
   - Silicosis
   - Gastrectomy
   - Recent immigrant (≤ 5 yrs) from high-prevalence country
   - Resident/employee of high-risk setting
   - Children/adolescent
   - Prison inmate
   - Medical caregiver
   - TB lab personnel
3. Reactions > 15 mm are classified as positive in all other persons.

*Sources:* American Thoracic Society/Centers for Disease Control. Diagnostic standards and classifications of tuberculosis in adults and children. *Am J Respir Crit Care Med* 161: 1376–1395, 2000; and ATS/CDC. Targeted tuberculin testing and treatment of latent tuberculosis infection. *Am J Respir Crit Care Med* 161 (4 Pt 2): S221–47, 2000.

## I. Fungal Pneumonias

### 1. Histoplasmosis

▶ **H&P Keys**

Mostly asymptomatic, can have abrupt onset of flulike illness, with fever, chills, substernal chest pain, nonproductive cough with myalgias, arthralgias, and headache.

▶ **Diagnosis**

Chest roentgenogram: acute disease often normal, hilar adenopathy with lower-lobe alveolar infiltrates, leading to chronic calcification). Progressive form mimics tuberculosis. Diagnosis with sputum culture. Progressive disseminated histoplasmosis: blood and bone marrow culture. Serologic testing (acute and convalescent titers; poor sensitivity).

▶ **Disease Severity**

Progressive and progressive disseminated more severe. Latter associated with T-cell dysfunction (AIDS).

▶ **Concept and Application**

Infection with *Histoplasma capsulatum.* Inhalation of spores from soil (bat and bird droppings) evolve into pathogenic yeast form. Endemic areas: Ohio and Mississippi River valleys and neighboring states.

▶ Treatment Steps

*Acute*—None needed.

*Progressive Cavitary Disease*
1. Itraconazole.
2. Alternative: ketoconazole.

*Progressive Disseminated Disease*—Amphotericin B.

*Chronic Suppression (for Patients with AIDS)*—Itraconazole.

2. Blastomycosis

▶ H&P Keys

Abrupt fever, chills, cough with mucopurulent sputum, arthralgias, and myalgias. Signs of consolidation, erythema nodosum.

▶ Diagnosis

KOH preparation of expectorated sputum; culture, complement fixation. Chest roentgenogram (round densities, may cavitate).

▶ Disease Severity

Chest roentgenogram, evidence of extrapulmonary involvement.

▶ Concept and Application

Infection with *Blastomyces dermatitidis*. Yeast form pathogenic. Manifestations vary: asymptomatic to severe, life-threatening, disseminated illness. Midwest and south central United States, midwestern Canada.

▶ Treatment Steps

*Progressive Pulmonary, Nonsevere*
1. Itraconazole.
2. Alternative: ketoconazole.

*Disseminated or Severe Disease*—Amphotericin B.

3. Coccidioidomycosis

▶ H&P Keys

Cough, fever, pleuritic chest pain, headache (may be indicative of meningitis); erythematous rash, "valley fever": erythema nodosum, erythema multiforme, arthralgias.

▶ Diagnosis

Chest roentgenogram (patchy pneumonitis, hilar adenopathy, "coin lesions," cavitary lesions), KOH preparation of sputum, lung biopsy, complement fixation, skin test.

▶ Disease Severity

Disseminated disease (meningitis, skin lesions, bone, etc). Dissemination more common in AIDS, steroids, malignant disease, African Americans, Native Americans, Mexicans.

▶ Concept and Application

Infection with *Coccidioides immitis*. Spherules are pathogenic form. Mostly mild, self-limited, but can be life threatening and disseminated. Southwestern United States and California valley regions, northern Mexico.

▶ Treatment Steps

*Nonmeningeal Disease*
1. Fluconazole or amphotericin B.
2. Alternative: ketoconazole, itraconazole.

*Disseminated Disease or Meningitis*
1. Fluconazole, miconazole, or amphotericin B.
2. Intrathecal amphotericin if fluconazole fails.

4. Cryptococcus

▶ H&P Keys

*Pneumonia*—Usually asymptomatic, but may have fever, malaise, chest pain, cough.

*Meningitis*—Subacute fever, confusion, headache. May be fulminant. Cranial nerve palsies.

▶ Diagnosis

Cerebrospinal fluid (CSF) examination (India ink stain, latex particle agglutination), lung biopsy, chest roentgenogram (variable, large and small round lesions).

▶ Disease Severity

Disseminated disease (CNS), presence of meningitis, chest roentgenogram.

▶ Concept and Application

*Cryptococcus neoformans,* found in bird droppings and soil. Increased risk in AIDS, corticosteroid use, Hodgkin's disease, other immunocompromised states.

▶ Treatment Steps

1. None needed in noncompromised host with isolated pulmonary disease.

*Immunocompromised Host or Disseminated Disease*
1. Amphotericin B plus flucytosine.
2. Alternatives: fluconazole, itraconazole.

5. Invasive Aspergillosis

▶ H&P Keys

Immunosuppressed patient on multiple antibiotics, high fever, pleuritic chest pain, pleural friction rub.

▶ Diagnosis

Cultures of sputum and nasal swab (suggestive, not diagnostic), lung biopsy.

▶ Disease Severity

Chest roentgenogram (lobar, peripheral wedge-shaped infiltrates, often cavitary), pulse oximetry, ABG.

▶ Concept and Application

Opportunistic infection with *Aspergillus fumigatus* causing pneumonia, pulmonary infarction.

▶ Treatment Steps

1. Amphotericin B; use liposomal preparation if renal dysfunction. Alternatives: voriconazole or caspofungin (if amphotericin refractory).
2. Add flucytosine if metastatic infection.
3. Consider surgical resection if focal but severe disease.

6. Phycomycosis

▶ H&P Keys

Occurs in diabetic ketoacidosis, with glucocorticosteroids, cytotoxic agents, burn victims. Rhinocerebral disease, acute pneumonia with pleuritic chest pain and hemoptysis.

▶ Diagnosis

Chest roentgenogram (multiple wedge-shaped infiltrates), tissue biopsy.

▶ Disease Severity

Life-threatening disease.

▶ Concept and Application

Infection with *Mucor* (most common), also *Rhizopus* or *Absidia*.

▶ Treatment Steps

1. Amphotericin B and aggressive resectional surgery.
2. Prognosis extremely poor.

## II. OBSTRUCTIVE PULMONARY DISEASES

### A. Pulmonary Function Tests

See Table 16–2.

*Obstruction*—Low forced expiratory volume in one second ($FEV_1$), low or normal forced vital capacity (FVC), reduced $FEV_1$:FVC ratio (< 75%), normal total lung capacity (TLC).

*Restriction*—Defined by reduced TLC. Pure restriction will also have low $FEV_1$, FVC with normal or elevated $FEV_1$:FVC ratio.

*Combined Obstruction and Restriction*—Reduced $FEV_1$, FVC, and $FEV_1$:FVC ratio with reduced TLC.

### B. Asthma

▶ H&P Keys

Acute onset of dyspnea, wheezing, cough that remit spontaneously or with treatment.

### 16-2 CHARACTERISTIC CHANGES IN LUNG VOLUMES AND FLOW RATES IN PATIENTS WITH RESTRICTIVE AND OBSTRUCTIVE VENTILATORY DISORDERS

| Test | Restrictive | Obstructive | Combined |
|---|---|---|---|
| Forced vital capacity (FVC) | Decreased | Decreased or normal | Decreased |
| Total lung capacity (TLC) | Decreased | Increased | Decreased |
| FEV-1 | Decreased | Decreased | Decreased |
| FEV-1/FVC ratio | Increased or normal | Decreased | Decreased or normal |

▶ Diagnosis

Pulmonary function testing (PFT) (obstructive), response to bronchodilators, response to bronchoconstricting provocational agents.

▶ Disease Severity

PFT, use of accessory muscles, ABG, paradoxical pulse, respiratory rate, pulse oximetry, symptoms, mentation.

▶ Concept and Application

Bronchospasm, inflammation, hyperreactivity to inhaled antigens and irritants, mucus plugging. Obstruction may improve to normal with treatment (Fig. 16–1).

▶ Treatment Steps

1. Acute Asthma

    *Bronchodilators*
    1. Inhaled β-agonist, inhaled ipratropium bromide.
    2. If fails, consider subcutaneous epinephrine, and/or intravenous aminophylline.

    *Anti-inflammatory Agents*—Systemic corticosteroids; use if severe.

2. Chronic Asthma

    a. Anti-inflammatory Agents
    1. Inhaled corticosteroids, cromolyn sodium, nedocromil sodium, or oral anti-leukotriene blocker (montelukast, zafirlukast).
    2. Choose one as "controller"; may add a second for poor control. Combining inhaled steroid with long-acting inhaled β-agonist improves control.

    b. Bronchodilator Agents
    β-Agonists (inhaled, subcutaneous, oral) as "rescue," theophylline.

    c. Avoidance of Causative Agents

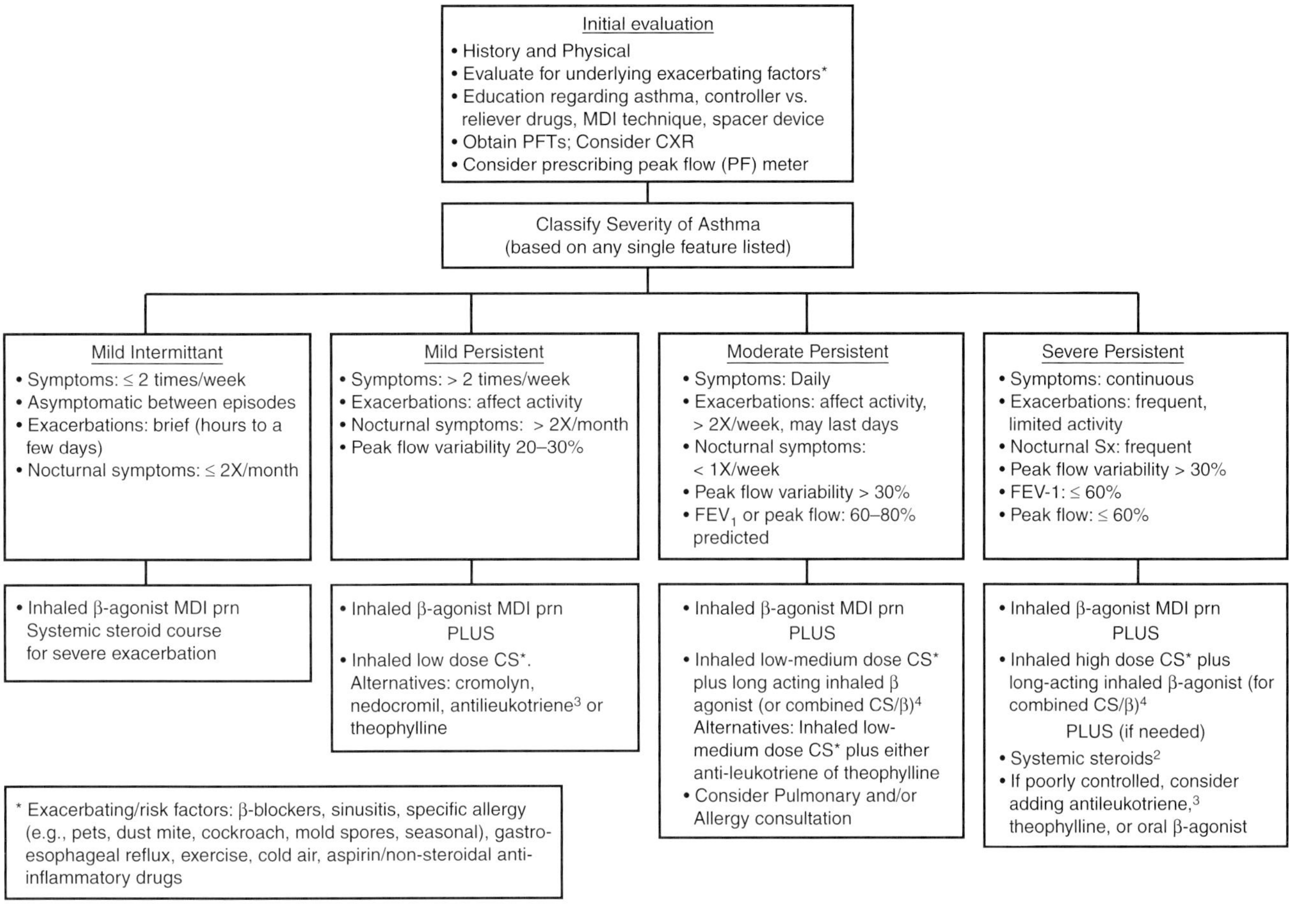

```
                        ┌─────────────────────────────────────────┐
                        │           Initial evaluation            │
                        │  • History and Physical                 │
                        │  • Evaluate for underlying exacerbating factors* │
                        │  • Education regarding asthma, controller vs.   │
                        │    reliever drugs, MDI technique, spacer device │
                        │  • Obtain PFTs; Consider CXR            │
                        │  • Consider prescribing peak flow (PF) meter │
                        └─────────────────────────────────────────┘
                                         │
                        ┌─────────────────────────────────────────┐
                        │        Classify Severity of Asthma      │
                        │   (based on any single feature listed)  │
                        └─────────────────────────────────────────┘
```

| Mild Intermittant | Mild Persistent | Moderate Persistent | Severe Persistent |
|---|---|---|---|
| • Symptoms: ≤ 2 times/week<br>• Asymptomatic between episodes<br>• Exacerbations: brief (hours to a few days)<br>• Nocturnal symptoms: ≤ 2X/month | • Symptoms: > 2 times/week<br>• Exacerbations: affect activity<br>• Nocturnal symptoms: > 2X/month<br>• Peak flow variability 20–30% | • Symptoms: Daily<br>• Exacerbations: affect activity, > 2X/week, may last days<br>• Nocturnal symptoms: < 1X/week<br>• Peak flow variability > 30%<br>• $FEV_1$ or peak flow: 60–80% predicted | • Symptoms: continuous<br>• Exacerbations: frequent, limited activity<br>• Nocturnal Sx: frequent<br>• Peak flow variability > 30%<br>• FEV-1: ≤ 60%<br>• Peak flow: ≤ 60% |
| • Inhaled β-agonist MDI prn Systemic steroid course for severe exacerbation | • Inhaled β-agonist MDI prn PLUS<br>• Inhaled low dose CS*. Alternatives: cromolyn, nedocromil, antileukotriene[3] or theophylline | • Inhaled β-agonist MDI prn PLUS<br>• Inhaled low-medium dose CS* plus long acting inhaled β agonist (or combined CS/β)[4] Alternatives: Inhaled low-medium dose CS* plus either anti-leukotriene of theophylline<br>• Consider Pulmonary and/or Allergy consultation | • Inhaled β-agonist MDI prn PLUS<br>• Inhaled high dose CS* plus long-acting inhaled β-agonist (for combined CS/β)[4]<br>PLUS (if needed)<br>• Systemic steroids[2]<br>• If poorly controlled, consider adding antileukotriene,[3] theophylline, or oral β-agonist |

* Exacerbating/risk factors: β-blockers, sinusitis, specific allergy (e.g., pets, dust mite, cockroach, mold spores, seasonal), gastroesophageal reflux, exercise, cold air, aspirin/non-steroidal anti-inflammatory drugs

Figure 16–1. Chronic Asthma Management. Adapted, with permission, from Sherman ES. Chronic asthma management. In Sherman MS, Schulman ES, eds. *The Pocket Doctor*, 2001, Educational Communications, Mt. Kisko, NY, 2001 and www.pocketdoctor.com.

## C. Chronic Obstructive Pulmonary Diseases

Commonly used term with no agreed-upon definition. Term is usually applied to patients with chronic bronchitis or emphysema who have obstruction on PFTs. The obstruction may be partially reversible.

### 1. Chronic Bronchitis

▶ H&P Keys

Defined as presence of chronic productive cough for *3 months in 2 successive years* without other discernible cause. Dyspnea, recurrent productive cough, "blue bloater"; cyanosis with edema, wheezes.

▶ Diagnosis

PFTs (obstructive), history, chest roentgenogram (usually clear or hyperinflated). Sputum cultures for acute exacerbations.

▶ Disease Severity

PFTs, pulse oximetry, ABG.

▶ Concept and Application

In pure form, pathologic conditions in bronchi and airways, not alveoli. Tobacco smoke a causative agent. Bacterial infections may exacerbate (pneumococcus, *Haemophilus,* others).

*Simple Chronic Bronchitis*—Symptoms fit criteria for chronic bronchitis but no obstruction on PFTs (therefore not truly a form of COPD).

*Obstructive Chronic Bronchitis*—Symptoms fit criteria for chronic bronchitis, reduced $FEV_1$ percent with no or partial bronchodilator response (this is a form of COPD). Obstruction caused by hypertrophic glands in airway, mucous hypersecretion.

▶ Treatment Steps
1. Smoking cessation.
2. Ipratropium bromide.
3. Add inhaled β-agonist bronchodilator if needed (combined product now available).
4. Influenza and pneumococcal vaccination.
5. Antibiotics for acute bacterial exacerbation.
6. Oxygen if $Po_2 < 55$ (or $\leq 60$ with cor pulmonale).
7. Corticosteroids if severe.

2. Emphysema

▶ H&P Keys

Dyspnea, wheezing, cough. "Pink puffer": thin, not cyanotic, tachypneic. Diminished breath sounds, hyperinflated chest, hyperresonant to percussion.

▶ Diagnosis

Obstructive PFTs (TLC may be increased), chest roentgenogram, history, and physical. Serum protein electrophoresis or $\alpha_1$-protease inhibitor level if deficiency suspected.

▶ Disease Severity

PFTs, ABG, exercise tolerance.

▶ Concept and Application

Defined pathologically: enlarged respiratory air spaces beyond terminal bronchioles, with destruction of alveoli. Smoking a major risk factor; $\alpha_1$-protease inhibitor deficiency a rare cause.

▶ Treatment Steps
1. Smoking cessation.
2. Ipratropium bromide.
3. Add inhaled β-agonist bronchodilator if needed (combined product now available).
4. Influenza and pneumococcal vaccination.
5. Oxygen if $Po_2 < 55$ (or $\leq 60$ with cor pulmonale).
6. Corticosteroids if severe and patient responsive. $\alpha_1$-Protease inhibitor for deficient patients.

3. Cystic Fibrosis

   ▶ H&P Keys

   Persistent cough, recurrent pneumonia and bronchitis, recurrent abdominal pain, meconium ileus, failure to thrive, steatorrhea, infertility, diabetes, family history. Usually diagnosed in childhood.

   ▶ Diagnosis

   Sweat chloride test (60 mEq/L before age 20; 80 in adults) diagnostic. Genetic testing available for more common genotypes of CF. *Pseudomonas* lung infection, unexplained azoospermia, and obstruction on PFTs suggests diagnosis. Chest roentgenogram (hyperinflation, enlarged pulmonary arteries, bronchiectasis, cystic areas).

   ▶ Disease Severity

   PFTs, pulse oximetry, ABG, chest roentgenogram.

   ▶ Concept and Application

   Autosomal recessive disorder; CF gene locus located on long arm of chromosome 7; genetic defect in chloride permeability in exocrine glands due to cystic fibrosis transmembrane regulator protein (CFTR); affects all exocrine secretions; frequent *Pseudomonas* and *Staph* infections.

   ▶ Treatment Steps
   1. Chest physiotherapy.
   2. Inhaled β-agonist and mucolytic agents (DNase, acetylcysteine).
   3. Antibiotics prn; aerosol tobramycin for chronic *Pseudomonas*.
   4. Influenza vaccine.
   5. Pancreatic enzymes (experimental: genetic replacement therapy with CFTR).
   6. Lung transplant in selected cases.

4. Bronchiectasis

   ▶ H&P Keys

   Chronic cough, copious purulent sputum, recurrent fever, weakness, weight loss, hemoptysis, clubbing, cyanosis, edema.

   ▶ Diagnosis

   History, chest roentgenogram, high-resolution computerized tomographic (CT) scan, bronchography (rarely used), sputum culture.

   ▶ Disease Severity

   PFTs (obstructive), stigmata of cor pulmonale.

   ▶ Concept and Application

   Abnormal dilatation of bronchi from inflammation and destruction of bronchial wall. Often associated with infection, bronchial obstruction, immotile-cilia syndrome, cystic fibrosis, allergic bronchopulmonary aspergillosis, immunoglobulin deficiency.

▶ Treatment Steps
1. Chest physiotherapy.
2. Antibiotics for infection.
3. Steroids for allergic bronchopulmonary aspergillosis if present.
4. Surgery or bronchial artery embolization for severe hemoptysis.

## III. RESTRICTIVE PULMONARY DISEASES

### A. Idiopathic

1. Sarcoidosis

    ▶ H&P Keys
    May be asymptomatic. Dyspnea, cough, wheezing, hemoptysis, skin lesions (erythema nodosum, nodules, plaques), eye pain, arthralgias, cardiac arrhythmias, cranial nerve palsies. More common in African Americans, Scandinavians.

    ▶ Diagnosis
    Chest roentgenogram (bilateral hilar adenopathy, interstitial lung disease), tissue biopsy (noncaseating granuloma). Elevated serum calcium or angiotensin-converting enzyme suggestive. Exposure history to rule out occupational granulamatous disease or intravenous injection of foreign matter (ie, talc).

    ▶ Disease Severity
    PFTs (restriction, low diffusion), chest roentgenogram, gallium scan (reflects disease activity); presence of CNS and cardiac involvement.

    ▶ Concept and Application
    Granulomatous disorder of unknown etiology.

    ▶ Treatment Steps
    1. May be self-limited.
    2. Corticosteroids for significant pulmonary, CNS, or cardiac disease.
    3. Hydroxychloroquine sulfate (Plaquenil Sulfate) or topical steroids for skin involvement.
    4. Alternative agents include methotrexate, azathioprine.

2. Idiopathic Pulmonary Fibrosis

    a. Usual Interstitial Pneumonitis (UIP)

    ▶ H&P Keys
    Insidious onset of dyspnea (may progress over many years), nonproductive cough, clubbing, fine crackles, cyanosis, stigmata of cor pulmonale, Raynaud's phenomenon.

▶ Diagnosis
Chest roentgenogram (diffuse interstitial infiltrates), lung biopsy, PFTs (restriction, low diffusion), low positive antinuclear antibodies (ANA) titer.

▶ Disease Severity
PFTs, high resolution chest CT scan, ABG, exercise capacity.

▶ Concept and Application
Pulmonary fibrosis of unknown etiology leading to hypoxia and cor pulmonale. Also called fibrosing alveolitis.

▶ Treatment Steps
1. Corticosteroids.
2. If fails—azathioprine or cyclophosphamide.
3. Treat cor pulmonale with diuretics, oxygen.
4. Lung transplant only definitive therapy.

b. Desquamative Interstitial Pneumonitis (DIP)—Predominant alveolar component, more responsive to drugs, mostly in smokers.

▶ Diagnosis
Chest roentgenogram (diffuse interstitial infiltrates), lung biopsy, PFTs (restriction, low diffusion).

▶ Disease Severity
PFTs, high resolution chest CT scan, ABG, exercise capacity.

▶ Treatment Steps
1. Stop smoking.
2. Corticosteroids.
3. If fails—cyclophosphamide.
4. Treat cor pulmonale with diuretics, oxygen.

B. Pneumoconiosis

1. Silicosis

▶ H&P Keys
Sandblasters, miners, stoneworkers. Asymptomatic, or progressive dyspnea, cough.

▶ Diagnosis
Exposure history, chest roentgenogram (upper lobe nodules, "eggshell calcification" of hilar nodes), PFTs (restriction), lung biopsy only if diagnosis in doubt.

▶ Disease Severity
Chest roentgenogram and PFTs. Progressive massive fibrosis: coalescence of small nodules into larger conglomerate lesions.

▶ Concept and Application
Inhalation of quartz particles damages alveolar cells and causes reactive fibrosis. Increased risk for tuberculosis.

▶ Treatment Steps
1. Avoidance of further exposure.
2. No medical treatment known to be effective.
3. Lung transplantation in severe cases.

2. Asbestosis

▶ H&P Keys

History of asbestos exposure (mining, shipbuilding, insulation workers, construction). Asymptomatic, or progressive dyspnea, persistent cough, basilar inspiratory crackles, clubbing.

▶ Diagnosis

Clinical diagnosis: interstitial disease with exposure history. Chest roentgenogram (lower-lobe linear infiltrates, pleural plaques and thickening); high resolution chest CT scan, PFTs (restriction), ferruginous bodies (hemosiderin-coated asbestos fibers) in sputum, alveolar lavage fluid, or lung tissue suggestive but not diagnostic.

▶ Disease Severity

Chest roentgenogram, PFTs.

▶ Concept and Application

Inhalation of asbestos fibers releases damaging enzymes and inflammatory mediators; direct damage to epithelial cells, leading to inflammation, fibrosis, and interstitial lung disease. Increased risk of lung cancer, especially in smokers.

▶ Treatment Steps
1. Avoidance of further exposure.
2. Stop smoking.

a. Other Asbestos-Related Diseases

*Mesothelioma*—Malignant tumor of the mesothelial cells of the pleura. Usually associated with severe chest wall pain.

*Pleural Plaques*—Benign, asymptomatic fibrous plaques detected on chest roentgenogram. Most common finding in asbestos exposure.

*Pleural Thickening*—Asymptomatic, detected on chest roentgenogram.

*Acute Benign Pleural Effusions*

3. Coal Workers' Pneumoconiosis

▶ H&P Keys

Coal miners, carbon manufacturers.

*Simple Coal Workers' Pneumoconiosis*—Asymptomatic radiographic finding.

*Complicated Coal Workers' Pneumoconiosis (Progressive Massive Fibrosis—PMF)*—Dyspnea, signs of cor pulmonale, hemoptysis.

*Chronic Obstructive Lung Disease*—Dyspnea, wheezing, productive cough.

▶ Diagnosis

Occupational exposure, chest roentgenogram (small round opacities, usually upper lobes), PFTs. X-ray findings are not necessary for the diagnosis.

▶ Disease Severity

PFTs (usually normal in simple disease; restrictive in PMF, obstructive in COPD), chest roentgenogram. Simple has small round opacities; PMF has enlarging, irregular nodular infiltrates, which may cavitate.

▶ Concept and Application

Pulmonary nodules resulting from exposure to coal dust. PMF probably caused by an immunologic response. Effects of coal dust inhalation and concomitant smoking are additive on COPD severity. Increased risk for tuberculosis. COPD from coal dust exposure may be present even absent radiographic findings.

▶ Treatment Steps
1. Avoidance.
2. Surveillance for COPD, PMF, tuberculosis.
3. Stop smoking.
4. Treatment of COPD if present.

4. Hypersensitivity Pneumonitis

▶ H&P Keys

*Acute*—Fever, chills, dyspnea, malaise 4–6 hours after exposure to antigen, lasting 18–24 hours.

*Subacute*—Insidious onset of cough, progressive dyspnea, fatigue, and weight loss, diffuse crackles.

*Chronic*—Insidious onset of progressive dyspnea over years.

▶ Diagnosis

Exposure history key to diagnosis. Common antigens include: Thermophilic *Actinomyces* (farmer's lung: moldy hay; bagassosis: moldy sugar cane); avian secretory proteins (pigeon breeder's disease). Serum precipitins can help identify agent but are not diagnostic of disease. High resolution CT pattern suggestive.

▶ Disease Severity

Chest roentgenogram (interstitial and alveolar infiltrates); PFTs (restriction, decreased diffusion).

▶ Concept and Application

Immune-complex-mediated and cell-mediated hypersensitivity responses to inhaled antigen.

▶ Treatment Steps
1. Removal and avoidance of offending antigen.
2. Corticosteroids for severe attacks or if symptoms persist.

## IV. PLEURAL DISEASES

### A. Pleural Effusion

▶ H&P Keys

Asymptomatic or signs and symptoms of underlying cause. Dyspnea, pleuritic chest pain. Decreased breath sounds, dullness to percussion.

▶ Diagnosis

Chest roentgenogram with lateral decubitus views. Pleural fluid chemistries (LDH, protein, glucose) (Table 16–3), cell count, cultures.

▶ Disease Severity

Chest roentgenogram.

▶ Concept and Application

*Transudate*—Increased hydrostatic pressure or decreased systemic oncotic pressure.

*Diagnosis*—Pleural protein:serum protein < 0.5, pleural LDH:serum LDH < 0.6, pleural LDH less than two thirds of the upper limit of normal for serum LDH.

*Examples*—Congestive heart failure, nephrotic syndrome.

*Exudate*—Intrapulmonary or abdominal inflammation adjacent to pleura.

*Diagnosis*—Pleural:serum protein > 0.5, pleural:serum LDH > 0.6, pleural LDH greater than two thirds upper limit of normal for serum LDH.

*Examples*—Parapneumonic effusion, empyema, malignant disease, collagen vascular diseases.

▶ Treatment Steps
1. Treatment of underlying disease.
2. Drainage of fluid with thoracentesis or chest tube if symptomatic or infected.
3. Sclerosis with doxycycline or talc for recurrent effusions.

**16-3 CHARACTERISTIC CHEMISTRIES OF PLEURAL EFFUSIONS**

|  | Exudate | Transudate |
|---|---|---|
| Protein | > 3 g/dL | < 3 g/dL |
| Pleural/serum protein | > 0.5 | < 0.5 |
| LDH | > 200 | < 200 |
| Pleural/serum LDH | > 0.6 | < 0.6 |

## B. Pleurisy (Pleuritis)

▶ **H&P Keys**

Pleuritic chest pain (sharp pain on inspiration), usually rapid onset, dyspnea, low-grade fever.

▶ **Diagnosis**

Chest roentgenogram, history and physical.

▶ **Disease Severity**

Usually self-limited.

▶ **Concept and Application**

Inflammation of pleura.

*Pleurodynia*—Epidemic infection with coxsackie B or ECHO virus.

*Pleuritis*—Pleural inflammation, which may be due to infection, pulmonary infarction, collagen vascular disease, etc.

▶ **Treatment Steps**
1. Nonsteroidal anti-inflammatory agents.
2. If fails—corticosteroids if indicated.

## C. Pneumothorax

▶ **H&P Keys**

Chest pain, dyspnea, enlarged hemithorax, hyperresonance to percussion, absent or reduced breath sounds and fremitus on involved side, tracheal shift away from involved side.

▶ **Diagnosis**

Chest roentgenogram (air in pleural space).

▶ **Disease Severity**

Chest roentgenogram, pulse oximetry and ABG, pulse rate, respiratory rate, blood pressure.

▶ **Concept and Application**

Communication between lung or atmosphere and pleural space.

*Spontaneous Pneumothorax*—Rupture of subpleural blebs or bullae; also seen with COPD and interstitial lung diseases.

*Traumatic Pneumothorax*—Result of direct or indirect chest trauma.

*Tension Pneumothorax*—Intrapleural pressure exceeds atmospheric pressure, decreases venous return, which drops cardiac output and blood pressure.

▶ **Treatment Steps**
1. Observation if stable.
2. Chest tube if large, symptomatic, or if tension pneumothorax is present or suspected.

## V. DISEASES OF PULMONARY CIRCULATION

### A. Cardiogenic Pulmonary Edema (Congestive Heart Failure)

▶ H&P Keys

Dyspnea, diapheresis, wheezing, tachycardia, cyanosis, diffuse crackles or rales, edema, cough with frothy sputum, fine and coarse crackles, S3, displaced point of maximal impulse (PMI), peripheral edema.

▶ Diagnosis

History and physical, chest roentgenogram (diffuse alveolar infiltrates, enlarged heart, Kerley's B lines), echocardiogram or nuclear multiple-gated arteriography (MUGA) scan, electrocardiogram (ECG) (ischemic changes), pulmonary artery catheterization (elevated pulmonary artery and pulmonary artery occlusion pressures).

▶ Disease Severity

ABG, clinical appearance, vital signs, pulmonary artery occlusion pressure.

▶ Concept and Application

Increased hydrostatic pressure from left ventricular failure (ischemia, myocardial infarction [MI]) or fluid overload.

▶ Treatment Steps

1. Oxygen.
2. Diuresis (furosemide, low-dose dopamine).
3. Venodilators (nitroglycerin, morphine), afterload reduction agents (intravenous nitroglycerin, sodium nitroprusside; angiotensin converting enzyme inhibitors).
4. Dobutamine.
5. Pulmonary arterial catheter to monitor therapy may be helpful.
6. Treatment of ischemia if present.

### B. Adult Respiratory Distress Syndrome

▶ H&P Keys

Acute onset of severe dyspnea, tachypnea, cough productive of frothy sputum, diffuse rales and rhonchi, cyanosis, signs and symptoms of underlying process (sepsis and trauma most common).

▶ Diagnosis

Chest roentgenogram (bilateral alveolar infiltrates), ABG (hypoxemia $PaO_2 < 50$ mm Hg with $FIO_2 > 0.6$), pulmonary artery catheterization (pulmonary artery occlusion pressure > 18) in setting of known risk factor.

▶ Disease Severity

Chest roentgenogram and ABG.

▶ Concept and Application

Pulmonary edema from increased permeability across the alveolar and capillary walls. Risk factors: sepsis, diffuse pulmonary infection, trauma, aspiration, drowning, toxic inhalations, hypertransfusion, others.

▶ Treatment Steps
1. Treatment of underlying cause (eg, antibiotics for sepsis).
2. Supportive measures: mechanical ventilation, oxygen, and positive end-expiratory pressure (PEEP).
3. Use of low tidal volumes on ventilator (5–8 mL/kg) improves outcome.

## C. Newborn Respiratory Distress Syndrome (Hyaline Membrane Disease)

▶ H&P Keys

Neonate, usually premature, with dyspnea, tachypnea, poor air movement; chest wall retractions occur shortly after birth.

▶ Diagnosis

Chest roentgenogram (diffuse granular or ground-glass infiltrate), pulse oximetry, ABG.

▶ Disease Severity

Clinical appearance of respiratory distress, ABG.

▶ Concept and Application

Decreased pulmonary surfactant leading to reduced lung compliance and atelectasis.

▶ Treatment Steps
1. Prevention of premature labor and use of prenatal steroid therapy to reduce incidence of disease.
2. Oxygen.
3. Continuous distending airway pressure (CDAP or CDP).
4. Mechanical ventilation.
5. Surfactant replacement therapy.

## D. Pulmonary Embolism

▶ H&P Keys

Acute onset of dyspnea and pleuritic chest pain. Cough, hemoptysis, tachypnea, tachycardia; look for pleural rub, edema, or tenderness in lower extremity (Fig. 16–2).

▶ Diagnosis

ABG (acute respiratory alkalosis, usually decreased $P_{O_2}$), chest roentgenogram (clear, or wedge-shaped infiltrate, effusion), ECG (sinus tach, or S1, Q3, T3 inversion pattern), ventilation perfusion lung scan (perfusion defect with normal ventilation), noninvasive (eg, duplex ultrasound) or venogram studies for deep venous thrombosis (DVT) in lower extremities, pulmonary angiogram, contrast helical "spiral" CT, quantitative D-dimer levels (if < 500 ng/mL, PE unlikely).

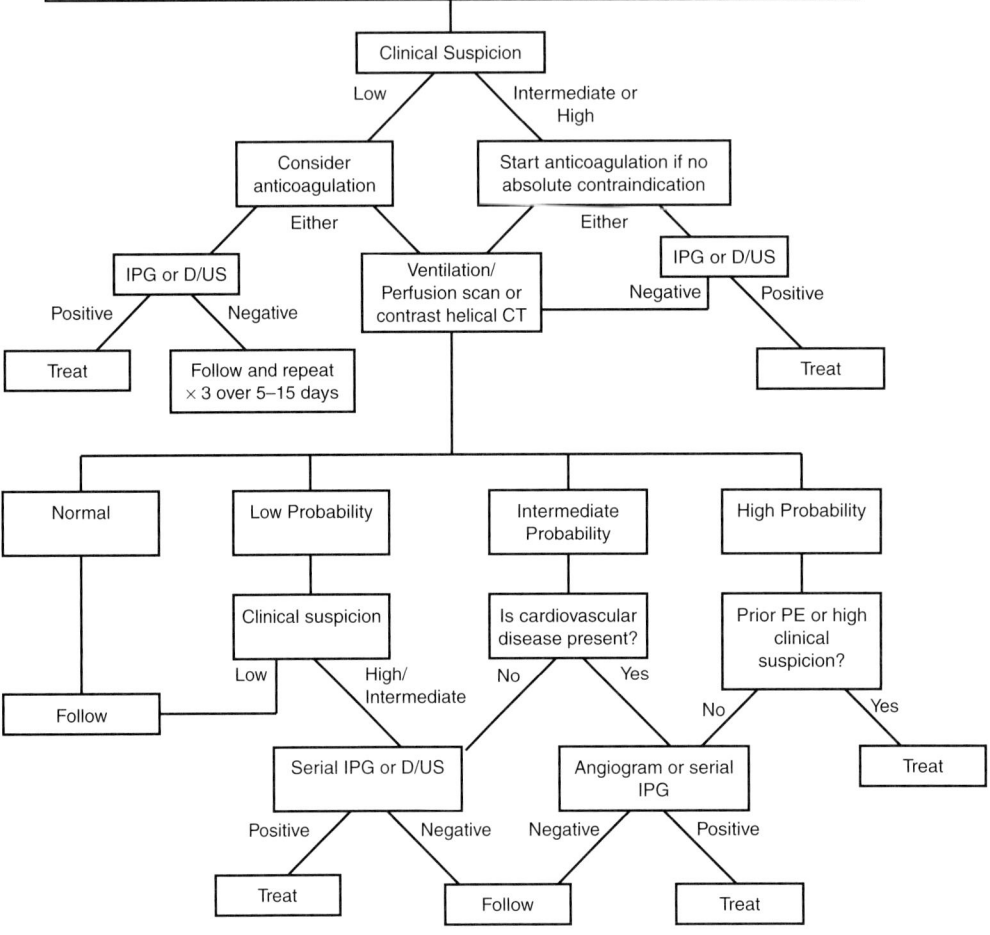

Figure 16–2. Management of Acute Pulmonary Thromboembolism. Adapted, with permission, from Schulman ES. Management of acute pulmonary thromboembolism. In: Sherman MS, Schulman ES, eds. *The Pocket Doctor 2001*. Educational Communications, Mt. Kisko, NY, 2001 and www.pocketdoctor.com.

▶ Disease Severity

ABG, vital signs.

▶ Concept and Application

Venous thrombus, usually from lower extremity, embolizes to pulmonary artery. Pregnancy, use of birth control pills, smoking, malignant disease, obesity, immobilization (hip fracture) at highest risk for DVT.

▶ Treatment Steps

1. Anticoagulation (heparin, then warfarin for 3–6 months).
2. Thrombolytic agents for massive embolism with shock.
3. Embolectomy in unresponsive cases.

4. Vena caval interruption if anticoagulation is contraindicated (vena caval clip, Greenfield filter, others).
5. Prophylaxis of high-risk patients with subcutaneous low-dose heparin, warfarin, or compression boots.

## E. Pulmonary Vasculitis

▶ H&P Keys

Dyspnea; symptoms of underlying disease process.

▶ Diagnosis

Chest roentgenogram, ABG, urinalysis, creatinine, serologic studies for systemic vasculitic processes (ANA, ANCA, hepatitis B and C, rheumatoid factor, cryoglobulins, complement). Tissue biopsy usually required for diagnosis (open lung biopsy or biopsy of other affected organs).

▶ Disease Severity

ABG, exercise tolerance, serologic studies of underlying disease.

▶ Concept and Application

Inflammation of pulmonary blood vessels.

*Leukocytoclastic Vasculitis*—Neutrophilic inflammation caused by drugs, neoplasms, infection.

*Granulomatous Vasculitis*—Lymphocytic infiltration, eg, Wegener's granulomatosis (renal involvement), allergic granulomatosis (asthma, eosinophilia; "Churg–Strauss syndrome").

*Collagen Vascular Diseases*—Rheumatoid arthritis, systemic lupus erythematosus, progressive systemic sclerosis, polymyositis, dermatomyositis, mixed connective tissue disease.

▶ Treatment Steps

*Leukocytoclastic Vasculitis*
1. Usually self-limited.
2. Steroids if hypoxemia present.

*Wegener's Granulomatosis*—Cyclophosphamide with or without corticosteroids.

*Allergic Granulomatosis, Collagen Vascular Diseases*
1. Corticosteroids; azathioprine or cyclophosphamide in severe cases.
2. Progressive systemic sclerosis usually does not respond.

## F. Vasculitis: Goodpasture's Syndrome

▶ H&P Keys

Hemoptysis, hematuria, fever, dyspnea. Pulmonary involvement associated with smoking.

▶ Diagnosis

Antiglomerular basement membrane antibodies, renal biopsy (linear immunofluorescence pattern).

▶ Disease Severity
Amount of hemoptysis, chest roentgenogram, blood urea nitrogen (BUN), creatinine, ABG.

▶ Concept and Application
Circulating glomerular basement membrane antibodies damage glomerular and alveolar basement membranes.

▶ Treatment Steps
Corticosteroids plus cyclophosphamide or azothioprine; plasmapheresis.

### G. Cor Pulmonale
Defined as right-ventricular failure secondary to pulmonary disease.

▶ H&P Keys
Breathlessness, hepatic discomfort, symptoms of underlying disease. Right-ventricular heave, loud split S2, peripheral edema, ascites.

▶ Diagnosis
Chest roentgenogram (large pulmonary artery, right-ventricle hypertrophy [RVH]); ECG (RVH, pulmonale), echocardiogram (RVH, elevated pulmonary artery pressures), PFTs (reflect underlying disease).

▶ Disease Severity
ABG, cardiac catheterization (direct measurement of pulmonary artery pressures), symptoms, and exercise tolerance.

▶ Concept and Application
Hypoxic vasoconstriction leads to pulmonary hypertension and hypertrophy of right ventricle. Occurs in severe primary pulmonary diseases, including COPD, interstitial lung diseases, and sleep apnea.

▶ Treatment Steps
1. Oxygen, diuretics.
2. Treatment of underlying disease.
3. Endothelin receptor antagonist (Bosentan) in selected cases (ie, primary pulmonary hypertension or scleroderma pulmonary vasculopathy).

## VI. PULMONARY NEOPLASTIC DISEASES

### A. Bronchogenic Carcinoma

▶ H&P Keys
Smoking, asbestosis produce highest risk. Asymptomatic or cough, hemoptysis, dyspnea, chest pain, fever, weight loss, hoarseness, focal wheezing or decreased breath sounds, adenopathy.

▶ Diagnosis

Chest roentgenogram (coin lesion or mass, adenopathy), CT scan, bronchoscopic or percutaneous needle biopsy or cytologic aspiration.

▶ Disease Severity

Severity depends on stage, cell type, and patient's general condition.

▶ Concept and Application

*Adenocarcinoma*—Usually peripheral; glandlike structure on path.

*Squamous Cell*—Usually central, often cavitates, best prognosis.

*Oat Cell (Small Cell)*—Usually central, high metastatic potential.

*Alveolar Cell*—Subtype of adeno, originates in terminal bronchioles or alveoli, peripheral. Mimics pneumonia on chest x-ray.

*Large Cell*—Poorly differentiated, tends to be peripheral, rapid-growing with high metastatic potential.

▶ Treatment Steps

*Non–Small Cell*
1. Staging, surgery if resectable.
2. Radiation for palliation.

*Small Cell*
1. Chemotherapy.
2. Rarely resectable (usually metastatic when discovered).

*All*
1. May metastasize to other lung, mediastinum, brain, adrenal glands, other organs.
2. Watch for superior vena cava syndrome, hypercalcemia.

## B. Carcinoid Tumors

▶ H&P Keys

Asymptomatic or wheezing, cough, hemoptysis, obstruction. Carcinoid syndrome (episodic flushing, bronchospasm, and diarrhea) is rare.

▶ Diagnosis

Chest roentgenogram (clear, mass, or obstructive pneumonia). Lung biopsy, urine 5-hydroxyindoleacetic acid.

▶ Disease Severity

Metastatic workup.

▶ Concept and Application

Tumors are slow-growing with low metastatic potential. Classified as "neurosecretory," but cellular origin is now unclear.

▶ Treatment Steps
1. Surgical resection.
2. Chemotherapy or radiation for recurrent or metastatic disease.

### C. Metastatic Malignant Tumors

▶ H&P Keys

Often asymptomatic, or cough, hemoptysis, wheezing, dyspnea, pain, symptoms of obstructive pneumonia. Signs and symptoms of primary malignant disease.

▶ Diagnosis

Chest roentgenogram (single or multiple masses or nodules, pleural effusion, hilar or mediastinal adenopathy), biopsy of pulmonary lesion or primary lesion.

▶ Disease Severity

Metastatic workup.

▶ Concept and Application

Metastatic tumor cells enter via hematogenous or lymphatic route. Colon, breast, lymphoma, testicular, kidney, thyroid, melanoma, others.

▶ Treatment Steps

1. Surgical excision for single metastases if possible.
2. Otherwise, systemic therapy determined by primary tumor cell type and site.

## VII. ILL-DEFINED SYMPTOM COMPLEX

### A. Cough

▶ H&P Keys

Smoking history, sputum characteristics (color, viscosity), postnasal drip, throat clearing, reflux symptoms, wheezing, occupational history, medication history help pinpoint cause.

▶ Diagnosis

History and physical, PFTs, bronchoprovocation challenge tests, chest roentgenogram, sputum culture, trial of medication. Common causes of cough:

*Postnasal Drip*—History of rhinitis, frequent throat clearing.

*Asthma*—Wheezing may not be present. Diagnose by history, bronchoprovocation challenge.

*COPD*—Diagnose by history and physical. Cough may be productive.

*Gastroesophageal Reflux*—Worse at night and recumbent.

*Others*—Recurrent aspiration, lung carcinoma, congestive heart failure, medications (β-blockers, angiotensin-converting enzyme [ACE] inhibitors), bronchiectasis, others.

▶ Disease Severity

Cough intensity and number.

### ▶ Concept and Application
Nonspecific symptom caused by (1) direct stimulation of cough receptors (foreign body, tumor); (2) increased sensitivity of cough receptors (asthma); (3) inadequate glottic closure (aspiration, reflux); or (4) altered mucus quantity or quality (chronic bronchitis, bronchiectasis).

### ▶ Treatment Steps
1. Treatment of underlying disorder if identified.
2. Therapeutic trials of bronchodilators, antacids, antihistamines, proton pump inhibitors, or decongestants may be diagnostic.
3. Guaifenesin, dextromethorphan, or codeine may alleviate symptoms.

## B. Dyspnea

### ▶ H&P Keys
Shortness of breath, chest tightness, air hunger, signs and symptoms of underlying disease.

### ▶ Diagnosis
History and physical examination, PFTs, exercise testing, ECG, chest roentgenogram. Differential diagnosis of dyspnea includes pulmonary diseases, congestive heart failure (CHF), neuromuscular disease, anemia, hyperventilation disorders (eg, metabolic acidosis, psychogenic).

### ▶ Disease Severity
Exercise tolerance, symptom scores. Usually dyspnea correlates with degree of pulmonary dysfunction.

### ▶ Concept and Application
Sensation of increased respiratory effort.

### ▶ Treatment Steps
1. Specific treatment of underlying disease (bronchodilators for COPD, diuretics for CHF, etc).
2. General supportive measures include oxygen for hypoxia, nutritional and psychologic support.
3. Pulmonary rehabilitation.

## C. Chest Pain

### ▶ H&P Keys
Quality of pain, location, and relationship to breathing keys to diagnosis. Signs and symptoms of underlying disease.

### ▶ Diagnosis
*Breathing-associated Pain*—Pleuritis, lung infection, pulmonary embolism, pneumothorax, musculoskeletal pain, pericarditis.

*Pain Not Associated with Breathing*—Pulmonary hypertension, airway, or mediastinal inflammation, cardiac ischemia, dissecting aortic aneurysm, esophagitis, costochondritis.

### ▶ Disease Severity
Symptoms, exercise test, chest roentgenogram, PFTs, ECG.

▶ Concept and Application

Sensation of pain resulting from tissue injury or inflammation.

▶ Treatment Steps
1. Diagnostic workup to identify source of pain.
2. Specific therapy of underlying disease.
3. Analgesics, therapeutic trial of antacids, nitrates, nonsteroidal anti-inflammatory drugs when diagnostic work-up is unrevealing.

## D. Hemoptysis

▶ H&P Keys

Cough productive of bloody or blood-tinged sputum.

▶ Diagnosis

Differential diagnosis (common causes).

- *Tracheobronchial disorders:* Acute or chronic bronchitis, bronchogenic carcinoma, bronchiectasis, cystic fibrosis, trauma, telangiectasia.
- *Cardiovascular disorders:* Pulmonary infarction, mitral stenosis, CHF, atrioventricular malformation, aneurysm, others.
- *Hematologic disorders:* Anticoagulation, thrombocytopenia, hemophilia, disseminated intravascular coagulation.
- *Parenchymal lung disorders:* Bacterial pneumonia, tuberculosis, paragonimiasis, contusion.
- *Vasculitic disorders:* Systemic lupus erythematosus, Goodpasture's syndrome, Wegener's granulomatosis.

▶ Disease Severity

Massive hemoptysis: > 600 mL blood/24 hr.

▶ Concept and Application

Damage to pulmonary parenchyma, tracheobronchial tree, or pulmonary vasculature; defects in coagulation, increased hydrostatic pressure. Mechanism depends on underlying etiology.

▶ Treatment Steps
1. Diagnostic workup (chest roentgenogram, complete blood count [CBC], platelet count, prothrombin time [PT], partial thromboplastin time [PTT], sputum culture, cytology, acid-fast bacilli [AFB] smear, cytology).
2. Quantitate hemoptysis.
3. Bronchoscopy to localize source.
4. Treatment of coagulation abnormalities and CHF if present.
5. Cough suppressant (codeine).
6. Antibiotic if infection present.
7. Surgical excision of bleeding segment or angiographic embolization if persists.

## E. Wheezing and Stridor

▶ H&P Keys

Audible, continuous, musical adventitial sound. Location and timing to respiratory cycle help in diagnosis.

▶ Diagnosis

PFT, flow volume loop, bronchoprovocation challenge, chest roentgenogram, soft-tissue neck films, bronchoscopy.

*Stridor*—Inspiratory "wheeze" heard best over trachea and upper airway (eg, epiglottitis, croup, tracheal stenosis, angioedema, laryngeal ("psychogenic") asthma.

*Focal Inspiratory and Expiratory Wheeze*—Bronchogenic tumor, foreign body.

*Diffuse Expiratory Wheeze*—Asthma, COPD, CHF.

▶ Disease Severity

Clinical symptoms, PFT.

▶ Concept and Application

Sound caused by vibrations of airway narrowed by bronchospasm, inflammation, mass, or edema.

▶ Treatment Steps

Treatment of underlying disease, bronchodilators, oxygen if hypoxic.

## F. Solitary Pulmonary Nodule (Coin Lesion)

▶ H&P Keys

Asymptomatic, or cough and hemoptysis. Smoking history, occupational exposures, previous malignant disease help in diagnosis.

▶ Diagnosis

Chest roentgenogram (single round lesion 1–6 cm), old chest roentgenogram, CT scan, bronchoscopic or transthoracic needle biopsy or aspirate, open biopsy.

▶ Disease Severity

Lung biopsy.

▶ Concept and Application

Round mass may be benign or malignant tumor, tuberculoma, granuloma, artifact, cyst, resolving pneumonia, others.

▶ Treatment Steps

1. Locate old films: if lesion unchanged more than 2 years, probably benign. If unavailable or new lesion, CT scan and biopsy mass. Unless a firm benign diagnosis can be made, surgical excision usually required. Laminated or solid calcification suggests benign granuloma. A negative PET scan also suggests a benign lesion.
2. Consider periodic chest roentgenography over 2 years if nonsmoker, age < 45, with nonspiculated lesion < 2.2 cm.

## G. Sleep Apnea Syndrome

▶ H&P Keys

Daytime sleepiness, restlessness, unrefreshed sleep, morning headaches, neuropsychiatric changes, signs and symptoms of cor pulmonale. Hypothyroidism, use of sedatives, ethanol should be ruled out.

▶ Diagnosis

Physical examination (obesity, narrowed pharyngeal opening); polysomnography.

▶ Disease Severity

Polysomnography, degree of nocturnal oxygen desaturation.

▶ Concept and Application

*Central Sleep Apnea*—Defective central drive causing transient apneic periods.

*Obstructive Sleep Apnea*—Occlusion of oropharyngeal upper airway during sleep.

▶ Treatment Steps

*Central Sleep Apnea*—Oxygen, respiratory stimulants (acetazolamide), noninvasive mechanical ventilation (BiPAP).

*Obstructive Sleep Apnea*—Nasal continuous positive airway pressure (CPAP), tracheostomy, weight reduction, avoidance of sedatives and alcohol.

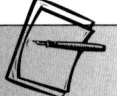

▶ on rounds

### BACTERIAL AND OTHER PNEUMONIA

#### Pneumococcal Pneumonia
- Acute onset of rigors, fever, and "rusty sputum."
- Lobar infiltrate on CXR.
- Caused by *Streptococcus pneumoniae*.
- Is the most common cause of community-acquired pneumonia.

#### Staphylococcal Pneumonia
- Fever, cough, and purulent sputum.
- Multifocal infiltrates, abscess, and effusions on CXR.
- Caused by *Staphylococcus aureus*.

#### *Haemophilus influenzae* Pneumonia
- Fever, cough, and purulent sputum.
- Found in young children, alcoholics, COPD patients.
- Multilobar, patchy infiltrates on CXR.

#### Mycoplasma Pneumonia
- Fever, chills, sore throat, nonproductive cough, and headache.
- Common in young adults.
- Interstitial or diffuse alveolar infiltrate on CXR.

#### *Pneumocystis carinii* Pneumonia
- Opportunistic infection, often HIV related.
- Fever, dyspnea, tachypnea, tachycardia, rales, nonproductive cough.
- CXR may be clear or demonstrate diffuse infiltrates.

# BIBLIOGRAPHY

American Thoracic Society/Centers for Disease Control. Diagnostic standards and classifications of tuberculosis in adults and children. *Am J Respir Crit Care Med* 161:1376–1395, 2000.

Fishman AP, ed. *Pulmonary Diseases and Disorders*. 3rd ed. New York: McGraw-Hill Book Co; 2002.

Light RW. *Pleural Diseases*. 4th ed. Philadelphia: Williams & Wilkins; 2001.

Murray JF, Nadel JA, eds. *Textbook of Respiratory Medicine*. 3rd ed. Philadelphia: WB Saunders Co; 2000.

NHLBI/WHO workshop report: Global Strategy for Asthma Management and Prevention 2002 update NIH Pub No. 02-3659.

# Diseases of the Renal and Urologic Systems 17

I. **INFECTIOUS DISEASES AND INFLAMMATORY CONDITIONS / 529**
   A. Urinary Tract Infection / 529
   B. Painful Bladder and Urethral Syndromes / 529
   C. Prostatitis / 530
   D. Epididymitis / 530
   E. Urethritis / 531
   F. Orchitis / 531
   G. Gonorrhea / 532
   H. Syphilis / 532
   I. Chlamydia / 532
   J. Herpes / 533
   K. Human Immunodeficiency Virus (HIV/AIDS) / 533

II. **BENIGN CONDITIONS OF THE GENITOURINARY TRACT / 534**
   A. Cryptorchidism / 534
   B. Testicular Torsion / 534
   C. Intersex / 534
   D. Infertility / 535
   E. Hydrocele and Varicocele / 536
   F. Benign Urethral Stricture / 536
   G. Peyronie's Disease / 537
   H. Erectile Impotence / 537
   I. Hypospadias / 538
   J. Vesicoureteral Reflux / 538
   K. Urolithiasis / 539
   L. Neurogenic Bladder / 539
   M. Stress-related Urinary Incontinence / 540
   N. Enuresis / 540
   O. Ureteropelvic Junction Obstruction / 540
   P. Urologic Trauma / 541

III. **NEOPLASIAS OF THE GENITOURINARY TRACT / 542**
- A. Benign Prostatic Hyperplasia / 542
- B. Prostate Cancer / 542
- C. Bladder Carcinoma / 543
- D. Renal Cell Carcinoma / 544
- E. Wilms' Tumor / 544
- F. Testicular Carcinoma / 545
- G. Penile, Urethral, and Scrotal Carcinoma / 545

IV. **RENAL DISORDERS / 546**
- A. Pyelonephritis / 546
- B. Acute Renal Failure / 546
- C. Chronic Renal Failure / 547
- D. Tubulointerstitial Disease / 548
- E. Renal Transplant Rejection / 548
- F. Nephrotic Syndrome / 549
- G. Glomerulonephritis / 549
- H. Diabetic Nephropathy / 550
- I. Renal Osteodystrophy / 550
- J. Papillary Necrosis / 550
- K. Renovascular Hypertension / 551
- L. Preeclampsia / 551
- M. Eclampsia / 552
- N. Polycystic Kidney Disease / 552
- O. Nephrosclerosis / 552
- P. Lupus Nephritis / 553

V. **ELECTROLYTE AND ACID–BASE DISORDERS / 553**
- A. Hyponatremia / 553
- B. Hypernatremia / 554
- C. Hypokalemia / 554
- D. Hyperkalemia / 554
- E. Volume Depletion / 555
- F. Volume Excess / 555
- G. Metabolic Alkalosis / 555
- H. Respiratory Alkalosis / 556
- I. Metabolic Acidosis / 556
- J. Respiratory Acidosis / 556
- K. Hypomagnesemia / 557
- L. Hypercalcemia / 557
- M. Hypocalcemia / 558

**BIBLIOGRAPHY / 559**

## I. INFECTIOUS DISEASES AND INFLAMMATORY CONDITIONS

### A. Urinary Tract Infection

▶ H&P Keys

Dysuria, urgency, frequency, nocturia, suprapubic pain, back or flank pain, tenesmus, voiding of small volumes of urine, urethral discomfort.

▶ Diagnosis

Urinalysis: pyuria, white blood count/high-power field, bacteriuria, hematuria. Urine culture, dip-slide method. Cystoscopy, voiding cystourethroscopy, intravenous (IV) urography in chronic cases.

▶ Disease Severity

Gross hematuria, pain, ascending infection, fever and chills, initial or persistent or recurrent infection, pregnancy status, renal function.

▶ Concept and Application

Male-female difference because of anatomy; bacterial-mucosal adherence principal reason for recurrent infection. Urinary stasis, *Escherichia coli* is principal pathogen. Fecal flora are primary source during in-dwelling or short-term catheterization. Asymptomatic bacteriuria in pregnant females (3–15%).

▶ Treatment Steps

1. Uncomplicated: TMP-SMZ for 5–7 days, also nitrofurantoin monohydrate macrocrystals 100 mg twice a day BID for 7–10 days. Three-day regimens effective. Persistent/recurrent infection: chronic or prophylactic use of antibiotics.
2. Timed voiding, urodynamics, and imaging for complicated cases.
3. Rule out nonbacterial causes such as TB, chlamydia, and yeast.

### B. Painful Bladder and Urethral Syndromes

▶ H&P Keys

Urinary urgency and frequency or dysuria, absence of documented chronic urinary tract infection (UTI), negative neurologic findings, absence of carcinoma.

▶ Diagnosis

Cystoscopy: hydrodistention, urodynamics, bladder biopsy. Diagnosis of exclusion.

▶ Disease Severity

Degree of *urinary* frequency, level of pain, and bladder capacity and deterioration of quality of life.

▶ Concept and Application

Etiology undefined; grouping of syndromes rather than specific disease. Theories of mast-cell activity and glycosaminoglycan layer defects. Epithelial permeability.

▶ Treatment Steps
1. Cystoscopy, hydrodistention.
2. Pentosan polysulfate 100 mg TID.
3. Anticholinergics.
4. Therapies for chronic pain.

## C. Prostatitis

▶ H&P Keys

Slow or sudden onset, perineal discomfort, voiding dysfunction, prostate tenderness on digital rectal exam. UTI.

▶ Diagnosis

Urine culture and sensitivity, extraprostatic secretion culture, urinalysis (pyuria).

▶ Disease Severity

Fever or rigors, urinary retention, constant or intermittent discomfort, degree of voiding dysfunction.

▶ Concept and Application

Distinguish true bacterial prostatitis (acute and chronic) from nonbacterial (inflammatory states, chlamydia) and prostatodynia. Acute bacterial prostatitis responds dramatically to antibiotics. Fifty percent empiric response to antibiotics in other conditions. Prostatodynia associated with pelvic floor or sphincter spasm.

▶ Treatment Steps
1. Acute bacterial infection requires culture-appropriate antibiotics.
2. Chronic bacterial or nonbacterial infection requires ciprofloxacin or levafloxin or tetracyclines for 4- to 6-week course.
3. Warm soaks and nonsteroidal anti-inflammatory drugs (NSAIDs).
4. Chronic pain evaluation for prostatodynia.

## D. Epididymitis

▶ H&P Keys

Pain, tenderness, discomfort distinct from testis parenchyma. Normal testis, palpable epididymal discomfort. Slow or sudden onset. No trauma, sexual activity, voiding symptoms, genitourinary (GU) instrumentation.

▶ Diagnosis

Pyuria; culture and sensitivity are usually negative. Scrotal ultrasound or Doppler good flow state, inflammation of epididymis.

▶ Disease Severity

Fever or rigors, testis and epididymis are indistinguishable, scrotal induration, incapacitation.

▶ Concept and Application

Rule out torsion or tumor in young men (Prehn's sign is unreliable). Bacterial infection in older men with voiding dysfunction; chlamydia in younger men. Irritative urine reflux in acute or chronic states. Most respond to antibiotics in 3–6 weeks.

▶ Treatment Steps
1. Intermediate course of antibiotics (ciprofloxacin or tetracyclines).
2. NSAIDs.
3. Warm soaks, elevation.

### E. Urethritis

▶ H&P Keys
Purulent or mucoid discharge. Dysuria and frequency during urination. History of sexual activity.

▶ Diagnosis
Gonococci (GC) culture in Thayer–Martin media, Gram stain (–) diplococci, or specific chlamydia culture.

▶ Disease Severity
Ranges from painless discharge to severe voiding symptoms, epididymal and testicular involvement, systemic illness.

▶ Concept and Application
Generally gonococcal and nongonococcal (*Chlamydia trachomatis, Ureaplasma urealyticum, Trichomonas*) complications of urethral stricture or Reiter's syndrome.

▶ Treatment Steps
1. Gonococcal infection: ceftriaxone, 250 mg intramuscularly (IM); levafloxin 500 mg, one dose.
2. Nongonococcal infection: tetracycline 500 mg 4 times/day QID; doxycycline, 100 mg BID for 7–10 days, or levafloxin 250 mg, 300 mg BID for 7–10 days.
3. Metronidazole for *Trichomonas*. Acyclovir for herpes.

### F. Orchitis

▶ H&P Keys
Rapid or slow onset, fever and malaise, absence of trauma. Scrotal contents can be normal, inflamed, or distorted (torsion). Sexual or voiding dysfunction. Child or adolescent versus adult.

▶ Diagnosis
Pyuria, scrotal ultrasound, urine culture.

▶ Disease Severity
Scrotal induration, fistula, abscess on ultrasound, rule out torsion-hyperemic blood flow and systemic infection.

▶ Concept and Application
Rule out torsion in young men; bacterial infection in older men and sexually transmitted disease (STD) in younger men. Mumps orchitis in children and adolescents. Chronic orchalgia can be present without infection.

▶ Treatment Steps
1. Four to six weeks of ciprofloxacin, levafloxin, doxycycline.
2. NSAIDs, warm soaks, and elevation.

### G. Gonorrhea

▶ H&P Keys

Sexual exposure; thick, creamy urethral discharge; urethritis. May involve epididymis.

▶ Diagnosis

Gram-negative diplococcus. GC culture in Thayer–Martin media.

▶ Disease Severity

Severity of pain and discharge; associated epididymitis or orchitis.

▶ Concept and Application

β-Lactamase plasmid-penicillin resistance. Pili contribute to virulence. Different infection rate per exposure (male 20%, female 90%). Coexisting chlamydial infection.

▶ Treatment Steps

Ceftriaxone, 125 mg IM, ciprofloxacin 500 mg PO, single dose, plus azithromycin 1 gm PO single dose, and doxycycline, 100 mg BID for 7 days.

### H. Syphilis

▶ H&P Keys

Sexual activity. Painless genital ulcer, lack of vesicles. Negative travel history.

▶ Diagnosis

Rapid plasma reagin and fluorescent treponemal antibody-absorption test for syphilis, patient's history.

▶ Disease Severity

Primary, secondary, or tertiary disease; systemic symptoms, neurosyphilis; cardiovascular changes.

▶ Concept and Application

*Treponema pallidum* or spirochete family of bacteria. Three stages of disease with different systemic findings.

▶ Treatment Steps

1. Benzathine, 2.4 million units IM, one dose.
2. Erythromycin base 2 g/day for 2 weeks.
3. Late latent benzathine 2.4 million units IM weekly for 3 weeks.

### I. Chlamydia

▶ H&P Keys

Sexual activity, younger age group, clear or mucoid discharge.

▶ Diagnosis

No routine culture; tissue culture 8–10 days, fluorescent antibody stains, history.

▶ Disease Severity
Pain, spread to testis or prostate.

▶ Concept and Application
Obligate intracellular parasite. Cannot produce adenosine triphosphate. Antibiotics effective. Neonatal infection is serious—conjunctivitis or pneumonitis. Think of mycoplasma and ureaplasma in differential diagnosis.

▶ Treatment Steps
Doxycycline, tetracycline, quinolones, azithromycin 1 g PO, single dose.

## J. Herpes

▶ H&P Keys
Genital ulcer, painful vesicles, multiple lesions.

▶ Diagnosis
Tzanck test with Wright or Giemsa stain and cell culture.

▶ Disease Severity
Pain, coalesced vesicles, persistence or recurrence of infection.

▶ Concept and Application
Double-strand DNA virus. Subclinical infections, systemic complications—aseptic meningitis, fever, urinary retention in women, and, in rare cases, hepatitis or pneumonia.

▶ Treatment Steps
1. Oral acyclovir, 200 mg 5 times/day for 10 days. Topical application for pain relief.
2. Suppressive treatment, acyclovir 400 mg PO BID.

## K. Human Immunodeficiency Virus (HIV/AIDS)

▶ H&P Keys
Night sweats, fever, adenopathy, weight loss, opportunistic infections.

▶ Diagnosis
HIV antibody test. Western blotting.

▶ Disease Severity
HIV positivity versus systemic disease.

▶ Concept and Application
RNA virus, AZT therapy. Lymphocyte counts.

▶ Treatment Steps
1. Per current therapy.
2. Evaluation of GU symptoms as per uninfected patients. Minimize invasive procedures in immunocompromised patients.

## II. BENIGN CONDITIONS OF THE GENITOURINARY TRACT

### A. Cryptorchidism

▶ H&P Keys

Immature birth, absence of testis on scrotal exam. If hypospadias is present, consider sex ambiguity.

▶ Diagnosis

Physical exam. In adults, consider CT scan.

▶ Disease Severity

Retractile testis; inguinal canal versus intra-abdominal, unilateral, or bilateral.

▶ Concept and Application

Maldescent of testes hormonally controlled. Gubernaculum provides path of descent with or without mechanical assistance. Rule out retractile, ectopic, or absent testis (blind-ending vas deferens at exploration).

▶ Treatment Steps
1. Surgical correction at 6–12 months of age.
2. Hormonal manipulation.

### B. Testicular Torsion

▶ H&P Keys

Common scrotal swelling in children. Acute severe onset. Possible nausea and vomiting, abdominal pain.

▶ Diagnosis

Negative urinalysis, distorted or rotated gonad, Doppler ultrasound, nuclear flow scan.

▶ Disease Severity

Degree of pain and scrotal swelling. Duration (less than or more than 5 hours). Absence of contralateral testis.

▶ Concept and Application

Twisting of spermatic cord with mechanical ischemia. Congenital tunica vaginalis attachment is irregular; thus favors twisting (bell-clapper deformity). Contralateral side at risk.

▶ Treatment Steps

Surgical correction in 5 hours. Bilateral orchiopexy with permanent suture.

### C. Intersex

▶ H&P Keys

Salt loss, salt retention. Phallic enlargement. Precocious pubic hair, early masculinization, early epiphyseal closure (congenital adrenal hyperplasia [CAH]). Sparse axillary and pubic hair (testicular feminization). Penile scrotal hypospadias and bilateral cryptorchidism. Groin mass (gonad).

▶ Diagnosis
Buccal smear, karyotype. Metabolic studies for congenital adrenal hyperplasia. Genitography, ultrasound gonadal histology.

▶ Disease Severity
Degree of underdevelopment or ambiguity of genitalia. Neonatal versus pubertal diagnosis. Reproductive and gender role dysfunction.

▶ Concept and Application
Four major groups:

1. Female pseudohermaphrodites, normal ovaries, 46,XX, virilization (CAH).
2. Male pseudohermaphrodites, normal testis, 46,XY, failure to masculinize (testicular feminization), androgen insensitivity (receptor block, other 5-α-reductase deficiency.
3. True hemaphrodites, testicular and ovarian tissue. Appearance and karyotype variable.
4. Dysgenetic gonads, replaced by fibrous stroma, mosaicism with XY,XX (Turner's syndrome) and XO lines.

▶ Treatment Steps
1. Variable. Treatment depends on specific syndrome and time of recognition.
2. Possible gender reassignment usually male to female.
3. Support in assigned role (testicular feminization).

D. Infertility

▶ H&P Keys
Failure to conceive after 1 year of unprotected intercourse. Asymmetric or undescended testicles. Testicular mass. Varicocele. Secondary sexual characteristics. Drug and chemical exposure. Stress.

▶ Diagnosis
Semen analysis (> 20 million/cc, 1.5–5 cc volume). Urinalysis, semen fructose (obstruction/dysfunction of seminal vesicles). Luteinizing hormone (LH), follicle-stimulating hormone (FSH), and testosterone level. Sperm function tests.

▶ Disease Severity
Mild disorders of semen parameters (motility or morphology) to azoospermia (total absence of sperm).

▶ Concept and Application
Need to distinguish treatable (blockage, varicocele) from untreatable (gonadal failure, FSH three times normal) conditions.

▶ Treatment Steps
1. Varicocele repair.
2. Repair of anatomic blockage.

3. Clomiphene citrate administration (idiopathic infertility).
4. Assisted reproductive techniques.
5. Adoption.

### E. Hydrocele and Varicocele

▶ H&P Keys

*Hydrocele*—Painless scrotal mass; fluid accumulation in tunical layer of testis; symmetrical swelling, occasionally bilateral; transillumination.

*Varicocele*—Spermatic venous varices; "bag of worms" palpation; commonly occurs on left side; occasionally, painful or heavy sensation.

▶ Diagnosis

Physical exam, urinalysis, scrotal ultrasound. Check tumor marker in young men if diagnosis is questionable.

▶ Disease Severity

*Hydrocele*—Cosmetic deformity.

*Varicocele*—Deformity, pain, testicular atrophy, infertility problems.

▶ Concept and Application

*Hydroceles*—Benign; membranes actively secrete serumlike fluid. Reaccumulation with simple drainage.

*Varicoceles*—Gonadal venous valve insufficiency; occasionally subclinical on right side. Unclear mechanisms for effect on fertility in some men. Most men with varicoceles do not have fertility problems. Sperm parameters improve after procedure in two thirds of infertile men.

▶ Treatment Steps

*Hydrocele*
1. Drainage with sclerotherapy or surgical correction (5–15% recurrence).
2. Observation.

*Varicocele*
1. Venous ligation or embolization.
2. Observation.

### F. Benign Urethral Stricture

▶ H&P Keys
Prior history of STD or urinary instrumentation, decreased force of stream, meatal stenosis.

▶ Diagnosis
Physical exam, urinalysis, retrograde urethrogram, cystoscopy.

▶ Disease Severity
Blood urea nitrogen (BUN) and creatinine, degree of voiding dysfunction, dysuria.

▶ Concept and Application

Usually occurs at meatus, fossa navicularis (glans–shaft border), or bulbar urethra; bulbar is site for most STD infections. Ischemia from instrumentation or catheterization while on cardiopulmonary bypass.

▶ Treatment Steps
1. Dilatation.
2. Optical internal urethrotomy.
3. Plastic staged repair. Biopsy irregular stricture to rule out neoplasia.

## G. Peyronie's Disease

▶ H&P Keys

Painless, firm, nonindurated area on penile shaft.

▶ Diagnosis

Physical exam. Color-flow Doppler ultrasound.

▶ Disease Severity

Firm area, degree of pain with erection, deformity of erection, impotence.

▶ Concept and Application

Idiopathic fibrosis of tunic of corpora cavernosa. Asymmetric thickening leads to erectile thickening and pain. Natural history is unclear. Ten percent are associated with Dupuytren's contracture.

▶ Treatment Steps
1. Observation.
2. Oral antioxidants.
3. Surgical excision and graft repair.

## H. Erectile Impotence

▶ H&P Keys

Neurological disease, diabetes, peripheral vascular disease, medications, radical pelvic surgery, Peyronie's plaque, psychological factors.

▶ Diagnosis

History and physical exam, color-flow Doppler ultrasound, nocturnal penile tumescence studies, hormone profile (testosterone), LH, FSH, prolactin.

▶ Disease Severity

Occasional or permanent inability to attain erection sufficient for vaginal penetration.

▶ Concept and Application

Vascular, muscular, or neurologic etiology is the site of primary dysfunction; psychogenic issues much less common.

▶ Treatment Steps
1. Sildenafil 25 to 100 mg PO.
2. Intracavernosal injection (prostaglandin $E_1$ or papaverine–regitine).
3. Vacuum suction device.
4. Penile prosthesis.

### I. Hypospadias

▶ H&P Keys
Ectopic position of urethral meatus on ventral shaft of penis. Lack of ventral foreskin. Check for undescended testicles.

▶ Diagnosis
Physical examination.

▶ Disease Severity
Glandular position to more proximal location on shaft (penile or scrotal). Associated anomalies.

▶ Concept and Application
Occurs at the rate of 1 in 300 live male births. Failure of mesothelial folds to close in the midline. Epispadias (dorsal urethral opening) is extremely rare. Associated with midline closure defects.

▶ Treatment Steps
Surgical correction.

### J. Vesicoureteral Reflux

▶ H&P Keys
Associated family history. Occurs in 50% of infant UTIs and 30% of childhood UTIs; recurrent UTIs in infancy and childhood.

▶ Diagnosis
Ultrasound, IV urography, renal nuclear scan.

▶ Disease Severity
Grades 1–5, international classification.

▶ Concept and Application
Ectopic ureteral bud leading to lateral placement of ureter in bladder. Decreased flap-valve mechanism. May improve with maturity. High-pressure voiding states also can overwhelm normal anatomy. Goal is to preserve upper tracts. Avoid renal scarring and hypertension.

▶ Treatment Steps
1. Prophylactic antibiotics: trimethoprim–sulfamethoxazole, nitrofurantoin. Initial medical management of grades 1–3; grade 4, medical or surgical; grade 5, surgery. Cohen reimplant.
2. Breakthrough infection, noncompliance, reflux persistent at puberty are indications for surgery.

### K. Urolithiasis

▶ **H&P Keys**
Prior history of stone, geography, metabolic disorders, flank or groin tenderness.

▶ **Diagnosis**
Urinalysis, IV urogram, ultrasound.

▶ **Disease Severity**
Stone burden on imaging studies; degree of urinary obstruction or renal impairment; pain, nausea, vomiting.

▶ **Concept and Application**
Most stones are "idiopathic" calcium oxalate. Struvite stones are associated with infections *(Proteus)* and uric acid; cysteine is less common.

▶ **Treatment Steps**
1. Small calculi: hydration, pain control, spontaneous passage.
2. Upper tract: extracorporal shockwave lithotripsy.
3. Lower tract: ureteroscopic extraction or lithotripsy.

### L. Neurogenic Bladder

▶ **H&P Keys**
Neurologic exam, palpable bladder, rectal exam. Rule out stricture disease.

▶ **Diagnosis**
Urodynamics: pressure-flow, cystometrogram, electromyography, uroflowmetry, cystoscopy.

▶ **Disease Severity**
Voiding dysfunction versus complete retention, total incontinence, chronic urinary tract infection, deterioration of renal function.

▶ **Concept and Application**
Several classification schemes: (1) failure to empty versus failure to store is most functional scheme, (a) emptying failure resulting from decompensated detrusor mechanical obstruction or overactive sphincters (smooth and striated), (b) failure to store because of overactive detrusor or incompetent sphincters; and (2) motor versus sensory. Classification of uninhibited versus autonomous is used least often.

▶ **Treatment Steps**
1. Failure to empty (detrusor): clean intermittent catheterization; bethanechol is ineffective.
2. Failure to empty (mechanical): cystoscopy to rule out stricture or enlarged prostate.
3. Failure to empty (sphincter dyssynergia): α-blockage, bladder neck incision, sphincterotomy. Failure to store (detrusor): anticholinergics, surgical bladder augmentation. Failure to store

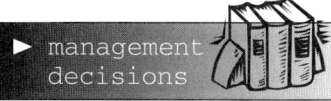

▶ management decisions

**GENITOURINARY TRACT**

**Urolithiasis**
Size and location of stone. Observe with spontaneous passage, extracorporeal shock wave lithotripsy (ESWL), ureteroscopy for lower ureter. Chronic/recurrent stones—medical management.

**Prostate Cancer**
Patient age, disease stage and performance status: Local disease: younger patients (< 70) surgery > radiation, older patients radiation > surgery. Androgen ablation in advanced disease.

**Vesicoureteral Reflux**
Initial antibiotic therapy (grades 1–3), surgery (ureteral reimplant) higher grade or failed medical therapy.

**Enuresis**
Reassurance with spontaneous resolution, behavioral modification, intranasal DDAVP.

(sphincter incompetence): bladder sling surgery, collagen injections, artificial sphincter placement.

*Note:* Diabetes can induce a sensory neurogenic bladder. Initial good motor function can be maintained with *timed* voiding. Chronic overdistention creates dilated myopathy with motor decompensation as well. Treatment involves intermittent catheterization.

### M. Stress-related Urinary Incontinence

▶ H&P Keys

Childbirth, pelvic surgery (total abdominal hysterectomy), loss of urine with cough or movement.

▶ Diagnosis

Incontinence cystogram, urodynamics, cystoscopy.

▶ Disease Severity

Occasional leakage to gravity incontinence.

▶ Concept and Application

Forms of failure to store: type 1, hypermobility of urethra and mild leakage; type 2, descensus of bladder and cystocele; type 3, nonfunctional bladder neck.

▶ Treatment Steps

1. Initial management is conservative: pelvic floor strengthening exercises, possible biofeedback training, use of α-agonists to tighten bladder neck (phenylpropanolamine, 50 mg daily).
2. Then consider bladder neck suspension. Type 3 is treated with collagen injections or bladder sling surgery.

### N. Enuresis

▶ H&P Keys

Lack of neurologic history, structural disorder that precludes normal toilet training, polyuria.

▶ Diagnosis

Urinalysis and culture and sensitivity. Radiography if infection is present, wetting is diurnal and present beyond age 12 years.

▶ Disease Severity

Frequency and persistence into adolescence.

▶ Concept and Application

Persistence of immature reflex pattern of bladder emptying.

▶ Treatment Steps

1. Reassure patient about spontaneous resolution. Restrict fluids in evening.
2. 1-deamino-8-D-arginine vasopressin, 10–40 μg intranasally.

### O. Ureteropelvic Junction Obstruction

▶ H&P Keys

Flank pain or abdominal pain or mass.

▶ Diagnosis
Renal ultrasound, cystoscopy as indicated, retrograde pyelogram.

▶ Disease Severity
Renal function, preserved renal parenchyma. Can occur with or without dilation of collecting system.

▶ Concept and Application
A dynamic segment of ureter, patent but functionally obstructive. Can occur at ureteral vesical junction (megaureter). Severe prostatism, neurogenic bladder, or ureteral reflux can cause general hydronephrosis.

▶ Treatment Steps
1. Surgical correction, open or endoscopic, of ureteropelvic junction.
2. Megaureter: observation or surgery. Treat prostatism or reflux according to recommendations.

## P. Urologic Trauma

▶ H&P Keys
Cardiovascular stability, hematuria, pelvic stability, prostate location on rectal exam. Penile and scrotal ecchymosis, blood at urethral meatus, blunt or penetrating trauma.

▶ Diagnosis
Urinalysis, CT scan, IV urogram, retrograde urethrogram, cystogram. Ultrasound for oliguria.

▶ Disease Severity
Mild contusions treated with observation. Renal fracture involving collecting system, ureteral disruption, intra- versus extraperitoneal bladder extravasation. Penile or testicular fracture.

▶ Concept and Application
Much renal trauma can be managed conservatively; ureteral injuries usually iatrogenic (ureteroscopy or gynecologic); urethral disruption and pelvic hematoma mitigate against immediate repair. Diagnosis of genital injury is aided by ultrasound.

▶ Treatment Steps
Renal (stable):

1. Observation and bed rest, serial imaging; renal (unstable). Diversion of urine with stent; ureteral (major). Catheter drainage; bladder (extraperitoneal). Drainage and later repair in most cases. Debridement and repair.
2. Surgery or angiography. Ureteral (minor). Early or immediate repair (major, delayed diagnosis). Open repair. Urethra (suprapubic): Penile-testicular.
3. Urine diversion with later repair. Bladder (intraperitoneal).

## III. NEOPLASIAS OF THE GENITOURINARY TRACT

### A. Benign Prostatic Hyperplasia

▶ H&P Keys

Hesitancy, decreased force of stream, postvoid dribbling, nocturia, urgency, frequency. Enlarged prostate. Rule out palpable bladder.

▶ Diagnosis

Uroflowmetry, postvoid residual urine, urinalysis, pressure-flow urodynamics if indicated, cystoscopy if indicated, serum prostate-specific antigen (PSA).

▶ Disease Severity

American Urological Association symptom score of 0–35. UTIs, renal deterioration, urinary retention.

▶ Concept and Application

Testosterone and aging are principal factors in enlargement. Static component is enlarged gland; dynamic component is smooth muscle tone in prostate, prostate capsule, and bladder neck.

▶ Treatment Steps
1. Expectant management.
2. Decrease tone α-blocker (several) hs.
3. Medical bulk reduction with finasteride.
4. Surgical bulk reduction with TURP.

### B. Prostate Cancer

▶ H&P Keys

Digital rectal exam and serum PSA. Ultrasound is not part of routine exam. Hematuria and obstruction symptoms are less specific.

▶ Diagnosis

Needle biopsy of prostate. Staging: Bone scan. Endorectal coil magnetic resonance imaging (eMRI) investigational. Computed tomography (CT) scan and MRI of body are not useful.

▶ Disease Severity

Tumor grade and stage (Jewett–Whitmore, A-D, TMN system). (A/T1) local, PSA, or incidental biopsy, nonpalpable disease; (B/T2) palpable organ, confined disease; (C/T3) extracapsular disease; (D/T4, $N^+$, $M^+$) lymph node or distant metastasis.

▶ Concept and Application

There are 31,900 cancer-related deaths per year. Etiology is unknown. Adenocarcinoma. Disparity in racial incidence: high in African-American men, low in native Asians. PSA plus digital rectal exam detects more cancer than either test alone. True value of screening awaits long-term follow-up, indirect data supports it. Androgen-sensitive and androgen-resistant tumor.

▶ Treatment Steps

Prostate cancer is a progressive disease. Slow rate of progression suggests that active observation is an option in patients with local disease and expected lifespan of < 10 years. *Local disease:* Radical prostatectomy or radiation therapy. *Extracapsular disease:* Radiation therapy. *Advanced disease:* Androgen ablation (orchiectomy, LH-releasing hormone agonists with or without antiandrogen). Brachytherapy and cryosurgery for local disease is investigational. Palliative therapy for hormone-refractory disease.

## C. Bladder Carcinoma

▶ H&P Keys

Gross or microscopic hematuria. Irritative voiding symptoms. Occasionally, pelvic pain. Exposure to tobacco, cyclophosphamide, analine dyes.

▶ Diagnosis

IV urogram, cystoscopy, barbitage cytology. Transurethral resection biopsy of bladder lesion.

▶ Disease Severity

Key determinant is presence or absence of muscle invasion by the tumor. Degree of hematuria does not correlate with tumor stage. TNM staging system. Patients with gross nodal and distant disease do poorly.

▶ Concept and Application

Cancer-related deaths per year, 10,000. Two thirds of tumors are superficial and treated by resection; two thirds of these will recur, and 10–20% progress to muscle-invasive disease. Associated carcinoma in situ is a bad prognostic feature regarding recurrence and progression. Tumor grade is strong indicator of recurrence.

▶ Treatment Steps

*Superficial*
1. Resect initial tumor and observe, on standard schedule (see below), multiple tumors or recurrence. Treat with intravesical bacillus Calmette–Guérin (BCG).
2. Mitomycin. Decreases papillary recurrence, decreases recurrence and progression in carcinoma in situ.

*Cysto Schedule*—Every 3 months for 1 year, every 6 months for 1 year, yearly thereafter. Recurrence resets schedule.

*Muscle Invasive*
1. Radical cystectomy and urinary tract reconstruction (ileal conduit or continent neobladder).
2. Radiation therapy, and chemotherapy used in combination.
3. Transurethral resection.

*Advanced Disease*
1. Methotrexate, vinblastine, Adriamycin, and cisplatin (MVAC), with 40–50% response and 15% sustained complete remission.
2. Paclitax or combinations.

## D. Renal Cell Carcinoma

▶ H&P Keys

Classically called "internists' tumor" because it was found after workup for general weight loss, fatigue, and so on. Now, it is usually discovered as incidental mass on an imaging study. Classic hematuria, flank pain, and mass are present in only 11% of patients.

▶ Diagnosis

Mass on IV urogram, ultrasound, CT, or MRI. Angiography rarely performed now. CT criteria: Mass with slight increase in Hounsfield units after contrast: Paraneoplastic effect of hypercalcemia and elevated liver function tests (LFTs) (Stauffer's syndrome) does not indicate metastases. Anemia is more common than erythrocytosis.

▶ Disease Severity

Robeson or TNM tumor stage. Weight loss, fatigue, and large-mass organ-confined disease easily treated with surgery. Metastatic disease responds poorly to therapy.

▶ Concept and Application

Annual mortality rate is 12,000. Arises from proximal tubule. Exposure to tobacco increases the relative risk twofold. Surgical disease; not responsive to irradiation, chemotherapy.

▶ Treatment Steps
1. Radical nephrectomy is treatment of choice if no evidence of metastatic disease.
2. Interleukin-2 or 5-fluorouracil (FUDR), or research protocol.
3. Progesterones are used for palliation and have few side effects. Some positive results with biological response modifiers.

## E. Wilms' Tumor

▶ H&P Keys

Pediatric tumor. Noticed as flank mass on exam. Hematuria.

▶ Diagnosis

History and physical exam, CT scan or ultrasound, IV urogram.

▶ Disease Severity

Clinical staging, performance status.

▶ Concept and Application

Arises from metanephric blastema tissue. Occurs in young children (peak age 3 years); rarely presents in adolescents and adults.

▶ Treatment Steps
1. Radical nephrectomy for localized or regional disease and chemotherapy (actinomycin and vincristine).
2. Radiation therapy for advanced disease.

### F. Testicular Carcinoma

▶ H&P Keys

Painless testis mass, testis rupture after mild trauma. Advanced disease includes gynecomastia, shortness of breath, adenopathy, abdominal mass.

▶ Diagnosis

Scrotal ultrasound, tumor markers (beta human chorionic gonadotropin and α-fetoprotein [AFP]). Diagnosis by radical orchiectomy (inguinal incision).

▶ Disease Severity

Marker level, retroperitoneal CT scan, organ confined versus subdiaphragmatic lymph nodes versus pulmonary/visceral disease.

▶ Concept and Application

Annual mortality rate, 350. Major distinction: seminoma versus nonseminomatous lesion (eg, embryonal, teratoma, choriocarcinoma). Nonseminoma: any elevated AFP and more than twice the normal β-human chorionic gonadotropin (β-hCG). Tumors sensitive to platinum-based chemotherapy.

▶ Treatment Steps

Radical orchiectomy. Staging. Seminoma (local): 2,500 cGy of radiation; seminoma (node positive): chemotherapy. Nonseminoma (local): retroperitoneal lymph node dissection (RPLND); nonseminoma (advanced, 6 positive nodes or > 2.5 cm): Chemotherapy followed by salvage RPLND. Bleomycin, etopiside, and cisplatin (BEP).

*Seminoma*
1. Radical orchiectomy and radiation.
2. Chemotherapy.

*Nonseminoma*
1. Radical orchiectomy.
2. Retroperitoneal lymph node dissection (RPLND) for localized.
3. Chemotherapy and RPLND etoposide; advanced: (BEP) cisplatin Bleomycin, usually 3 cycles.

### G. Penile, Urethral, and Scrotal Carcinoma

▶ H&P Keys

If patient is not circumcised, check under foreskin and look for bloody urethral stricture and scrotal mass. Check for inguinal adenopathy.

▶ Diagnosis

Physical exam and biopsy.

▶ Disease Severity
Degree of penile shaft destruction, adenopathy, weight loss.

▶ Concept and Application
Rare cancer in developed world; usually squamous in origin. Adenopathy may be secondary to infection.

▶ Treatment Steps
1. Local excision.
2. Inguinal lymph node disection.
3. Bleomycin-based chemotherapy.

## IV. RENAL DISORDERS

### A. Pyelonephritis

▶ H&P Keys
History of UTIs, voiding dysfunction, flank pain, fever, malaise. Differentiate acute from chronic pyelonephritis.

▶ Diagnosis
Urine culture, urinalysis (pyuria, white blood cell casts), renal ultrasound to rule out obstruction by stone or other cause.

▶ Disease Severity
Discomfort to frank sepsis. Acute infection versus chronic deterioration (renal scarring, insufficiency, proteinuria, hypertension).

▶ Concept and Application
Ascending urinary tract infection can cause significant initial damage in pediatric population (usually associated with reflux). Infection and obstruction enhance renal damage. Can be associated with stone disease. Usually standard pathogens.

▶ Treatment Steps
1. Rule out obstruction and calculus.
2. Treat with culture-appropriate antibiotics.
3. Monitor renal function in chronic patients.

### B. Acute Renal Failure

▶ H&P Keys
Increased creatinine and BUN, edema, hypertension, toxicity exposure, rhabdomyolysis, hemolysis.

▶ Diagnosis
Urine diagnostic indexes, renal failure index, electrolyte measurements, possible renal biopsy.

▶ Disease Severity
Acute progression versus rapid progression; oliguric versus nonoliguric. Rate of improvement and associated pathology.

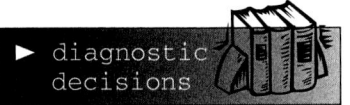

## RENAL DISORDERS

**Polycystic Kidney Disease**
Positive family history in 75%, clinical (bilateral flank masses, elevated BP, uremia).

**Alport's Syndrome**
Hematuria, proteinuria, hearing loss, ocular disorders.

**Acute Scrotum**
Patient age: torsion in younger patients, hyperacute onset, orchitis in older patients gradual onset. Orchitis in younger patients due to chlamydia, *E. coli* in older population. Rule out trauma or chronic mass; varicocele, hydrocele.

**Flank Pain**
Acute obstruction—stone, papillary necrosis, fungus ball. Rule out pyelonephritis or renal abscess; consider vascular occlusion, renal vein thrombosis, or arterial emboli.

**Voiding Dysfunction**
Failure to empty/failure to store, irritative versus obstructive symptoms. Look for associated neurologic disease or history of infection.

▶ Concept and Application

Prerenal, 55%; intrinsic, 40%; and postrenal causes, 5%. Conversion of oliguric to nonoliguric state improves management and may improve outcome. Prerenal conditions include congestive heart failure (CHF), hypovolemia, plasma protein deficiency. Hepatorenal syndrome probably reflects renal response to prerenal circulatory environment. Intrinsic disease caused by restricted blood flow to glomeruli, decreased basement membrane permeability, tubular plugging, disrupted tubules. Intrinsic disease; also acute glomerular nephritis and allergic interstitial nephritis. Acute anuria suggests urologic origin. Also consider solitary kidney. Acute tubular necrosis. Mortality can range between 25% and 70%.

▶ Treatment Steps

Assess clinical and laboratory parameters.

*Prerenal*
1. Restore adequate circulating plasma volume.
2. Correct nonrenal pathology.

*Renal*
1. Convert to nonoliguric state, remove toxins, dialyze as needed.
2. Urologic evaluation (ultrasound, cystoscopy, retrograde stent placement) as needed.

## C. Chronic Renal Failure

▶ H&P Keys

Diabetes, hypertension, pericarditis, glomerulopathy, obstructive uropathy, edema, anemia, puritis, osteodystrophy (osteitis fibrosa).

▶ Diagnosis

Shrunken kidneys on imaging, uremia, creatinine clearance, edema, hyperkalemia normochromic, normocytic anemia.

▶ Disease Severity

Creatinine clearance, edema, electrolyte derangement, neurologic complications of uremia.

▶ Concept and Application

Multiple causes, majority of cases involve hypertension, diabetes mellitus, and glomerulonephritis. Early reduction of glomerular filtration (GFR) (30–50%) compensated. Azotemia between 20% and 35% GFR and overt renal failure below 20% of normal.

▶ Treatment Steps
1. Initial dietary restriction of protein.
2. Control hypertension.
3. Correct electrolyte imbalances.
4. Dialysis and transplantation.

## D. Tubulointerstitial Disease

▶ H&P Keys

Toxin exposure (analgesics, heavy metal), immune disorders, neoplasia, vascular disease, family history of renal disorders.

▶ Diagnosis

Electrolyte irregularities, eosinophilia, impaired creatine clearance, renal biopsy.

▶ Disease Severity

Acute or chronic, tubular defects versus marked GFR deterioration.

▶ Concept and Application

Pathology is morphologically in tubules and interstitium, not glomerulus. *Acute disease:* inflammation, tubule necrosis, edema. *Chronic forms:* fibrosis is common. Condition has many causes. Look for dysfunction in tubular transport. Proteinuria usually not severe. Eventual GFR dysfunction.

▶ Treatment Steps
1. Remove offending agent.
2. Compensate tubular defect.
3. Treat primary disease.

## E. Renal Transplant Rejection

▶ H&P Keys

Oliguria, azotemia, graft tenderness, fever, proteinuria.

▶ Diagnosis

Ultrasound to rule out obstruction, urine output, proteinuria, renal scan, renal biopsy.

▶ Disease Severity

Mild azotemia, frank renal failure, rapidity of onset and progression.

▶ Concept and Application

Immunologic reaction, cellular and humoral. Hyperacute, acute accelerated, acute, and chronic rejection.

▶ Treatment Steps

*Hyperacute and Acute Accelerated*—Rare, nephrectomy.

*Acute*
1. Immunosuppression.
2. Methylprednisolone.
3. Cyclosporine.

*Chronic*
1. Rule out obstruction, no treatment.
2. Kidney-sparing diet.

## F. Nephrotic Syndrome

▶ H&P Keys

Edema.

▶ Diagnosis

Urinalysis, proteinuria, 24-hr collection, hypoalbuminemia, renal biopsy.

▶ Disease Severity

Rapid versus chronic course. Degree of proteinuria/renal insufficiency.

▶ Concept and Application

Albuminuria, hypoalbuminemia, hyperlipidemia, and edema. Minimal change disease, mesangial proliferative IgA glomerulonephritis (Berger's disease), focal and segmental glomerulosclerosis, membranous Berger's disease.

▶ Treatment Steps

Treatment with combination of steroids, cytotoxic drugs, cyclosporine.

## G. Glomerulonephritis

▶ H&P Keys

Infectious disease, primary renal disease, multisystem disease. Abrupt azotemia, oliguria, edema, hypertension.

▶ Diagnosis

Serum electrolytes, proteinuria, urinalysis for hematuria, red cell casts.

▶ Disease Severity

Degree of edema, renal insufficiency, acute versus rapidly progressing disease.

▶ Concept and Application

Glomerular damage, capillary wall damage (anionic charge/pore size), vascular changes resulting from vessel damage and surrounding inflammation.

▶ Treatment Steps

*Acute Supportive Disease*
1. Diuresis.
2. Bed rest.
3. Antihypertension drugs as needed.

*Rapidly Progressing Disease*
1. Glucocorticoid
2. Pulse treatment.
3. Cytotoxic agents.
4. Plasma exchange.

## H. Diabetic Nephropathy

▶ H&P Keys

History of diabetes, diabetic stigmata, edema, hypertension.

▶ Diagnosis

BUN and creatinine, creatinine clearance, oliguria.

▶ Disease Severity

Degree and duration of diabetes, level of renal impairment.

▶ Concept and Application

Microangiopathy of renal system and glomeruli (Kimmelstiel–Wilson lesions), nodular deposits in glomeruli.

▶ Treatment Steps

1. *Early:* compensate for electrolyte-fluid derangement.
2. *Later:* dialysis or transplantation.

## I. Renal Osteodystrophy

▶ H&P Keys

Renal insufficiency, growth retardation, rickets. Bone pain or proximal muscle weakness in adults.

▶ Diagnosis

Calcium and phosphorus levels. Parathyroid activity. Plain film findings.

▶ Disease Severity

Renal dwarfism versus growth retardation or maturation, degree of orthopedic disability in adults. Extent of calcium imbalance, pathologic calcification.

▶ Concept and Application

Impaired vitamin D metabolism, parathyroid hormone overproduction. Dialysis accelerates bone pathology secondary to aluminum deposition. Osteitis fibrosa cystica, renal rickets, osteosclerosis.

▶ Management

Early treatment to reduce morbidity.

1. Reduce dietary phosphate with calcium carbonate as phosphate binder.
2. Balanced dialysate. Keep $PO_4$ at 4.5 mg/dL and Ca at 10 mg/dL.

## J. Papillary Necrosis

▶ H&P Keys

Hematuria and flank pain, patient may be asymptomatic, disease often associated with severe infection and other conditions.

▶ Diagnosis

Urinalysis, culture, filling defect on urogram; ring shadow may be present.

▶ Disease Severity
Asymptomatic or flank pain infection, obstructive uropathy with papillary sloughing.

▶ Concept and Application
Infection or microangiopathy of renal pyramids. Associated with diabetes, alcoholism, sickle cell anemia.

▶ Treatment Steps
1. Asymptomatic finding: treat primary disease.
2. Mechanical removal of obstruction.

## K. Renovascular Hypertension

▶ H&P Keys
Hypertension, rapid onset, poorly controlled, epigastric bruit.

▶ Diagnosis
Renal vein renin sampling (ratio > 1.5); angiography (classic, digital, MRI); occasionally, IV urogram (not a screening test).

▶ Disease Severity
Pharmacologic control, severity of stenosis on imaging.

▶ Concept and Application
Usually secondary to atherosclerotic vascular disease; several forms of fibromuscular hyperplasia.

▶ Treatment Steps
1. Medical.
2. Angioplasty.
3. Surgical repair.

## L. Preeclampsia

▶ H&P Keys
Pregnancy related, edema, proteinuria, and hypertension after 24th week of pregnancy.

▶ Diagnosis
Blood pressure 140/90, proteinuria, 30 mm Hg systolic or 15 mm Hg diastolic relative to earlier pregnancy readings.

▶ Disease Severity
Progression to eclampsia; need for intervention beyond bed rest.

▶ Concept and Application
Etiology unknown. Glomerular capillary endotheliosis is major pathologic alteration.

▶ Treatment Steps
1. Bed rest.
2. Antihypertensives (hydralazine), delivery.
3. Magnesium sulfate 4–6 g, then 1–2 g/hr.

### M. Eclampsia

▶ H&P Keys
Preeclampsia and seizures.

▶ Diagnosis
Preeclampsia and seizure evaluation.

▶ Disease Severity
Proteinuria, level of hypertension and degree of seizure activity.

▶ Concept and Application
Etiology unknown.

▶ Treatment Steps
Control blood pressure and seizures.

### N. Polycystic Kidney Disease

▶ H&P Keys
Flank mass, renal insufficiency, family history.

▶ Diagnosis
Azotemia, uremia, CT scan, proteinuria.

▶ Disease Severity
Age of onset, infection, hypertension, rate of renal deterioration, abdominal distension.

▶ Concept and Application
Ten percent of end-stage renal failure. Cortical and medullary cysts. Hepatic cysts, cerebral aneurysms. Presents in third and fourth decade. Hypertension in 75%. Autosomal dominant disease (usually adult, wide range and penetrance). Two genes identified. Autosomal recessive, infancy or childhood (renal failure or portal fibrosis) medullary ductal ectasia.

▶ Treatment Steps
1. Hypertension control.
2. Dialysis or transplantation.

### O. Nephrosclerosis

▶ H&P Keys
Mild, moderate, or malignant hypertension; neurologic signs; papilledema.

▶ Diagnosis
Urinalysis, proteinuria, renal imaging (size).

▶ Disease Severity
Mild sclerosis with mild-to-moderate physiologic changes (slight azotemia, exaggerated natriuresis with fluid challenge versus malignant hypertension, neurologic symptoms.

▶ Concept and Application

Mild-to-moderate secondary changes of essential hypertension, vascular atherosclerotic changes (afferent arterioles). Severe disease with fibrinoid necrosis and hyperplastic arteriolitis.

▶ Treatment Steps

Control hypertension (acute and chronic).

## P. Lupus Nephritis

▶ H&P Keys

Associated history of systemic lupus erythematosus (SLE) and physical exam, edema.

▶ Diagnosis

Urinalysis, azotemia, low $C_3$ and $C_4$ concentrations. Positive double-stranded DNA antibody, proteinuria, nephrotic syndrome, renal biopsy.

▶ Disease Severity

Asymptomatic, clinical SLE, mild-to-severe renal status.

▶ Concept and Application

Renal involvement in 35–90% of SLE patients, deposition of circulating immunocomplexes, autoantibody activity.

▶ Treatment Steps

1. Steroids.
2. Cyclophosphamide.
3. Azathioprine.

## V. ELECTROLYTE AND ACID–BASE DISORDERS

### A. Hyponatremia

▶ H&P Keys

Nausea, confusion, lethargy, coma, seizures, decreased deep-tendon reflexes.

▶ Diagnosis

Serum sodium < 130 mg/dL.

▶ Disease Severity

Abnormal laboratory value to severe clinical derangement.

▶ Concept and Application

Free-water retention, exogenous free water, TURP or water intoxication, syndrome of inappropriate secretion of antidiuretic hormone (SIADH), renal and cardiac decompensation.

▶ Treatment Steps

Restrict free water, replace salt.

## B. Hypernatremia

▶ **H&P Keys**

Dehydration, hyperpnea, oliguria, thirst, hypotension.

▶ **Diagnosis**

Serum sodium > 145 mg/dL.

▶ **Disease Severity**

Laboratory finding to severe clinical derangement.

▶ **Concept and Application**

Impaired thirst mechanism, excessive water loss, solute and free-water loss (diabetic ketoacidosis).

▶ **Treatment Steps**

Slow replacement of free water to avoid cerebral edema.

## C. Hypokalemia

▶ **H&P Keys**

Dysrhythmia, rhabdomyolysis, muscle weakness or cramps.

▶ **Diagnosis**

Serum potassium < 3.5 mg/dL. Changes in electrocardiogram (ECG): wide decrease in T wave, U wave, atrioventricular block.

▶ **Disease Severity**

Laboratory finding to severe clinical derangement.

▶ **Concept and Application**

Inappropriate gastrointestinal (GI) or GU loss, cellular sequestration, decreased intake. Because of body stores, small decrease in serum value can indicate significant total-body depletion.

▶ **Treatment Steps**

1. Oral replacement for chronic loss (diuretic use).
2. IV replacement is not advised except in monitored situation (keep below 20 mEq/hr).

## D. Hyperkalemia

▶ **H&P Keys**

Renal insufficiency, diarrhea, weakness.

▶ **Diagnosis**

Laboratory findings, ECG: widened QRS waves and peaked T waves.

▶ **Disease Severity**

Laboratory value or severe clinical derangement.

▶ **Concept and Application**

Reduced renal excretion of potassium; adrenal insufficiency, excessive intake; hyperchloremic acidosis.

▶ Treatment Steps
1. Limit exogenous potassium.
2. Correct underlying acidosis.
3. Exchange resin, insulin/$D_{50}$ glucose.
4. Dialysis.

### E. Volume Depletion

▶ H&P Keys
Decreased skin turgor, orthostasis, thirst, coma, sunken eyes.

▶ Diagnosis
Serum electrolytes, increased sodium, BUN, osmolality increased.

▶ Disease Severity
Laboratory derangement to severe clinical compromise.

▶ Concept and Application
Third spacing, insufficient replacement of free water, excessive loss of free water.

▶ Treatment Steps
1. Slow replacement of free water.
2. Replace sodium as needed.

### F. Volume Excess

▶ H&P Keys
Renal insufficiency, CHF, pathologic freewater consumption (water intoxication), syndrome of inappropriate antidiuretic hormone secretion (SIADH), nausea, seizures, weakness, coma.

▶ Diagnosis
Serum electrolytes, clinical scenario.

▶ Disease Severity
Mild electrolyte disturbance to severe clinical derangement.

▶ Concept and Application
Excessive exogenous free water or poor elimination of free water.

▶ Treatment Steps
Restrict fluids.

### G. Metabolic Alkalosis

▶ H&P Keys
GI loss, renal loss, H⁺ translocation (hypokalemia), $NaHCO_3$ administration.

▶ Diagnosis
Elevation of arterial pH, increase in plasma $HCO_3$, compensatory hypoventilation (up $P_{CO_2}$).

▶ Disease Severity
Compensated disturbance or severe metabolic derangement.

▶ Concept and Application

Generally a loss of H⁺, retention of bicarbonate, or contraction alkalosis.

▶ Treatment Steps
1. Correct primary cause.
2. Compensate electrolyte abnormality.

### H. Respiratory Alkalosis

▶ H&P Keys

Hypoxemia, CHF, pulmonary disease, severe anemia, gram-negative sepsis, hepatic failure.

▶ Diagnosis

Elevated arterial pH, hypocapnea, plasma $HCO_3$ decreased.

▶ Disease Severity

Mild compensated disorder or severe metabolic derangement.

▶ Concept and Application

Hyperventilation caused by hypoxemia or central stimulation of respiration. Primary respiratory disease and mechanical ventilation also a cause.

▶ Treatment Steps
1. Correct underlying medical defect.
2. Rebreathing (increase $P_{CO_2}$).

### I. Metabolic Acidosis

▶ H&P Keys

Low arterial pH, reduced plasma $HCO_3$ concentration, compensatory hyperventilation.

▶ Diagnosis

Electrolytes, blood gas, associated metabolic disorders.

▶ Disease Severity

Mild electrolyte disturbance to severe metabolic derangement.

▶ Concept and Application

Generally characterized as anion gap (ingestions, ketoacidosis, lactic acidosis, renal failure, rhabdomyolysis), and hyperchloremic (normal anion gap) renal dysfunction, GI loss of $HCO_3$, renal loss of $HCO_3$, ingestion.

▶ Treatment Steps
1. Correct primary etiology.
2. Replace $HCO_3$ with accompanying additional cation load (Na⁺).

### J. Respiratory Acidosis

▶ H&P Keys

Medications, acute cardiac arrest, obesity, upper-airway obstruction, chestwall pathology, adult respiratory distress syndrome, and chronic obstructive pulmonary disease.

---

▶ management decisions

**ELECTROLYTE AND ACID–BASE DISORDERS**

Metabolic Acidosis
Correct primary pathology (anion gap or nonanion gap causes), assess renal function and GI function, evaluate for lactic acidosis or ketoacidosis.

Hypercalcemia
Discern appropriate etiology—neoplasia, hyperparathyroidism, sarcoidosis; evaluate ECG; saline hydration and furosemide diuresis; calcitonin or bisphosphonates.

▶ **Diagnosis**
Blood gas and electrolytes. Elevated serum $HCO_3$, reduced arterial pH. Elevated $P_{CO_2}$.

▶ **Disease Severity**
Mild disorder to severe decompensation.

▶ **Concept and Application**
Inability to excrete respiratory $CO_2$, multiple mechanical and structural disorders.

▶ **Treatment Steps**
Correct primary ventilatory defect.

### K. Hypomagnesemia

▶ **H&P Keys**
Alcoholism, malnutrition, diuretics, diabetic ketoacidosis, lethargy, delirium, irritability of central nervous system.

▶ **Diagnosis**
Low serum magnesium (< 1.1 mEq/dL); electrocardiogram (ECG), prolonged QT waves; hypokalemia; hypocalcemia.

▶ **Disease Severity**
Electrolyte abnormality to severe neurologic decompensation.

▶ **Concept and Application**
Metabolism similar to calcium; generally difficult to deplete body stores.

▶ **Treatment Steps**
IV or IM exogenous replacement.

### L. Hypercalcemia

▶ **H&P Keys**
Carcinoma, hyperparathyroidism or hyperthyrosis, sarcoidosis, milk alkali syndrome.

▶ **Diagnosis**
Serum-free calcium > 2.9 mEq. ECG, short QT and long PR waves.

▶ **Disease Severity**
Abnormal electrolytes to tetany and cardiac arrest.

▶ **Concept and Application**
Inappropriate calcium storage mobilization, hormonal etiology, neoplasia. Excretion linked to sodium and state of hydration.

▶ **Treatment Steps**
1. Saline infusion, furosemide.
2. Diuresis.
3. Calcitonin, mithramycin.
4. Sodium etidronate.

## M. Hypocalcemia

▶ **H&P Keys**

Renal failure, hypoparathyroidism, vitamin D deficiency, malabsorption, Chvostek's sign, Trousseau's sign, perioral paresthesias, muscle cramps.

▶ **Diagnosis**

Serum calcium (free Ca < 2.2 mEq).

▶ **Disease Severity**

Electrolyte finding to tetany, neurologic, cardiovascular complications.

▶ **Concept and Application**

Secondary to parathyroid surgery, poor absorption, inability to access bone stores.

▶ **Treatment Steps**
1. Correct underlying defect.
2. Administer exogenous calcium and vitamin D.

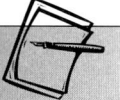

▶ on rounds

### UROLOGIC DISORDERS

**Prostate Cancer**
- Diagnosis by digital rectal exam and PSA followed by needle biopsy, bone scan.
- Staging: Jewett–Whitmore A–D.
  A = Local, nonpalpable
  B = Palpable, confined
  C = Extracapsular
  D = Lymph node or distant mets
- Treatment if local includes radical prostatectomy or radiation.
- Treatment if extracapsular is radiation.
- Treatment for advanced disease includes androgen ablation (orchiectomy, LH-releasing hormone agonists).

**Wilms' Tumor**
- Pediatric tumor (peak age 3), flank mass, hematuria.

**Bladder Cancer**
- Risk factors include exposure to tobacco, cyclophosphamide and analine dyes.

**Hydrocele**
- Painless scrotal mass, transillumination, fluid in tunical layer of testes, a cosmetic problem.

**Varicocele**
- Spermatic venous varicies, "bag of worms" feel, pain, infertility.

**Testicular Torsion**
- Scrotal swelling in children, acute severe onset, nausea, abdominal pain.

## BIBLIOGRAPHY

Gillenwater J, Grayhack J, Howards S, Duckett JW. *Adult and Pediatric Urology.* St. Louis: Mosby; 1996.

Walsh PC, Retik AB, Vaughn ED, Wein AJ (eds.). *Campbell's Urology.* 8th ed. Philadelphia: Saunders; 2002.

# Surgical Principles | 18

I.  **DISORDERS OF THE SKIN AND SUBCUTANEOUS TISSUE / 564**
   A. Cellulitis / 564
   B. Lipoma / 564
   C. Hemangioma / 564
   D. Neurofibroma / 565
   E. Sebaceous Cyst / 565
   F. Basal Cell Carcinoma / 566
   G. Squamous Cell Carcinoma / 566
   H. Melanoma / 567
   I.  Sarcoma / 568
   J. Decubitus Ulcer / 568
   K. Venous Ulceration / 569
   L. Arterial Ulcer / 569

II. **BREAST DISORDERS / 570**
   A. Benign Breast Mass / 570
   B. Breast Cancer / 570

III. **DISEASES OF THE ENDOCRINE SYSTEM / 572**
   A. Thyroid Neoplasm / 572
   B. Hyperparathyroidism / 572
   C. Cushing's Disease/Cushing's Syndrome / 573
   D. Pheochromocytoma / 574

IV. **DISORDERS OF THE KIDNEY AND URINARY TRACT / 575**
   A. Testicular Tumors / 575
   B. Carcinoma of the Bladder / 575
   C. Prostate Cancer / 576
   D. Renal Cell Carcinoma / 576
   E. Renal Calculi / 577
   F. Benign Prostatic Hypertrophy / 578

V. **TRAUMA / 578**
   A. Multiple Injuries / 578
   B. Cranial Injury / 580
   C. Abdominal Injury / 580

VI. **POSTOPERATIVE INFECTIONS / 582**
   A. Wound Infections / 582
   B. Urinary Tract Infections / 583
   C. Atelectasis and Pneumonia / 583

VII. **DISEASES OF THE CIRCULATORY SYSTEM / 584**
   A. Carotid Artery Disease / 584
   B. Renovascular Disease / 586
   C. Peripheral Arterial Occlusive Disease / 586
   D. Aneurysms of the Thoracic Aorta / 588
   E. Aortic Dissection / 589
   F. Abdominal Aortic Aneurysmal Disease / 590
   G. Thoracic Outlet Syndrome (TOS) / 591
   H. Infrainguinal Aneurysmal Disease / 592
   I. Arterial Embolism/Thrombosis / 593
   J. Deep Venous Thrombosis (DVT) / 594
   K. Varicose Veins / 595
   L. Superficial Thrombophlebitis / 595

VIII. **DISEASES OF THE GASTROINTESTINAL TRACT / 596**
   A. Zenker's Diverticulum / 596
   B. Midesophageal Traction Diverticulum / 596
   C. Achalasia / 597
   D. Esophageal Varices / 597
   E. Cancer of the Stomach / 598
   F. Gastric Volvulus / 598
   G. Appendicitis / 599
   H. Ulcerative Colitis / 599
   I. Crohn's Disease / 600
   J. Acute Mesenteric Ischemia / 600
   K. Small-bowel Obstruction / 601
   L. Large-bowel Obstruction / 603
   M. Diverticulitis / 603
   N. Rectal Tumor / 604
   O. Hemorrhoids / 604
   P. Perirectal Abscess / 605
   Q. Anorectal Fistula / 605
   R. Pilonidal Cyst / 605
   S. Benign Neoplasm of the Small Bowel / 606
   T. Benign Neoplasm of the Colon / 606
   U. Colon Cancer / 606
   V. Duodenal Atresia / 608

W. Malrotation / 608
X. Hirschsprung's Disease / 609
Y. Imperforate Anus / 609

## IX. DISEASES OF THE GALLBLADDER AND LIVER / 610
A. Biliary Atresia / 610
B. Acute Cholecystitis / 610
C. Choledochal Cyst / 611
D. Choledocholithiasis / 612
E. Carcinoma of the Gallbladder / 612
F. Hepatic Adenoma / 612
G. Focal Nodular Hyperplasia / 613
H. Primary Hepatobiliary Cancer / 613
I. Liver Metastasis / 614

## X. DISEASE OF THE PANCREAS / 615
A. Acute Pancreatitis / 615
B. Pancreatic Carcinoma / 616
C. Gastrinoma / 616

## XI. HERNIA / 617
A. Inguinal Hernia / 617
B. Femoral Hernia / 617
C. Umbilical Hernia / 618
D. Incisional Hernia / 618
E. Diaphragmatic Hernia / 619
F. Hernia with Obstruction / 619

## BIBLIOGRAPHY / 619

## I. DISORDERS OF THE SKIN AND SUBCUTANEOUS TISSUE

### A. Cellulitis

▶ H&P Keys

Skin trauma; pain; fever; tender, erythematous, and edematous skin; ulcer; surgical wound; skin puncture; red or tender streaks; indistinct advancing edge; history of venous or lymphatic insufficiency.

▶ Diagnosis

Physical examination, blood culture, biopsy of ulcers.

▶ Disease Severity

Malaise, fever, lymphangitis, bullae. Sepsis/bacteremia.

▶ Concept and Application

Injury to skin, bacterial invasion of skin and subcutaneous tissue (*Streptococci, Staphylococci,* anaerobes) spread by way of lymphatics.

▶ Treatment Steps
1. Warm packs, rest, elevation of limb.
2. Intravenous (IV) antibiotics.
3. Local wound care.
4. Remove the infective source (eg, IV line, infected bullae).

### B. Lipoma

▶ H&P Keys

Swelling, rarely painful; soft subcutaneous lobulated mass, "slipping sign."

▶ Diagnosis

Physical examination; excisional biopsy.

▶ Disease Severity

Hard mass, calcification, rapid growth.

▶ Concept and Application

Benign tumor of mature fat cells (malignant counterpart: liposarcoma).

▶ Treatment Steps
1. Observation.
2. Surgical excision (cosmesis, local symptoms, persistent growth).

### C. Hemangioma

▶ H&P Keys

Red or bluish, raised lesion; painless. Congenital forms are common and regress spontaneously.

▶ Diagnosis

Physical examination.

▶ Disease Severity
Rate of growth, degree of disfigurement, ulceration, infection, cardiac failure (arteriovenous shunting), intravascular coagulation.

▶ Concept and Application
True neoplasm or malformation of normal vascular structures, mostly capillaries. The most common head and neck tumor in children.

▶ Treatment Steps
1. Observation.
2. Corticosteroids, injection sclerotherapy.
3. Radiation.
4. Partial or complete surgical excision (do not biopsy secondary to hemorrhage risk).
5. Embolization.

## D. Neurofibroma

▶ H&P Keys
Mass, pain, sensory deficit, muscular weakness. If multiple, must consider von Recklinghausen disease (neurofibromatosis).

▶ Diagnosis
Physical examination, nerve conduction studies, electromyography, magnetic resonance imaging (MRI).

▶ Disease Severity
Peripheral nerve dysfunction, multiple lesions, recurrent lesions, malignant transformation, involvement of craniospinal axis, diffuse growth.

▶ Concept and Application
Neoplastic activity in nerve sheath, part of von Recklinghausen disease complex.

▶ Treatment Steps
1. Observation.
2. Surgical excision.

## E. Sebaceous Cyst

▶ H&P Keys
Asymptomatic swelling, spherical mass with punctum.

▶ Diagnosis
Physical examination.

▶ Disease Severity
Size of lesion, infection and abscess formation, ulceration.

▶ Concept and Application
Thin layer of epidermal cell lining, contains keratinous debris.

▶ Treatment Steps
1. Surgical excision including capsule.
2. Incision and drainage if infected.

## F. Basal Cell Carcinoma

▶ H&P Keys

Lesion on face or other sun-exposed areas; bleeding; pearly nodule; central ulceration; rolled, raised, or beaded edge. Most common skin cancer. Seen most commonly in elderly population.

▶ Diagnosis

Physical examination, biopsy.

▶ Disease Severity

Size and site of lesion, destruction of adjacent tissue, intracranial extension, ulceration.

▶ Concept and Application

Ultraviolet-B light exposure, fair-skinned persons. Slow growth and local invasion.

▶ Treatment Steps
1. Excision:
    a. Curettage and electrodesiccation.
    b. Surgical excision.
    c. Mohs' micrographic surgery (facial lesion).
2. Radiation, topical chemotherapy.
3. Close follow-up.

## G. Squamous Cell Carcinoma

▶ H&P Keys

Erythematous plaque or nodule, ulceration with raised edges, chronic ulcer, lymphadenopathy. Second most common form of skin cancer.

▶ Diagnosis

Physical examination; biopsy.

▶ Disease Severity

Burn-scar carcinoma (Marjolin's ulcer), fixed to surrounding structures, ulceration, lymphadenopathy (regional), histologic differentiation.

▶ Concept and Application

Invasive neoplasms devised from keratinocytes, ultraviolet exposure, irradiation, chronic irritation, chronic granulomas, burn scar, chronic sinus. Lower lip, ears, and genitalia have higher metastatic potential.

▶ Treatment Steps
1. Radiotherapy.
2. Surgical excision, en block dissection of lymph nodes.

## H. Melanoma

▶ H&P Keys

Increase in size or change in color of mole, or any pigmented nevus, bleeding, itching, pain, lymphadenopathy, family history, hepatomegaly. Associated with chromosomes 1, 6, 9; majority arises de novo; up to 50% in existing nevi; 90% skin, with other sites being eye, anus, and visceral sites. High risk for persons with over 50 moles. Mean age of diagnosis is 48 years.

▶ Diagnosis

Physical examination, excisional biopsy, chest x-ray (CXR), liver function tests (LFTs).

▶ Disease Severity

Worst prognosis with mole or moles on trunk, especially if congenital or dysplastic, thickness of tumor, Breslow's classification, ulceration, melanosis, satellitosis, lymphadenopathy, subungual lesions, pattern of growth, multiple nevi, location of the lesion. The most common sites of metastasis are liver and lung.

▶ Concept and Application

Malignant tumor of melanocytes; lymphatic and blood metastatic spread. Ultraviolet exposure, genetic predisposition, presence of dysplastic nevi. The four major histology types are: superficial spreading (70%), nodular melanoma (15–30%), lentigo maligna melanoma (< 10%), acral lentiginous melanoma (< 10%).

▶ Treatment Steps
1. Wide surgical excision, therapeutic nodal dissection.
2. Regional hyperthermic limb perfusion.
3. Chemotherapy, immunotherapy.

▶ cram facts

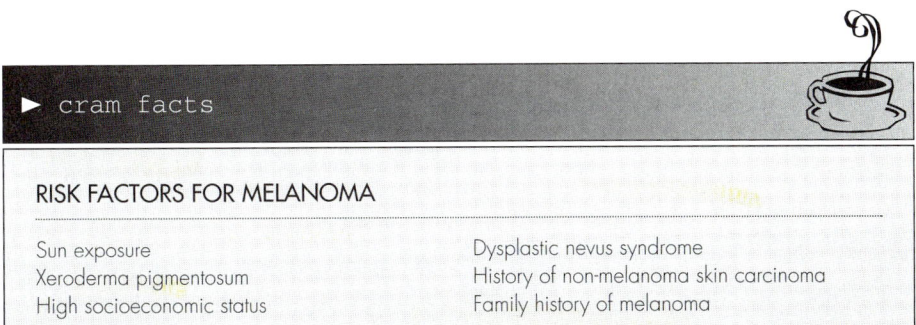

### RISK FACTORS FOR MELANOMA

| | |
|---|---|
| Sun exposure | Dysplastic nevus syndrome |
| Xeroderma pigmentosum | History of non-melanoma skin carcinoma |
| High socioeconomic status | Family history of melanoma |

> cram facts

**BRESLOW THICKNESS PROGNOSIS AND MARGIN OF EXCISION**

- < 0.76 mm—1-cm margin of excision—< 10% 10-year mortality.
- 0.76 mm—4-mm to 2-cm margins of excision—intermediate prognosis.
- > 4 mm—2-cm margins of excision—worst prognosis, > 50% 10-year mortality.

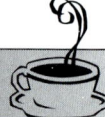

### I. Sarcoma

▶ H&P Keys

Painless discrete mass in limb, abdominal mass, hepatomegaly. Patient often gives an antecedent history of trauma.

▶ Diagnosis

MRI, computed tomography (CT) scan, needle biopsy, incisional biopsy, CXR.

▶ Disease Severity

Tumor size, depth, and site; histologic grade, presence of metastatic disease, recurrence of tumor. Rapid growth.

▶ Concept and Application

Invasive neoplasm derived from mesodermal connective tissue. Radiation exposure, oncogenic viruses. Arsenic, vinyl chloride, human immunodeficiency virus (HIV), neurofibromatosis. The most common site for metastasis is lung.

▶ Treatment Steps
1. En bloc resection.
2. Radiotherapy, chemotherapy.
3. Hyperthermic limb perfusion.

### J. Decubitus Ulcer

▶ H&P Keys

Blanching erythema, shallow or extensive dermal defects, contractures, fever, cellulitis. Immobilized patient (paralysis, cast).

▶ Diagnosis

Physical examination, x-ray of ulcer to assess osteomyelitis and subcutaneous extension (air).

▶ Disease Severity

Depth and size of defect, osteomyelitis, nutrition, albumin, associated cardiopulmonary disease.

▶ Concept and Application

Microcirculatory ischemia from prolonged pressure. Immobilization, incontinence of urine or feces, malnutrition, inadequate care.

▶ Treatment Steps

*Prevention*—Keep dry, turn patient frequently, use air or foam mattress, improve nutrition, optimize cardiovascular function.

*Definitive*—Drainage of infected spaces, antibiotics, debridement, musculocutaneous flaps or skin grafts.

## K. Venous Ulceration

▶ H&P Keys

Ulceration in leg, commonly over medial malleolus, varicose veins, history of deep vein thrombosis, saphenofemoral incompetence, perforator incompetence, brawny skin in distal medial one third of leg, scars from healed ulcers, hyperpigmentation, ichthyosis, dependent edema, fever, cellulitis (stasis dermatitis), lipodermatosclersosis; "inverted champagne bottle" legs.

▶ Diagnosis

Clinical examination, Doppler venous flow mapping, venogram. Impedance plethysmography (IPG) or photoplethysmography (PPG) study.

▶ Disease Severity

Cellulitis, subfascial perforators, obesity, cardiac failure, anemia, malnutrition.

▶ Concept and Application

High venous pressure, pericapillary fibrin deposition, hypoxia, loss of subcutaneous fat, frank ulceration of skin.

▶ Treatment Steps

*Conservative*—Elevation, ambulation, gradient-compression hosiery, compressive dressing, cleansing of wound (whirlpool for large wounds), antibiotics only if signs of infection, debridement.

*Surgical*
1. Ligation of perforators.
2. Skin graft.

## L. Arterial Ulcer

▶ H&P Keys

Smoking, increased low-density lipoprotein, diabetes. Intermittent claudication, pain at rest, cold feet, ulcer, pale or cold skin, gangrenous toes, absent pulses. Punched-out appearance of ulcer, extremely painful.

▶ Diagnosis

Ankle–brachial index (ABI), Doppler arterial flow mapping, arteriography, magnetic resonance angiography (MRA).

▶ Disease Severity

Pain at rest, established gangrene, infection, diabetes mellitus, previous amputation, cerebrovascular accident, myocardial infarction, or angina. Previous vascular surgery.

▶ Concept and Application
Skin ischemia resulting from atherosclerotic peripheral vascular disease.

▶ Treatment Steps
Angiography, angioplasty, arterial bypass surgery, debridement, skin graft, closure procedure (if needed) after revascularization, antibiotics only if signs of infection.

## II. BREAST DISORDERS

### A. Benign Breast Mass

▶ H&P Keys
Breast lump; mastalgia; menstrual history; pregnancy; lactation. Bloody nipple discharge (ductal papilloma or cancer). Any discrete mass in a postmenopausal woman, or that persists through the follicular phase of the menstrual cycle in a premenopausal woman, requires evaluation to rule out cancer.

▶ Diagnosis
Women should self-examine the breasts regularly. Physical examination is not sufficient to exclude malignancy. (Premenopausal women should be reexamined in 2–4 weeks.) Bilateral mammograms further define lesion features and assess other areas, including contralateral breast. Fine-needle aspiration cytology; ultrasound; core biopsy; excisional biopsy.

▶ Disease Severity
A mass that is discrete, hard, fixed, irregular, or associated with lymphadenopathy or skin changes is suggestive of breast cancer. Fever and fluctuation indicate abscess.

▶ Concept and Application
Benign breast findings are noted in > 80% of women; most in the category of "fibrocystic disease."

▶ Treatment Steps
1. Fluid-filled, cystic lesions are aspirated and followed clinically.
2. Fibrocystic disease is treated conservatively.
3. Discrete nodules require close follow up or excisional biopsy.
4. Careful follow up needed—for nonimproving mastitis, consider "inflammatory cancer."

### B. Breast Cancer

▶ H&P Keys
History of previous breast or other cancer; family history of breast cancer (first- and second-degree relatives); early menarche; late menopause; nulliparity; environmental (eg, radiation exposure)

and dietary (eg, alcohol use) factors. Palpable breast mass, hard, irregular; dimpling of the skin; nipple retraction; brawny, edematous, indurated skin (inflammatory carcinoma); lymphadenopathy (axillary, supraclavicular, cervical); hepatomegaly (metastatic disease).

▶ Diagnosis
Annual screening mammography recommended for women over age 50. Bilateral mammogram; fine-needle cytology; stereotactic core biopsy; excisional biopsy; tumor markers.

▶ Disease Severity
Inflammatory carcinoma; skin ulceration; chest wall invasion; metastasis to regional lymph nodes; distant metastasis (most common: bone, lung, liver, adrenals, pleura). Staging: **I,** tumor < 2 cm diameter, no spread; **II,** movable regional lymph node metastasis; **III,** fixed axillary lymph node metastasis; **IV,** distant metastasis.

▶ Concept and Application
Malignant transformation of breast epithelial cells is strongly influenced by hormones—breast cancer is more than 150 times more common in women than men. Mutations in tumor-suppressor genes such as p53, BRCA-1, and BRCA-2 have been implicated in approximately 10% of breast cancers. Ten percent of lifetime breast cancer risk. Four percent of American women die of breast cancer.

▶ Treatment Steps
1. Stages I and II, either modified radical mastectomy (MRM) or lumpectomy with axillary dissection and postoperative radiotherapy.
2. Stage III, MRM or radical mastectomy.
3. Stage IV, palliative procedures.
4. Adjuvant chemotherapy in premenopausal women, and tamoxifen in postmenopausal; however, adjuvant therapy remains controversial.
5. Consider prophylactic bilateral mastectomy for patients at highest risk. — *Virchow's node*
6. Sentinel node biopsy; it allows for a more precise surgical intervention in breast cancer and decreasing morbidity. If sentinel node is positive for tumor then an axillary dissection is indicated because the negative predictive value is exceedingly low in experienced hands. It is not 100% accurate and is not good for medial breast lesions.

*Note:* NSABP-04 (National Surgical Adjuvant Breast and Bowel Project) determined: no survival difference among MRM, lumpectomy with radiation, or lumpectomy alone; lumpectomy alone yielded a higher local recurrence rate than the other two treatments.

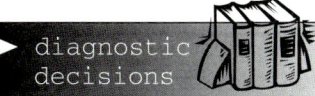

▶ diagnostic decisions

**BREAST MASS**

**Cystic**
If aspirate is bloody, cytology is suspicious, or cyst does not resolve, excisional biopsy is indicated.

**Solid**
If clinical breast examination, mammogram, and fine-needle aspiration *all* are negative, can be followed clinically ("triple diagnosis"). Otherwise, excisional biopsy—the "gold standard" for diagnosis of breast cancer—is mandatory.

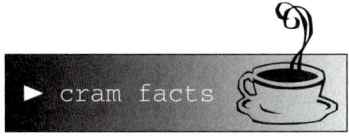

▶ cram facts

**TNM STAGING OF BREAST CANCER**

Tis = CA in situ or Paget's
T1 = < 2 cm
T2 = 2–5 cm
T3 = > 5 cm
T4 = Invade chest wall or inflammatory carcinoma
N1 = Ipsilateral axillary nodes
N2 = N1 + matted or fixed
N3 = Ipsilateral, + internal maxillary nodes
M1 = Distant metastases or + supraclavicular nodes

## III. DISEASES OF THE ENDOCRINE SYSTEM

### A. Thyroid Neoplasm

▶ H&P Keys

Neck mass, dysphagia, dysphonia, respiratory difficulty, hoarseness, hard or fixed mass, vocal cord paralysis, bony pain, lymphadenopathy. Female patient, childhood neck irradiation, lymphadenopathy, goiter. Medullary cancer, multiple endocrine neoplasia (MEN) syndrome.

▶ Diagnosis

History and physical, thyroid tests (and calcitonin if suspect medullary thyroid cancer), thyroid function tests, four primary types of thyroid cancer: papillary (85%), follicular (10%), medullary (4%), and anaplastic (1%), fine-needle aspiration cytology, thyroid suppression trial; high-resolution ultrasound, radioisotope scan, CT scan, MRI.

▶ Disease Severity

Papillary, follicular cancer—good prognosis. Symptoms of local invasion, metastatic disease, older age, gender, size of tumor, histology, lymphadenopathy, cellular differentiation. Anaplastic carcinoma has dismal prognosis.

▶ Concept and Application
1. Genetic predisposition, neck radiation, preexisting goiter.
2. Etiology of goiter: environmental (iodine deficiency), immunologic, genetic, viral, neoplastic, and drug induced [lithium, amiodarone]).
3. Differential diagnosis of thyroid nodule: multinodular goiter (50%), adenoma (33%), carcinoma (10%), cyst, inflammatory thyroid disease, and developmental abnormalities.

▶ Treatment Steps
1. Lobectomy, total thyroidectomy, cervical lymph node dissection.
2. Thyroxine, radioiodine, radiation, chemotherapy.

### B. Hyperparathyroidism

▶ H&P Keys

Lethargy, confusion, depression, peptic ulcer, anorexia, muscle weakness, recurrent nephrolithiasis, renal insufficiency, constipation.

▶ Diagnosis

Hypercalcemia, elevated parathyroid hormone (PTH), hypophosphatemia, ultrasonography, CT scan, MRI, thallium–technetium scan, sestamibi scan.

▶ Disease Severity

Renal failure; primary, secondary, tertiary disease.

---

▶ cram facts

**INDICATION FOR SURGERY IN A THYROID NODULE**

- Malignant lesions
- Indeterminate on biopsy
- Hypofunctioning lesions
- Local symptoms
- Neck disfigurement

▶ Concept and Application
Excess PTH production, from parathyroid adenoma, hyperplasia (all four glands), and rarely parathyroid carcinoma.

▶ Treatment Steps
- Surgical management (up to 25% require surgery).
1. Adenoma resection.
2. Three and one-half gland excision for hyperplasia, consider MEN evaluation.

- Medical management
1. IV fluids
2. Furosemide
3. Stop thiazide or vitamin D
4. Severe cases:
    - Bisphosphonates
    - Estrogen/progesterone

### C. Cushing's Disease/Cushing's Syndrome

▶ H&P Keys
Cushing's syndrome is a condition caused by an excess of adrenocortical hormones from all causes. Cushing's disease is Cushing's syndrome caused by pituitary hypersecretion of ACTH.

Alteration in appearance, "mooning" of face, truncal obesity, acne, hirsutism, buffalo hump, bruising, weakness of shoulders or thighs, purple striae, back pain, impotence or amenorrhea, hypertension, diabetes.

▶ Diagnosis
Plasma cortisol/adrenocorticotropic hormone (ACTH) levels (high levels indicate pituitary or ectopic ACTH tumor), 24-hour urine cortisol confirms Cushing's syndrome, dexamethasone suppression test (low-dose suppression test normal test follows 1 mg of dexamethasone resulting in feedback inhibition, which suppresses ACTH and cortisol and an abnormal test results in no ACTH suppression); high-dose dexamethasone suppression test distinguishes between pituitary and ectopic sources of ACTH secretion, metyrapone test, cortisol-releasing hormone test, isotope-scanning, CT scan of abdomen, angiography, venous sampling, MRI, NP.59 (iodocholesterol scanning).

▶ Disease Severity
Hypertension, stroke, diabetes mellitus, muscle wasting, osteoporosis (pathologic fractures), duration of disease.

▶ Concept and Application
1. Excess cortisol production, pituitary adenoma producing ACTH, adrenal adenoma or carcinoma, ACTH-secreting tumors.
2. Ectopic ACTH secretion results from bronchial carcinoid, thymic carcinoid, and adenocarcinoma or small-cell carcinoma of the lungs.
3. High ACTH indicates pituitary or ectopic ACTH tumor.
4. Low ACTH indicates hypersecretion from adrenal source.

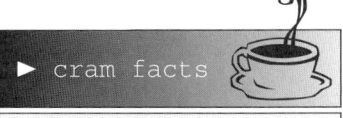

### ETIOLOGY OF HYPERPARATHYROIDISM

Primary: Adenoma 80%
Secondary:
- Renal failure
- Carcinoma with bone metastases
- Multiple myeloma
- Osteogenesis imperfecta
- Paget disease

Tertiary: Renal transplant patients

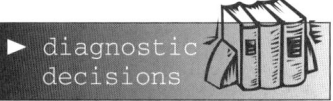

### CUSHING'S SYNDROME

**Adrenal Hyperplasia**
High plasma adrenocorticotropic hormone (ACTH), secondary to pituitary hypersecretion, pituitary tumor magnetic resonance imaging (MRI) with gadolinium enhancement (useful in diagnosis), or ectopic tumor.

**Adrenal Adenoma**
Low plasma ACTH. Abdominal computed tomography (CT) scan or MRI to localize.

**Adrenal Carcinoma**
Low ACTH. Look for palpable abdominal mass. Markedly elevated urinary 17-ketosteroids and plasma dehydroepiandrosterone (DHEA).

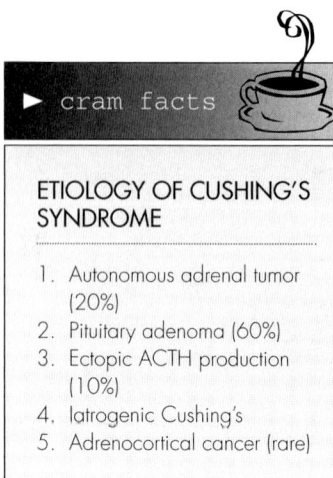

### cram facts

**ETIOLOGY OF CUSHING'S SYNDROME**

1. Autonomous adrenal tumor (20%)
2. Pituitary adenoma (60%)
3. Ectopic ACTH production (10%)
4. Iatrogenic Cushing's
5. Adrenocortical cancer (rare)

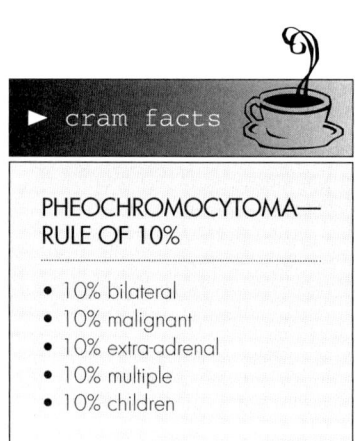

### cram facts

**PHEOCHROMOCYTOMA—RULE OF 10%**

- 10% bilateral
- 10% malignant
- 10% extra-adrenal
- 10% multiple
- 10% children

▶ Treatment Steps

*Medical*
1. Irradiation used in children with pituitary tumors.
2. Mitotane for metastatic adrenal cancer (blocks $\beta_2$ hydroxylation, reversible adenolytic).
3. Lifelong mineralo- and glucocorticoid replacement after bilateral adrenalectomy.
4. Temporary steroid replacement after unilateral adrenalectomy (because of contralateral atrophy).

*Surgical*
1. Pituitary ablation (transsphenoidal), adrenalectomy.
2. Postoperative corticosteroid therapy, removal of source of ectopic ACTH.

### D. Pheochromocytoma

▶ H&P Keys

Classic triad—hypertension, palpitation, diaphoresis. Also, patients may experience episodic headache, blurred vision, weight loss, flushing, anxiety, tachycardia.

▶ Diagnosis

Twenty-four-hour urine vanillylmandelic acid (VMA), serum catecholamine, glucagon stimulation test, phentolamine suppression test, CT scan of abdomen, metaiodobenzylguanidine (MIBG) isotope scanning, venous sampling.

▶ Disease Severity

Myocardial infarction, arrhythmias, renal failure, pregnancy, stroke.

▶ Concept and Application

There are four adrenergic receptors: $\alpha_1$, $\alpha_2$, $\beta_1$, and $\beta_2$. Tumors of adrenal medulla and chromaffin tissue, associated multiple endocrine neoplasia type II (MEN II); excess catecholamine production (1/1,000 of hypertensives have pheochromocytoma). Extra-adrenal pheochromocytoma do not produce epinephrine.

▶ Treatment Steps

*Preoperative*
1. α-Adrenergic blocker first (phenoxybenzamine).
2. Then β-adrenergic blocker.
3. Volume replacement.
4. Blood pressure control (nitroprusside, calcium channel blockers).

*Note:* Preoperative vasodilation allows for intravascular volume re-expansion and decreases hypotension following removal of the tumor. If the β-blocker is administered first, a hypertensive crisis may result because of unopposed α-adrenergic vasoconstriction.

*Surgical*—Adrenalectomy with hemodynamic monitoring, fluid therapy, nitroprusside and propranolol.

## IV. DISORDERS OF THE KIDNEY AND URINARY TRACT

### A. Testicular Tumors

▶ H&P Keys

Asymptomatic painless swelling (85%), or nodularity and more common on the right side, associated hydrocele (5%).

▶ Diagnosis

Physical examination, ultrasound, surgical exploration by way of inguinal approach.

▶ Disease Severity

*Staging*—CT scan (chest, abdomen), cavogram, lymphangiogram, tumor markers (β-human chorionic gonadotropin [β-hCG], and α-fetoprotein [α-FP]).

▶ Concept and Application

Seminomatous versus nonseminomatous.

▶ Treatment Steps

1. Orchiectomy by way of inguinal approach.
2. For seminoma, radiation to retroperitoneum.
3. For nonseminoma germ-cell tumor, retroperitoneal lymphadenectomy, adjuvant chemotherapy.

### B. Carcinoma of the Bladder

▶ H&P Keys

Hematuria, pyuria, frequency; tobacco, β-naphthylamine and para-aminodiphenyl exposure. *Risk factors for bladder squamous cell carcinoma:* chronic indwelling catheter or infection, bladder stone/strictures, infection with *Schistosoma hematobium*. *Risk factors for bladder transitional cell carcinoma:* exposure to aromatic amines, benzidine, naphthylamine, dyes, rubber, textiles, and plastics, cigarette smoking, dietary nitrosamines, cytoxan exposure.

▶ Diagnosis

Urinary cytology; cystoscopy with biopsy; CT scan and MRI to detect local invasion, nodal lesions, and distant metastases; CXR, bone scan.

▶ Concept and Application

*Staging*—Cell type (transitional, squamous, adenomatous), grade, and depth of invasion.

▶ Treatment Steps

*Carcinoma in situ*
1. Intravesical therapy (bacillus Calmette–Guérin [BCG], doxorubicin, mitomycin C).
2. Intravesical fulguration.

*Superficial*
1. Intravesical chemotherapy, local immunotherapy.
2. Transurethral endoscopic resection.
3. Recurrence common, may require cystectomy.

*Invasive*—Radical cystectomy is treatment of choice, chemotherapy.

### C. Prostate Cancer

▶ H&P Keys

Often asymptomatic; average age, 73 years. Dysuria, urinary frequency or retention, hematuria. Most common malignant tumor in men, incidence of 10% over age 65, 65% of men age 80 or over. *Risk factors:* age, race (African Americans two-fold increase), family history.

▶ Diagnosis

Digital rectal examination; prostate-specific antigen (PSA). Confirmation by needle biopsy; staging; transrectal ultrasound, CT scan, MRI. Metastatic disease—CXR, intravenous pyelogram (IVP), bone scan, CT scan.

▶ Concept and Application

Adenocarcinoma (95%). At diagnosis, 40% of tumors have metastasized; in 40% of patients, tumor extends beyond capsule. *Common site for metastasis:* obturator lymph nodes (lymphatic pathway), bone (lumbar spine most frequent).

▶ Treatment Steps

*Stages A and B (Confined to Prostate)*
1. Treat with radical prostatectomy or interstitial/external radiation.
2. Impotence seen in 50%, incontinence 10% to 30%.

*Stage C (Disease Outside Capsule)*—Treat with radiation.

*Metastatic Carcinoma*
1. Castration.
2. Estrogen administration, chemotherapy, luteinizing hormone–releasing hormone (LHRH), flutamide.

### D. Renal Cell Carcinoma

▶ H&P Keys

Flank mass, pain, gross hematuria (40% of patients with classic triad), hypertension, fever, anemia, erythrocytosis.

▶ Diagnosis

Excretory urography with nephrotomograms, ultrasound with needle biopsy, CT scan, renal angiogram.

▶ Concept and Application

Staging by way of tumor–node–metastasis (TNM) system; cavogram, bone scan, MRI; elevated renin and erythropoietin.

▶ Treatment Steps
1. Stages I and II, radical nephrectomy.
2. Stage III, radical nephrectomy with lymphadenectomy and possible adjuvant immuno/chemotherapy.
3. Stage IV, still radical nephrectomy; if lung or brain metastatic disease is isolated, surgical excision is optimal; immuno/chemotherapy.
4. Advanced disease may be treated with α-interferon or interleukin-2 (IL-2).

## E. Renal Calculi

▶ H&P Keys

Excruciating pain (upper back to testicle or vulva) secondary to dilation of urinary tract, hematuria, nausea, vomiting, urinary frequency or urgency, no comfortable position, decreased bowel sounds (reflex ileus).

▶ Diagnosis

*Urinalysis*—Hematuria, crystals; ultrasound: hydronephrosis or acoustic shadow.

▶ Disease Severity

Recurrent calculi, hyperparathyroidism, decreased renal function, hydronephrosis. *Indications for surgical intervention:* infection, complete obstruction, intractable pain, debilitating condition (diabetes mellitus/immune compromised), progressive renal damage.

▶ Concept and Application

Infection related to calculi, struvite stones, urea-splitting bacteria (eg, *Proteus*); uric acid calculi, 5–10%, radiolucent (uric acid + xanthine); cystine calculi, decreased reabsorption of dibasic amino acids. Calcium-oxalate stones (three times more in men than women), calcium metabolism, hyperparathyroidism. *Three theories of ureteric stone formation:* nucleation theory, stone matrix theory, decreased urinary crystallization inhibitors.

▶ Treatment Steps

*Surgical*
1. Shock wave lithotripsy.
2. Transurethral extraction if < 4 mm (90% chance of success) to 6 mm (50% chance of success).
3. Nephrostomy (percutaneous, open).

*Medical*
1. Half may pass spontaneously, analgesics imperative.
2. Treat cause.
3. Diuretics, cholestyramine (oxalate-binding resin).
4. Fluids, low-purine diet, alkali, and allopurinol for uric acid stones.

### F. Benign Prostatic Hypertrophy

▶ H&P Keys

Frequency, nocturia, hematuria, dribbling, decreased force of stream (retention), difficulty initiating stream. Degree of obstruction relates to gland's size.

▶ Diagnosis

Digital rectal examination, urinalysis, endoscopy, biopsy, cystometry.

▶ Disease Severity

Indication for biopsy of BPH prostate: PSA > 4.

▶ Concept and Application

Obstruction of outflow in the aging male, stromal and epithelial hyperplasia.

▶ Treatment Steps

*Medical*
1. α-Blockade—decreases smooth muscle tone; 5 α-reductase blockade (Proscar).
2. Hormonal manipulations; antiandrogen, LHRH agonist.

*Surgical*—Transurethral resection of the prostate (TURP) or open prostatectomy.

*Note:* Postoperative TURP syndrome is due to opening of venous sinuses and excess absorption, and is characterized by seizure, sodium loss, cerebral edema, and hypervolemia.

## V. TRAUMA

### A. Multiple Injuries

▶ H&P Keys

*Blunt Trauma*—Mechanisms (compression, crushing, deceleration); alcohol and drug use; prehospital care; multiple victims; localized pain or neurologic deficit; bruises; swelling; deformities.

*Penetrating Trauma*—Type of agent and energy (missile caliber and velocity, stab weapon characteristics, occupational injury); proximity to vital structures; associated blunt trauma; delay from injury to medical care; suicide attempt; entrance and exit wounds.

▶ Diagnosis

*Primary Survey (Includes Initiating Appropriate Treatment)*—ABCs—**A**irway, with control of cervical spine; **B**reathing and ventilation; **C**irculation with control of obvious bleeding and insertion of IV lines; **D**isability (alert, responds to verbal stimuli, responds to painful stimuli, or unresponsive); Glasgow Coma Scale; **E**xposure and control of environmental factors.

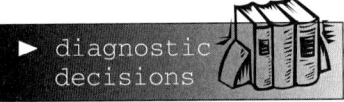

### ▶ diagnostic decisions

**GLASGOW COMA SCALE**

| Eye opening | (4) Spontaneous |
| | (3) To voice |
| | (2) To pain |
| | (1) None |
| Verbal response | (5) Oriented |
| | (4) Confused |
| | (3) Inappropriate words |
| | (2) Incomprehensible sounds |
| | (1) None |
| Motor response | (6) Obeys commands |
| | (5) Localizes pain |
| | (4) Withdrawal, to pain |
| | (3) Flexion, to pain |
| | (2) Extension, to pain |
| | (1) None |

*Secondary Survey*—**AMPLE**—**A**llergies, **M**edications, **P**ast illness and surgery, **L**ast meal, **E**vents related to the trauma. Complete physical examination; diagnostic tests (complete cervical spine and other x-rays, CT scan, ultrasound, peritoneal lavage, blood test results).

▶ Disease Severity

Immediately life-threatening conditions; old age; preexisting diseases; use of anticoagulants; intoxication (alcohol, drugs); requirement of blood transfusions; multiple systems affected; hypothermia; severe neurologic deficit.

▶ Concept and Application

Death and sequelae may result from initial injury (eg, aortic transection with exsanguination, severe brain damage) or complications (eg, brain edema, sepsis, renal failure). Aims of trauma care are to restore appropriate function of injured systems and prevent complications.

▶ management decisions

## LIFE-THREATENING CONDITIONS REQUIRING IMMEDIATE TREATMENT

### Airway Obstruction
Respiratory distress; cyanosis; use of accessory muscles; noisy breathing, or no breath. Avoid tongue drop (most common cause), remove blood, foreign body (eg, teeth, piece of food). If face, oropharynx, or larynx severely damaged or edematous, emergency surgical airway is required (cricothyroidotomy or tracheostomy).

### Tension Pneumothorax
Respiratory distress, cyanosis, hypotension, tracheal deviation, unilateral absence of breath sounds, neck vein distention. Insert large-bore needle into the chest, followed by tube thoracostomy.

### Open Pneumothorax
"Sucking chest wound," occurs when a chest wall defect is greater in diameter than two thirds of the trachea. Requires closure of the defect and insertion of water-sealed chest tube.

### Flail Chest
Unstable chest wall from sternum or rib fractures. Intubation and ventilation. Treat associated hemo- or pneumothorax.

### Exsanguinating Hemorrhage
Stop obvious bleeding by applying direct pressure. Establish large-bore intravenous (IV) lines. Massive hemothorax—shock, loss of breath sounds, shifting of mediastinum—require chest tube drainage and urgent thoracotomy.

### Cardiac Tamponade
Usually, penetrating parasternal or upper abdominal trauma. Cyanosis, hypotension, distended neck veins, and muffled heart sounds. Needle pericardiocentesis for temporary relief; sternotomy or thoracotomy for definitive treatment.

▶ Treatment Steps
1. ABC (airway, breathing, circulation), oxygen, fluid replacement, warming; transfusion of blood products, tetanus toxoid, antibiotics, mannitol for brain edema.
2. Priority is treatment of life-threatening conditions.
3. Surgical management according to specific injuries.

### B. Cranial Injury

▶ H&P Keys

Loss of consciousness, amnesia, headache, lethargy, irritability, seizures, weakness of extremities, scalp laceration or hematoma, hemotympanum, rhinorrhea, otorrhea, periorbital or mastoid ecchymosis. History of alcohol or drug use.

▶ Diagnosis

Neurologic examination, CT scan of the head, cervical spine x-rays. Subdural hemorrhage is venous in origin, occurs in elderly, and shows a smooth semilunar white density on the head CT scan. Epidural hemorrhage is arterial in origin and is marked by a concave focal white density on the head CT scan.

▶ Disease Severity

Age, Glasgow coma scale (eye opening, verbal and motor responses), amnesia longer than 24 hours, focal neurologic deficits, hypoxia, associated injuries, hypertension, bradycardia, Cheyne–Stokes respiration, loss of gag or cough reflex.

▶ Concept and Application

Sudden movement of brain relative to skull (deceleration injury), cerebral laceration, diffuse axonal injury, intracranial hemorrhage, brain edema, raised intracranial pressure.

▶ Treatment Steps
1. Secure airway; correct hypoxia; restore blood pressure; hyperventilate (controversial).
2. Administer hyperosmolar agents, antibiotics, anticonvulsant prophylaxis.
3. Appropriate surgical intervention, suture scalp laceration; perform craniotomy; intraventricular bolt to monitor intracranial pressure, hypothermia.
4. Barbituric coma (controversial).

### C. Abdominal Injury

▶ H&P Keys

Abdominal pain, distention, tenderness, guarding, or rigidity; tachycardia, hypotension, tachypnea, narrowed pulse pressure, cool extremities; associated injuries, mechanism of injury.

▶ Diagnosis

Serial physical examinations; serum amylase, urinalysis, upright CXR, abdominal ultrasound, abdominal x-ray, CT scan of abdomen and pelvis, diagnostic peritoneal lavage (DPL), selective arteriography.

### ▶ Disease Severity
Indicators of surgical injury: persistent hypotension, no response to therapy, peritonitis, associated injuries, evisceration, blood on nasogastric aspirate or rectal examination, positive DPL.

### ▶ Concept and Application
Blunt or penetrating (missile, stab) injury to abdomen or lower chest.

### ▶ Treatment Steps
Secure airway; fluid resuscitation, close monitoring, blood transfusion; exploratory laparotomy: address all intra-abdominal organs.

*Spleen*
1. Splenorrhaphy, splenectomy.
2. Can manage nonoperatively if blood pressure and hematocrit stable with serial CT scans (Fig. 18–1).

*Liver*
1. Pringle maneuver, direct ligation of bleeding vessels, hepatic lobectomy, insertion of atriocaval shunt, drainage, packing.
2. Nonoperative management with red cell replacement and serial CT scans in hemodynamically stable patients.

*Biliary Tract*—Cholecystectomy, T-tube in common bile duct, choledochojejunostomy.

*Pancreas*
1. Drainage, Whipple procedure; debridement of devitalized pancreas, ligation of main duct if visualized, internal drainage.
2. Can also manage expectantly with serial CT scans in stable patient without evidence of ductal injury.

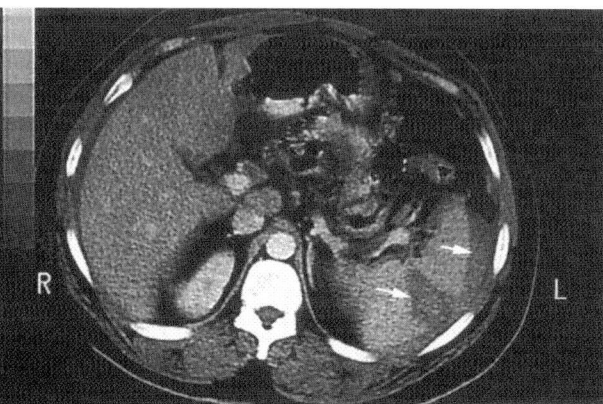

Figure 18–1. Computed tomography (CT) scan showing ruptured spleen following abdominal trauma in patient with human immunodeficiency virus (HIV) infection and splenomegaly. Note intra- and perisplenic hematoma (*arrows*).

*Gastrointestinal (GI) Tract*—Primary repair, drainage, exteriorization of injury less common. Colon resection and colostomy with gross contamination.

*Kidney*
1. Observation, serial imaging.
2. Partial or total nephrectomy.

## VI. POSTOPERATIVE INFECTIONS

### A. Wound Infections

▶ H&P Keys

Fever, wound pain, malaise, anorexia, tachycardia, local redness, tenderness, crepitance, swelling, discharge (bloody, serous, or purulent), postoperative days 3 to 7 most commonly.

▶ Diagnosis

Physical examination, wound exploration, culture.

▶ management decisions

### POSTOPERATIVE INFECTIONS

**Wound**
Erythema, edema, pain/tenderness, drainage, fever, and leukocytosis. Open and pack the wound. Antibiotics if extensive cellulitis present or patient immunocompromised. Rule out foreign body and fistula.

**Respiratory Tract**
Productive cough, yellow or green sputum; fever, tachycardia, tachypnea. Leukocytosis; infiltrate on chest x-ray (CXR). Treat with intensive respiratory physiotherapy and intravenous (IV) antibiotics (empirically, a cephalosporin).

**IV Lines**
*Superficial phlebitis (erythema, and tenderness over IV line insertion area):* Remove line; treat with warm compresses and analgesic anti-inflammatory drugs. *Central venous catheter infection (positive blood cultures):* remove line and give antibiotics if infection persists or patient immunocompromised.

**Intra-abdominal**
Peritonitis requires exploratory laparotomy or laparoscopy. Abscess may be drained percutaneously. Both require IV antibiotics that cover enteric gram-negatives and anaerobes.

**Genitourinary**
History of catheterization or instrumentation of urinary tract. Remove catheters if possible. Maintain diuresis. Oral or IV antibiotics depending on severity of infection.

**Gastrointestinal**
Fever, leukocytosis, and diarrhea. Stool culture and *Clostridium difficile* (*C. difficile*) toxin assay. Treat with metronidazole or vancomycin.

**Prosthetic device**
Fever, leukocytosis, and bacteremia. Computed tomography (CT) scan, magnetic resonance imaging (MRI), radionuclide scan, blood cultures. Give IV antibiotics. Definitive treatment is removal of prosthesis.

▶ Disease Severity

Fever, mentation changes, abscess, fascial dehiscence, evisceration, nutritional status, associated disease.

▶ Concept and Application

Contamination of wound at surgery, postoperative formation of hematoma or seroma, foreign body, wound-tissue ischemia, classification of surgical wound.

▶ Treatment Steps
1. Evacuate pus, debridement.
2. Antibiotics.
3. Local wound care.
4. Optimize nutrition/hemodynamics.

## B. Urinary Tract Infections

▶ H&P Keys

Dysuria, frequency, suprapubic or flank pain and tenderness, fever.

▶ Diagnosis

Urinalysis, urine Gram stain and culture, blood cultures.

▶ Disease Severity

High fever, mentation changes. Response to therapy.

▶ Concept and Application

Contamination of urinary tract, urine stasis, urinary tract instrumentation.

▶ Treatment Steps
1. Adequate hydration and catheter care.
2. Remove catheter, if possible.
3. Antibiotics.

## C. Atelectasis and Pneumonia

▶ H&P Keys

Early postoperative period; pain; shallow breathing. Fever, dyspnea, cough, tachycardia, tachypnea, cyanosis, decreased breath sounds. Purulent sputum suggests pneumonia.

▶ Diagnosis

Physical examination, arterial blood gases (ABGs), sputum culture, CXR, complete blood count.

▶ Disease Severity

Cyanosis, tracheal deviation, dyspnea at rest, mentation, ABGs, mentation.

▶ Concept and Application

Obstruction of tracheobronchial airway, abnormality of surfactants, loss of lung volume atelectasis, secondary bacterial infection (pneumonia). Increased work of breathing. Pain-induced decreased lung volumes.

▶ Treatment Steps
1. Deep breathing or coughing exercises, ambulation, bronchodilator therapy, physical therapy for the chest, intermittent positive-pressure breathing, antibiotics, bronchoscopy, nasotracheal suctioning.
2. Pain control is mandatory.

## VII. DISEASES OF THE CIRCULATORY SYSTEM

### A. Carotid Artery Disease

▶ H&P Keys

*Definitions*—Transient ischemic attacks (TIA): brief paresis or numbness of an arm or leg contralateral to the affected carotid territory—< 24 hours. Resolving ischemic neurologic deficits (RIND): deficit of the contralateral carotid territory > 24 hours, but that resolves within 7 days. Amaurosis fugax (AF): transient episode of monocular or partial blindness. Stroke: permanent neurologic deficit.

*Symptoms*—Many patients have significant disease without exhibiting symptoms. Symptomatic patients experience TIAs, blindness, or resolving or permanent neurologic deficit. Unstable symptoms may result from crescendo TIAs, stroke in evolution, or waxing and waning neurologic deficits.

Vertebral–basilar artery symptoms result from ischemia to the cerebellum and brain stem and consist of vertigo, drop attacks, dizziness, and clumsiness.

*Signs*—Carotid bruits, presence of Hollenhorst plaques (nonspecific). Significant disease, including occlusions of the internal carotid artery, high-grade stenosis, and ulceration without stenosis, can exist without signs.

▶ Diagnosis

*Noninvasive Testing*—Duplex ultrasound for initial investigation; 95% accurate and 90% sensitive.

*Arteriography*—The gold standard for analyzing cerebral vascular disease (Fig. 18–2). Not obtained unless operative intervention is contemplated. Not obtained in all patients and is still used selectively.

*Magnetic Resonance Angiography (MRA)*—Also done to evaluate carotid vascular disease, particularly in patients with renal insufficiency, as well as the intracranial segments and three-dimensional reconstruction.

▶ Disease Severity

Patients with symptoms and a stenosis of ≥ 70% of the internal carotid arteries benefit from endarterectomy. Asymptomatic patients with ≥ 60% stenosis benefit from prophylactic carotid endarterectomy.

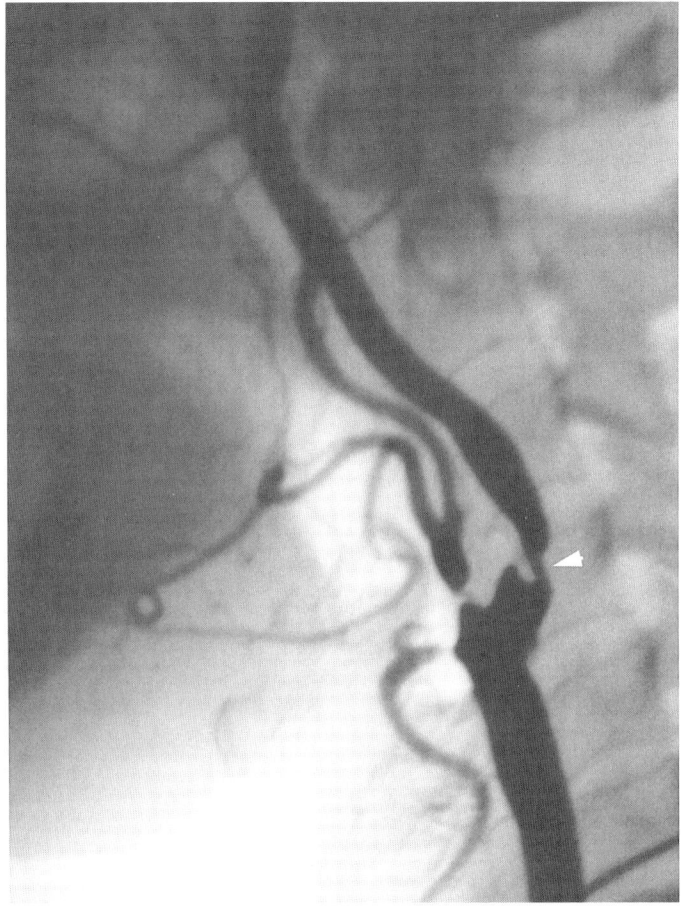

Figure 18-2. Carotid angiogram showing a high-grade stenosis of the origin of the internal (arrow) as well as the external carotid artery. This study is currently reserved for recurrent carotid artery stenosis (atherosclerotic or radiation therapy related), high carotid bifurcation, stenotic "string sign" lesion of the internal carotid artery, or if the patient is being considered for carotid angioplasty and stenting.

▶ Concept and Application

Ulceration of atherosclerotic plaque results in the release of microemboli (usually platelets), resulting in ischemia and infarct of cerebral parenchyma.

▶ Treatment Steps
1. Medical therapy is indicated for patients with stenosis < 60% whether symptomatic or asymptomatic (acetylsalicylic acid, Plavix).
2. Surgery is beneficial for symptomatic patients with stenosis of 70% or more, asymptomatic ≥ 60% stenosis.
3. Accepted combined morbidity and mortality of carotid endarterectomy is 2% to 4%.
4. Carotid stenting is new alternative (controversial).

   *Indications for Operation*—TIA, resolution of stroke, symptoms, high-grade stenosis.

   *Contraindication to Operation*—Fixed dense stroke, total occlusion of carotid.

## B. Renovascular Disease

▶ H&P Keys

Two percent to 7% of patients with hypertension have renovascular disease. In more than three quarters of these, renal artery lesions are secondary to atherosclerosis. The second most common cause is fibrodysplasia. Family history of hypertension early onset, accelerated hypertension, resistance to antihypertensive drugs, deterioration of renal function, upper abdominal bruit are all signs of renovascular hypertension. Worsening renal function with start of angiotensin-converting enzyme (ACE) inhibitor is a telltale sign.

▶ Diagnosis

*Renal Vein Renins*—Ratio of renin from involved compared to uninvolved kidney is > 1.5.

*Renal Arteriography*—For deteriorating renal function or persistent diastolic hypertension > 110 mm Hg.

▶ Disease Severity

Surgery is effective in 90% of patients with fibromuscular dysplasia, and in 60% with atherosclerotic disease. Factors suggesting potential renal salvage include urographic visualization of the kidney, renal length of ≥ 9 cm, retrograde filling of the distal arterial tree, lateralizing renal vein renins. Generally, angioplasty for FMD lesions and bypass for atherosclerotic lesions (in a low-risk patient).

▶ Concept and Application

Unilateral renal artery stenosis leads to release of renin. Increased renin causes an increase of angiotensin I and, subsequently, of angiotensin II with vasoconstriction and sodium retention.

▶ Treatment Steps

*Medical*—Attempt to control hypertension with antihypertensive drugs, especially β-blockers.

*Surgical*
1. Percutaneous arterial dilatation (with or without stenting) is most successful in fibromuscular dysplasia. Focal lesions more amenable to interventions.
2. Aortorenal, hepatorenal, splenorenal, or iliorenal bypass.
3. Endarterectomy or reimplantation also may be used for atherosclerotic lesions.

## C. Peripheral Arterial Occlusive Disease

▶ H&P Keys

*Definitions*—*Claudication* is a deep ache or cramping (most commonly in the calf) secondary to muscle ischemia during exercise. *Rest pain* is a burning pain usually confined to the forefoot and is indicative of severe disease. *Tissue loss* is necrosis secondary to inadequate blood flow, or inadequate perfusion for healing an open wound. *Distal aortic occlusion (Leriche's syn-*

*drome*) is characterized by claudication of the hip, thigh, and buttock muscles; atrophy of the leg; impotence, and diminished or absent femoral pulses.

*Risk Factors*—Smoking, hypertension, diabetes, hyperlipidemia, history of myocardial infarction or stroke, family history of atherosclerotic cardiovascular disease.

▶ Diagnosis

*Physical Examination*—Diminished or absent pulses distal to the point of stenosis. Bruits, pallor on elevation, rubor with dependency, temperature change, loss of hair.

*Arterial Pressure Ankle–Brachial Index (ABI)*—Normal 1.0–1.2, abnormal < 0.95, claudication ≤ 0.8, rest pain ≤ 0.4, tissue loss, ≤ 0.5.

*Noninvasive Vascular Tests*—Segmental pressure measurements with segmental pulse volume recordings or Doppler waveforms, and arterial duplex ultrasound.

*Imaging Studies*—Invasive studies reserved for preoperative patients. Arteriography defines the site and severity of arterial obstruction and delineates proximal and distal arterial anatomy. Complications include hematoma, arteriovenous fistula, false aneurysm, distal embolization of clot, or atheromatous plaque. MRA provides arterial anatomy without the risks of contrast agents, but may overestimate stenosis.

▶ Disease Severity

Heart disease, previous amputations, small-vessel disease (limits revascularization attempts).

▶ Concept and Application

Atherosclerotic narrowing (stenosis), distal loss of vasomotor tone and vasodilation. Capillary dilatation produces a purple rubor, characteristic of disease progression.

▶ Treatment Steps

*Medical*
1. Reduction of risk factors, improvement of collateral circulation, avoidance of foot trauma, exercise program.
2. Antiplatelet and vasodilatory agents.

*Surgical*
1. For incapacitating claudication or limb salvage (rest pain, tissue loss with inadequate perfusion for healing).
2. Aortoiliac or aortofemoral reconstruction: patency is 80% at 5 years; operative mortality is 5%. For patients with poor cardiopulmonary reserve, an extra-anatomic bypass (femorofemoral, iliofemoral, or axillobifemoral) can be used. Iliac angioplasty with or without stenting also has good results.
3. Femoropopliteal reconstruction is indicated in claudication and in patients with rest pain and tissue loss. The optimal graft is autogenous greater saphenous vein; other alter-

natives include polytetrafluoroethylene (PTFE), alternate site vein, and composite grafts. Reconstructions to the tibial, peroneal, or pedal arteries is mostly indicated for limb salvage.

4. Infrainguinal angioplasty and stenting also are treatment options.

### D. Aneurysms of the Thoracic Aorta

▶ H&P Keys

Majority are asymptomatic chest pain and pressure are main symptoms; also, hoarseness, superior vena caval syndrome, and cough and dyspnea from tracheobronchial obstruction. Hemoptysis is indicative of erosion into the trachea and main-stem bronchus.

▶ Diagnosis

Plain x-ray of specific location; involvement of surrounding structure requires angiography. CT scan and MRI are helpful. Echocardiography and anteriography may be diagnostic. Transesophageal echo is a sensitive diagnostic method.

▶ Disease Severity

*Ascending Aortic*—Excellent surgical results—mortality < 10%.

*Aortic Arch*—Reimplantation of brachiocephalic vessels. Mortality rate, 10–15%; neurologic complications, 10%.

*Descending Aortic*—Mortality, 10%; paraplegia, 5–30%.

▶ Concept and Application

*Etiology*—Atherosclerosis, cystic medial degeneration, myxomatous degeneration, dissection, infection, trauma, and poststenotic dilatation. Syphilitic aortitis is rare. Incidence of aneurysm increases with age. Rupture is the most common cause of death.

▶ Treatment Steps

1. Aneurysms > 6 cm should be resected even if asymptomatic.
2. Documented enlargement is indication for surgery.

*Ascending Aortic*—Replacement with Dacron graft, and repair of aortic valve, if necessary.

*Aortic Arch*

1. Reconstruction with Dacron graft.
2. Deep hypothermic circulatory arrest on cardiopulmonary bypass.

*Descending Aortic*

1. Replacement with Dacron graft.
2. Partial bypass used in attempt to lower complications of paralysis and organ failure.

## E. Aortic Dissection

### ► H&P Keys

Pain is severe and of sudden onset, and may radiate to the back, abdomen, and extremities. Patients may have neurologic deficit, dyspnea, pulmonary edema, nausea, and vomiting. Three times more frequent in males; frequent between the ages of 45 and 70 years. Hypertensive history in 80–90% of patients. Shock, pulmonary edema, and a murmur of aortic insufficiency may be noted. Blood pressure difference between contralateral extremities; unequal pulses.

*Differential Diagnosis*—Myocardial infarction, cerebrovascular accident, pulmonary embolism, aortic thrombosis, and acute abdominal disorders.

### ► Diagnosis

CXR may show a dilated aorta, widened mediastinum, pulmonary edema, or mass effect with or without pleural effusion (rupture). CT (Fig. 18–3A), MRI, and transesophageal echocardiogram. Aortogram is test of choice; usually shows splitting of contrast column (Fig. 18–3B), distortion of column, or aortic insufficiency.

### ► Disease Severity

Dissections classified as ascending (involve the entire aorta in 90% of the cases) or descending (involve the aorta distal to the left subclavian artery). May be managed medically or require immediate surgical intervention. Mortality rate is 10%, dependent on the location and status of the dissection.

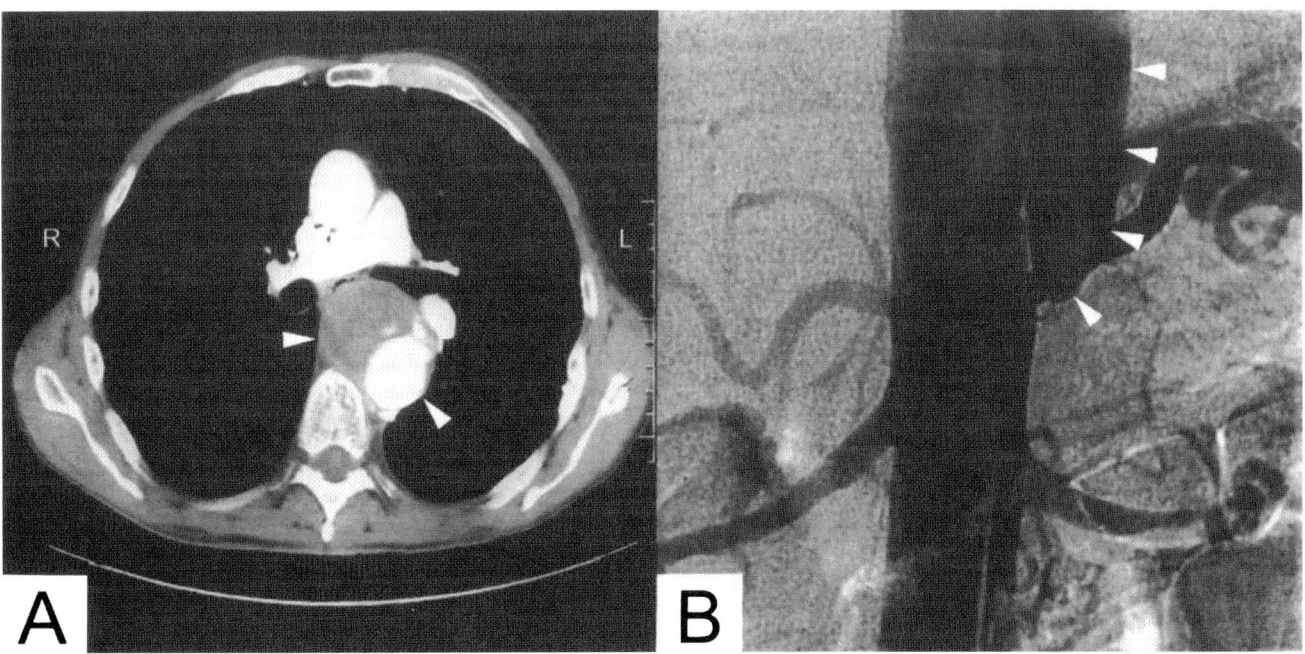

Figure 18-3. Dissecting thoracoabdominal aneurysm in a 70-year-old man with history of hypertension. **A.** Contrasted computed tomography (CT) scan of descending thoracic aorta showing dilatation (arrowheads), double lumen, and mural thrombus. **B.** Aortogram demonstrating true and false lumina, separated by a septum. The dissection column (*arrowheads*) extends to the suprarenal portion of the aorta. (Courtesy of Dr. Oswaldo Yano, Mount Sinai School of Medicine, New York, NY)

▶ Concept and Application

Degeneration of medial layer can be caused by hypertension, atherosclerosis, coarctation, endocrine factors, Marfan's syndrome, trauma, and pregnancy-induced hypertension. Hemodynamic forces, shear stress, and weakened arterial wall lead to the development of an intimal tear. A hematoma forms within the torn aorta and dissects distally as well as proximally within the media.

▶ Treatment Steps

*Ascending Dissections*
1. Should be managed surgically.
2. Approach through median sternotomy with cardiopulmonary bypass.

*Immediate Operation*—Free rupture, aortic insufficiency, pericardial tamponade.

*Descending Dissections*
1. Control blood pressure with nitroprusside.
2. Propranolol and Methyldopa administered after stabilization.
3. One third of patients require surgery for enlarging aneurysm.
4. Immediate surgery indicated for failure to control hypertension, expansion of the aneurysm, rupture into the pleural space, development of a neurologic deficit, or visceral or lower extremity ischemia.

## F. Abdominal Aortic Aneurysmal Disease

▶ H&P Keys

Most patients are asymptomatic; some may be aware of a pulsatile abdominal mass. Sudden onset of severe abdominal pain radiating to the back and associated with hypotension indicative of ruptured aneurysm. On physical examination, palpable mass in the supraumbilical area. In obese patients or those with tortuous aortas, physical examination may disclose no abnormalities. Abdominal bruit may be present.

▶ Diagnosis

Ultrasound to assess size of aneurysm (least expensive, least invasive, most rapid diagnosis). Plain x-rays to detect calcification of the aneurysmal wall, if present (suggestive, not diagnostic). CT scan to assess size of aneurysm as well as extent above and below the renal and iliac vessels (Fig. 18–4). Aortography preoperatively to determine suprarenal involvement, suspected renovascular disease, visceral arterial involvement, possible distal occlusive or aneurysmal disease.

▶ Disease Severity

Risk of rupture increases with increasing diameter. Majority of aneurysms continue to enlarge. Twenty percent of aneurysms $\leq 6$ cm rupture, compared with 40% of aneurysms $> 6$ cm. Coexistent coronary and carotid atherosclerotic disease common.

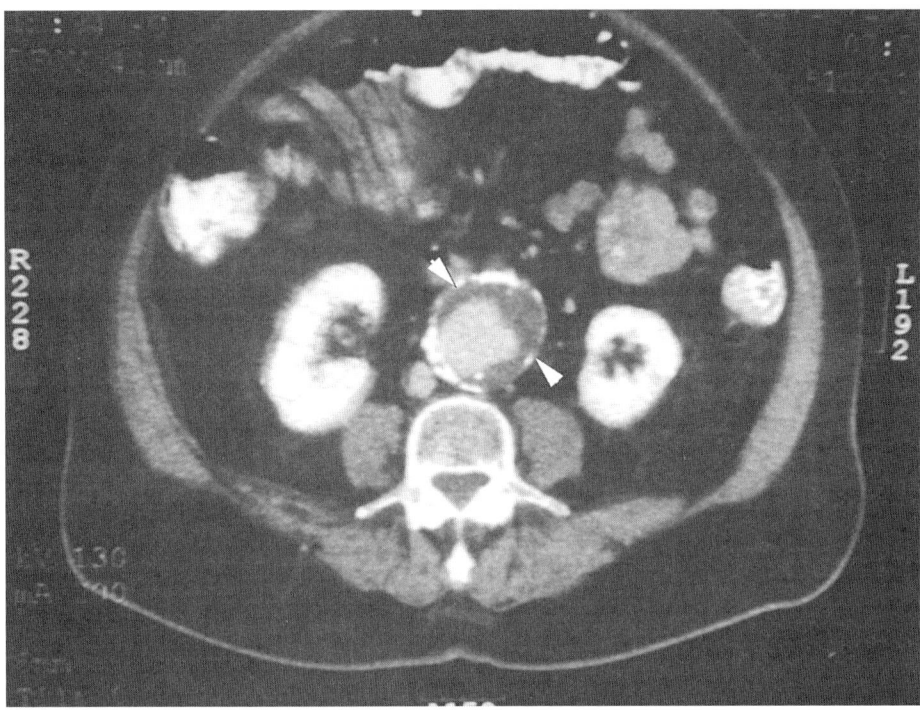

Figure 18–4. Abdominal CT scan with intravenous contrast showing an abdominal aortic aneurysm (arrows). Note the white inner lumen surrounded with a darker mural thrombus and an outer white ring of calcification around the aneurysm.

▶ Concept and Application

Aneurysmal dilatation secondary to atherosclerotic changes. Inability to withstand increased wall tension secondary to damage of elastic fibers of media. Hereditary deficiency of collagen cross-linking or abnormal copper metabolism.

▶ Treatment Steps
1. Recommend repair of all aneurysms ≥ 5 cm in diameter.
2. Aortic replacement with PTFE or Dacron grafts.
3. Complications of surgery include renal failure, myocardial infarction, stroke, graft infection, limb loss, bowel ischemia, impotence.

### G. Thoracic Outlet Syndrome (TOS)

▶ H&P Keys

History of clavicle or rib trauma or fracture, exercise or occupational injury, poor posture. Must rule out cervical disk disease and carpal tunnel syndrome. Symptoms of thoracic outlet syndrome dependent on compression of brachial plexus, axillary or subclavian artery or vein. Neurologic symptoms include weakness, paresthesia, pain, and numbness, usually in the fingers and hands with ulnar distribution. Late manifestations include motor weakness, atrophy, and sensory loss. Symptoms of arterial compression include ischemic pain, numbness, fatigue, paresthesia, coldness, and weakness in the hand or arm. Symptoms are intensified by exercise. Arterial embolization or thrombosis may occur. Symptoms of vein compression are edema of arm, pain, and cyanosis. Arterial signs include absent or weak brachial and radial pulses, delayed capillary refill, distal gangrene. Venous signs include distention of veins of chest, arm, or hand; edema; cyanosis.

▶ Diagnosis

*Adson Maneuver*—While palpating pulse, ask patient to inhale deeply and turn head to examine side with neck extended. Positive if bruit is heard or pulse lost. Costoclavicular compression maneuver, hyperabduction maneuver, elevated-arm stress test. Diagnostic studies include plain x-rays to assess cervical ribs, abnormal first ribs, prominent transverse processes, abnormalities of the clavicle; plethysmography to demonstrate obstruction to arterial flow; phlebograms to demonstrate compression or obstruction of the axillary or subclavian veins; arteriograms to show partial or complete arterial occlusion. Electromyography may detect compression of peripheral nerves (conduction delay). Somatosensory evoked potentials may provide objective evidence of nerve dysfunction. Duplex also can be useful to evaluate arterial and venous anatomy.

▶ Disease Severity

*Three Basic Types of TOS*—Neurogenic (95%); venous (2%); and arterial (1%).

▶ Concept and Application

Compression areas include interscalene triangle, scalenus anticus space (between the first rib and clavicle), costocoracoid fascia, and pectoralis minor tendon. In addition, compression may be associated with cervical ribs, long transverse process of C7, scalene muscle fiber variants with degenerative changes and increased intramuscular fibrosis.

▶ Treatment Steps

1. Intensive physical therapy if no evidence of vascular occlusion, distal embolization, or poststenotic aneurysm.
2. Surgical treatment can be resection of the first rib, anterior scalenectomy, middle scalenectomy; removal of a cervical rib if present.
3. Improvement noted in 60–75%, no change in symptoms in 10–15%, and deterioration in 5–10%.

### H. Infrainguinal Aneurysmal Disease

▶ H&P Keys

Femoral and popliteal aneurysms are often asymptomatic. They may appear as a groin or popliteal mass. Ischemia of foot and toes can precipitate symptoms. Fifty percent of popliteal and 74% of femoral arterial aneurysms are bilateral. Thirty percent of patients with popliteal aneurysms have abdominal aortic aneurysms, and 85% of patients with femoral aneurysms have other associated aneurysms.

▶ **Diagnosis**

Ultrasound delineates size of the aneurysm. Angiography is indicated in all patients in whom surgical correction is considered. Because of the high incidence of coexistent aortic, iliac, and femoral aneurysms, evaluation must include assessment of the entire arterial tree.

▶ **Disease Severity**

Immediate treatment indicated when acute thrombosis causes ischemia. Early surgery indicated for recurrent embolization. Asymptomatic aneurysms also should be repaired.

▶ **Concept and Application**

Cause can be atherosclerosis, previous surgery, trauma (blunt or penetrating); infection, especially associated with femoral aneurysm from IV drug abuse; and associated with femoral catheterization or angiography.

▶ **Treatment Steps**

*Femoral Artery Aneurysm*
1. Excision and replacement.
2. Preferable to use autologous artery or vein, but prosthetic material can be used.

*Popliteal Artery Aneurysm*—Proximal and distal ligation of native popliteal artery, with bypass using autogenous saphenous vein.

## I. Arterial Embolism/Thrombosis

▶ **H&P Keys**

*Acute Occlusion*—Six Ps—pulselessness, pallor, paresthesia, pain, paralysis, and poikilothermia. Irreversible limb loss may occur within 6–8 hours. Previous history of claudication and physical findings of vascular disease may be absent. Normal pulses in the unaffected extremity.

▶ **Diagnosis**

Clinical assessment includes echocardiography because cardiac system is most common source of emboli. Noninvasive vascular evaluation with ABI. Arteriogram used if diagnosis is in question and no immediate threat to limb viability.

▶ **Disease Severity**

Embolism usually secondary to cardiac source. Therapy initiated (ie, atrial fibrillation, myocardial infarction, congestive heart failure). Severity depends on degree of medical comorbidities.

▶ **Concept and Application**

Embolic occlusion is more common than thrombotic. Thrombosis generally occurs in area of atherosclerotic disease. Compromise of oxygenation leads to anaerobic metabolism, acidosis, membrane destabilization, and cellular edema and death.

► Treatment Steps
1. Heparinization.
2. Embolectomy.
3. Thrombolytic agents (urokinase, streptokinase) are used when thrombus has progressed into small vessels.
4. Fasciotomy is recommended with prolonged ischemia or excessive swelling.
5. Maintenance of urine output and alkalinization recommended to prevent renal injury.

### J. Deep Venous Thrombosis (DVT)

► H&P Keys

Patient can be asymptomatic or exhibit the classic findings of calf swelling and tenderness, elevated temperature, and a Homan's sign (leg pain on dorsiflexion of the foot). Phlegmasia cerulea dolens may occur when there is complete iliofemoral venous occlusion, with massive swelling, pain, and cyanosis of the leg, which may progress to venous gangrene. Symptoms are unilateral; patient often gives a history of previous DVT or superficial thrombophlebitis. Others at risk: post-trauma, immobilization, cancer, and post-surgery.

► Diagnosis

Clinical findings on examination are incorrect in approximately 50% of the patients. Doppler ultrasound is accurate 80–85% of the time. Duplex ultrasound can be used to assess for thrombosis. Sensitivity and specificity for above-the-knee thrombi is 90–100%. Duplex scan has become the standard test for diagnosis. Venograms are still used and accepted as the gold standard.

► Concept and Application

Thrombosis is related to three factors—endothelial abnormalities, blood stasis, and hypercoagulability (Virchow's triad). Platelet aggregation and procoagulants compromise the venous endothelium and result in a hypercoagulable state.

► Treatment Steps
1. Prevention is the best management. Attempts to overcome venous stasis include exercise, leg elevation, elastic or pneumatic stockings, and early ambulation after surgery.
2. Bed rest with leg elevation reduces the edema associated with DVT.
3. Drug therapy consists of IV unfractionated heparin to prevent propagation of the thrombus and pulmonary embolus. The partial thromboplastin time should be extended to 1.5 times the normal value. LMWH (low-molecular-weight heparin) is an alternative. Warfarin therapy is then initiated, and continued for 3–6 months.
4. Vena cava filter placement is indicated when anticoagulation is contraindicated, or patient has pulmonary embolism or recurrent DVT on adequate anticoagulation, multiple small emboli creating chronic pulmonary insufficiency, septic emboli refractory to treatment, or has undergone a pulmonary embolectomy.

5. Thrombolytic therapy also is used in cases of iliofemoral DVT to abate the late sequelae of venous thrombosis, namely valvular incompetence, and development of chronic venous insufficiency.
6. Rarely, surgical thrombectomy or a bypass is performed.

## K. Varicose Veins

▶ H&P Keys

It is estimated that 10–20% of the population has some difficulty with varicose veins. Patients may have no symptoms or may complain of aching, swelling, heaviness, cramps, itching, and disfigurement. Dry, scaling skin; edema and brawny induration; and, occasionally, hemorrhage may be noted. Physical examination shows dilated, tortuous, subcutaneous veins of the thigh and leg (often involving the greater and lesser saphenous systems). Pitting edema of the ankles and legs, as well as brawny discoloration of the medial lower leg, is noted.

▶ Diagnosis

Valvular competence of the deep, superficial, and perforating veins between deep and superficial systems must be determined. The Brodie–Trendelenburg test should be used to determine competence of valves in the greater saphenous vein and perforating veins, duplex ultrasound and venous refill times.

▶ Concept and Application

Fundamental abnormality is sequential incompetence of the valves. Secondary varicosities result from obstruction of deep veins.

▶ Treatment Steps

1. Nonoperative management consists of improving venous return and reducing venous pressure by elevation and graduated elastic stockings.
2. Surgical therapy is indicated for severe symptoms, large varicosities, attacks of superficial phlebitis, hemorrhage from a ruptured varix, or ulceration from venous stasis or for cosmetic reasons.
3. Sclerotherapy is used for small and "spider" varicosities.

## L. Superficial Thrombophlebitis

▶ H&P Keys

History of IV catheters or drug abuse. Lower extremity thrombophlebitis is associated with varicose veins, thromboangiitis obliterans, or cellulitis. Cancer may cause recurrent or migratory superficial thrombophlebitis (Trousseau's sign). Signs include erythema, pain, induration, heat, tenderness along the course of a superficial vein, fever, and leukocytosis.

▶ Diagnosis

History and physical examination.

▶ Disease Severity
Disease usually is self-limited, with a short and uncomplicated time course. Recurrent superficial phlebitis is an indication for venous stripping.

▶ Concept and Application
Introduction of bacteria with either IV catheters or IV drug abuse. Local infection and inflammatory response result in thrombosis.

▶ Treatment Steps
1. Conservative measures include analgesia, nonsteroidal anti-inflammatory agents, local heat, and elastic compression bandages.
2. If inflammation of saphenous vein involves the saphenofemoral junction, pulmonary embolism may result, and ligation of the greater saphenous vein or anticoagulation is indicated.
3. In cases of suppuration, surgical excision of involved vein is indicated.

## VIII. DISEASES OF THE GASTROINTESTINAL TRACT

### A. Zenker's Diverticulum

▶ H&P Keys
Dysphagia, regurgitation of undigested food, coughing, mass on the left side of the neck, foul breath.

▶ Diagnosis
Barium swallow.

▶ Disease Severity
Pulmonary complications, poor nutrition, weight loss, size of pouch, presence of carcinoma is rare. This is the most common esophageal diverticulum.

▶ Concept and Application
Incoordination of the cricopharyngeal muscle at its junction with the thyropharyngeus causing a posterior pharyngeal mucosal herniation.

▶ Treatment Steps
1. Pulmonary care.
2. Diverticulectomy, cricopharyngeal myotomy.

### B. Midesophageal Traction Diverticulum

▶ H&P Keys
Often associated with mediastinal granulomatous disease. Most commonly asymptomatic and incidentally discovered.

▶ Diagnosis
Barium esophagogram.

▶ Disease Severity
Only dependent on associated symptoms.

▶ Concept and Application
Mediastinal adenopathy from tuberculosis (TB) or histoplasmosis adheres to the esophagus, "dragging" its wall and creating a diverticulum.

▶ Treatment Signs
Only in symptomatic patients is excision indicated. This is a true diverticulum.

## C. Achalasia

▶ H&P Keys
Dysphagia, regurgitation of undigested food, weight loss, dyspnea, cough.

▶ Diagnosis
Barium esophagogram ("bird's beak"), panendoscopy, esophagomanometry.

▶ Disease Severity
Aspiration, pneumonia, old age, recurrent dysphagia. Increased risk for squamous cell carcinoma.

▶ Concept and Application
Dilatation, absent esophageal peristalsis, and incomplete relaxation of lower esophageal sphincter, hypertensive lower esophageal sphincter, decreased ganglion cells in Auerbach's plexus.

▶ Treatment Steps

*Medical*—Calcium channel blockers, esophageal balloon dilatation.

*Surgical*—Distal esophagomyotomy (Hellar myotomy) and antireflux procedure (laparoscopic or open).

## D. Esophageal Varices

▶ H&P Keys
Asymptomatic, or hematemesis, melena, signs of liver failure (ascites, encephalopathy, clonus, gastrointestinal bleeding, caput medusa, jaundice, hepatomegaly, palmar erythema, cachexia). Patient with history of alcohol abuse.

▶ Diagnosis
Esophagogram and esophagogastroduodenoscopy.

▶ Disease Severity
Recurrent bleeding. Child's classification, ascites, encephalopathy, nutritional status, degree of coagulopathy.

▶ Concept and Application
Significant elevation of portal pressures. Majority of patients have cirrhosis or had extrahepatic portal obstruction in childhood.

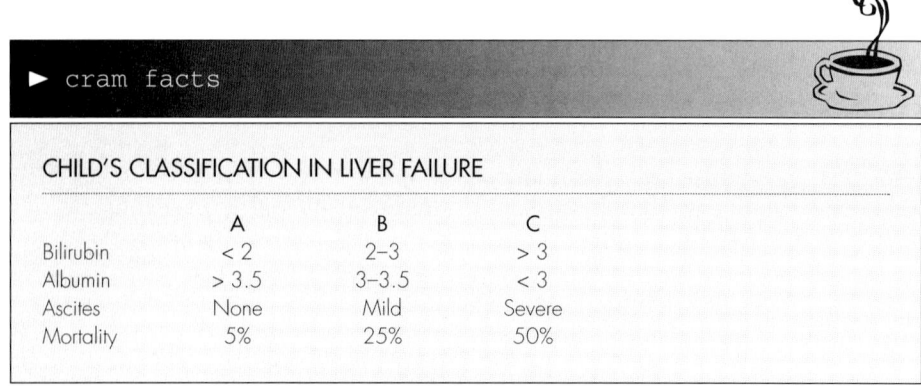

### cram facts

**CHILD'S CLASSIFICATION IN LIVER FAILURE**

|  | A | B | C |
|---|---|---|---|
| Bilirubin | < 2 | 2–3 | > 3 |
| Albumin | > 3.5 | 3–3.5 | < 3 |
| Ascites | None | Mild | Severe |
| Mortality | 5% | 25% | 50% |

▶ Treatment Steps
1. If bleeding is acute, fluid resuscitation, vasopressin, β-blockers, sclerotherapy, balloon tamponade, endoscopic banding.
2. Transjugular intrahepatic portosystemic shunts (TIPS).
3. Portosystemic shunt used most commonly in an urgent or elective status to relieve portal hypertension.

### E. Cancer of the Stomach

▶ H&P Keys

Anorexia, epigastric pain, weight loss, dysphagia (esophagogastric junction), vomiting, hematemesis, epigastric mass, ascites, hepatomegaly, anemia.

▶ Diagnosis

Barium meal, CT scan of abdomen, gastroscopy, fecal occult blood.

▶ Disease Severity

Weight loss, tumor histology, depth of invasion, cachexia, ascites, abdominal pain, peritonitis secondary to perforation, degree of local extension, associated adenopathy, and previous gastric surgery.

▶ Concept and Application

Malignant changes of the gastric epithelium. Premalignant conditions are atrophic gastritis, intestinal metaplasia, dysplastic gastric polyp, and pernicious anemia.

▶ Treatment Steps
1. Radical gastric resection.
2. Chemotherapy.

### F. Gastric Volvulus

▶ H&P Keys

Retching, inability to vomit; epigastric distention; inability to pass nasogastric tube; chronic crampy abdominal pain.

▶ Diagnosis

Upper gastrointestinal (UGI) series, endoscopy.

▶ Disease Severity

Duration of symptoms, perforation or gangrene of stomach or shock.

▶ Concept and Application

Presence of paraesophageal hiatus hernia. Eventration of left hemidiaphragm, rotation around the longitudinal axis (organo-axial volvulus), or mesenteric axial volvulus.

▶ Treatment Steps

*Acute*—IV fluids, antibiotics, derotation, anterior gastropexy, and gastrostomy.

*Chronic*—Anterior gastropexy and antireflux procedure (open or laparoscopic).

## G. Appendicitis

▶ H&P Keys

Periumbilical pain shifting to right lower quadrant, anorexia, nausea and vomiting, low-grade fever, tender right lower quadrant, tender on rectal examination.

▶ Diagnosis

History and physical, leukocytosis, ultrasound (especially in children). Fecalith, ileus, mass effect on plain x-rays, CT scan with oral or rectal contrast.

▶ Disease Severity

Marked leukocytosis, high fever, peritonitis, elderly, pregnancy, morbidity from delayed diagnosis. Perforation and abscess.

▶ Concept and Application

Obstruction of appendix lumen and bacterial invasion.

▶ Treatment Steps

1. Fluid resuscitation, antibiotics.
2. Appendectomy (open or laparoscopic).

## H. Ulcerative Colitis

▶ H&P Keys

Abdominal cramps, tenesmus, bloody diarrhea, weight loss, abdominal tenderness, fever.

▶ Diagnosis

Colonoscopy, barium enema; rectum always involved.

▶ Disease Severity

Dehydration, malnutrition, cecal perforation, massive lower GI bleeding, frequent relapses, systemic manifestations, total colonic involvement, failure of medical treatment. Increased risk of colon carcinoma.

▶ Concept and Application

Immunologic injury to colon mucosa, defect of suppressor T cells in gut wall. Possible infectious cause.

▶ Treatment Steps

*Acute*
1. Bed rest, sulfasalazine, steroids, nothing by mouth.
2. Total parenteral nutrition.
3. Subtotal colectomy and ileostomy (if fails medical management, persistent gastrointestinal bleeding, or toxic megacolon).

*Chronic* — Sulfasalazine, steroids, immunosuppressive agents, proctocolectomy with ileoanal pull-through and J-pouch.

### I. Crohn's Disease

▶ H&P Keys

Recurrent, crampy abdominal pain, diarrhea, perianal fistula and abscess, extraintestinal manifestations, abdominal mass, rectal bleeding less common than with ulcerative colitis.

▶ Diagnosis

Small-bowel series, colonoscopy, barium enema.

▶ Disease Severity

Severe anal disease, extraintestinal manifestations, malnutrition, abdominal mass, intra-abdominal abscesses, failure of medical treatment, amount of small bowel and colon involved.

▶ Concept and Application

Possible immunologic mechanism that leads to inflammatory reaction and damage transmural.

▶ Treatment Steps

*Medical*
1. Bed rest.
2. Low-residue, high-protein diet.
3. Sulfasalazine, metronidazole, aminosalicylates delivered orally or rectally.
4. 6-Mercaptopurine and cyclosporin in refractory cases.

*Surgical*
1. Small-bowel resection, segmental colectomy, stricturoplasty.
2. Surgery is indicated only for complications (obstruction, perforation, bleeding, failure of medical therapy, malignancy).
3. Unlike ulcerative colitis, surgery is not definitive treatment.

### J. Acute Mesenteric Ischemia

▶ H&P Keys

Abdominal pain, rectal bleeding, atrial fibrillation, minimal abdominal findings (pain out of proportion to physical findings). Abdominal pain in the setting of low cardiac output.

▶ Diagnosis

Elevated white blood cell (WBC) count, ABG, lactic acid, angiography (definitive).

▶ Disease Severity

Fever, abdominal tenderness, guarding, hypotension, leukocytosis, base deficit, elevated lactic acid, disseminated intravascular coagulation, pulmonary dysfunction, diffuse peritonitis, associated cardiac comorbidity.

▶ Concept and Application

Embolic and thrombotic occlusion of mesentery vessels, severe splanchnic vasoconstriction, low-flow state, or mesenteric vein thrombosis (Fig. 18–5).

▶ Treatment Steps
1. IV fluids, antibiotics, thromboembolectomy, bowel resection, anticoagulation, intra-arterial papaverine.
2. Treatment of cardiac etiologic findings with arrhythmia control.
3. Long-term anticoagulation.

## K. Small-bowel Obstruction

▶ H&P Keys

Colicky abdominal pain, vomiting, failure to pass flatus or feces; abdominal distention, visible peristalsis, high-pitched bowel sounds, dehydration, previous surgery.

▶ Diagnosis

Plain abdominal x-rays (distended small bowel with air-fluid levels) (Fig. 18–6), barium small-bowel follow through, CT scan (can determine the site and degree of obstruction).

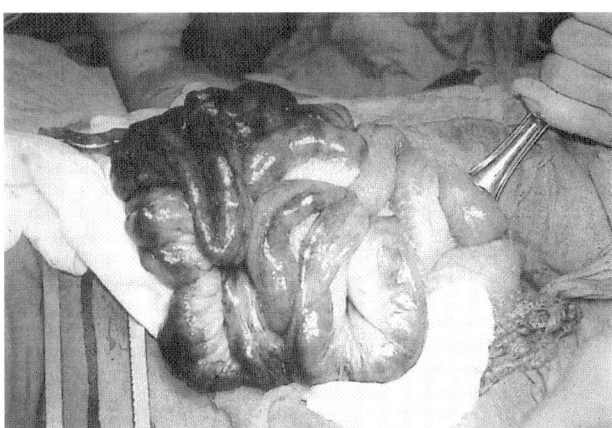

Figure 18–5. Acute mesenteric ischemia in a 74-year-old man with history of atrial fibrillation and heart failure, who developed acute abdominal pain and shock. Exploratory laparotomy disclosed extensive areas of intestinal necrosis and embolic occlusion of the superior mesenteric artery.

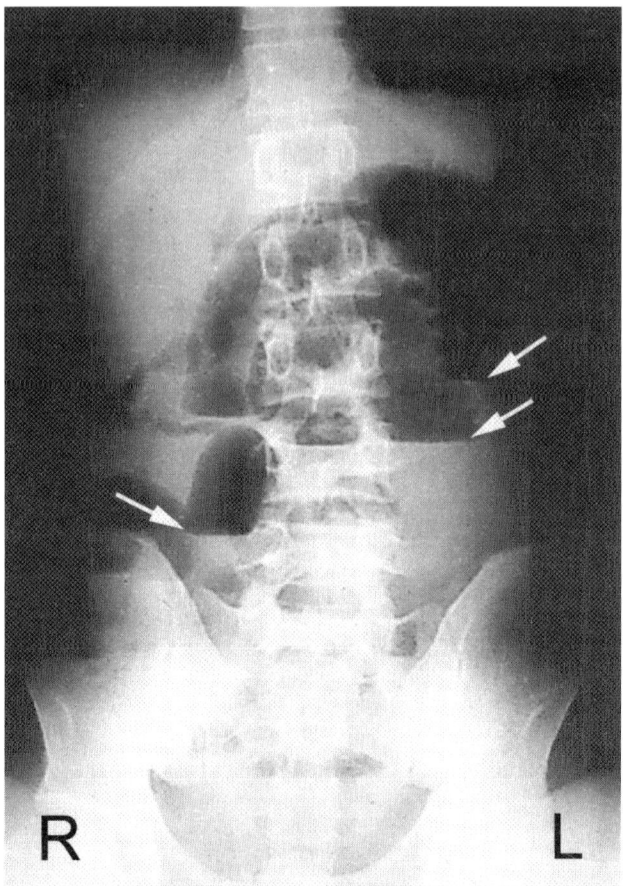

Figure 18–6. Upright abdominal x-ray showing small-bowel obstruction secondary to Crohn's disease. Note distended loops of small-bowel and multiple air–fluid levels (arrows).

▶ Disease Severity

Poor urine output, leukocytosis, unremitting pain, high fever, peritonitis.

▶ Concept and Application

Narrowing or occlusion of bowel lumen, proximal bowel distention with gas and fluid. Distension leads to increased intestinal wall pressure, ischemia, and gangrene. Adhesions, hernia, and tumor are the most common causes.

▶ Treatment Steps
1. Fluid and electrolyte resuscitation, nasogastric decompression, monitor urine output.
2. Laparotomy, with correction of cause with or without bowel resection.

## L. Large-bowel Obstruction

▶ H&P Keys

Crampy abdominal pain, nausea, vomiting, and obstipation; abdominal distention; visible peristalsis; high-pitched, frequent bowel sounds; abdominal tenderness; palpable mass; cachexia.

▶ Diagnosis

Plain x-ray of abdomen, Gastrografin enema, colonoscopy. Rule out volvulus.

▶ Disease Severity

Poor urine output, leukocytosis, high fever, obstructing tumor, peritonitis.

▶ Concept and Application

Narrowing or occlusion of bowel lumen, or volvulus, with proximal bowel distention with gas and fluid; gangrenous bowel resulting from vascular compromise.

▶ Treatment Steps

*Medical*
1. Fluid and electrolyte resuscitation, nasogastric decompression, monitoring urine output.
2. Endoscopic decompression (volvulus, partially obstructing lesion).

*Surgical*
1. Decompression (colostomy or cecostomy).
2. Colectomy with colostomy or primary anastomosis.

## M. Diverticulitis

▶ H&P Keys

Abdominal pain, left lower quadrant tenderness, constipation, low-grade fever, mild abdominal distention, mucus per rectum. History of constipation.

▶ Diagnosis

CT scan of the abdomen and pelvis, colonoscopy is rarely needed in the acute setting.

▶ Disease Severity

High WBC count, perforation, abscess formation, fecal peritonitis, septic shock.

▶ Concept and Application

Raised intracolonic pressure leading to pulsion diverticulum; entrapped fecalith causes obstruction of the diverticulum and resulting inflammation with potential perforation.

▶ Treatment Steps

*Medical*—Systemic antibiotics, fluid–electrolyte resuscitation, bowel rest.

*Surgical*
1. Drainage of abscess.
2. Colectomy (Hartman's procedure).
3. Colectomy with primary anastomosis done less frequently in an acute setting.

### N. Rectal Tumor

▶ **H&P Keys**

Rectal bleeding, mucous discharge, change of bowel habits, tenesmus, rectal mass, hepatomegaly, ascites.

▶ **Diagnosis**

Colonoscopy, barium enema, flexible sigmoidoscopy, endorectal ultrasound, MRI, CT scan of pelvis and abdomen.

▶ **Disease Severity**

Anemia, abnormal LFTs, destruction, lymph node involvement, tumor differentiation, fixed tumor.

▶ **Concept and Application**

Malignant change in adenoma, genetic predisposition, mutation of genes by carcinogenic agents.

▶ **Treatment Steps**
1. Local excision for superficial lesions.
2. Low anterior resection or abdominoperineal resection.
3. Radiation, chemotherapy.

### O. Hemorrhoids

▶ **H&P Keys**

Rectal bleeding, mucous discharge, prolapse spontaneously or with defecation, anal verge normal or hypertrophic, visible prolapsed hemorrhoids. Rule out portal hypertension.

▶ **Diagnosis**

Rectal examination, proctosigmoidoscopy.

▶ **Disease Severity**

Degree of hemorrhoidal prolapse, thrombosis, failure of conservative measures.

▶ **Concept and Application**

Prolapse of normal mucosal cushion, increased anal canal pressure. In portal hypertension, increased pressure in the inferior mesenteric vein.

▶ **Treatment Steps**
1. Rule out coexistent rectal or sigmoid pathology (eg, cancer), sigmoidoscopy.
2. High-fiber diet, warm sitz baths.
3. Sclerotherapy.
4. Rubber band ligation.
5. Cryosurgery.
6. Hemorrhoidectomy.

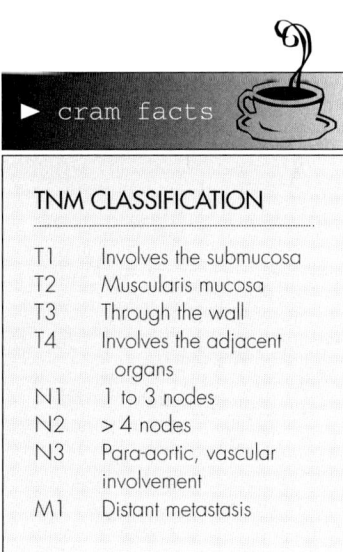

▶ cram facts

**TNM CLASSIFICATION**

| | |
|---|---|
| T1 | Involves the submucosa |
| T2 | Muscularis mucosa |
| T3 | Through the wall |
| T4 | Involves the adjacent organs |
| N1 | 1 to 3 nodes |
| N2 | > 4 nodes |
| N3 | Para-aortic, vascular involvement |
| M1 | Distant metastasis |

## P. Perirectal Abscess

▶ H&P Keys

Deep buttock or rectal pain, fever, perianal mass.

▶ Diagnosis

Rectal–perianal examination, CT scan sometimes indicated.

▶ Disease Severity

Coexisting Crohn's disease, diffuse spread of abscess, extension into adjacent anatomic space, presence of complex fistula.

▶ Concept and Application

Invasion of perirectal spaces by pathogenic organisms; infection of anal crypts, hair follicles, or sebaceous cysts. Supralevator, perianal, intersphincteric, and ischioanal abscesses.

▶ Treatment Steps
1. Examination under anesthesia.
2. Incision and drainage.
3. Antibiotics.
4. Warm sitz baths and local wound care.

## Q. Anorectal Fistula

▶ H&P Keys

Chronic purulent discharge from perianal opening, history of perianal abscess.

▶ Diagnosis

Rectal examination, anoproctoscopy, rectal ultrasound, fistulography.

▶ Disease Severity

Coexisting Crohn's, complex or high fistulas, TB, incontinence, HIV disease.

▶ Concept and Application

Injury or infected anal crypts. Epithelialization of fistulous tract.

▶ Treatment Steps
1. Examination under anesthesia.
2. Lay open the fistula and use seton; if associated with diverticulitis, perform colon resection, Goodsall's rule.

## R. Pilonidal Cyst

▶ H&P Keys

Purulent drainage from sacrococcygeal sinus; pain, tender mass, induration, hair emerging from opening.

▶ Diagnosis

Physical examination.

▶ Disease Severity

Hirsutism, multiple tracts, multiple recurrence, poor postoperative course.

▶ Concept and Application
Macerated skin, suction effect of buttock when walking, loose hair embedded in skin. Possibly congenital.

▶ Treatment Steps
1. Incision and drainage of abscess; wide local excision of sinus tract, down to sacral fascia.
2. Healing by primary closure (if not infected), secondary intention, local flaps.

### S. Benign Neoplasm of the Small Bowel

▶ H&P Keys
Asymptomatic, occult GI bleeding, bowel obstruction (crampy abdominal pain, bloating, vomiting).

▶ Diagnosis
Small-bowel follow through, CT scan of the abdomen and pelvis.

▶ Disease Severity
Massive GI bleeding, intussusception, obstruction.

▶ Concept and Application
Benign smooth-muscle (leiomyoma) or mucosal tumor.

▶ Treatment Steps
Enucleation, wedge excision, depending on size and symptomatology.

### T. Benign Neoplasm of the Colon

▶ H&P Keys
Rectal bleeding, altered bowel habits, mucus discharge from rectum, rectal mass, heme-positive stools, family history, anemia.

▶ Diagnosis
Colonoscopy, barium enema (Fig. 18–7).

▶ Disease Severity
Family history of polyposis or colon cancer, size of polyp, histological variant, degree of dysplasia, multiple adenomas.

▶ Concept and Application
Neoplasia of intestinal epithelium (tubular, villous), abnormal mixture of normal tissue (hamartomas), other benign growths (eg, lipoma).

▶ Treatment Steps
Polypectomy, bowel resection, panproctocolectomy and J-pouch (for familial polyposis).

### U. Colon Cancer

▶ H&P Keys
Familial polyposis, inflammatory bowel disease, adenomatous polyps. Fatigue, anemia, changes in bowel habits, weight loss. Palpable abdominal mass (right colon, sigmoid) or rectal mass.

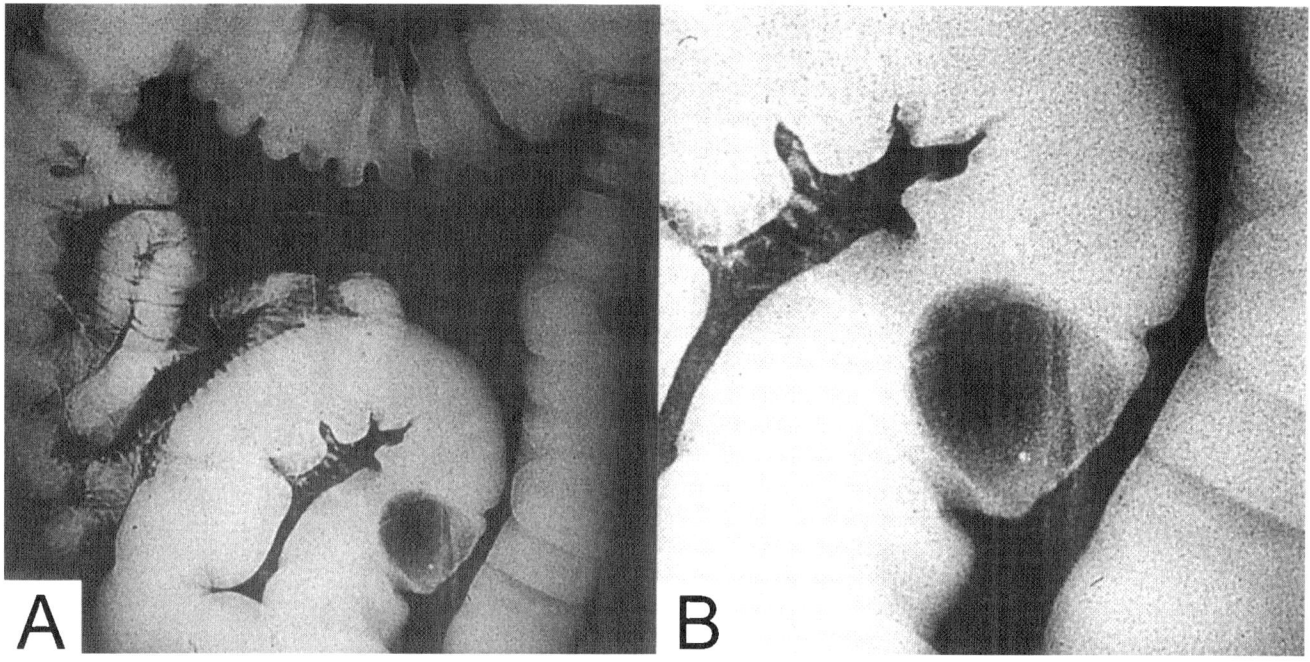

Figure 18–7. Benign tumor of sigmoid colon (submucosal lipoma) in a 35-year-old man. Note regular and smooth appearance of the lesion, and normal distensibility of the colonic wall.

▶ Diagnosis

*Proximal Colon*—Anemia, bulky tumor, and palpable mass.

*Distal Colon*—Luminal narrowing and obstruction. Digital rectal examination; occult fecal blood; barium enema; colonoscopy with biopsy. Carcinoembryonic antigen (CEA) is useful to detect recurrence after resection.

▶ Disease Severity

Depth of tumor according to a modified Dukes' classification—A, muscularis propria; B, serosa; C, regional lymph nodes; D, liver metastasis.

▶ Concept and Application

Prolonged exposure of colonic mucosa to carcinogens, concentrated after water is absorbed in the colon. Polyp–cancer sequence—villous adenomas more prone to malignant transformation than tubular adenomas.

▶ Treatment Steps

1. Surgical resection usually indicated—segment of colon along with regional lymph nodes.
2. Resection of liver metastases can contribute to cure.
3. Radiotherapy useful for rectal tumors.
4. Chemotherapy indicated for Dukes' C stage or distant metastasis.

### V. Duodenal Atresia

▶ **H&P Keys**

Bile-stained vomiting, post-feeding vomiting, distended upper abdomen, passage of meconium, antepartum polyhydramnios, stigmata of Down's syndrome (30%).

▶ **Diagnosis**

Plain x-ray ("double-bubble" sign), UGI series and follow-through, barium enema, evaluate cardiac system with echocardiography.

▶ **Disease Severity**

Prematurity, associated anomalies (eg, congenital heart disease), low birth weight, trisomy 21.

▶ **Concept and Application**

Hypoplasia or atresia of duodenum at level of ampulla. Rule out annular pancreas.

▶ **Treatment Steps**
1. Elevate head of bed, nasogastric decompression.
2. Correct fluid and electrolyte imbalance.
3. Duodenoduodenostomy, decompression gastrostomy; correct associated malrotation.
4. Chromosomal studies; genetic counseling.

### W. Malrotation

▶ **H&P Keys**

Biliary vomiting, hematemesis, heme-positive nasogastric aspirate, failure to thrive, mild abdominal distention, passage of meconium.

▶ **Diagnosis**

Plain x-ray of abdomen, UGI series, barium enema.

▶ **Disease Severity**

Hematemesis, bloody stools, peritonitis, heart rate, blood pressure, leukocytosis, ABG, mental changes.

▶ **Concept and Application**

Abnormality of usual embryonic intestinal rotation and fixation.

*Types*—(1) Nonrotation (midgut suspended by superior mesenteric vessels); (2) incomplete rotation (narrow small-bowel mesentery, adhesive Ladd's bands); (3) reversed rotation (retro-arterial cecal rotation); and (4) anomalous fixation of mesentery.

▶ **Treatment Steps**
1. Fluid and electrolyte correction, nasogastric decompression, antibiotics.
2. Surgical derotation of bowel, division of Ladd's bands, widen base of mesentery, fixation of cecum, appendectomy.

## X. Hirschsprung's Disease

▶ H&P Keys

Failure to pass meconium, chronic constipation, bile-stained vomiting, reluctance to feed, diarrhea, irritability, abdominal distention, palpable stool in lower abdomen, stool expulsion after rectal examination, male infant.

▶ Diagnosis

Plain abdominal x-ray, barium enema, rectal biopsy, and rectal manometry.

▶ Disease Severity

Diarrhea, abdominal guarding, distention; malnutrition; length of bowel involved.

▶ Concept and Application

Absence of cephalocaudal growth of parasympathetic myenteric nerve cells, functional obstruction, rectum always involved.

▶ Treatment Steps
1. Rectal tube and colonic washing.
2. Colostomy, endorectal pull-through.

## Y. Imperforate Anus

▶ H&P Keys

Anal dimple but no orifice; ectopic anal opening or fistula; meconium in vagina, urethra, or urine.

▶ Diagnosis

Physical examination, test urine for meconium, Rice–Wangensteen radiographic technique, ultrasound of kidneys and heart, sacrum x-ray. Seventy percent associated with other abnormalities.

▶ Disease Severity

Associated anomalies—VACTERL (vertebral, anorectal, cardiac, tracheal, esophageal, renal, limb), acidosis, neurologic deficit, agenesis of sacral vertebrae, incontinence.

▶ Concept and Application

Abnormal growth and fusion of embryonic anal hillocks, faulty division of the cloaca by urorectal septum.

▶ Treatment Steps
1. Posterior sagittal anoplasty, sigmoid colostomy, division of fistula.
2. Repeated anal dilation.

## IX. DISEASES OF THE GALLBLADDER AND LIVER

### A. Biliary Atresia

▶ H&P Keys

Jaundice, dark urine, pale-colored stools, hepatomegaly, splenomegaly, usually in 2- to 4-week-old infants.

▶ Diagnosis

Rose Bengal nuclear scan, hepatoiminodiacetic acid (HIDA) scan, serum lipoprotein X, abdominal ultrasound; needle biopsy of liver, exploratory laparotomy, cholangiography. Must rule out α-antitrypsin deficiency.

▶ Disease Severity

Jaundice, fever, cirrhosis, sepsis, esophageal varices, liver failure, delayed diagnosis, age (< 12 weeks).

▶ Concept and Application

Absence of patent bile ducts, periportal fibrosis, cirrhosis.

▶ Treatment Steps
1. IV fluids, vitamin K.
2. Roux-en-Y hepaticojejunostomy, liver transplantation.

### B. Acute Cholecystitis

▶ H&P Keys

Right upper-quadrant pain, radiation to subscapular area, nausea and vomiting, anorexia, fever, history of fatty food intolerance. Right upper quadrant tenderness and guarding, palpable gallbladder.

▶ Diagnosis

Plain x-ray of abdomen (radiopaque stones), ultrasound, HIDA scan, LFTs.

▶ Disease Severity

Unremitting fever; leukocytosis; elevated amylase; free perforation; palpable gallbladder, suggesting empyema or pericholecystic abscess; chills; common duct stones; diabetes mellitus; response to therapy.

▶ Concept and Application

Obstruction of cystic duct with stone, secondary bacterial invasion.

▶ Treatment Steps

*Acute*
1. IV fluids, nasogastric tube, antibiotics, and cholecystectomy.
2. Cholecystostomy if patient is too ill for cholecystectomy (Fig. 18–8).

*Chronic*—Cholecystectomy.

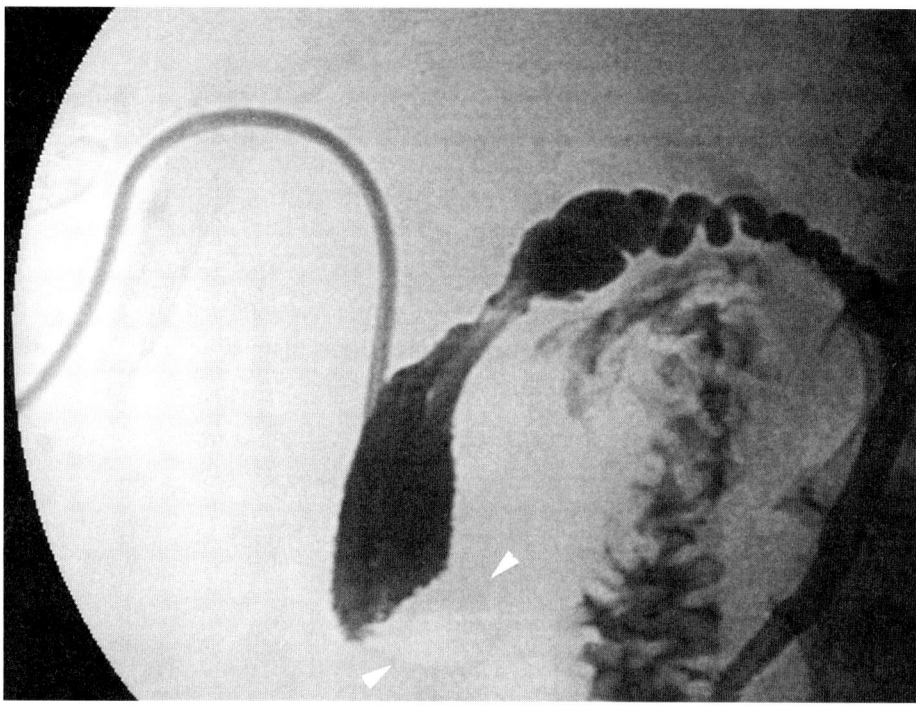

Figure 18–8. A cholecystostomy tube cholangiogram showing a somewhat decompressed gallbladder filled with gallstones. Arrows point to the portion of the gallbladder containing stones. This patient had calculus cholecystitis in the setting of severe hemodynamic instability and was too sick for an open cholecystectomy.

## C. Choledochal Cyst

### ▶ H&P Keys
Abdominal pain, episodic jaundice, mass in right upper quadrant, fever, dark urine, pale stools.

### ▶ Diagnosis
Ultrasound and CT scan of abdomen, endoscopic retrograde cholangiopancreatography (ERCP), percutaneous transhepatic cholangiography (PTC).

### ▶ Disease Severity
Fever, jaundice, recurrent pancreatitis.

### ▶ Concept and Application
Persistence of embryonic hepaticopancreatic duct, regurgitation of pancreatic juice in bile duct, cystic changes in bile duct, fibrosis, inflammation. If untreated, risk of carcinoma is increased.

### ▶ Treatment Steps
1. Excision of choledochal cyst.
2. Cholecystectomy and biliary reconstruction with a Roux-en-Y limb.

### D. Choledocholithiasis

▶ H&P Keys

Biliary colic, pruritus, chills, fever, jaundice, dark urine, pale stools, right upper quadrant tenderness, nausea and vomiting.

▶ Diagnosis

LFTs, ultrasound, ERCP, PTC, amylase, lipase.

▶ Disease Severity

Heart rate, leukocytosis, amylase, presence of hepatic abscess, biliary cirrhosis, liver failure, portal hypertension, coexistent diabetes mellitus, sepsis, confusion.

▶ Concept and Application

Stones originating in gallbladder; primary stones arising in intrahepatic duct or common bile duct.

▶ Treatment Steps

*Acute*
1. IV fluids, IV antibiotics.
2. ERCP and sphincterotomy, cholecystectomy and common bile duct exploration, with possible transduodenal sphincteroplasty, or choledochoduodenostomy.

*Chronic*
1. Antibiotics.
2. Drainage procedures as above.

### E. Carcinoma of the Gallbladder

▶ H&P Keys

Right upper quadrant pain, jaundice, weight loss, right upper quadrant mass.

▶ Diagnosis

LFTs, ultrasound, CT scan of abdomen and pelvis.

▶ Disease Severity

Weight loss, malnutrition, age, depth of tumor invasion, incidental finding, nonresectability.

▶ Concept and Application

Eighty percent of cases associated with gallstones. Porcelain gallbladder may be present.

▶ Treatment Steps

1. Cholecystectomy, radical regional lymphadenectomy and wedge excision of gallbladder bed.
2. Surgery most often is palliative.

### F. Hepatic Adenoma

▶ H&P Keys

Right upper quadrant pain, asymptomatic, palpable liver mass, hemoperitoneum, hypotension, use of oral contraceptives, female gender.

▶ Diagnosis
Ultrasound, CT scan of the abdomen, technetium colloid sulfur scan, MRI, aspiration biopsy.

▶ Disease Severity
Abdominal distention, guarding, large adenoma, spontaneous rupture.

▶ Concept and Application
Encapsulated homogeneous mass of hepatocyte, no bile ducts or central vein present.

▶ Treatment Steps
1. < 6 cm: observation, discontinue oral contraceptive.
2. > 6 cm: surgical resection.

## G. Focal Nodular Hyperplasia

▶ H&P Keys
Most often asymptomatic, much less tendency to hemorrhage than adenomas.

▶ Diagnosis
Ultrasound, CT scan, biopsy.

▶ Disease Severity
Extension, compression of adjacent structures, symptoms.

▶ Concept and Application
Histologically normal-appearing hepatocytes, bile ducts, Kupffer cells.

▶ Treatment Steps
Conservative, observation with imaging follow-up.

## H. Primary Hepatobiliary Cancer

▶ H&P Keys
Fatigue, weight loss, abdominal discomfort, jaundice. Palpable liver mass, signs of cirrhosis and portal hypertension.

▶ Diagnosis
Elevated AFP, alkaline phosphatase, direct bilirubin. Ultrasound, CT scan, or MRI. Percutaneous or laparoscopic needle biopsy.

▶ Disease Severity
Hepatocellular carcinoma (HCC) can undergo spontaneous rupture. Invasion of diaphragm and adjacent organs. Metastases to lymph nodes, lung, bone, adrenals, and brain.

▶ Concept and Application
HCC is the most common fatal cancer worldwide, and has many risk factors (eg, hepatitis, cirrhosis, and aflatoxin exposure). Cholangiocarcinoma involves the biliary tree and is often unresectable. Hepatoblastoma is a distinctive tumor of infants and children.

► Treatment Steps
1. Liver resection, radiotherapy, chemotherapy.
2. Liver transplantation may be indicated in select patients with HCC and other tumors.

### I. Liver Metastasis

► H&P Keys

History of cancer, especially GI (portal drainage). Anorexia, fatigue, weight loss, abdominal and shoulder pain. Jaundice, hepatomegaly (firm liver, nodular border), ascites. May be asymptomatic.

► Diagnosis

High alkaline phosphatase. Ultrasound, CT scan (Fig. 18–9), needle biopsy.

► Disease Severity

Multiplicity, involvement of both liver lobes. Prognosis depends on the primary tumor type.

► Concept and Application

Large size of liver and portal and systemic blood supply contribute to metastatic seeding.

► Treatment Steps
1. Palliative chemotherapy and moderate-dose radiation.
2. Resection is only curative method, most often indicated for select patients with colorectal or endocrine tumors.

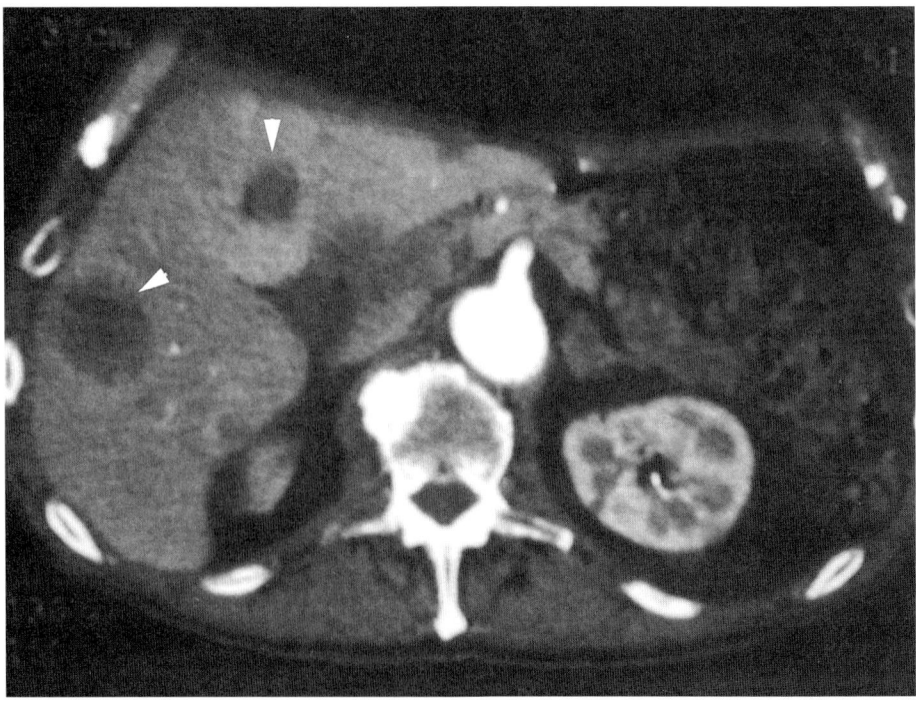

Figure 18–9. Abdominal CT scan of a cachectic patient showing bilobar liver metastatic lesions (arrows). This patient will be managed nonsurgically.

## X. DISEASE OF THE PANCREAS

### A. Acute Pancreatitis

▶ H&P Keys

Epigastric and back pain, nausea and vomiting, retching, hypotension, fever, left pleural effusion, abdominal tenderness, abdominal mass, jaundice, abdominal distention, Cullen's sign, Grey Turner's sign. Alcohol abuse.

▶ Diagnosis

Amylase, lipase, ultrasound, CT scan, plain x-ray, ERCP.

▶ Disease Severity

Age, blood glucose, WBC, lactic dehydrogenase, aspartate transaminase, calcium level, urea, hematocrit, excess base, arterial $Po_2$. Estimated fluid sequestered > 6 L. Fibrinogen, methemalbumin, respiratory rate, urine output, persistent fever, abdominal mass, jaundice, hematemesis, and hemoperitoneum.

▶ Concept and Application

Enzymatic digestion of gland, duct obstruction (gallstones and protein), chemical injury to the gland.

▶ Treatment Steps
1. Fluid replacement, GI rest, calcium and magnesium replacement.
2. ERCP, analgesia, cholecystectomy, biliary drainage, debridement of necrotic pancreatic tissue.

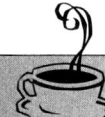

▶ cram facts

### RANSON'S CRITERIA (PREDICTING THE SEVERITY OF ACUTE PANCREATITIS)

On Admission:
| | | |
|---|---|---|
| W | WBC | > 16,000/mm³ |
| A | Age | > 55 yr |
| G | Glucose | > 200 mg/dL |
| A | AST | > 250 IU/dL |
| L | LDH | > 350 IU/L |

At 48 hrs:
| | | |
|---|---|---|
| B | Base deficit | > 4 mEq/L |
| E | Estimated fluid gain | > 6 L |
| C | Calcium | < 8 mg/dL |
| H | Hct fall | > 10% |
| U | Urea rise | > 5 mg/dL |
| P | $PaO_2$ | < 60 mm Hg |

Mortality rate in acute pancreatitis closely related to the number of positive Ranson signs (1% if up to 2 signs, 15% if 3–4, 40% if 5–6, and 100% if 7–8 signs present).
**NOTE:** Amylase is not part of the Ranson's criteria.

## B. Pancreatic Carcinoma

▶ H&P Keys
Vague abdominal pain, back pain, weight loss, pruritus, jaundice, abdominal mass, hepatomegaly, migratory thrombophlebitis.

▶ Diagnosis
Ultrasound, CT scan (Fig. 18–10), ERCP, endoscopy, MRCP, aspiration biopsy of pancreatic mass, angiography, lymph node involvement, distant metastasis, vascular invasion.

▶ Concept and Application
Malignant change in ductal epithelium, increased risk with severe smoking.

▶ Treatment Steps

*Curative*—Pancreaticoduodenectomy, total pancreatectomy, distal pancreatectomy, external-beam radiation, multidrug chemotherapy.

*Palliative*—Bilioenteric bypass, biliary stent, analgesia, celiac plexus nerve block.

## C. Gastrinoma

▶ H&P Keys
Severe peptic ulcer symptoms, diarrhea, previous ulcer operation.

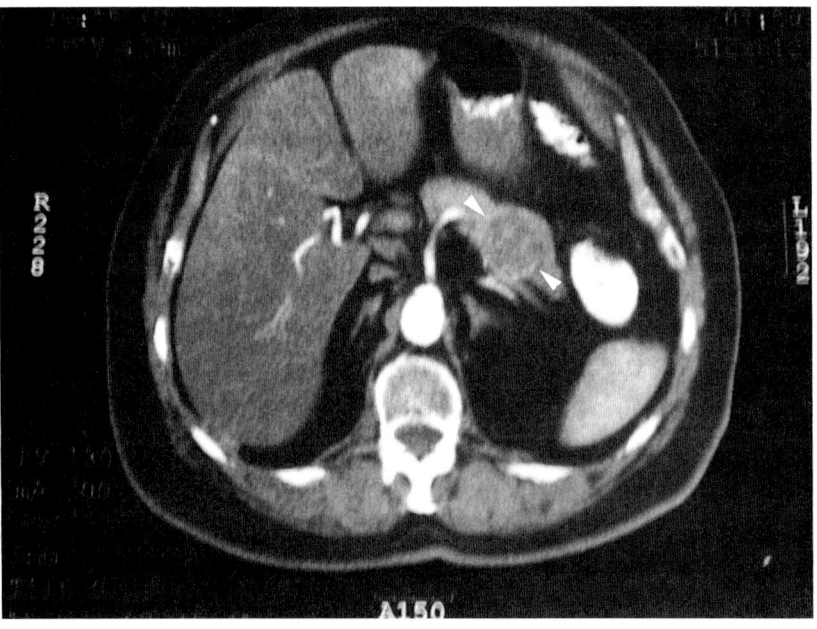

Figure 18–10. Abdominal CT scan showing an oval-shaped, distal pancreatic mass (arrows). This patient will be managed with a distal pancreatectomy and possible adjuvant therapy depending on the stage of the tumor.

▶ Diagnosis
Basal acid output/maximal acid-output ratio, serum gastrin level, secretin provocative test, UGI endoscopy, CT scan, transhepatic portal vein sampling, intraoperative endoscopic ultrasound, gastrinoma triangle (cystic duct, junction of second and third portions of the duodenum and junction of the head and neck of the pancreas).

▶ Disease Severity
Refractory peptic ulcer disease, hemorrhage, perforated ulcer, extremely high gastrin levels, multiple tumors, associated MEN type I. Malignant potential reported in 50–70%.

▶ Concept and Application
Hypersecretion of gastric acid caused by excessive production of gastrin by tumor.

▶ Treatment Steps
1. Omeprazole, $H_2$-receptor antagonist, streptozocin and 5-fluorouracil (for malignancy), gastrectomy.
2. Resection of the tumor, with pancreaticoduodenectomy common.

## XI. HERNIA

### A. Inguinal Hernia

▶ H&P Keys
Aching in groin; bulge or lump in groin, with or without one in the scrotum, mass in the groin. Symptoms may be precipitated by exercise and/or straining.

▶ Diagnosis
Physical examination; herniography (rarely needed; children).

▶ Disease Severity
Uncorrected chronic cough; prostatism or constipation; large, indirect hernia; nonreducible hernia; abdominal distention; recurrent hernia; leukocytosis; fever; tenderness; history of chronic obstructive pulmonary disease (COPD); incarceration or strangulation.

▶ Concept and Application
Persistent peritoneal diverticulum, increased intra-abdominal pressure, weakness of transversalis fascia, patent process vaginalis.

▶ Treatment Steps
Standard or laparoscopic herniorrhaphy.

### B. Femoral Hernia

▶ H&P Keys
Groin discomfort; lump in the groin; mass below inguinal ligament, medial to femoral vessels. Rule out lymphadenopathy.

▶ Diagnosis
Physical examination, ultrasound.

▶ Disease Severity
Intestinal obstruction, tender and irreducible hernia, compression and/or thrombosis of femoral vein.

▶ Concept and Application
Protrusion of intra-abdominal contents through femoral canal.

▶ Treatment Steps
1. Excision of sac, closure of femoral canal.
2. For intestinal obstruction, exploratory laparotomy, and possible bowel resection.

### C. Umbilical Hernia

▶ H&P Keys
Bulge in umbilicus; fascial defect felt.

▶ Diagnosis
Physical examination.

▶ Disease Severity
Associated diseases such as cirrhosis and intra-abdominal tumor; pregnancy.

▶ Concept and Application
Gradual yielding of the umbilical scar tissue.

▶ Treatment Steps
1. Younger than 6 years, observation.
2. Older than 6 years, repair fascial defect.

### D. Incisional Hernia

▶ H&P Keys
Pain; swelling adjacent to scar.

▶ Diagnosis
History and physical examination.

▶ Disease Severity
Large multiple defects, intercurrent disease, bowel obstruction, age, sepsis, general debility, steroids, nutrition; history of COPD.

▶ Concept and Application
Disruption of fascial suture resulting from surgical technique, wound infection, age, general debility, type of incision or suture material, nutrition.

▶ Treatment Steps
1. Weight reduction to correct intercurrent disease, improved nutrition.
2. Fascial repair—direct or with mesh placement.

### E. Diaphragmatic Hernia

▶ H&P Keys

Gasping respiration, cyanosis, heart sound displaced to right, absent breath sound on left, bowel sounds on affected hemithorax, scaphoid abdomen.

▶ Diagnosis

CXR, antenatal ultrasound, UGI series.

▶ Disease Severity

Associated anomalies, ABG, cyanosis, respiratory rate, prolonged mechanical ventilation, response to therapy.

▶ Concept and Application

Incomplete diaphragm, persistence of pleuroperitoneal hiatus, impaired pulmonary development.

▶ Treatment Steps
1. Nasogastric tube decompression, mechanical ventilation, arterial line, Priscoline (pulmonary vasodilator), extracorporeal membrane oxygenation (ECMO).
2. Surgery to reduce herniated bowel and repair diaphragmatic defect.

### F. Hernia with Obstruction

▶ H&P Keys

Pain at site of hernia, abdominal pain, vomiting, obstipation, fever, tachycardia, prostration, abdominal distention, hypoactive bowel sounds, oliguria.

▶ Diagnosis

Physical examination, leukocytosis, plain x-ray, high-resolution ultrasound scan.

▶ Disease Severity

Fever, urine output, heart rate, blood pressure, abdominal guarding, mentation changes, age.

▶ Concept and Application

Intra-abdominal contents present within hernial sac, fascial neck compromises blood supply. Edematous intestinal segment.

▶ Treatment Steps
1. IV fluids, nasogastric tube decompression, monitoring of urine output, antibiotics, correction of electrolyte imbalance.
2. Surgery to release hernia content, resect bowel, repair hernia.

## BIBLIOGRAPHY

Cameron J. *Current Surgical Therapy.* 7th ed. Philadelphia: Mosby; 2001.

Greenfield LJ. *Surgery: Scientific Principles and Practice.* 3rd ed, Philadelphia: Lippincott-Raven Publishers; 2001.

Sabiston D. *Textbook of Surgery: The Biological Basis of Modern Surgical Practice.* 17th ed. Philadelphia: WB Saunders Company; 2001.

Schwartz SI. *Principles of Surgery.* 8th ed. New York: McGraw-Hill; 2000.

# Ill-Defined Symptom Complex 19

I. **SYMPTOMS REFERABLE TO THE CIRCULATORY SYSTEM / 622**
    A. Palpitations / 622
    B. Murmurs / 622

II. **SYMPTOMS REFERABLE TO THE RESPIRATORY SYSTEM / 623**
    A. Dyspnea / 623
    B. Stridor / 624
    C. Cough / 624
    D. Hemoptysis / 625

III. **SYMPTOMS REFERABLE TO THE GENITOURINARY SYSTEM / 626**
    A. Renal Colic / 626
    B. Dysuria / 626
    C. Oliguria and Anuria / 627
    D. Proteinuria / 628

IV. **ILL-DEFINED PRESENTATIONS / 629**
    A. Lymphadenitis / 629
    B. Dizziness / 629
    C. Malaise and Fatigue / 630
    D. Septic Shock / 631
    E. Enlarged Lymph Nodes / 631
    F. Chest Pain / 632
    G. Gastrointestinal Hemorrhage / 633
    H. Diarrhea / 634
    I. Reye's Syndrome / 635
    J. Dyspepsia / 636
    K. Abdominal Pain / 637
    L. Nausea and Vomiting / 638
    M. Dysphagia / 639
    N. Jaundice / 640
    O. Ascites / 641
    P. Weight Loss / 642

**BIBLIOGRAPHY / 643**

## I. SYMPTOMS REFERABLE TO THE CIRCULATORY SYSTEM

### A. Palpitations

▶ H&P Keys

Onset, duration, timing, and frequency of palpitations; precipitating and alleviating factors; associated symptoms of chest pain, dyspnea, light-headedness; history of heart disease or murmur, diabetes, or thyroid disease; risk factors for coronary artery disease; medication use; tachycardia, hypotension, fever; evidence of congestive heart failure; evidence of thyroid disease; murmur or rub; environmental exposures, caffeine use, illicit drug use.

▶ Diagnosis

Studies: electrocardiogram (ECG); serum electrolytes, complete blood count (CBC), urine drug screen, drug levels, thyroid studies if indicated; Holter monitor and echocardiography if cardiac cause is suspected. Cardiac causes include arrhythmias; valvular heart disease; cardiomyopathy, pericarditis, congestive heart failure. Other causes include anxiety, fever, thyrotoxicosis, pregnancy, hypoglycemia, drugs (alcohol, nicotine, cocaine, caffeine, decongestants, theophylline, epinephrine), and pheochromocytoma.

▶ Disease Severity

Cardiac arrhythmia associated with hypotension, chest pain, or shortness of breath.

▶ Concept and Application

Palpitations are often a normal physiologic response to emotional or physical activity. Palpitations in a patient with a history of cardiac disease warrant further workup for arrhythmia.

▶ Treatment Steps
1. Remove precipitating factors.
2. Treat underlying disease.
3. Reassure patient if process is benign.

### B. Murmurs

▶ H&P Keys

Associated symptoms of chest pain, palpitations, dyspnea, dizziness; history of hypertension, rheumatic or cardiac disease, anemia or thyroid disease; fever, wide pulse pressure; nature of carotid upstroke; other heart sounds; timing, location, quality, intensity, and radiation of murmur; evidence of congestive heart failure; history of intravenous drug abuse.

▶ Diagnosis

Studies: ECG, chest roentgenogram, echocardiography if cardiac workup is appropriate. Cause can be innocent or physiologic, valvular heart disease, or septal defects.

▶ Disease Severity

Severity depends on nature and extent of underlying cardiac etiology and associated symptoms such as chest pain or shortness of breath.

▶ Concept and Application

Results from vibrations in heart and great vessels caused by turbulent blood flow.

▶ Treatment Steps
1. Treat underlying cardiac disease.
2. Reassure patient if etiology is benign.

## II. SYMPTOMS REFERABLE TO THE RESPIRATORY SYSTEM

### A. Dyspnea

▶ H&P Keys

Associated symptoms of chest pain, palpitations, cough, fever, weight loss; duration, timing, and frequency of dyspnea; relation of dyspnea to exertion and position; smoking history; occupational or environmental exposures; past or present history of pulmonary or cardiac disease; patient's general appearance with regard to respiratory difficulty; abnormal vital signs; lung percussion and auscultation; abnormal cardiac rhythm or auscultation; signs of congestive heart failure; abdominal mass or distention; mental status assessment.

▶ Diagnosis

History and physical exam findings key to making diagnosis. Chest roentgenogram, ECG, arterial blood gases, pulmonary function tests, exercise stress testing, echocardiography, ventilation-perfusion scan only if indicated. Pulmonary causes include asthma or emphysema; bronchitis, pneumonia, or lung abscess; pneumothorax; pulmonary embolism; malignancy (primary lung cancer or lung metastases); interstitial lung disease; pulmonary hypertension; large pulmonary effusion. Cardiac causes are ischemic heart disease, left-sided heart failure, arrhythmias, pericardial tamponade. Other causes include neurologic or muscular disorders affecting the respiratory muscles, abdominal distention from ascites or marked obesity, anxiety, deconditioning, and upper-airway infection or obstruction.

▶ Disease Severity

Decreased mentation, tachycardia, hypotension; signs of congestive heart failure; hypoxemia, hypercarbia, ECG or chest roentgenogram abnormalities.

▶ Concept and Application

Sensation of dyspnea is produced by differing mechanisms depending on the specific underlying disease.

▶ Treatment Steps
1. Treat underlying disease process.
2. Provide supplemental oxygen or mechanical ventilation if needed.

### B. Stridor

▶ H&P Keys

Associated symptoms of fever, cough, dyspnea, dysphagia, odynophagia, hoarseness, weight loss; neck and oropharynx exam, gag reflex, indirect mirror exam, if possible.

▶ Diagnosis

Arterial blood gases or pulse oximetry, lateral roentgenogram of neck if infection is suspected. In adults, flexible fiber-optic endoscopy of airway. Infectious causes of intralaryngeal lesions are acute bacterial epiglottitis and laryngotracheobronchitis (croup). Other types of intralaryngeal lesions are caused by malignancy, foreign body, trauma, benign tumors, and smoke inhalation.

▶ Disease Severity

Patient's inability to handle oral secretions, coupled with dyspnea or hypoxemia, indicates near-complete airway obstruction and requires emergency intubation or tracheotomy.

▶ Concept and Application

Stridor indicates *marked* upper airway obstruction, inspiratory stridor indicates airway obstruction above the vocal cords, and mixed or expiratory stridor usually indicates an obstruction below the vocal cords.

▶ Treatment Steps
1. Control airway.
2. Remove obstructing lesion if possible.
3. Provide supplemental oxygen.
4. Intravenous (IV) antibiotics (third-generation cephalosporin) if etiology is infectious.
5. IV steroids if airway edema and swelling are suspected.

### C. Cough

▶ H&P Keys

Frequency, duration, and timing of cough; color and nature of sputum; other upper respiratory tract symptoms; fever, dyspnea, orthopnea, anorexia, weight loss, vomiting; associated heartburn or postnasal drip; smoking history; environmental or occupational precipitants; past or present history of pulmonary, cardiac, sinus, or allergic disease; exposure to tuberculosis (TB); medications; tachypnea; evidence of otitis, pharyngeal erythema or exudates, sinus tenderness; lymphadenopathy; percussion and auscultation of lungs; signs of congestive heart failure.

▶ Diagnosis

Studies: emphasis on history and physical exam. Chest roentgenogram if abnormal pulmonary exam or if pneumonia, malignancy, pulmonary edema, TB, bronchiectasis, or sarcoidosis is suspected.

If sputum is purulent, Gram stain and culture. If chest roentgenogram is negative, consider pulmonary function tests. If malignancy still suspected, CT scan of chest followed by bronchoscopy. Pulmonary causes include pneumonia or tracheobronchitis, asthma, irritants (pollutants, cigarette smoke), chronic obstructive pulmonary disease, lung cancer, tuberculosis, pulmonary edema, bronchiectasis, or sarcoidosis. Other causes are reflux; postnasal drip or rhinitis; pharyngitis, otitis, sinusitis, impacted cerumen; and angiotensin-converting enzyme (ACE) inhibitors.

▶ Disease Severity

Presence of dyspnea, fever, tachypnea, weight loss; evidence of congestive heart failure; worsening bronchospasm; or hypoxia.

▶ Concept and Application

Afferent cough receptors located in the nose, larynx, lungs, stomach, sinuses, pharynx, or auditory canals respond to mechanical, inflammatory, chemical, and thermal stimulants. Therapy is directed at removing these stimulants.

▶ Treatment Steps

1. Treat underlying etiology.
2. Initiate trial of $H_2$-blockers if reflux is suspected.
3. Administer antihistamines or inhaled steroids if allergic rhinitis is suspected.
4. Use antitussives if cough is bothersome to the patient.

D. Hemoptysis

▶ H&P Keys

Duration of symptoms and appearance of expectorated blood and sputum; associated symptoms of chest pain, fever, weight loss, hematuria; exposure to tuberculosis; smoking history or asbestos exposure; history of rheumatic fever or heart murmur; history of bleeding disorder, anticoagulant use, or blunt trauma; history of aortic repair; lymphadenopathy; chest wall exam and lung auscultation; heart murmur; signs of congestive heart failure.

▶ Diagnosis

Studies: chest roentgenogram, coagulation studies, culture and stain for acid-fast bacilli if TB is suspected. Bronchoscopy if abnormal CXR, history of tobacco use, age > 40 yrs or persistent hemoptysis. Infectious causes include bronchitis, TB (with cavitary disease), aspergilloma, lung abscess, and necrotizing pneumonia. Pulmonary causes include pulmonary embolism (with infarction), malignancy, foreign body, bronchiectasis, arterial or venous malformations, bronchial adenoma, pulmonary contusion, pulmonary edema (usually just blood-streaked sputum, not gross hemoptysis), and pulmonary vasculitis (Goodpasture's, Wegener's). Other cause is bleeding diathesis, including excessive anticoagulant therapy; aortobronchial fistula, mitral valve prolapse, mitral stenosis.

▶ Disease Severity

Massive hemoptysis is defined as cough producing more than 600 cc of blood in 24 hours. Minor amounts of hemoptysis can accompany cough associated with a respiratory infection.

▶ Concept and Application

Inflammation, ulceration, or injury to any part of the tracheobronchial mucosa can result in hemoptysis. Pulmonary vascular injury also causes hemoptysis. Bleeding disorders associated with hemoptysis are usually accompanied by an underlying bronchopulmonary lesion.

▶ Treatment Steps

1. Ensure protection of the airway.
2. Establish the diagnosis.
3. Treat the underlying cause.

## III. SYMPTOMS REFERABLE TO THE GENITOURINARY SYSTEM

### A. Renal Colic

▶ H&P Keys

Onset, location, duration, and radiation of pain; associated symptoms of nausea or vomiting, hematuria, dysuria, inability to void, or fever; past history of nephrolithiasis, systemic illness, or urinary infections; dietary and medication history; family history of nephrolithiasis; lymphadenopathy or organomegaly.

▶ Diagnosis

Studies: urinalysis; serum blood urea nitrogen (BUN), creatinine, calcium, and uric acid; kidney, ureter, and bladder roentgenogram; and IV pyelogram. Causes include nephrolithiasis, pyelonephritis, renal embolic infarction, abdominal or pelvic mass or infection, papillary necrosis.

▶ Disease Severity

Severity of pain, nausea, and vomiting. Presence of fever.

▶ Concept and Application

Nonradiating pain usually indicates upper-tract disease, and pain radiating to the groin usually indicates ureteral disease. Ureteral obstruction causes hyperperistalsis (mechanism of pain).

▶ Treatment Steps

1. Control pain.
2. Administer intravenous hydration.
3. Treat underlying disease process.

### B. Dysuria

▶ H&P Keys

Duration and timing of dysuria; associated symptoms of urinary frequency, hematuria, nocturia, fever, flank or abdominal pain, vaginal or urethral discharge, nausea and vomiting, or dyspareunia; risk factors for sexually transmitted disease (STD); history of diabetes, sickle cell disease; recurrent urinary tract infections, or renal calculi; abnormal vital signs; costovertebral angle tenderness; suprapubic tenderness; pelvic or prostatic examination.

▶ Diagnosis

Studies: urinalysis; urine gram stain; and urine culture if pyuria is present. Cervical cultures in women if urine analysis negative; urethral cultures in men. Urologic evaluation with cystoscopy, IV pyelogram, or ultrasound if no evidence of infection. Causes include acute bacterial cystitis or pyelonephritis; urethritis; vulvovaginitis; renal calculi; urethral irritant, stricture, tumor, or foreign body; and trauma.

▶ Disease Severity

Fever and severe costovertebral angle tenderness. Need to rule out obstruction associated with infection.

▶ Concept and Application

Irritation or inflammation of bladder or urethral mucosa leads to intense burning sensation.

▶ Treatment Steps

1. Antibiotics if infection suspected by exam and urinalysis.
2. Provide STD counseling.
3. Treat underlying disease.

## C. Oliguria and Anuria

▶ H&P Keys

Associated qualitative changes in the urine; associated symptoms of fever, rash, vomiting, diarrhea, blood loss, weight loss, travel; past or present history of renal, cardiac, hepatic, pelvic, vascular, or neurologic disease; family history of renal disease; history of trauma or surgical procedures; recent radiologic procedures; medication use; volume depletion or overload; elevated blood pressure or hypotension; retinopathy; signs of congestive heart failure; abdominal or pelvic mass; prostatic enlargement; abnormal mental status.

▶ Diagnosis

Oliguria is < 400 mL/day; anuria is < 50 mL/day of urine output. Urinalysis (macro- and microscopic evaluation); urinary indexes (sodium, creatinine, and osmolality); serum electrolytes, glucose, BUN, creatinine, CBC; ultrasound, IV pyelogram, cystoscopy, and voiding cystourethrogram if needed to evaluate site of obstruction. Prerenal causes include decreased fluid intake, hemorrhage, gastrointestinal (GI) losses, renal losses; vasodilatation secondary to drugs, sepsis, or anaphylaxis; and "third-spacing" of fluids (congestive heart failure, burns, hypoalbuminemia, pancreatitis). Renal causes include acute tubular necrosis, vascular disease, glomerulonephritis or interstitial nephritis, end-stage renal disease, bilateral cortical necrosis, hemolytic–uremic syndrome, and paraprotein or crystal-mediated disease. Postrenal causes include bilateral ureteral obstruction, bladder outlet obstruction, urethral obstruction, prostatic obstruction, anticholinergic medications, and congenital malformation of the kidney.

▶ Disease Severity

Malignant hypertension or congestive heart failure.

▶ Concept and Application

Anuria should not be attributed to primary renal disease without evaluating the patency of the bladder, ureters, urethra, renal veins and arteries, and any urinary catheters.

▶ Treatment Steps

1. Catheterize bladder or flush existing catheter.
2. Alleviate any obstruction if possible.
3. Discontinue nephrotoxic drugs.
4. Administer fluids if needed.
5. Optimize arterial blood volume and cardiac status.
6. Treat hypertension aggressively.
7. Measure intake and output.
8. Hemodialyze if volume overload, electrolyte abnormalities, or acid–base disturbance is life-threatening.
9. Treat underlying disease.

### D. Proteinuria

▶ H&P Keys

Associated urinary symptoms; associated systemic symptoms: recent sore throat, rash, joint pain, fever, fatigue, anorexia; past or present history of renal disease or urinary tract infections; history of HIV infection, hypertension, or diabetes; medication use (particularly analgesics); family history of renal disease; elevated blood pressure; rash, lymphadenopathy, or joint effusions; edema; retinopathy; heart murmur; organomegaly or abdominal mass.

▶ Diagnosis

Studies: urinalysis (dipstick evaluation), followed by microscopic examination. Twenty-four-hour urine protein measurement. Serum electrolytes, glucose, BUN, creatinine, albumin, cholesterol, CBC. Serum complement levels, antinuclear antibody (ANA), and antistreptococcal antibodies and serum and urine protein electrophoresis. Renal ultrasound, intravenous pyelogram (IVP), or biopsy if indicated. Renal causes include exercise induced or orthostatic proteinuria; urinary tract infection; glomerular, interstitial, or tubular disease; and polycystic kidney disease. Proteinuria also is associated with the following systemic illnesses: diabetes mellitus, malignancy, systemic lupus erythematosis, preeclampsia, amyloidosis, sarcoidosis, cryoglobulinemia, HIV infection, infectious endocarditis and hepatitis, syphilis, and drug-induced illness (ACE inhibitors, cephalosporins, heroin, penicillamine).

▶ Disease Severity

Massive proteinuria (> 3.5 g/day).

▶ Concept and Application

Glomerular proteinuria secondary to injury of basement membrane leads to increased protein permeability. Tubular proteinuria secondary to decreased tubular protein reabsorption.

▶ Treatment Steps

1. Benign, transient, or exercise-induced proteinuria requires no further work-up.
2. Discontinue drug associated with proteinuria.
3. Treat underlying renal or systemic illness responsible for the condition.

## IV. ILL-DEFINED PRESENTATIONS

### A. Lymphadenitis

▶ H&P Keys

Pain at site of recent trauma or wound; associated symptoms of fever, malaise, anorexia; contact with cats; immunocompromised patient; tachycardia; enlarged tender regional lymph nodes; nearby erythema, rash, or abscess.

▶ Diagnosis

Studies: CBC with differential; blood and wound cultures. Causes include superficial thrombophlebitis, cellulitis, and cat-scratch fever.

▶ Disease Severity

Systemic manifestations (fever, malaise).

▶ Concept and Application

Lymph node inflammation.

▶ Treatment Steps

1. Heat and analgesics.
2. Antibiotics (vary with the clinical situation but should include both grampositive and negative coverage).
3. Incision and drainage if abscess is present or does not respond to antibiotics.

### B. Dizziness

▶ H&P Keys

Onset, duration, frequency, and intensity of episodes; associated symptoms of nausea, ear pain, tinnitus, hearing loss, dysphagia, diplopia, dysarthria, hemiparesis; precipitating and relieving factors; history of anemia or cardiac, cerebrovascular, thyroid, or psychiatric disease; recent viral illness; medication use; orthostatic hypotension or tachycardia; nystagmus; evidence of cerumen impaction, middle-ear disease, or hearing loss; carotid bruit; aortic stenosis murmur; abnormal neurologic exam; evidence of congestive heart failure or arrhythmia.

▶ Diagnosis

Studies: provocative testing; CBC and electrolytes if metabolic abnormality is suspected; audiological evaluation and electronystagmography if vestibular disorder is suspected; and magnetic resonance imaging (MRI), if further testing indicated. Vestibular disorders include benign postural vertigo, otitis, Ménière's disease, tumors, and vestibular neuronitis and ototoxic drugs. Systemic causes include arrhythmia and aortic stenosis; cerebellar ischemia or stroke and basilar insufficiency; anxiety, depression, and psychoses; multiple sclerosis; anemia; hypoglycemia; hypoxia; and drug side effects. Other causes are carotid sinus hypersensitivity, hyperventilation, and orthostatic hypotension.

▶ Disease Severity

Depends on specific etiology, degree of associated symptoms, and whether patient is incapacitated by dizziness.

▶ Concept and Application

Vestibular disorders result from interruption of vestibular nerve, frequently at its endpoint in the inner ear.

▶ Treatment Steps
1. Treat underlying disease.
2. Avoid precipitating factors.
3. Treat symptoms with meclizine and antiemetics if needed.
4. Reassure patient if etiology is benign.

### C. Malaise and Fatigue

▶ H&P Keys

Duration, associated symptoms of fever, arthralgias, dyspnea, weight loss; recent illness; changes in lifestyle, occupation, or sleep; history of anemia, malignancy, cardiac, pulmonary, renal, or endocrine disease; psychiatric history of depression or anxiety disorder; history of medication; pharyngeal erythema or exudates; lymphadenopathy; rash, pallor, or jaundice; thyroid enlargement; evidence of arrhythmia or congestive heart failure; abdominal tenderness or mass; focal findings on neurologic exam; and slow deep tendon reflexes.

▶ Diagnosis

Studies: CBC, electrolytes, BUN, creatinine, glucose; thyroid function tests. Causes include overexertion or inadequate sleep; anxiety or depression; side effect of medication; mononucleosis, tuberculosis, hepatitis, HIV infection, or endocarditis; anemia; hypothyroidism; chronic cardiopulmonary disease, connective tissue, or renal disease; malignancy; and chronic fatigue syndrome.

▶ Disease Severity

Accompanying symptoms if depression is suspected, and severity and extent of underlying organic etiology.

▶ Concept and Application

Malaise and fatigue accompany most illnesses, both organic and emotional.

---

▶ diagnostic decisions

**OLIGURIA AND ANURIA**

When patients are oliguric or anuric, think:
1. High—both kidneys are not functional secondary to acute tubular necrosis, hypotension, chronic hypertensive damage, etc.
2. Medium—ureters are obstructed secondary to retroperitoneal mass or fibrosis or bladder mass obstructing both ureters.
3. Low—urethra obstructed by an enlarged or infected prostate, urethral mass, or stone.

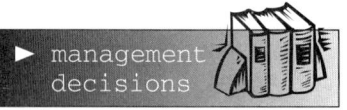

▶ management decisions

**OLIGURIA AND ANURIA**

When patients are oliguric or anuric:
1. In males, evaluate the prostate first.
2. Place a Foley catheter into the bladder to get an accurate measurement of output.
3. Image the GU tract without contrast—ultrasound is ideal.
4. Obtain blood for BUN, creatinine, electrolytes, and CBC. Obtain urine for urinalysis, culture, and electrolytes.

▶ Treatment Steps
1. Treat underlying etiology.
2. Educate patient.

## D. Septic Shock

▶ H&P Keys

Recent skin, respiratory, gastrointestinal, urinary tract infections; immunocompromised condition; decreased urine output; fever, tachypnea, tachycardia, hypothermia, or hypotension; change in mental status; cool extremities; and decreased or absent peripheral pulses.

▶ Diagnosis

Blood, urine, sputum cultures; electrolytes, BUN, creatinine, CBC, coagulation studies; arterial blood gases; chest roentgenogram, ECG; lactate level, liver function tests.

▶ Disease Severity

Hypotension, inadequate response to volume, requirement of pressors, high lactate level, and prolonged oliguria.

▶ Concept and Application

Results from interactions between microbes, leukocytes, humoral mediators, and vascular endothelium. Endotoxins cause activation of complement system, coagulation cascade, and numerous other mediators that lead to marked vasodilatation and myocardial depression.

▶ Treatment Steps
1. Place patient in Trendelenburg position.
2. Replace volume.
3. Monitor urinary output—place urinary catheter if needed.
4. Monitor cardiac rhythm and central venous pressure.
5. Administer broad-spectrum antibiotics until organism identified.
6. Support blood pressure with vasopressors, such as dopamine.
7. Provide supplemental oxygen.
8. Treat electrolyte and acid–base abnormalities.

## E. Enlarged Lymph Nodes

▶ H&P Keys

Associated symptoms are fever, anorexia, sore throat, weight loss, cough, dyspnea, night sweats, edema, red eye, and rash; history of malignancy, connective tissue disease, or immunocompromised condition; exposure to cats or TB; risk factors for HIV infection; smoking history; location and physical characteristics of peripheral nodes; joint effusion or inflammation; rash; and hepatomegaly or splenomegaly.

▶ Diagnosis

Studies: CBC with differential. Throat culture; monospot if pharyngitis or cervical or submandibular adenopathy is present. Rapid plasma reagin, HIV, ANA, rheumatoid factor. Chest roentgenogram. Lymph node biopsy if there is still no diagnosis and if suspicion of malignancy or serious infectious process is still high. Causes of generalized disorder are mononucleosis, HIV, and syphilis; malignancy; connective tissue disease; lipodoses; and drug reaction to dilantin, hydralazine, or allopurinol. Causes of regionalized disorder include local infection; reactive hyperplasia; pharyngitis, syphilis, herpes, chancroid, cat-scratch fever, rubella; malignancy; and granulomatous disease.

▶ Disease Severity

Extent and etiology of underlying disease govern severity. Nodes in excess of 3 cm or in patients older than 50 years often indicate malignancy.

▶ Concept and Application

Mechanisms responsible for lymph node enlargement include antigenic response of lymphocytes and macrophages, infectious infiltration of inflammatory cells, proliferation of malignant lymphocytes or macrophages within the lymph node, and invasion of lymph node by malignant cells.

▶ Treatment Steps
1. Identify underlying process.
2. Remove entire node if malignancy suspected.
3. Treat underlying disease.

## F. Chest Pain

▶ H&P Keys

Quality, location, radiation, and duration of pain; associated symptoms such as dyspnea, diaphoresis, fever, cough, dizziness, aggravating and relieving factors; history of recent trauma or surgical procedure; relation to meals; past or present history of cardiac, pulmonary, esophageal, or rheumatologic disease; risk factors for ischemic heart disease; current medication or alcohol use; signs of anxiety or depression; evidence of tachycardia, arrhythmia, tachypnea, hypotension, hypertension, fever, or weight loss; chest auscultation; localized tenderness and pain with movement; and asymmetric leg edema.

▶ Diagnosis

Studies: history and physical examination are keys. Chest roentgenogram, rib films, ECG, barium swallow. Cardiac causes include myocardial ischemia or infarction and pericarditis. Pulmonary causes include pulmonary embolism, pneumonia or tracheobronchitis, pneumothorax, and pleurisy. Vascular cause is aortic aneurysm or dissection. And gastrointestinal (GI) causes include esophagitis or gastroesophageal reflux; aspirin or nonsteroidal anti-inflammatory drugs (NSAIDs) related gastritis; peptic ulcer disease, gallbladder, or pancreatic disease; costochondritis or muscle, bone, or ligament strain; panic attacks, anxiety, or somatization disorder; breast disease; and herpes zoster.

▶ Disease Severity

Dependent on specific disease etiology and associated symptoms.

▶ Concept and Application

Scientific concepts are listed under specific disease etiology.

▶ Treatment Steps

1. Identify etiology of pain.
2. Treat underlying disease.
3. Administer pain medication if needed.

## G. Gastrointestinal Hemorrhage

▶ H&P Keys

Presence of hematemesis, vomiting of "coffee ground" material; melanotic stools, hematochezia; onset and duration of symptoms; accompanying symptoms of dizziness, tachycardia, weakness, weight loss, nausea, anorexia; predisposing conditions; medications (especially aspirin, NSAIDs, glucocorticoids); alcohol abuse; liver disease; history of previous GI bleeding or malignancy, diverticulitis, vomiting, or inflammatory bowel disease. Pallor and cool skin may be present if patient is in shock.

Pulse will reveal tachycardia; blood pressure may be elevated, normal, or low, depending on degree of blood loss. Oral cavity may contain blood or be pale in color, abdomen may be tender or rigid if perforation is present, rectal exam may reveal melanotic stool, hematochezia or hemoccult positive stool.

▶ Diagnosis

For upper GI hemorrhage: CBC, prothrombin time/partial thromboplastin time (PT/PTT). Nasogastric tube localizes bleeding to upper GI tract. If bleeding is rapid, may need emergency upper endoscopy; otherwise, upper endoscopy when stable. Angiography or radiolabeled red blood cell scan if bleeding is rapid and site is still unknown. Causes include esophagitis, esophageal cancer, esophageal tear (Mallory–Weiss), esophageal varices, gastric ulcer, gastritis, gastric cancer, gastric varices, and duodenal ulcer. For lower GI hemorrhage: CBC, PT/PTT, anoscopy, sigmoidoscopy. If bleeding is rapid, angiography and radiolabeled red blood cell scan. If patient stabilizes, colonoscopy to detect underlying lesion. Causes include hemorrhoids, anal fissures, anal fistulas, diverticulosis, infectious proctitis, trauma to rectal vault, colonic cancer, Meckel's diverticulum, colonic angiodysplasias, infectious diarrhea, ischemic colitis, and inflammatory bowel disease.

▶ Disease Severity

Degree of volume loss, assessed by orthostasis, hypotension, signs of shock (end-organ failure), tachycardia, hemoglobin, and hematocrit.

▶ Treatment Steps

*Acute GI Bleeding*
1. Establish IV access for rapid delivery of fluid if necessary.
2. Central venous access may be required in the presence of hemodynamic compromise.

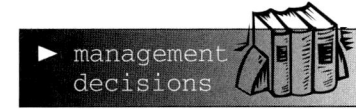

▶ management decisions

### GASTROINTESTINAL HEMORRHAGE

1. Assess severity of process. Does patient have massive hemorrhage, hypotension, and tachycardia?
2. If the patient has massive hemorrhage, then urgent surgical evaluation is needed.
3. Hemodynamic instability requires large bore IV access and potentially central venous access with careful monitoring of blood pressure, heart rate, and hemoglobin.

3. Replacement of blood loss with normal saline or blood products (whole blood if available or primarily pRBCs plus platelets and plasma).
4. Regular monitoring of hemoglobin and hematocrit and vital signs to detect ongoing or recurrent bleeding.

*Rapid Upper GI Bleeding*
1. Upper endoscopy with sclerosis of varices.
2. Coagulation of bleeding ulcers with laser, thermocoagulation, or electrocautery.
3. If bleeding persists and is severe, use of arterial vasoconstrictors can be attempted.
4. Angiography with local vasoconstrictors or embolization of bleeding site may also be attempted.
5. Depending on the rate of bleeding and the site, surgery may be indicated.

*Rapid Lower GI Bleeding*
1. Colonoscopy to identify the site of bleeding is usually not helpful.
2. Arteriography followed by infusion of vasoconstrictors at the bleeding site may be necessary.
3. Emergency surgery may also be necessary.

*Less Severe Acute Bleeding*
1. Watchful waiting is indicated for most GI bleeding because most episodes are self-limited.
2. Replacement of blood may be indicated if the patient's underlying medical condition will not tolerate waiting for the bone marrow to replenish the blood supply (eg, coronary artery disease).
3. Long-term therapy includes iron replacement.
4. Patients should not be fed orally until their condition is stable.

*Chronic GI Bleeding*
1. Radiologic and endoscopic evaluation to determine the source of bleeding.
2. Replace iron.

## H. Diarrhea

▶ H&P Keys

General medical history; onset, duration, and pattern of symptoms (establish whether acute or chronic); relationship of diarrhea to food intake; stool characteristics (color, quantity, formed, excessive odor, presence of blood or mucus); other GI symptoms accompanying diarrhea (nausea, vomiting, abdominal pain, flatulence, bloating); weight loss; medication history (especially recent use of antibiotic); dietary history (especially lactose, sorbitol use, fat substitutes, unusual or raw meats); history of substance abuse; psychological and psychiatric history (stressors, eating disorder); previous abdominal surgery; travel history; and risk factors for HIV disease. Complete physical exam, including vital signs (fever, blood pressure, orthostatic changes), weight, oral mucosa (moist or dry), axillary sweat, abdominal exam (tenderness, distention, mass), rectal exam (blood, mucus, fecal impaction).

▶ Diagnosis

Causes of acute diarrhea (< 2 weeks) include viral, bacterial, or parasite infection; medications; diverticulitis; ischemic colitis; and inflammatory bowel disease. If patient looks ill, has high fever, bloody diarrhea, or dehydration, studies include CBC, serum electrolytes, stool exam for white blood cells, ova, and parasites; stool culture; *Clostridium difficile* toxin; and liver function tests (if elevated, check viral serology). In the elderly, radiologic studies may be indicated for acute diverticulitis and ischemic colitis. For chronic diarrhea, most patients should have CBC, serum electrolytes, total protein, albumin, pancreatic enzymes, liver function tests, stool exam for ova and parasites, and thyroid stimulating hormone. Further testing may include colonoscopy, upper endoscopy with biopsy, fecal fat quantification if malabsorption is suspected, specific tests for type of malabsorption, and blood levels of secreted substances that could cause diarrhea. Causes include inflammatory bowel disease; malabsorption from pancreatic insufficiency, lactose intolerance, bacterial overgrowth, amyloidosis, celiac sprue, intestinal bypass surgery, Whipple's disease; secretory substances from carcinoid tumor, Zollinger–Ellison syndrome, villous adenoma, medullary carcinoma of thyroid, vasoactive intestinal peptide secreting adenoma; changes in bowel motility (diabetes mellitus, irritable bowel syndrome, scleroderma); obstruction (fecal impaction, malignant tumor); medications; and hyperthyroidism.

▶ Concept and Application

Many mechanisms are possible for this symptom. For example, damage to intestinal mucosa from infection, toxins, inflammatory diseases, irradiation, or vascular disease. Medications also cause diarrhea by a variety of mechanisms. Malabsorption causes undigested solute to be delivered to the intestine, stimulating secretory function of the bowel. Neurologic, endocrine, or idiopathic conditions may cause changes in intestinal motility.

▶ Treatment Steps

1. Identify underlying cause of diarrhea.
2. Avoid antidiarrheals if infection is suspected while workup is underway.
3. Treat symptoms with psyllium, loperamide, diphenoxylate with atropine, and/or cholestyramine once infection is ruled out.
4. Clonidine for diabetic diarrhea.
5. Octreotide for VIPomas and carcinoid tumors.

## I. Reye's Syndrome

▶ H&P Keys

Age of patient (most likely in children ages 2–16 years); recent viral illness (upper respiratory, GI, varicella); nausea and vomiting; depressed mental status; seizures. Examine patient for increased respiratory rate, hepatomegaly, and altered mental status (from lethargy to agitation to decorticate posturing to decerebrate posturing to flaccid).

▶ **Diagnosis**

Serum electrolytes (metabolic acidosis with respiratory alkalosis), liver function tests (extremely high aspartate transaminase, alanine transaminase, and lactic dehydrogenase [LDH]; moderate increases in bilirubin), elevated arterial ammonia levels, prolonged PT/PTT, low serum glucose. CT or MRI scan of head to rule out other causes of change in mental status, and liver biopsy if diagnosis is uncertain.

▶ **Disease Severity**

Arterial ammonia > 300 µg/dL. Prognosis is worse with increasing degree of depressed mental status on admission.

▶ **Concept and Application**

Pathology is unknown. Epidemiologically associated with use of aspirin with a viral infection. Involves mitochondria of brain or liver causing cerebral edema.

▶ **Treatment Steps**
1. Reduce cerebral edema by:
   - Increasing serum osmolarity with hyperosmolar solutions.
   - Elevating patient's head 30 degrees.
   - Intubation and hyperventilation if patient is posturing.
2. Administer osmotic agents and barbiturates.
3. Monitor serum electrolytes, glucose, PT/PTT, and ammonia levels.
4. Follow serial EEGs.
5. Treat seizures if needed.
6. Avoid lumbar puncture if possible.

## J. Dyspepsia

▶ **H&P Keys**

Onset, severity, pattern, duration of symptoms; abdominal pain and pressure; gassiness or bloating; excessive belching; burning sensation in chest; weight loss; bowel movements; psychological stressors; dietary history (symptoms often follow ingestion of food or specific foods); early satiety; medication history. Physical exam is usually nonspecific.

▶ **Diagnosis**

In patients younger than 40 years, diagnostic testing reserved for those who do not respond to symptomatic and dietary therapy.

In older patients, especially those with abdominal pain, imaging studies of the upper and lower GI tracts, pancreas, and biliary tract by endoscopy or radiologic studies should be done as directed by history and physical exam. If no etiology for the symptoms can be uncovered after directed set of exams, dyspepsia becomes a likely diagnosis.

GI disease or systemic disease may generate similar symptoms, but dyspepsia is a diagnosis of exclusion.

▶ **Disease Severity**

Determined by the patient's complaints. No study is available to quantitate severity.

▶ Concept and Application

Unknown and likely multifactorial. Hypotheses include a functional illness secondary to a psychological disorder or a subtle motility disorder.

▶ Treatment Steps
1. Restrict patient's diet on the basis of the dietary history.
2. Trial of $H_2$-blockers or antacids.
3. Trial of medications to improve gastric motility.
4. Counsel patient on nature of symptoms.

## K. Abdominal Pain

▶ H&P Keys

Onset, character, location, pattern, duration, intensity of pain; maneuvers that elicit or relieve pain; nausea, vomiting, melena, bright red blood per rectum, constipation, diarrhea; weight loss, anorexia; concurrent or recent infections; history of trauma, peptic ulcer disease, alcohol use, pancreatitis, biliary disease, previous abdominal surgeries, malignancy, or kidney stones; medications; dietary history; gynecologic history; general medical illness (especially diabetes, vascular disease, sickle cell anemia). Physical exam includes general appearance of patient and vital signs. Inspection of abdomen for signs of distention and retroperitoneal hemorrhage (eg, flank ecchymoses); palpation to localize tenderness, detect rebound tenderness, and identify masses and organomegaly; auscultation to detect presence and character of bowel sounds and percussion to detect shifting dullness of ascites; cough test for peritoneal inflammation. Rectal exam to check for pain suggesting pelvic peritonitis and for obvious or occult blood. Gynecologic exam to check for pain suggesting pelvic peritonitis, purulent cervical discharge, and cervicitis.

▶ Diagnosis

Studies: depend on patient's clinical status and which diagnoses seem most likely after the history and physical exam. Initially, CBC, electrolytes, BUN and creatinine, pancreatic enzymes, liver function tests, and urinalysis. Further blood testing would depend on outcome of previous tests and clinical picture. Other studies may include obstruction series, abdominal ultrasound, water-soluble contrast or barium enema, angiography, CT scan of abdomen and pelvis, endoscopy of GI tract, radionuclide studies, laparoscopy, aspiration of peritoneal fluid.

▶ Concept and Application

Abdominal pain has multiple causes, including the following: traumatic rupture of abdominal organs, inflammatory bowel disease, abdominal abscess, irritable bowel disease, trauma to abdominal musculature, peptic ulcer disease (with or without perforation), pancreatitis, appendicitis, hepatitis, ruptured viscus or diverticuli, acute cholecystitis, ascending cholangitis, intestinal obstruction, ureteral obstruction (extrinsic or intrinsic), aortic aneurysm rupture, intestinal ischemia, bowel infarction, ectopic pregnancy, pelvic inflammatory disease, ruptured ovarian cyst, torsion of ovary or testicle, diabetic ketoacidosis, sickle-cell crisis, porphyria, C1 esterase deficiency, familial Mediterranean fever, embolic disease, vasculitis, and toxins.

▶ Disease Severity

Acute onset, autonomic stimulation (tachycardia, tachypnea), hemodynamic instability, signs of peritoneal inflammation, signs of perforation, severity of pain, metabolic acidosis, signs of obstruction.

▶ Treatment Steps

1. Radiologic and laboratory evaluation as outlined above.
2. Avoid pain medications that might mask the underlying condition (until a diagnosis is established).
3. Administer antibiotics if infection is at all possible.
4. For chronic abdominal pain, an outpatient evaluation on the basis of symptoms and exam can be done if no acceleration of the symptoms occurs.

## L. Nausea and Vomiting

▶ H&P Keys

Onset and duration of symptoms (acute versus chronic), character of vomitus (color, contents, blood, or "coffee grounds"), relationship to eating, history or symptoms of eating disorders, accompanying GI symptoms (diarrhea, abdominal pain, constipation), weight loss, signs of infection (fever, myalgias, cough, dysuria, frequency), medication history, substance abuse history, pregnancy, vertigo, tinnitus, history or symptoms of central nervous system disease, chest pain, history of cardiac disease, psychological stressors, previous surgical history (especially GI surgery). Physical exam includes general appearance, vital signs, signs of dehydration (orthostasis, dry mucous membranes, absence of axillary sweat), abdominal exam, complete exam for systemic disease that may cause nausea and vomiting.

▶ Diagnosis

Studies: serum electrolytes, BUN and serum creatinine, CBC, liver function tests, pancreatic enzymes, urine or serum pregnancy test. Further tests depend on results of history and physical; may include endoscopy and radiologic studies of GI tract, ultrasound of abdomen, obstruction series, stool examination for pathogens, CT of abdomen, gastric emptying study, ECG. GI causes include gastric outlet obstruction, gastroparesis, peptic ulcer disease, upper GI tract bleeding, appendicitis, intestinal obstruction, cholecystitis, pancreatitis, peritonitis, perforation, and infection (viral or bacterial or parasitosis). Other causes include renal failure, cardiac disease (myocardial infarction), CNS disease (tumor, encephalitis, meningitis, hydrocephalus), migraine headaches, labrynthitis, Ménière's disease, endocrine disease (diabetic ketoacidosis, adrenal insufficiency, hyperthyroidism), pregnancy, medications, toxins, psychiatric disease and psychological stress.

### ▶ Concept and Application

Vomiting center, in lateral reticular formation, controls acts of vomiting. Inputs to this center arise from chemoreceptor trigger zone in floor of fourth ventricle, GI tract, cerebral cortex, higher midbrain, labrynthine apparatus, and other parts of body. Output from vomiting center goes to phrenic nerve, spinal nerves, and vagus nerve to larynx, pharynx, esophagus, and stomach.

### ▶ Treatment Steps

1. Identify underlying condition.
2. Treat symptoms with dopamine antagonists (eg, metoclopramide) or serotonin $5\text{-HT}_3$-receptor antagonists (eg, ondansetron).
3. Antihistamines and anticholinergics are useful for motion sickness and labrynthitis.
4. Corticosteroids and lorazepam are useful in severe nausea and vomiting.

## M. Dysphagia

### ▶ H&P Keys

Difficulty swallowing (solids, liquids, or both) or moving foods from mouth to esophagus; pain on swallowing (odynophagia); symptoms of gastroesophageal reflux; coughing or choking on swallowing; sensation of food or medications getting stuck in middle of chest or at xyphoid process; course of dysphagia (onset, duration: did difficulty swallowing solids precede difficulty swallowing liquids? Are symptoms progressive or intermittent?), weight loss; history of aspiration of a foreign body, aspiration pneumonia, neurologic disease, ingestion of caustic substances (eg, lye), cigarette smoking, iron deficiency anemia, or irradiation of head, neck, or mediastinal structures; hoarseness of voice; or substance abuse. Physical symptoms include inflammatory or exudative lesions of mouth and/or tongue, cervical adenopathy, thyromegaly, neck mass, fine or coarse extra-breath sounds. Neurologic exam to detect cerebrovascular accident or neuromuscular disease.

### ▶ Diagnosis

Diagnostic tests should include ear, nose, and throat exam, with laryngoscopy, cineradiographic barium swallow, upper endoscopy, esophageal motility studies, chest roentgenogram, CT of chest as indicated by history and physical exam. Causes include oropharyngeal dysphagia (difficulty moving food from mouth to pharynx to esophagus as result of neurologic disease such as cerebrovascular accident or upper and lower motor neuron disease), myopathy, cricopharyngeal achalasia, Zencker's diverticulum, or tumors; esophageal dysphagia (difficulty swallowing within the esophagus) caused by obstructing lesions such as strictures, benign tumors, malignant tumor, neuromuscular disease, achalasia of lower esophageal sphincter, motility disorders, or lesion of upper stomach.

▶ Disease Severity

Dysphagia for solids progressing to dysphagia for liquids suggests an expanding obstructive lesion. Weight loss suggests significant impairment or underlying malignancy.

▶ Concept and Application

Swallowing is complex process involving cerebral cortex; input from GI tract, brain stem swallowing center, and cranial nerves V, VII, IX, X, XII, and smooth and striated muscles. Neuromuscular lesions, inflammatory conditions, tumors, esophageal diverticulum, and infiltrative disease can cause difficulty swallowing.

▶ Management

Dependent on underlying cause of the symptom. Achalasias and strictures may be treated with dilatation; achalasia may require myotomy. Esophageal cancers may be treated by resection, radiation therapy, or chemotherapy, depending on the stage; palliation is by laser therapy or bougienage. Neurologic conditions may respond to rehabilitation or may require nasogastric, gastric, or jejunal feedings.

## N. Jaundice

▶ H&P Keys

Onset and duration of symptoms; presence of yellow coloring of skin or sclera and darkening of urine; abdominal pain; fever; pruritus; acholic stools; weight loss; changes in bowel movements; anorexia; arthralgias; medications; substance abuse (especially alcohol); or history of congestive heart failure, malignancy, cholelithiasis, liver disease, or travel to areas where hepatitis is endemic. Physical exam should include color of skin (yellow to green), skin excoriations, and skin stigmata of hepatic cirrhosis (spider angiomata, gynecomastia, palmar erythema), vital signs (fever), lymphadenopathy, signs of congestive heart failure (jugular venous distention, pulmonary congestion, enlarged heart, pedal edema), and abdominal exam (liver size may be small, normal, or enlarged; edge of liver may be smooth or nodular; liver may be tender or nontender); pancreatic mass or gallbladder may be palpable; splenomegaly may be present with cirrhosis.

▶ Diagnosis

Studies: bilirubin levels (direct = conjugated, indirect = unconjugated); liver function tests (increased alkaline phosphatase and γ-glutamyl transferase suggest obstruction; increased aminotransferases suggest hepatocellular disease). CBC and PT/PTT; viral serology and drug screen if indicated by history and physical exam. Ultrasound of liver, CT scan of abdomen, liver biopsy, percutaneous cholangiography, endoscopic retrograde cholangiopancreatography may be indicated. Serum bilirubin usually equal to or greater than 2.0 mg/dL for detectable jaundice. Unconjugated bilirubinemia (80–90% of total bilirubin) is associated with hemolysis, absorption of hematoma, ineffective erythropoiesis, Gilbert syndrome, neonatal jaundice, Crigler–Najjar syndrome, and medications. Conjugated bilirubinemia (50% of total bilirubin) is associated with hepatitis, cirrhosis, biliary cirrhosis, medications, alcoholic liver disease, sepsis, Dubin–Johnson syndrome, Rotor's syndrome, cholestatic jaundice of pregnancy, cholelithiasis, sclerosing cholangitis, pancreatitis, malignancy, biliary atresia, biliary stricture, postoperative, and benign recurrent cholestasis.

▶ Disease Severity

May be reflected by degree of liver enzyme elevation but is not always directly correlated. Normal enzyme levels may reflect decreased synthetic activity that is seen in significant liver damage.

▶ Concept and Application

Increased unconjugated bilirubin is secondary to increased production, diminished uptake into liver, or diminished conjugation. Increased conjugated bilirubinemia is the result of hepatocellular damage or intrahepatic or extrahepatic cholestasis or obstruction.

▶ Treatment Steps

1. Identify etiology of jaundice.
2. Treat underlying process.

## O. Ascites

▶ H&P Keys

Onset and duration of abdominal swelling or distention, abdominal pain, weight loss, anorexia, shortness of breath, orthopnea, pedal edema, symptoms of reflux and burning, malaise and weakness, alcohol intake, or history of malignancy, heart, liver, or renal disease. Physical exam includes vital signs, check for orthostasis. Skin exam for spider angiomata and palmar erythema. Neck exam for jugular venous distention and supraclavicular adenopathy. Lung exam for rales or dullness to auscultation, percussion, or both, suggesting pulmonary edema or pleural effusion. Heart exam for enlargement, S3, and irregular rhythm. Abdominal exam to inspect for distention, auscultation for bowel sounds, and palpation for fluid wave, shifting dullness, abdominal mass, tenderness, liver size, and splenic enlargement. Gynecologic exam for pelvic masses and tenderness.

▶ Diagnosis

Studies: Establish ascites if uncertain from physical exam; ultrasound or CT scan of abdomen. Once ascites is confirmed, paracentesis of abdominal fluid to check for protein, albumin, lactic dehydrogenase (LDH), cell count, Gram stain and culture, cytology, and triglycerides (if indicated to differentiate transudate from exudative effusion). Peritoneal biopsy may be indicated for tuberculosis (TB). CBC, liver function tests, serum electrolytes, BUN, and creatinine; PT/PTT, albumin, and chest roentgenogram. Additional studies such as liver biopsy, Doppler ultrasound, laparoscopy, and angiography may be indicated to establish etiology. Causes include cirrhotic liver disease, congestive heart failure, nephrotic syndrome, malignancy (either primary or secondary), spontaneous bacterial peritonitis, trauma, TB, parasites, hepatic vein thrombosis, benign ovarian tumors, pancreatic pseudocyst, and peritoneal carcinomatosis.

▶ Concept and Application

Ascites fluid can be secondary to increased hydrostatic forces such as hepatic congestion from congestive heart failure or decreased oncotic pressure from hypoalbuminemia. Both mechanisms result in transudative ascites. Exudative ascites fluid is usually secondary to disease affecting peritoneum directly, such as tumor or infection.

▶ Treatment Steps

1. Identify etiology of ascites once presence is confirmed.
2. Treat underlying cause if possible (eg, congestive heart failure or ovarian cancer).
3. Salt and fluid restriction.
4. Administer potassium-sparing diuretics.
5. Add loop diuretics if needed.
6. Therapeutic paracentesis if patient is not intravascularly volume depleted and has symptoms such as shortness of breath.
7. Large-volume paracentesis requires careful hemodynamic monitoring and possibly intravascular fluid replacement (albumin).
8. Consider shunting in recurrent cirrhotic ascites unresponsive to medical management.

## P. Weight Loss

▶ H&P Keys

Documentation or confirmation of weight loss (intentional or involuntary); food history; associated symptoms of anorexia, nausea or vomiting, dysphagia, diarrhea, abdominal pain, fever, night sweats, polyuria; life stressors; history of malignancy, thyroid problem, diabetes, depression, or cardiac, pulmonary, thyroid, or GI disease; recent travel; medication and alcohol use; poor dentition; lymphadenopathy; thyroid mass or enlargement; jaundice or rash; abnormal abdominal exam; peripheral neuropathy.

▶ Diagnosis

Studies: electrolytes, glucose, BUN, creatinine. Stool hemoccult, chest roentgenogram, liver function tests if malignancy is suspected. Stool samples if GI loss is suspected, and thyroid function tests if thyroid disease is suspected. Causes include decreased intake resulting from malignancy, depression or anxiety, anorexia nervosa, inadequate access to food, drug or alcohol intake, HIV infection, liver disease, hypercalcemia, or severe infection, dementia, cardiopulmonary, or renal disease. Normal or increased intake resulting from malignancy, diabetes, hyperthyroidism, fever, GI disease (malabsorption), or anxiety.

▶ Disease Severity

Depends on underlying etiology. In the elderly, involuntary weight loss exceeding 5% within 1 year.

▶ Concept and Application

Principal mechanisms are inadequate intake, excessive metabolic needs, or nutrient losses.

▶ Treatment Steps
1. Treat underlying disease.
2. Administer mineral and vitamin supplements if needed.
3. In HIV- and malignancy-related weight loss, megestrol acetate is helpful to stimulate appetite.
4. Enteral or parenteral nutrition supplements if needed.

## BIBLIOGRAPHY

Carey CF, Lee H. *The Washington Manual of Medical Therapeutics.* 30th ed. Philadelphia: Lippincott Williams & Wilkins; 2001.

Fauci AS, Braunwald E, Isselbacher KJ, Martin JB. *Harrison's Principles of Internal Medicine.* 15th ed. New York: McGraw-Hill; 2001.

Tierney LM Jr., McPhee SJ, Papadakis MA, eds. *Current Medical Diagnosis and Treatment.* 42nd ed. New York: McGraw-Hill; 2003.

# Otolaryngology and Respiratory System Diseases | 20

I. **DISEASES OF THE EAR / 647**
   A. Infectious Otitis Externa / 647
   B. Malignant Otitis Externa / 647
   C. Acute Otitis Media / 648
   D. Chronic Otitis Media / 649
   E. Otitis Media with Effusion (Serous Otitis Media) / 650
   F. Cerumen (Earwax) Impaction / 651
   G. Vertigo / 651
   H. Otalgia / 653
   I. Hearing Loss / 653
   J. Sudden Hearing Loss / 655
   K. Barotrauma / 656
   L. Tinnitus / 657

II. **DISEASES OF THE MOUTH AND THROAT / 657**
   A. Herpes Simplex of the Orocavity / 657
   B. Oral Thrush (Candidiasis, Monoliasis) / 658
   C. Masses in the Nasopharynx / 658
   D. Malignant Neoplasms of the Oropharynx and Hypopharynx / 659
   E. Hoarseness / 660
   F. Strep Throat (Acute Tonsillitis/Pharyngitis) / 660
   G. Cancer of the Larynx / 661

III. **DISEASES OF THE RESPIRATORY SYSTEM / 662**
   A. Acute Sinusitis / 662
   B. Chronic Sinusitis / 662
   C. Fungal Sinusitis / 663
   D. Chronic Rhinitis / 664
   E. Allergic Rhinitis / 664
   F. Epistaxis (Nosebleed) / 665

G. Disorders of Olfaction and Taste / 667
H. Acute Upper Respiratory Infection (Most Common in Winter Months) / 667
I. Wegener's Granulomatosis / 668
J. Cystic Fibrosis / 669

**BIBLIOGRAPHY / 669**

## I. DISEASES OF THE EAR

### A. Infectious Otitis Externa

▶ H&P Keys

Pain in the external canal that can be enhanced by tragal pressure or by tugging on the auricle. Erythema of the ear canal and evidence of debris and swelling within the canal on otoscopy, occasional erythema of the pinna, and swelling in the postauricular space. History of mild ear canal trauma, exposure to high humidity, or swimming. Sensations of fullness, tinnitus, and hearing loss; occasional sensations of disequilibrium, itching of external canal.

▶ Diagnosis

Direct examination, identification of offending organism by Gram stain and/or culture.

▶ Disease Severity

Pain, fever, degree of swelling, closure of ear canal, regional soft-tissue swelling and erythema, and lymphadenopathy.

▶ Concept and Application

Contamination of the external canal by contaminated water or trauma of the ear canal by manipulation permits invasion of offending organism; organisms are usually mixed, bacterial, or fungal. Implies failure of the piloapocrine system and the protective effect of cerumen.

▶ Treatment Steps

1. Acute: Cleansing of ear canal, inspect eardrum to rule out middle-ear disease, place a wick to carry otic drops to the canal and maintain in place; otic drops usually containing 2% acetic acid to change pH of canal, hydrocortisone to reduce inflammation and swelling, and a specific topical antibiotic usually to cover gram-positive as well as gram-negative organisms; pain management is important, and antibiotics should be administered if the infection has extended beyond the confines of the canal to produce lymphadenopathy, soft-tissue involvement, and fever.
2. Subsequent prophylaxis requires keeping the ear dry and using prophylactic (acetic acid or alcohol) drops to decontaminate the ear after bathing or swimming in the future.

### B. Malignant Otitis Externa

▶ H&P Keys

Auricular pain, discharge, hearing loss, feeling of fullness, granular tissue within the external auditory canal. Usually a history of immunocompromise such as diabetes mellitus, old age, or HIV infection. Presence of lymphadenopathy and evidence of infiltration into surrounding soft tissues; loss of cranial function, including facial nerve (VII) and cranial nerves X, XI, XII.

▶ **Diagnosis**

Should include culturing the external auditory canal for offending organism, computed tomography (CT) scan to determine extent of bony destruction and infiltration into surrounding soft tissues. Possibly, subsequent magnetic resonance imaging (MRI) to evaluate presence of intracranial disease, and gallium and technetium scans to detect presence of bony involvement of surrounding structures.

▶ **Disease Severity**

Expanding soft-tissue involvement with intracranial spread and decreased function of cranial nerve.

▶ **Concept and Application**

Severe infection of periauricular soft tissue and bone in immunocompromised host, with rapidly expanding and infiltrating infection with potential for cranial nerve destruction, central nervous system (CNS) involvement. Most common organism is *Pseudomonas aeruginosa*.

▶ **Treatment Steps**

1. Intravenous antibiotics, with judicious debridement as necessary.
2. Despite aggressive treatment, still significant percentage of mortality.

## C. Acute Otitis Media

▶ **H&P Keys**

This infection usually occurs in all age groups but is more prevalent in children ages 3 months to 7 years of age. Occurs more frequently during winter months and is associated with upper respiratory tract and viral infections. Symptoms and signs normally include hyperemia of the tympanic membrane with erythema, exudate within the middle-ear space, and, at times, purulent discharge from the external canal as well as pain and dizziness with decreased appetite in young children. Other signs and symptoms are hearing loss, tinnitus, and, on occasion, imbalance; fever also is a key point.

▶ **Diagnosis**

Direct inspection via otoscopy, culture of any purulent debris from the external canal, and tympanocentesis in infants under 3 months of age.

▶ **Disease Severity**

Degree of fever, pain, hearing loss, and duration of otorrhea when present. Postauricular swelling indicates spread of disease process to mastoid air cell system; the presence of adenopathy within the parotid and upper neck indicates extension into soft tissues in surrounding regions. Necrotizing otitis media, β-hemolytic streptococci seen in patients with concomitant disease process or immunocompromise.

▶ Concept and Application

The basic etiology is eustachian tube dysfunction with bacterial spread through the eustachian tube from the nasopharynx into the middle-ear space. Most common organisms include strep pneumonia and *Haemophilus influenzae;* also *Branhamella catarrhalis,* streptococcus and staphylococcus, but less commonly; in infants gram-negative organisms such as *Escherichia coli* must be identified during tympanocentesis (most common in infants younger than 6 weeks).

▶ Treatment Steps

1. Systemic antibiotics, usually amoxicillin (30–40 mg/kg per day for uncomplicated infections and for children under age 12; other antibiotics used are amoxicillin–clavulanate, erythromycin, sulfa for children allergic to penicillin, and trimethoprim–sulfamethoxazole and cephalosporins as necessary.
2. Myringotomy may be indicated to determine bacteriology as well as tympanocentesis (as mentioned).
3. When purulent discharge and tympanic membrane perforation exist, topical antibiotic drops in addition to systemic antibiotics are useful.
4. Acute otitis media may benefit from prophylactic antibiotics as well as possible myringotomy and tube placement.

## D. Chronic Otitis Media

▶ H&P Keys

Chronic otitis media is a rare complication of acute otitis media. It is manifested by the presence of a tympanic membrane perforation or development of a cholesteatoma in the middle-ear space, particularly in the area of the pars flaccida. The physical findings are drum perforations with persistent otorrhea, hearing loss, tinnitus, presence of retraction pockets with epithelial debris, and occasional sensations of disequilibrium and vertigo.

▶ Diagnosis

Diagnostic studies include direct otoscopy, with careful cleansing of tympanic membrane area to identify presence or absence of perforation, its position and size. The character of the middle-ear mucous membrane is seen through the perforation and the presence or absence of epithelial debris either within the middle ear or in the pars flaccida area. Tuning-fork studies will suggest the reversal of the Rinne, with lateralization to the side of greatest conduction loss; and audiogram, tympanogram, CT scans of temporal bone, both axial and coronal views without contrast, help delineate the degree and severity of disease and location of bone destruction and cholesteatoma if present. Cultures are helpful in determining antibiotic therapy; chronic otitis media is produced most commonly by *P. aeruginosa* and staphylococcal organisms; not uncommonly *Proteus mirabilis* and *E. coli* may be present. Culture sensitivity is needed to determine the offending organism.

▶ Disease Severity

Degree of perforation and otorrhea, vertigo, degree of hearing loss, presence of facial nerve paralysis, or headache indicate the possibility of intracranial extension of middle-ear and mastoid disease.

▶ Concept and Application

Recurrent acute otitis media or single episode of acute necrotizing otitis media produce obstruction of tympanic membrane and chronic changes in the mucous membrane of the middle ear and mastoid concomitant with eustachian tube obstruction. Organisms involved are *P. aeruginosa* (most commonly) and *Staphylococcus aureus;* occasionally, *Proteus* species as well as *E. coli* may be isolates. In immunocompromised patients, acid-fast and fungal disease must be considered.

▶ Treatment Steps

1. Antibiotics directed at gram-negative organisms; treatment with antibiotics for 3–6 weeks; concomitant use of otic drops with broad-spectrum antibiotics, acidifying agents (2% acetic acid), and often steroids to reduce inflammation.
2. In patients with perforation, the ear must be kept dry during washing and bathing; swimming is not allowed.
3. If cholesteatoma is present, this is a surgical disease requiring extirpation of the cholesteatoma and sealing of the eardrum by means of tympanoplasty, with or without reconstruction of the ossicular chain if it is involved.

E. Otitis Media with Effusion (Serous Otitis Media)

▶ H&P Keys

History is associated with multiple bouts of acute otitis media with slow resolution. Condition also should be suspected in children with language delay and decreased response to auditory cues. Signs and symptoms include decreased hearing, retracted eardrum, dullness to the tympanic membrane, and straw-colored fluid with bubbles within the middle-ear space.

▶ Diagnosis

Direct visualization via otoscopy and insufflation during pneumatic otoscopy; also tympanometry and audiometry.

▶ Disease Severity

Degree of hearing loss, as noted on audiometry, and disability in response to auditory cues.

▶ Concept and Application

Eustachian tube blockage, with subsequent negative pressure within the middle-ear space changing the surface tension and producing metaplasia of epithelium of middle ear to a secretory epithelium migrating from the eustachian tube orifice of the middle ear.

▶ Treatment Steps
1. Initial management should be observation for approximately 3 months, during which 90% resolve.
2. Generally, antibiotics are offered initially; some suggest that antihistamine decongestants are not uniquely helpful. In adults with serous otitis media, if unilateral, one must pay careful attention to the nasopharynx to rule out nasopharyngeal lesions—again, particularly in immunocompromised hosts.
3. If the serous otitis media does not resolve and hearing loss persists after a period of careful observation and treatment, myringotomy with aspiration of the middle ear content and subsequent placement of ventilation tubes is the treatment of choice. In adults, attempts at autoinflation with Valsalva's maneuver is often effective in resolving serous otitis media; in children with recurrent nonresolving serous otitis media, adenoidectomy with or without tonsillectomy is often recommended.

## F. Cerumen (Earwax) Impaction

▶ H&P Keys

The patient will often complain of a history of feeling of fullness in the ear; decreased hearing, often after washing; pressure in the ear; and occasional pain in the external ear.

▶ Diagnosis

Direct visualization via otoscopy.

▶ Disease Severity

Quality of hearing loss and degree of cerumen impaction. Rule out foreign body within the external canal, particularly in children and retarded patients.

▶ Concept and Application

Often occurs with physical manipulation of the ear canal, particularly with the use of cotton applicators and digging in the ears. Narrow canal with increased cerumen production and possible foreign body.

▶ Treatment Steps

Removal of cerumen by mechanical irrigation when an intact tympanic membrane is known, or use of instruments, suction, or both as appropriate to degree of impaction and quality of cerumen.

## G. Vertigo

▶ H&P Keys

Vertigo is a complex complaint; it must be determined whether the vertigo is otologic, central, or medical in origin. Determining whether the disease is peripheral is made easier by the symptom of definite sensation of movement, most often rotary. When the vertigo is paroxysmal and severe, it is more likely to be peripheral; attacks may last minutes to hours (seldom longer) and may be associated with vegetative signs such as sweating, nausea, and vomiting. Patient never loses consciousness. Conversely, central vertigo is more often mild and described as a sensation of light-headedness or unsteadiness. It is vague, without specific onset or termination, and may be constant; attacks may last weeks or months, often without an obvious nystagmus. Associated symptoms of vertigo may be nystagmus (with peripheral pathology, the nystagmus can often be seen); with irritative lesions, nystagmus is often to the side of involved ear; nystagmus with changing of direction is more often central than peripheral. Causes of vertigo of otologic origin are acute otitis media, serous otitis media, head trauma with involvement of labyrinthine apparatus, and trauma to middle ear by penetrating wound, with dislocation of ossicles and production of vertigo and hearing loss, Cogan's syndrome, vestibular neuronitis, temporal bone fractures, acute barotrauma with perilymph fistulas, and endolymphatic hydrops (Ménière's disease). Ménière's disease is a disease process involving abnormal absorption or production of endolymph, which produces a quadrad or triad of symptoms of tinnitus, vertigo, fluctuant hearing loss, and sensations of fullness or blockage in the ear; the disease process may begin suddenly with tinnitus or any of the other symptoms; vertigo is severe and unrelenting for minutes to hours; nausea and vomiting are often present.

▶ Diagnosis

History of fluctuant hearing loss, tinnitus, vertigo, neurosensory hearing loss on audiometric evaluation, evidence of canal paresis with vestibular studies involving the affected ear, negative examinations with intracranial MRI with gadolinium for cranial nerve VIII and neurovascular bundles. Electronystagmography documenting canal paresis or hypoactivity of affected ear.

▶ Disease Severity

Severity of vertigo, length of episodes, frequency of attacks, degree of hearing loss.

▶ Concept and Application

Temporal bone studies indicate presence of hydrops of the endolymphatic space with destruction of neuroepithelium thought to be secondary to abnormality of stria vascularis, endolymphatic sac mechanism, or both.

▶ Treatment Steps

1. For acute cases, benzodiazepam-like drugs are effective if nausea and vomiting are not a problem.
2. For long-term management of Ménière's disease, diuretics and low-sodium diet are often effective.
3. In patients with continuing sensations of disequilibrium who fail to respond to medical therapy, endolymphatic sac decompression; cranial nerve VIII section; or, in patients who have nonfunctioning ears from auditory standpoint and unilateral disease for more than 5 years, labyrinthectomy is procedure of choice; diazepam and antihistamine group such as meclizine hydrochloride, diphenhydramine hydrochloride (Benadryl), or dimenhydrinate (Dramamine).

## H. Otalgia

▶ H&P Keys

Otalgia may represent pain of otologic origin or of distant disease referred to the ears, such as dental infection, pharyngitis, or tonsillitis. Symptoms include ear pain (sharp, constant, dull, or burning). Determination of duration of pain and exacerbating and remitting factors are essential. Physical examination includes inspection of the external ear, otoscopy with examination of external canal and tympanic membrane with middle ear; examination of the temporomandibular joints with direct pressure both externally and on the pterygoid muscles within the orocavity; and complete examination of the upper aerodigestive tract, nasopharynx, oropharynx, tongue, larynx, and hypopharynx.

▶ Diagnosis

If cause is not obvious, diagnostic studies such as CT scan and MRI of upper aerodigestive tract and neck are useful. Studies also include direct laryngoscopy, nasopharyngoscopy, audiologic testing, and tympanometry, as well as palpation of tonsillar fossae, tongue base, and neck. Direct laryngoscopy and cervical esophagoscopy also may be indicated.

▶ Disease Severity

Presence of tumors or lesions in the upper aerodigestive tract referring pain to the ear are of potentially great concern and may be life-threatening.

▶ Concept and Application

Direct stimulation of nerves supplying sensation to the ear via inflammatory process or direct pressure, transmission via the same nerves through the temporomandibular joint and mechanism of referred pain via myositis and muscle spasm from associated joint musculature. Referred pain from tongue base, larynx, or pyriform sinus occurs via the vagus or glossopharyngeal nerve.

▶ Treatment Steps

1. Management will vary, depending on underlying disease process.
2. It may be as simple as cerumen removal or as complex as cancer extirpation and adjunctive treatments.

## I. Hearing Loss

▶ H&P Keys

Obvious loss of hearing acuity is noted either by patient or by friends and family; may be associated with other otologic signs such as tinnitus or vertigo or with associated exposure to loud noise or head trauma. Hearing loss may be mild, moderate, or severe; patient may have congenital hearing loss as a result of either congenital or acquired disease, a history of head injury or recurrent ear infection, exposure to ototoxic drugs, exposure to loud noise, or infectious processes such as meningitis. Physical examination begins with an interview to determine degree of hearing loss; then otoscopy to rule out disease process in external canal or middle ear and tuningfork studies with Rinne and Weber studies as primary modalities.

▶ Diagnosis

Audiometry, including air, bone, and speech discrimination studies; brain stem evoked potential studies when indicated; tympanometry. In children with congenital losses or rapidly progressive neural losses, CT scan of temporal bone and serologic studies for autoimmune disease as well as congenital or acquired syphilis.

▶ Disease Severity

Careful evaluation of the individual's ability to communicate. Degree of hearing loss is evinced on audiometry.

▶ Concept and Application

Conductive hearing losses are manifested primarily by evidence of congenital findings of abnormal pinna and microtia, atresia, and periauricular tags and stenosis. Concomitant congenital abnormalities such as cleft palate, cardiac disease, and kidney abnormalities should trigger search for otic abnormality. Conductive hearing loss in children is most often of congenital or of traumatic origin in infancy. In acquired disease, acute otitis media and serous otitis media affect more than 30% of children at some point. Most common disease in young adults is otosclerosis, with gradual fixation of the stapes foot plate; it is a genetically determined disease process (Mendelian dominant with variable penetrance; Fig. 20–1). Other conductive hearing losses can occur as result of longitudinal fractures of the temporal bone and barotrauma with middle-ear bleeding; effusion also produces conduction hearing losses. Congenital sensorineural hearing losses may be of genetic origin (eg, Waardenburg's syndrome) or caused by congenital syphilis. Acquired neural losses may be secondary to head or ear trauma, meningitis, an autoimmune disease process, acoustic tumors, or syphilis. In the aging population, presbycusis or a gradual high-frequency sensorineural hearing loss is most often seen after age 60.

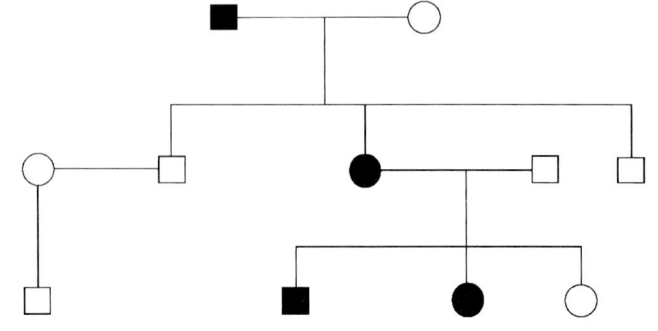

Figure 20–1. Pedigree of a typical family with autosomal dominant hearing loss. Note the multiple affected family members; transmission can be either maternal or paternal. ■, ● Affected male, female; □, ○ unaffected male, female.

▶ Treatment Steps
1. For sensorineural hearing losses of acquired type and of mild to moderate or even severe degree, amplification by means of hearing aid is available.
2. For profound losses not amenable to amplification, cochlear implant surgery is available.
3. For conductive hearing losses secondary to middle-ear disease, aspiration of fluid and myringotomy (as noted), ossicular reconstruction by means of stapes surgery or ossiculoplasty, and tympanoplasty for correction of tympanic membrane perforations.

### J. Sudden Hearing Loss

▶ H&P Keys

History of abrupt hearing loss for minutes to hours. Presence of tinnitus and vertigo and their severity should be determined by clinical history. History should include infection, trauma, vascular problem, otologic problem, neurologic problem, history of neurotoxic drugs, possible diabetes mellitus, autoimmune disorders, etc.

▶ Diagnosis

Audiometric testing, including air and bone conduction, electronystagmography (ENG) and calorics, testing of auditory brain responses, CT scan and MRI of the temporal bone, blood sugar, fluorescent treponemal antibody absorption (FTA-ABS) testing and sedimentation rate, and direct examination.

▶ Disease Severity

Degree of hearing loss as determined by audiogram; presence or absence of vertigo or tinnitus and patient's disability.

▶ diagnostic decisions

### SUDDEN HEARING LOSS

| Indications | Testing |
|---|---|
| All patients | Audiologic/tympanometric testing |
| Acoustic neuroma/skull base lesions | MRI or CT with contrast |
| Autoimmune inner-ear disease | Lymphocyte transformation testing |
| | Western blot immunoassay |
| Syphilis | FTA-ABS |
| | MHA-TP |
| Bacterial infections | Appropriate culture and Lyme disease titer |
| Viral infections | Appropriate titers |
| | HIV testing |
| Miscellaneous | ENG, ABR, ECoG, perilymphic fistula test, CBC, blood chemistries, metabolic studies |

ENG—electronystagmography; ABR—auditory brainstem evoked responses; ECoG—electrocochleography.

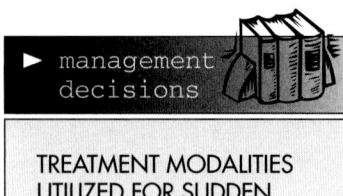

### management decisions

**TREATMENT MODALITIES UTILIZED FOR SUDDEN SENSORINEURAL HEARING LOSS**

**Anti-inflammatory and Immunologic Agents**
Steroids
Prostaglandin

**Antivirals**
Acyclovir

**Calcium Antagonists**
Nifedipine
Diuretics
Hydrochlorothiazide
Lasix

**Vasodilators**
Carbogen
Papaverine
Nicotinic acid
Pentoxifylline

**Volume Expanders**
Hydroxyethyl starch
Dextran

**Other Therapies**
Vitamins
Acupuncture
Procaine

▶ Concept and Application

Multiple etiologies with multiple mechanisms of disease: infection, including mumps; herpes zoster; syphilis; meningitis; otitis media encephalitis; vascular lesions, including embolic phenomenon, coagulopathy, cerebrovascular accident; trauma, including temporal bone fracture, barotrauma, or noise-induced trauma; otologic, including Ménière's disease, perilymph fistula, chronic otitis media, and acoustic neuroma; neurologic disease, including multiple sclerosis, Cogan's syndrome; and metabolic disorders, including diabetes mellitus, drug toxicity, and autoimmune disorders.

▶ Treatment Steps

1. After treatment of the underlying etiology when the hearing loss is idiopathic, high-dose steroids (60 mg Prednisone per day) tapered over 2 to 3 weeks may be beneficial.
2. Other numerous therapies have been employed depending on suspected etiology (see Management Decisions box).

### K. Barotrauma

▶ H&P Keys

History of recent scuba diving or air flight with inability to equalize pressure between external environment and middle ear; pain, tinnitus, hearing loss, and vertigo. Physical examination may reveal hemotympanum, eardrum perforation, nystagmus, nausea, vomiting, and hearing loss.

▶ Diagnosis

Direct inspection of ear via otoscopy and pneumatic otoscopy; audiologic and tympanometric testing; vestibular testing, including electronystagmography (ENG).

▶ Disease Severity

Degree of vertigo and patient's functioning, including hearing loss and duration of symptoms.

▶ Concept and Application

Acute changes in barometric pressure and failure of the eustachian tube to function properly. A large pressure gradient across the middle ear may result in trauma and the destruction of middle ear, inner ear, or both. Eustachian tube dysfunction may be a result of infectious, anatomic, or neoplastic abnormalities. The difference in barometric pressure may result in rupture of round or oval window seals, causing acute inner-ear abnormalities that lead to hearing loss or vertigo. Disruption of the tympanic membrane or vessels within middle ear may result in tympanic membrane perforation or hemotympanum.

▶ Treatment Steps

1. For uncomplicated barotrauma, appropriate nasal decongestants, systemic decongestants, and watchful waiting for resolution of hemotympanum or tympanic membrane perforation.
2. For inner-ear dysfunction, bed rest for 24 hours may result in resolution if no significant hearing loss or vertigo is present;

should these symptoms persist, middle-ear exploration with patching of oval and round windows is treatment of choice.
3. Prevention of barotrauma can be helped with appropriate use of nasal decongestants and systemic decongestants before scuba diving or flying. Patients' tolerance to these medications should be determined prior to use in conjunction with any diving activities!

## L. Tinnitus

▶ H&P Keys

History of noise in the ear, which is generated endogenously, not from the environment. Complaints are about continuous humming, hissing, or whistling. Pulsatile tinnitus that is synchronous with heartbeat may accompany hearing loss or vertigo.

▶ Diagnosis

Tinnitus that is bilateral, symmetrical, and of reasonably long standing is most often benign and requires audiometry. Unilateral tinnitus or pulsatile tinnitus requires workup with MRI, MRA, auscultation of the chest and neck to determine presence of transmitted or carotid bruits, auscultation within the ear to determine presence or absence of lesions, and CT scan to rule out vascular lesions of the ear.

▶ Disease Severity

Tinnitus may be extremely loud and produce inability to concentrate, sleep, or function. Tinnitus matching audiogram, CT scan, MRI, auscultation of neck, ultrasound, noninvasive studies of great vessels of neck, and transcranial Dopplers. Examination of the ear for vascular lesions involving middle ear.

▶ Concept and Application

Tinnitus may result from cochlear disease secondary to acoustic trauma, ototoxic drugs, viral or vascular disease of the cochlea, otosclerosis, conductive hearing loss such as ossicular discontinuity secondary to trauma, and serous otitis media. Tinnitus also may be of central origin, with brain stem lesions or eighth nerve lesions secondary to acoustic tumors. Patient should have temporomandibular joint examination as well.

▶ Treatment Steps
As per etiology.

# II. DISEASES OF THE MOUTH AND THROAT

## A. Herpes Simplex of the Orocavity

▶ H&P Keys

History of prodromal fever, headache, irritability, malaise, nausea, vomiting, halitosis, and tender adenopathy. Usually includes children ages 2–5 years.

▶ Diagnosis

Clinical examination with Giemsa stain evaluation of vesicular fluid revealing syncytial giant cells with intranuclear inclusions.

▶ Disease Severity

Degree of symptoms listed above.

▶ Concept and Application

Initial herpesvirus type I. Infection usually occurs in children ages 2–5 years.

▶ Treatment Steps

1. Symptomatic therapy includes salt water gargles and irrigations, soft diet, antipyretics and topical anesthetics as needed.
2. Intravenous (IV) hydration for severe debilitation.

## B. Oral Thrush (Candidiasis, Monoliasis)

▶ H&P Keys

Tends to occur in patients who are immunocompromised, debilitated, diabetic, or HIV positive; have used antibiotics or steroids for prolonged periods; or are receiving radiotherapy. Also seen in normal infants. Signs and symptoms include oral pain, odynophagia, and dysphagia. Physical examination reveals erythematous and edematous mucosa with soft, white exudate, which is easily scraped, revealing red, slightly ulcerated surface. Fever and adenopathy are unusual.

▶ Diagnosis

Physical examination, Gram's stain revealing yeast forms, culture on Saboraud's agar.

▶ Disease Severity

Depends on underlying etiology.

▶ Concept and Application

*Candida albicans* occurs on 25% of normal mucosa; a normal saprophytic organism becomes pathogenic in circumstances mentioned.

▶ Treatment Steps

1. Includes nystatin oral suspension (200,000 units per cc, 2–3 cc swish and swallow) every 4 hours until inflammation is controlled.
2. Mycelex troches or other antifungal agents also can be used.

## C. Masses in the Nasopharynx

▶ H&P Keys

History of nasal obstruction, bleeding, hearing loss, pain, and neck masses.

▶ Diagnosis

Direct examination of nasopharynx by anterior rhinoscopy, flexible intranasal endoscopy, rigid endoscopy, mirror laryngoscopy, lateral x-rays of the nasopharynx, CT scan, and MRI with gadolinium for more careful delineation. Biopsy of lesion when found with tissue diagnosis. Determination of presence or absence of immunocompromising disease process, AIDS, diabetes, post chemotherapy for malignancy.

▶ Disease Severity

Hearing loss, nasal obstruction, epistaxis, cranial nerve neuropathies and involvement, cervical lymphadenopathy, distant metastases.

▶ Concept and Application

Numerous lesions may involve nasopharynx, including lymphoepithelioma (poorly differentiated squamous cell carcinoma), chordoma, angiofibroma, lymphoma and other age-related tumors, serous otitis media secondary to eustachian tube blockage and infiltration by tumor. Tumor may invade skull base with third nerve palsy as well as other cranial nerve involvements; metastases to regional lymph nodes produces lymphadenopathies.

▶ Treatment Steps
1. Depends on type of lesion noted.
2. Benign processes respond most often to conservative management or surgical extirpation.
3. Malignancies may require extirpation and irradiation, chemotherapy, or both.
4. Lesions of the ear secondary to masses in the nasopharynx may require myringotomy and tube placement to correct serous otitis media.

## D. Malignant Neoplasms of the Oropharynx and Hypopharynx

▶ H&P Keys

Usual history of tobacco and ethanol use. More common in men than women; usually occurs between ages of 50 and 80 years. Symptoms may include globus sensation, odynophagia, dysphagia, irritation with foods, referred otalgia, lump in neck, alteration of voice, weight loss. More advanced lesions may include respiratory distress with stridor. Physical examination includes complete examination of upper aerodigestive tract, including indirect mirror examination and flexible fiber-optic nasopharyngolaryngoscopy as well as bimanual palpation of the orocavity and neck.

▶ Diagnosis

Careful clinical examination of upper aerodigestive tract, including direct laryngoscopy, cervical esophagoscopy, nasopharyngoscopy, and bronchoscopy, with appropriate histologic examination of biopsy material. Additional studies include CT scan and MRI of head and neck region.

▶ Disease Severity

TNM staging and extent of tumor with its location. Yielding extreme variation in disease severity.

▶ Concept and Application

Vast majority are squamous cell carcinoma of the involved mucosa and muscle, with varying degrees of tissue involvement based on stage and invasion. Initial spread of primary tumor tends to be in cervical lymph nodes, followed by distant metastasis should disease process continue.

▶ Treatment Steps

Combined treatment using surgery, irradiation, and chemotherapy as dictated by size and extent of tumor.

## E. Hoarseness

▶ H&P Keys

Presence of infectious disorder, local use/abuse, history of smoking and ethanol use, history of arthritis, history of trauma and intubation, possible endocrinopathy, benign and malignant neoplasms, functional disorders, reflux symptomatology; physical examination would include indirect mirror examination and direct laryngoscopy as well as complete physical examination of the upper aerodigestive tract; symptoms include hoarseness, possible referred otalgia, possible throat/laryngeal pain, dysphagia, dyspnea, cough, etc.

▶ Diagnosis

Thorough examination of the larynx using indirect and direct methods, complete examination of the upper aerodigestive tract; adjunctive radiologic studies would include CT scan, MRI scan, barium swallow, thyroid function tests, biopsy as appropriate.

▶ Disease Severity

Due to vast etiologic sources a large variety of disease severity occurs.

▶ Concept and Application

Disruption of normal mucosal wave of the vocal cords with creation of turbulent air flow resulting in hoarseness, edema, vocal masses and irregularities, as well as limited function or hyperfunctioning of the vocal cords may result in hoarseness.

▶ Treatment Steps

Directed toward etiology.

## F. Strep Throat (Acute Tonsillitis/Pharyngitis)

▶ H&P Keys

Sore throat, fever, malaise, anorexia, and odynophagia occurs more commonly in children. Physical findings include erythema of the pharynx and tonsils, purulent debris in tonsillar crypts and pharynx, malodorous purulence causing halitosis and bad taste, peritonsillar swelling and limited motion of the uvula and soft palate, dysphagia (with severe infections), and palpable and tender adenopathy with severe infections.

▶ Diagnosis

Direct physical examination with visualization of the tonsils and pharyngeal walls, culture of offending organisms.

▶ Disease Severity

Fever, tonsillar hypertrophy, dehydration, referred otalgia, odynophagia, dysphagia, dehydration, peritonsillar abscess, retropharyngeal abscess, and airway compromise. Response to therapy.

▶ Concept and Application

Bacterial infection involving the tonsils, pharynx, or both. Most common are β-hemolytic strep, *Streptococcus pyogenes*, *Haemophilus influenzae*, *Haemophilus parainfluenzae*, *Corynebacterium diphtheriae*, and *Streptococcus pneumoniae*. Other possibilities include viral diseases such as adenovirus and mononucleosis.

▶ Treatment Steps

1. Appropriate antibiotics, oral or IV hydration, incision and drainage of peritonsillar or retropharyngeal abscesses, if present.
2. IV hydration and antibiotics for recalcitrant infections.
3. Recurrent tonsillitis (six episodes per calendar year) is best treated with tonsillectomy.
4. Pain management, oral rinses, and antipyretics for fever are important.

G. **Cancer of the Larynx**

▶ H&P Keys

History of heavy tobacco and ethanol use or possible asbestos exposure. Occurs in males between the ages of 50 and 70 years. Symptoms include hoarseness, throat and neck pain, dysphagia, dyspnea, hemoptysis, weight loss, referred otalgia, neck mass. Physical examination may include visualization of tumor on indirect and flexible direct laryngoscopy, palpation of neck for masses, and detectable stridor, wheezing, and hoarseness.

▶ Diagnosis

Complete examination of the upper aerodigestive tract, including indirect and direct laryngoscopy, bimanual palpation, CT scan of neck and larynx, MRI.

▶ Disease Severity

Depends on TNM staging and extent of disease process.

▶ Concept and Application

Squamous cell carcinoma is most frequent malignant neoplasm of the larynx (95%). Tumor initially remains confined to the larynx, then spreads to cervical lymph nodes and ultimately metastasizes to distant areas.

▶ Treatment Steps

Management includes surgery, radiation therapy, and chemotherapy, depending on extent and stage of disease.

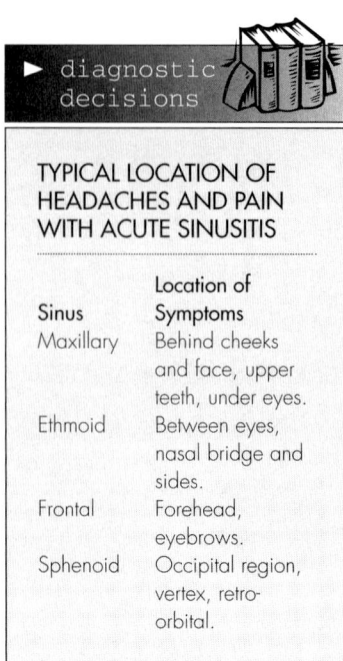

**TYPICAL LOCATION OF HEADACHES AND PAIN WITH ACUTE SINUSITIS**

| Sinus | Location of Symptoms |
|---|---|
| Maxillary | Behind cheeks and face, upper teeth, under eyes. |
| Ethmoid | Between eyes, nasal bridge and sides. |
| Frontal | Forehead, eyebrows. |
| Sphenoid | Occipital region, vertex, retro-orbital. |

## III. DISEASES OF THE RESPIRATORY SYSTEM

### A. Acute Sinusitis

▶ **H&P Keys**

History of recent upper respiratory tract infection associated with purulent rhinorrhea, headache, pain, and pressure over the affected sinus (cheek—maxillary, forehead—frontal, periorbital—ethmoid, and occipital—sphenoid). Other signs and symptoms include purulent postnasal drip, pressure and headache, nasal obstruction, referred otalgia, and orbital pain.

▶ **Diagnosis**

Nasal endoscopy, both standard and endoscopic; culturing of purulent discharge; sinus roentgenograms or CT scan of sinuses; sinus tap to determine presence of pus for culture and treatment.

▶ **Disease Severity**

Fever, chills, sinus pressure and pain; possible periorbital cellulitis, edema, proptosis, blindness, headache or intracranial complication such as meningitis, brain abscess, or cavernous sinus thrombosis.

▶ **Concept and Application**

Obstruction of ostea of sinuses in middle meatus (osteomeatal complex) leading to negative pressure, transudate followed by exudate, and acute infection. Presence of anatomic abnormalities such as septal deviation, concha bullosa, turbinate hypertrophy, nasal polyposis, and allergic rhinitis. Bacteriology is similar to that of acute otitis media, including *H. influenzae, S. aureus,* Group A β-streptococcus, pneumococcus, and more unusual organisms in immunocompromised hosts.

▶ **Treatment Steps**
1. Antibiotics such as amoxicillin or ampicillin or amoxicillin with clavulinic acid to cover suspected organisms; both systemic and topical decongestants to nasal mucosa.
2. Surgical drainage of affected sinuses as indicated by severity of disease and degree of patient's illness.
3. Steroids, antihistamines, or both for patients with a significant allergic component to their sinusitis.

### B. Chronic Sinusitis

▶ **H&P Keys**

Symptoms are persistent rhinorrhea, postnasal discharge, pressure, headache, foul smell or taste. Physical examination reveals presence of changes in nasal mucosa; history of allergy is predisposing factor; erythema and swelling of nasal mucosa and purulence are present.

▶ **Diagnosis**

Intranasal examination after careful vasoconstriction both by direct examination and by fiber-optic endonasal examination, with particular reference to middle meatus, osteomeatal complex to rule out presence of polypoid changes and presence or absence of occlusion of maxillary sinus and sphenoid ethmoid sinus complex. Plain roentgenograms are not as valuable as axial and coronal CT scans without contrast of sinuses to determine degree of sinus involvement, which sinuses are in fact involved, and presence of anatomic abnormalities. Cultures for offending organism.

▶ Disease Severity

Persistence of purulent rhinorrhea, pain, pressure, fatigue, halitosis; presence of complications of chronic sinusitis with orbital or intracranial complications.

▶ Concept and Application

Patients who have had poorly treated acute sinusitis and patients with allergic nasal disease with edema and polypoid changes of mucus membrane that block ostea outflow tracts are predisposed to sinusitis. Anatomic abnormalities such as septal deviations and pneumatization of turbinates with blockage of osteomeatal complex.

▶ Treatment Steps

Long-term antibiotics (3–6 weeks) with concomitant use of intranasal steroid sprays, nasal decongestants, and correction of intranasal anatomic abnormalities. In patients who fail conservative medical management, as described above; functional endoscopic sinus surgery (FESS) to remove the offending tissue blocking osteomeatal complex with ethmoidectomy, maxillary sinus antrostomy, sphenoidotomy, and frontal sinus duct reconstruction. Children refractive to conservative therapy should undergo adenoidectomy prior to consideration of endoscopic sinus surgery (see Management Decisions box).

## C. Fungal Sinusitis

▶ H&P Keys

Immunocompromised patients, patients with chronic sinusitis, or both; presence of unremitting sinusitis following vigorous local therapy; pain and swelling about the ethmoid and eyelid areas.

▶ Diagnosis

Diagnostic studies include biopsy, Gram stain and culture of suspicious material for septate versus nonseptate hyphae, CT scan for evidence of calcifications within the sinuses, and skin testing for *Aspergillus*.

▶ Disease Severity

Evidence of bone destructive, foul-smelling rhinorrhea, with swelling of soft tissues of cheek, eyelid, lateral face; involvement of infraorbital nerve; systemic manifestations of fatigue and debility.

▶ Concept and Application

Patients with immunocompromised states following chemotherapy for malignant disease or with diabetes or HIV infection have decreased ability to mount immunologic response to these sec-

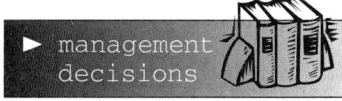

▶ management decisions

### INDICATIONS FOR FESS IN CHILDREN WITH CHRONIC SINUSITIS

1. Persistent symptoms despite adenoidectomy; *and*
2. CT evidence of chronic sinus disease, osteomeatal obstruction associated with sinusitis; *and*
3. Discussion of FESS with child's treating primary and speciality physicians; *and*
4. Committed postoperative follow-up for at least one year; *and*
5. Realistic parental expectations and understanding of potential complications.

FESS—function endoscopic sinus surgery.

ondary fungal infections; decreased ability also may be secondary to prolonged use of antibiotics with overgrowth of fungi as consequence.

▶ Treatment Steps
1. Surgical debridement.
2. Use of appropriate antifungal agents such as amphotericin.
3. Correction of underlying immunocompromising mechanism if possible.

### D. Chronic Rhinitis

▶ H&P Keys

Long-term nasal obstruction, postnasal discharge, sneezing, rhinorrhea, and possible purulence. Patients may complain of seasonal symptoms or have symptoms referable to emotional or temperature change. Physical examination reveals erythema of mucus membrane, often with crusting and bleeding and occasional purulence.

▶ Diagnosis

Gram stain of nasal smears for eosinophils or polymorphonuclear cells; sinus roentgenograms, CT scan, or both to rule out occult sinusitis. Allergy studies to rule out allergic disease as primary causative factor.

▶ Disease Severity

Persistence of nasal obstruction, postnasal discharge, pressure and pain, inability to sleep because of nasal obstruction, fatigue, loss of concentration, and loss of time from work.

▶ Concept and Application

Symptoms may be of allergic, infectious, or vasomotor origin. Determination of presence or absence of purulence by culture sensitivities. Presence of allergy by allergy studies and by history. Nasal obstruction secondary to temperature change mechanism, positioning of head, or emotional factors (fear, anger, passion, sadness); mechanism is endogenous release of vasoactive histamine-like substances that trigger vasodilatation and activation of goblet cells within the nasal and sinus mucous membranes.

▶ Treatment Steps

Determination of etiology and direction of therapy to allergic, infectious, or vasomotor disease process; also included in that therapy would be antihistamine decongestants, steroid nasal sprays, cromolyn sodium as a nasal spray, systemic steroids, and intranasal medicaments such as lubricating drops when indicated.

### E. Allergic Rhinitis

▶ H&P Keys

Nasal obstruction and congestion, nasal puritis, rhinorrhea, sneezing, and symptoms related to seasons. History of presence or absence of animals, specific plants, flowers, molds, and conditions (eg, feather pillows) that would support the growth of molds or allergies. Physical examination may reveal swollen, pale blue nasal mucosa and turbinates with nasal obstruction and generally clear rhinorrhea, and swollen (cobblestone-like) lymphoid tissue in the posterior pharyngeal wall.

▶ Diagnosis

Nasal smears to detect the presence of eosinophils, immunoglobulin E levels, and total eosinophil count. Allergic skin testing, RAST (radioallergosorbent test) testing, food diary with confirmation of symptoms related to specific food allergens.

▶ Disease Severity

Degree of function during allergic periods (ie, potential loss of school or work time).

▶ Concept and Application

The antigen/antibody reaction causing degranulation of mass cells and basophils releasing histamines, prostaglandins, and other vasoactive elements leading to symptoms of rhinorrhea, nasal congestion, puritis, and so on.

▶ Treatment Steps

1. If possible, avoiding specific allergen is most useful for mild to moderate symptoms.
2. Treatment with antihistamines, nasal steroids, systemic steroids, sympathomimetic medications as well as sodium cromolyn nasal spray are indicated.
3. Also, immunotherapy with allergy shots for desensitization as well as diet control are useful adjuncts.

## F. Epistaxis (Nosebleed)

▶ H&P Keys

Episode can be intermittent or acute; bleeding may be from anterior nares or may produce postnasal bleeding. Patient may give history of digital trauma to nose or history of nasal obstruction, particularly in boys younger than 15 years. Bleeding may respond to anterior nares pressure or may require intranasal packing, posterior nasal packing, or both.

▶ Diagnosis

Direct examination of nose after careful intranasal vasoconstriction and local anesthesia permits examination of anterior nares, particularly in area of Kiesselbach's (Little's) area (Figure 20–2). Postnasal space can be examined by fiberscope under local anesthesia; sinus roentgenograms or CT scans should be done to rule out intrasinus occult malignancies.

▶ Disease Severity

Minor intermittent bleeding stops spontaneously with gentle pressure. Severe postnasal bleeding is life-threatening and requires postnasal packing, hospitalization, and intensive care observation; necessity for blood transfusion and surgical intervention with ligation of sphenopalatine or maxillary artery.

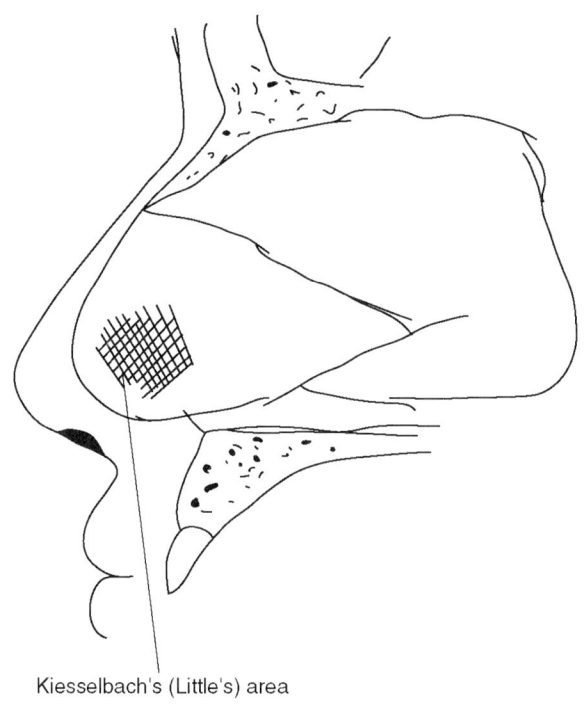

Figure 20-2. Epistaxis.

▶ Concept and Application

Most common cause is simple drying and crusting of nasal mucosa with neovascularization of Kiesselbach's area. Sphenopalatine artery bleeding is often associated with hypertension; patients may have Rendu–Osler–Weber disease or hereditary telangiectasia. Bleeding in young male children is produced by juvenile angiofibromas and other bleeding diatheses involving platelet or other coagulation deficit secondary to either primary platelet involvements or other blood dyscrasias.

▶ Treatment Steps

1. Bleeding from anterior Kiesselbach's area responds well to gentle pressure or, in recurrent involvements, to cauterization using trichloroacetic acid or other oxidizing agents such as silver nitrate in dilute solutions; significant bleeding requires anterior nasal packs.
2. Posterior bleeding requires posterior packing or intranasal balloons.
3. Unresponsive bleeding requires transfusion, ligation of offending vessels, hospitalization, and intensive care management.
4. For Rendu–Osler–Weber disease, bleeding from affected telangiectatic areas is controlled with cauterization or argon laser. Juvenile angiofibromas and neoplastic lesions of the sinuses require extirpation.

## G. Disorders of Olfaction and Taste

▶ H&P Keys

Anosmia (loss of sense of smell) and lack of taste and secondary to upper respiratory infection, nasal obstruction, trauma, viral infections, tumors, exposure to irritative fumes such as ammonia or other industrial pollutants.

▶ Diagnosis

Intranasal examination after careful intranasal vasoconstriction to rule out obstructive lesions of nasal cavity and nasal vault. CT scan of sinuses to rule out sinus and intranasal involvements and MRI with gadolinium to rule out involvements of the olfactory bulb and olfactory projections into the hypocampus and temporal lobe. Taste and smell testing and examination of the tongue to rule out atrophy or abnormality of taste buds.

▶ Disease Severity

Inability to function in environment because of inability to detect crucial odors, loss of appetite, malnutrition secondary to loss of appetite, psychic trauma because of loss of sense of taste and smell.

▶ Concept and Application

Olfactory fibers projected into the nose from the olfactory bulb through the area of the cribiform plate; lesions of nose that obstruct air flow to these critical fibers produce a relative anosmia. Head injury with a commotio injury in the brain case may result in forces that shear the olfactory fibers from the olfactory nerve. Viral infections most often produce reversible neuritic change in olfactory fibers, preventing their ability to respond to olfactory stimuli. Irritation secondary to industrial solvents and pollutants also may injure the neural epithelium in the same fashion. Loss of taste most often is olfactory in origin; majority of patients do not lose chorda tympani function, which monitors salty, sour, sweet, and bitter taste. Chorda tympani function can be lost following middle-ear or mastoid surgery or trauma to the temporal bone or head.

▶ Treatment Steps

1. Use of topical steroids for inflammatory process, removal of obstructive lesions of nose and nasal vault.
2. Removal from environment containing noxious and polluting substances.
3. Treatment of infectious processes when appropriate.
4. Return of olfactory function may take from 3 weeks to 18 months.

## H. Acute Upper Respiratory Infection (Most Common in Winter Months)

▶ H&P Keys

Manifested by coryza, rhinorrhea, nasal obstruction, pharyngitis, cough, conjunctivitis, headache. Physical examination reveals conjunctivitis, nasal obstruction with boggy, pale turbinates and, initially, clear rhinorrhea. Later, purulence may occur; pharynx is diffusely red without exudate; low-grade fever and, occasionally, small, mild to moderate cervical lymphadenopathy are present.

▶ Diagnosis

Physical examination, determination of febrile state.

▶ Disease Severity

Degree of nasal obstruction, ear discomfort, throat pain, dysphagia, musculoskeletal symptoms.

▶ Concept and Application

Acute upper respiratory infections are viral in origin in both adults and children, most commonly in winter months. More than 120 adenoviruses produce choryza-like symptoms; none confer any specific long-term immunity and none respond to antibiotic therapy.

▶ Treatment Steps

1. In acute phase, nasal and oral decongestants, steam or cool-mist vaporization, antihistamines, antipyretics, and antiinflammatory agents such as Tylenol in young children, and aspirin or nonsteroidal anti-inflammatory agents in adults.
2. Chicken soup and other fluids; bed rest when indicated.
3. Purulent phase lasts 3–5 days and should not require antibiotics. If it lasts longer, one must consider the possibility of sinusitis as a consequence of the acute upper respiratory infection; acute otitis medias may occur in conjunction as well.

## I. Wegener's Granulomatosis

▶ H&P Keys

Lesion of upper respiratory tract may involve ear, nose, sinus, soft palate, hard palate, tongue, and larynx—most often close to midline. Patients have generally systemic symptoms, including cough and often renal symptoms.

▶ Diagnosis

CT scans of sinuses and ear to determine presence of lesion, biopsy of specific lesions showing Wegener's granulomas and vasculitis chest roentgenogram. Biopsies of pulmonary lesions and renal biopsies also are indicated.

▶ Disease Severity

Wegener's granulomatosis may progress rapidly and may involve the ear, with both facial and auditory nerve involvement; may involve the sinuses and eyes, with changes in vision; and may involve the upper airway, with airway compromise.

▶ Concept and Application

Wegener's granulomatosis is a disease of unknown etiology manifested by the involvement of upper respiratory, pulmonary, and renal systems. Biopsies show classic granulomas and vasculitis.

▶ Treatment Steps

Use of cyclophosphamide and steroids in combination for long-term and supportive systemic therapy.

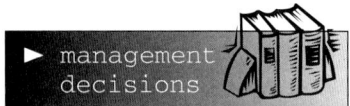
▶ management decisions

**RECOMMENDED MEDICAL TREATMENT FOR WEGENER'S GRANULOMATOSIS**

**Nonsystemic Localized Disease**
Upper airway: Nasal steroids, saline irrigations, antibiotics for superimposed bacterial infections
Lower airway: Systemic antibiotic therapy, systemic steroid therapy

**Systemic Disease**
Cyclophosphamide therapy
Steroid therapy
Systemic antibiotic therapy

## J. Cystic Fibrosis

▶ **H&P Keys**

Chronic recurrent upper and lower respiratory dysfunction with nasal obstruction, nasal purulence, loss of pulmonary function, dyspnea, chronic cough, production of purulent secretions with cough. Examination reveals debilitated child or adolescent; watery nasal polypoid tissue can be seen intranasally, often extending into the nasopharynx.

▶ **Diagnosis**

Direct examination shows multiple polypoid changes in young children; CT scans show polypoid and polycystic changes in all sinuses. Sweat colloid study and chest roentgenogram.

▶ **Disease Severity**

The degree of nasal obstruction and purulence and their impact on patient's pulmonary status with increased dyspnea, cough, cyanosis, and recurrent infection.

▶ **Concept and Application**

Mucous membrane abnormalities with loss of salivary function, mucous membrane reactivity with polypoid changes within the nose and sinuses, production of abnormal mucoid elements and increased tenacity and viscosity block sinus outflow tracts and involve pulmonary system.

▶ **Treatment Steps**

1. Systemic antibiotics.
2. Intranasal removal of polyps with recurrence and sinusitis, and functional endoscopic sinus surgery for recurrent sinusitis with polyp formation.
3. Supportive systemic therapy.

## BIBLIOGRAPHY

Cummings C, Fredrickson JM, Horker LA, Krause CA, Schuller DE. *Otolaryngology: Head and Neck Surgery.* 2nd ed. St. Louis: CV Mosby Co; 1993.

Lee KJ, ed. *Essential Otolaryngology: Head and Neck Surgery.* 8th ed. Stamford, CT: Appleton & Lange; 2003.

Seiden AM. *Otolaryngology: The Essentials.* 1st ed. Thieme Medical Publishers; 2002.

Wilson W. *Clinical Handbook of Ear, Nose and Throat Disorders,* 1st ed. Cre-Press-Parthenon Publishers; 2002.

# Index

Page numbers followed by *t* indicate tables. Page numbers followed by *f* indicate figures.

## A

Abacavir, 250
ABCs (airway, breathing, and circulation)
    alcohol, 230
    cocaine, 230
    epiglottitis, 435
    febrile seizures, 421
    hyaline membrane disease, 515
    poisoning and management overview, 232
    sedatives, 229
    shock, 239
    skull trauma/fracture, 218
    sleep apnea, 335, 524
    solvent sniffing, 231
    surgical principles, 578, 580
    transient tachypnea of the newborn, 429
    traumatic injury, 239
Abdominal and chest injury
    additional information, 223
    epidemiology and prevention of, 224
    epidemiology and prevention of chest/abdominal injury, 224
    flail chest, 223
    hemothorax, 222
    pelvic fractures, 224
    perforation of viscus, 223–224
    pneumothorax, 222
    rib cage, 221
    surgical principles, 580–582, 581*f*
Abdominal aortic aneurysms, 39–40
    mechanisms and disease diagnosis/treatment, 164
    surgical principles, 590–591, 591*f*
ABO group, 187, 431, 432
Abortion
    induced, 372
    septic, 372–373
    spontaneous, 371
Abruptio placentae
    mechanisms and disease diagnosis/treatment, 374
Abscesses
    anorectal, 142–143
    brain, 662
    breast, 355
    lactation, 368
    liver, 146
    mechanisms and disease diagnosis/treatment
        dermatology, 49–50
        neurology, 308–309
    pelvic inflammatory disease, 358
    perirectal, 605
    peritonsillar, 661
    strep throat, 661
    tubo-ovarian, 262, 358
    venous thrombosis, 322
*Absidia*, 503
Absolute neutrophil counts (ANCs), 195
Abuse syndromes
    child physical and sexual abuse
        attention-deficit hyperactivity disorder, 473
        domestic violence, 487
        epidemiology and prevention, 243
        mechanisms and disease diagnosis/treatment, 486–487
        somatization disorder, 469
    domestic violence, adult, 487–488
    elderly patients, 243, 488
    management principles, 240
Academic underachievement, 473
Acalculus, 144
Acanthosis nigricans, 84, 84*f*
Accidents. *See* Injuries/wounds/accidents; Trauma
Accolate, 199

Acetaminophen
    corneal ulcers, 411
    osteoarthritis, 274
    poisoning and mechanisms and
            disease
            diagnosis/treatment, 228
    rheumatoid arthritis, 283
    transfusion reactions, 187
    varicella (chickenpox), 46
Acetazolamide, 524
Acetic acid soaks, 77
Acetylcholine, 312, 327, 422
Acetylcholinesterase
    neural tube defects and central
            nervous system
            malformation in the
            fetus, 379
Acetylcysteine, 228, 507
Acetylgalactosamine, 335–336
Achalasia
    mechanisms and disease
            diagnosis/treatment, 113
    squamous cell carcinoma, 110
    surgical principles, 597
Achlorhydria, 173
Acid-base balance/disorders
    electrolyte and
        hypercalcemia, 557
        hyperkalemia, 554–555
        hypernatremia, 554
        hypocalcemia, 558
        hypokalemia, 554
        hypomagnesemia, 557
        hyponatremia, 553
        metabolic acidosis, 556
        metabolic alkalosis, 555–556
        respiratory acidosis, 556–557
        respiratory alkalosis, 556
        volume depletion, 555
        volume excess, 555
    intestinal obstruction, 138
    stomach
        mechanisms and disease
            diagnosis/treatment,
            115–117, 116$t$, 117$t$
Acid-fast bacteria (AFB), 308
*Acinetobacter*, 497
Acitretin, 54
Acne
    alcohol, 478
    mechanisms and disease
            diagnosis/treatment
            dermatology, 67
            pediatrics, 448

Acquired keratoderma
    mechanisms and disease
            diagnosis/treatment,
            76–77
Acromegaly
    overproduction syndromes
            (pituitary gland), 92, 93
    sleep apnea, 334
Actinic keratosis
    mechanisms and disease
            diagnosis/treatment, 69
    squamous cell carcinoma, 69
*Actinomyces*, 511
Actinomycin, 545
Activated protein C resistance
    mechanisms and disease
            diagnosis/treatment,
            191–192
Acute angle-closure glaucoma,
            414
Acute arterial occlusion
    mechanisms and disease
            diagnosis/treatment,
            35–36
Acute asthma, 504
Acute bacterial prostatitis, 530
Acute benign pleural effusions,
            510
Acute bronchiolitis
    mechanisms and disease
            diagnosis/treatment, 494
Acute bronchitis
    mechanisms and disease
            diagnosis/treatment, 494
Acute chest syndrome, 177
Acute cholecystitis
    mechanisms and disease
            diagnosis/treatment,
            144–145
    surgical principles, 610, 611$f$
Acute circulatory collapse. *See*
            Hypotension and acute
            circulatory collapse
            (shock)
Acute cutaneous candidiasis,
            48–49
Acute dacryocystitis
    mechanisms and disease
            diagnosis/treatment,
            400–401
Acute enteric infections
    mechanisms and disease
            diagnosis/treatment, 120,
            121$t$, 122–123, 124$t$

Acute epiglottitis
    mechanisms and disease
            diagnosis/treatment, 493
Acute exanthems
    varicella, 46
    varicella zoster, 46–47
Acute hepatitis, 146–147
Acute hypersensitivity
            pneumonitis, 511
Acute lupus erythematosus, 79
Acute lymphocytic leukemia
            (ALL)
    mechanisms and disease
            diagnosis/treatment,
            178–179
Acute mesenteric ischemia
    surgical principles, 600–601,
            601$f$
Acute myelogenous leukemia
            (AML)
    mechanisms and disease
            diagnosis/treatment,
            177–178
Acute otitis media, 650
Acute pancreatitis
    chylomicronemia, type 1
            familial, 99
    mechanisms and disease
            diagnosis/treatment,
            159–161
    surgical principles, 615
Acute pericarditis
    mechanisms and disease
            diagnosis/treatment, 20
Acute pharyngitis
    mechanisms and disease
            diagnosis/treatment,
            660–661
Acute pneumonia, 503
Acute pyelonephritis, 546
Acute renal failure
    mechanisms and disease
            diagnosis/treatment,
            546–547
Acute respiratory distress
            syndrome (ARDS)
    genitourinary tract infections,
            377
    mechanisms and disease
            diagnosis/treatment,
            514–515
    respiratory acidosis, 556
Acute rheumatic fever
    history and physical keys, 23

Acute sinusitis
    mechanisms and disease diagnosis/treatment, 662
Acute stress disorder, 466
Acute suppurative cholangitis
    mechanisms and disease diagnosis/treatment, 145–146
Acute tonsillitis
    mechanisms and disease diagnosis/treatment, 660–661
Acute tubular necrosis, 547
Acute upper respiratory infection, 667–668
Acute valvular diseases
    endocarditis, 23
    ischemic, 23
    rheumatic fever, 22
Acute venous thrombosis, 37
Acyclovir
    erythema multiforme, 62
    genital herpes, 264, 533
    herpes simplex virus, 52, 258, 304, 439
    ophthalmic herpes zoster, 413
    urethritis, 531
    varicella (chickenpox), 46, 265, 436
    varicella-zoster (shingles), 47
Adenocarcinoma
    bronchogenic carcinoma, 519
    mechanisms and disease diagnosis/treatment, 110
    prostate cancer, 542, 576
Adenoidectomy, 663
Adenoma sebaceum, 82, 82f
Adenomatous polyposis coli gene (APC), 131
Adenopathy
    bronchogenic carcinoma, 518
    HIV (human immunodeficiency virus), 533
    penile/urethral/scrotal carcinoma, 546
    syphilis, 260
    testicular carcinoma, 545
Adjustment disorders
    mechanisms and disease diagnosis/treatment, 467
Adolescence
    adjustment disorders, 467
    anorexia, 474

bipolar disorders, 461, 462
body dysmorphic disorder, 472
bulimia, 475
enuresis, 540
femur, fracture of neck of, 295
Osgood-Schlatter disease, 449
pregnancy
    mechanisms and disease diagnosis/treatment, 369–370
puberty, 538
slipped capital femoral epiphysis, 278
social phobia, 466
Adrenal gland
    disorders
        congenital adrenal hyperplasia, 98–99
        Cushing's syndrome, 96–97
        hirsutism, 97–98
        insufficiency, adrenal, 95–96
        pheochromocytoma, 98
Adrenal hyperplasia
    amenorrhea, 352
Adrenalin, 217
Adrenal insufficiency, 118
Adrenocorticotropic hormone (ACTH)
    Cushing's disease, 573–574
    Cushing's syndrome, 96
    overproduction syndromes (pituitary gland), 93
Adriamycin
    bladder carcinoma, 544
    endometrial cancer, 341
    Hodgkin's disease, 182
    multiple myeloma, 185
Adson maneuver, 592
Advair, 199
Advanced cardiac life support, 29
Adventitia, 42
Affective psychoses: mania and psychotic depression
    mechanisms and disease diagnosis/treatment, 454–455
Aflatoxin, 153
Afrin, 201
Agnogenic myeloid metaplasia
    mechanisms and disease diagnosis/treatment, 193–194
Agoraphobia, 464
Agranulocytosis, 195

AIDS (acquired immune deficiency syndrome)
    acute pericarditis, 20
    cryptococcal infection, 257–258
    cytomegalovirus, 253–254
    disseminated *Mycobacterium avium-intracellulare* complex, 255–256
    gastric cancer, 115
    herpes simplex virus, 258
    histoplasmosis, 500
    HIV (human immunodeficiency virus), 248–252
    lupus inhibitor, 189
    molluscum contagiosum, 51
    *Pneumocystis carinii* pneumonia, 252–253
    toxoplasma encephalitis, 256–257
    tuberculosis, 254–255
    ulcerative colitis, 134
Airbeds, 77
Airway control. See ABCs (airway, breathing, and circulation)
Akathisia, 324
Alanine aminotransferase (ALT), 138
    alcohol, 478
    cirrhosis, 155
    hepatitis, 150
    hepatitis B infection complicating pregnancy, 377
Albumin
    cirrhosis, 155
    hepatocellular carcinoma, 154
    Muehrcke's nails, 85
    neonatal hyperbilirubinemia, 432
    Terry's nails, 84
Albuterol
    allergic bronchopulmonary aspergillosis, 210
    anaphylaxis, 202
    bronchial asthma, 199, 200
    hypersensitivity pneumonitis, 211
Alcohol
    acute pancreatitis, 160
    adenocarcinoma, 110
    adolescent pregnancy, 370
    chronic pancreatitis, 161
    chylomicronemia, type 1 familial, 99

Alcohol *(continued)*
  colorectal carcinoma, 128
  dilated cardiomyopathy, 14
  Dupuytren's contracture, 288
  dysbetalipoproteinemia, type III, 100
  folic acid deficiency, 170
  gout, 280
  gram-negative bacillary pneumonias, 497
  *Haemophilus influenzae* pneumonia, 496
  hepatitis, 146, 149, 151
  hereditary nonpolyposis colorectal cancer, 130
  hoarseness, 660
  hyperlipoproteinemia, 33, 101
  hypoglycemia, 105
  hypomagnesemia, 557
  iron-deficiency anemia, 169
  larynx, cancer of the, 661
  liver disease, 146
  motor vehicle accidents, 242
  obsessive-compulsive disorder, 464
  oropharynx, malignant neoplasms of the, 659
  papillary necrosis, 551
  poisoning and mechanisms and disease diagnosis/ treatment, 230
  rosacea, 67
  sleep apnea, 524
  squamous cell carcinoma, 109
  substance-related disorders
    dementia, 480
    intoxication, 478–479
    Korsakoff's syndrome, 480
    mechanisms and disease diagnosis/treatment, 478–480
    Wernicke's encephalopathy, 480
    withdrawal syndromes, 479–480
  teratology, 367
  thiamine deficiency, 314
Aldesleukin, 205
Aldolase, 80, 282
Aldosteronism, 31
Alendronate, 279
Alkaline phosphatase
  alcohol, 479
  choledocholithiasis, 145
  cirrhosis, 156
  intestinal obstruction, 138
  metastases to bone, 287
  Paget's disease of bone, 289
  rickets, 280
Allegra, 201
Alleles and thalassemia-alpha, 171
Allergic bronchopulmonary aspergillosis (ABPA)
  bronchiectasis, 507
  mechanisms and disease diagnosis/treatment, 209–210
Allergic conjunctivitis, 393, 394
Allergic rhinitis
  atopic dermatitis, 207
  mechanisms and disease diagnosis/treatment, 200–202
Allergy injections, 199
Allergy patch testing, 208
Allopurinol, 180, 280
Alopecia, 79
Alopecia areata, 68–69
Alpha-antitrypsin deficiency, 150
Alpha-fetoprotein (AFP)
  hepatocellular carcinoma, 154
  neural tube defects, 379, 422
  prenatal diagnosis, 366
  testicular carcinoma, 545
Alport syndrome, 424, 425
Alprostadil, 485
Aluminum acetate solution, 209
Alveolar cell carcinoma, 519
Alzheimer's disease
  mechanisms and disease diagnosis/treatment, 327–328
  menopausal symptoms, 353
Amantadine
  influenza pneumonia, 499
  livedo reticularis, 81
  multiple sclerosis, 332
Ambiguous genitalia
  congenital adrenal hyperplasia, 98
  intersex, 535
Amblyopia, 399
  cataracts, 417
  congenital cataracts, 424
  mechanisms and disease diagnosis/treatment, 406–407
Amenorrhea
  ectopic pregnancy, 370
  mechanisms and disease diagnosis/treatment, 352
  overproduction syndromes (pituitary gland), 92
  prenatal care, 365
  Turner's syndrome, 446
  underproduction syndromes, 94
American Cancer Society, 129
American Diabetes Association (ADA), 103
American Fertility Society, 343
American Urological Association, 542
Amikacin, 256
Aminocaproic acid, 206
Aminoglutehimide, 97
Aminoglycosides, 422, 497
Aminopenicillins, 435
Aminophylline, 199
Aminosalicylates, 134, 135
Aminotransferase, 144
Amiodarone
  basic cardiac life support, 29
  tachyarrhythmias, 18
  ventricular tachycardia, 19
Amitriptyline, 286, 317
Amnesia
  concussion, 219
  contusions, 331
  thiamine deficiency, 314
Amniocentesis, 366, 380, 444
Amniotic fluid, 384, 431
  prenatal diagnosis, 366
Amobarbital, 471
*Amoeba*, 123
Amoxicillin
  acute otitis media, 649
  chancroid, 262
  drug reactions causing skin changes, 58
  Lyme disease, 268, 272, 309
Amphotericin
  aspergillosis, invasive, 503
  coccidioidomycosis, 502
  cryptococcal infection, 258, 502
  fungal meningitis, 307
  histoplasmosis, 501
  phycomycosis, 503
Ampicillin
  acute epiglottitis, 493
  genitourinary tract infections, 377
  *Haemophilus influenzae* pneumonia, 496
  pelvic inflammatory disease, 358
  septic meningitis, 307

Amprenavir, 250
Amputation
    chronic atherosclerotic
        occlusion, 35
    osteosarcoma, 286
    thermal injuries, 240
Amsler grid, 404
Amylase
    acute pancreatitis, 159
    bulimia, 476
    choledocholithiasis, 145
    intestinal obstruction, 138
    ischemic bowel disease, 137
Amyloid, 321, 327
Amyloidosis
    carpal tunnel syndrome, 311
    familial Mediterranean fever,
        141
    mechanisms and disease
        diagnosis/treatment, 81
    monoclonal gammopathy of
        undetermined
        significance, 185
    multiple myeloma, 184
    restrictive cardiomyopathy, 15
Amyotrophic lateral sclerosis
        (ALS)
    mechanisms and disease
        diagnosis/treatment, 328
Anagrelide, 193
Anal fissure
    mechanisms and disease
        diagnosis/treatment, 142
Analgesics. *See also specific drug*
    chronic pancreatitis, 161
    epistaxis, 217
    ingrowing nails, 67
    lumbar spine and spinal stenosis,
        333
    myocardial infarction, 5
    pain disorder, 470
    rib fracture, 221
    sickle cell anemia, 177
    varicella (chickenpox), 46
Analine dyes, 543
Anaphylaxis
    drug allergy, 213
    insect and snake bites, 238
    mechanisms and disease
        diagnosis/treatment,
        202–203, 239
    transfusion reactions, 187
Anastomosis, 135
*Ancylostoma*, 122

Androgens
    congenital adrenal hyperplasia,
        98, 99
    hereditary angioedema, 206
    hirsutism, 97, 98
    menopausal symptoms, 353
    prostate cancer, 542, 543
Anemia(s)
    acute enteric infections, 123
    agnogenic myeloid metaplasia,
        193
    anorexia, 475
    aplastic, 173–174
    blood-loss, 169–170
    celiac sprue, 124
    chronic disease
        mechanisms and disease
            diagnosis/treatment, 176
    chronic hemolytic, 170
    chronic lymphocytic leukemia,
        180
    chronic renal disease, 174, 547
    congenital syphilis, 438
    disseminated *Mycobacterium
        avium-intracellulare*
        complex, 255
    esophageal neoplasms, 109
    folic acid deficiency, 170–171
    gastric cancer, 114
    gastroesophageal reflux disease,
        110
    hemolytic, 171, 175
    hemolytic uremic syndrome,
        440
    iron-deficiency, 109, 124, 169
    lead-poisoning, 174
    lead toxicity, 323
    leiomyomata uteri, 342
    microangiopathic hemolytic, 31
    multiple myeloma, 184
    postpartum sepsis, 387
    respiratory alkalosis, 556
    rheumatoid arthritis, 283
    sickle cell, 176–177
    thalassemia-alpha, 171
    thalassemia-beta, 171–172
    venous thrombosis, 322
    vitamin$_{12}$ deficiency, 172–173
Anencephaly, 380
Aneuploidy, 366, 380
Aneurysms
    abdominal aortic, 39–40, 164
    infrainguinal aneurysmal
        disease, 592–593

    mechanisms and disease
        diagnosis/treatment, 39–40
    thoracic aorta
        surgical principles, 588–590,
            589*f*
Anger and sexual dysfunctions, 484
Angina pectoris
    abdominal aortic aneurysm, 164
    left-sided high output heart
        failure, 9
    stable, 6–7
    unstable, 3–4
Angiodysplasia, 169
Angioedema
    anaphylaxis, 202
    drug allergy, 213
    hereditary, 205–206
    urticaria, 57, 203
Angiography. *See also* mechanisms
        and disease diagnosis/
        treatment *and* surgical
        principles *under specific
        disease/disorder*
    atherosclerosis, 34*f*
    congenital anomalous disc
        elevation, 401
    diabetes mellitus with
        ophthalmologic
        manifestations, 410
    ischemic thrombotic strokes,
        319, 320*f*
    monocular defects, 405
    optic atrophy, 404
    papilledema, 402
    renovascular hypertension, 551
    subarachnoid hemorrhage, 322
    unstable angina, 3
    urologic trauma, 541
    variant angina, 5
    venous thrombosis, 322
    ventricular septic defect, 26
Angioplasty, 31, 35, 551
Angiotensin-converting enzyme
        (ACE) inhibitors
    congestive heart failure, 514
    diabetes mellitus, 104
    essential hypertension, 30
    left-sided low output heart
        failure, 8
    malignant hypertension, 31
    renovascular disease, 586
    right-sided heart failure, 10
    sarcoidosis, 508
    secondary hypertension, 31

Angiotensin II, 375
Anhedonia, 453, 459
Animal bites, 63–66, 203, 306. *See also* Insect/ectoparasite bites
Anion gap, 556
Anisometropia, 406
Ankle-brachial index (ABI)
    aortic occlusion, 41
    arterial ulcer, 569
    peripheral arterial occlusive disease, 587
Ankle injury, 237
Ankylosing spondylitis
    mechanisms and disease diagnosis/treatment, 283–284
    overview, 300
Ann Arbor staging system, 182, 183
Anoproctitis, 259
Anorectal abscess
    mechanisms and disease diagnosis/treatment, 142–143
Anorectal fistula
    mechanisms and disease diagnosis/treatment, 143–144
    surgical principles, 605
Anorexia
    acute lymphocytic leukemia, 178
    amenorrhea, 352
    anemia of chronic disease, 176
    bereavement, 488
    bulimia, 475
    lead toxicity, 323
    Legionnaire's disease, 497
    mechanisms and disease diagnosis/treatment, 474–475
    mononucleosis, 264
    mumps, 266
    obsessive-compulsive disorder, 464
    pancreatic carcinoma, 157
    poliomyelitis, 305
    rubella (German measles), 266
    strep throat, 660
Anoscopy, 350
Anovulation, 341, 344
Anoxia, 315
Antabuse, 478, 479
Antacids, 111, 116

Anterior cruciate ligament (ACL), 291
Anterior fontanelle, 423
Anterior pituitary disorders
    overproduction syndromes, 92–93
    underproduction syndromes, 94
Anterior superior spine, fracture of, 224
Anthracycline, 179
Anthralin, 54, 69
Antiarrhythmics, 10
Antibiotics
    acne, 67, 448
    acute dacryocystitis, 401
    acute enteric infections, 123
    acute epiglottitis, 493
    acute otitis media, 649
    acute pericarditis, 20
    acute respiratory distress syndrome, 515
    anorectal abscess, 143
    aspergillosis, invasive, 502
    atopic dermatitis, 56
    blepharitis, 396
    bronchiectasis, 507
    candidiasis, oral, 48
    chalazion, 397
    chlamydia, 533
    choledocholithiasis, 146
    chronic bronchitis, 506
    chronic otitis media, 650
    chronic sinusitis, 663
    conjunctivitis, 395
    contact dermatitis, 209
    corneal ulcers, 411
    cystic fibrosis, 669
    decubitus ulcer, 77
    distributive shock, 13
    diverticulitis, 139
    epididymitis, 530, 531
    epistaxis, 217
    facial fracture, 218
    follicular cyst, 76
    frostbite, 240
    genitourinary tract infections, 377
    gram-negative bacillary pneumonias, 497
    herpes simplex keratitis, 412
    humoral immunodeficiency, 204
    impetigo, 50
    infectious otitis externa, 647

    ingrowing nails, 67
    intussusception, 443
    ischemic bowel disease, 137
    lacerations, 225
    lactation, 368
    malignant otitis externa, 648
    necrotizing enterocolitis, 443
    neutropenia, 195
    ophthalmic herpes zoster, 413
    osteomyelitis, 271
    otitis media, 435
    pemphigus, 60
    peritonitis, 140
    pertussis, 495
    postpartum sepsis, 387
    prostatitis, 530
    pyelonephritis, 546
    septic abortion, 372
    septic arthritis, 272
    serous otitis media, 651
    shock, 239
    strep throat, 661
    swallowing (injury/accidents), 227
    teratology, 367
    transfusion reactions, 187
    urinary tract infections, 529
    varicella (chickenpox), 46
    venous thrombosis, 323
    vulva/vagina, candidiasis of the, 349
Anticentromere antibody, 80
Anticholinergics
    bladder, painful, 530
    delirium, 485
    irritable bowel syndrome, 128
    neurogenic bladder, 539
    obsessive-compulsive disorder, 465
    pelvic relaxation/urinary incontinence, 351
    tricyclic antidepressants, 228
Anticoagulants
    antithrombin III deficiency, 191
    cardioembolic strokes, 321
    gout, 280
    ischemic thrombotic strokes, 320
    lupus inhibitor, 190
    pulmonary embolism, 38, 516
    right-sided heart failure, 10
    venous thrombosis, 38
Anticonvulsants
    abscesses, 309
    bipolar disorders, 462

cyclothymia, 462
febrile seizures, 421
herpes simplex virus, 305
lumbar spine and spinal stenosis, 333
manganese toxicity, 324
meningioma, 326
metastases, 327
neurosyphilis, 310
panic disorder, 463
seizures, 316
subarachnoid hemorrhage, 322
Antidepressants
adjustment disorders, 467
affective psychoses: mania and psychotic depression, 455
anorexia, 475
delusional disorder, 456
depression, major (unipolar), 460
dysthymia, 461
generalized anxiety disorder, 464
pain disorder, 470, 471
panic disorder, 463
pelvic relaxation/urinary incontinence, 351
personality disorders, 469
somatization disorder, 470
Antidiarrheals, 126
Antidiuretic hormone (ADH), 8
Antifungals, 48
Antiglomerular basement membrane antibodies, 517, 518
Antihistamines
allergic rhinitis, 201, 665
anaphylaxis, 202
atopic dermatitis, 56, 207
chronic rhinitis, 664
conjunctivitis, 395
contact dermatitis, 56, 209
drug allergy, 213
eczema, 57
erythema multiforme, 62
fleas, 66
herpes gestationis, 59
insect and snake bites, 238
mosquitoes and flies, 66
pruritus, 62
scabies, 64
urticaria, 58, 203, 204
varicella (chickenpox), 46
vertigo, 652

Antihypertensives, 549, 551
Antikeratolytic agents, 448
Antimalarials, 80
Antimicrobial therapy, 436
Antimitochondrial antibodies (AMA), 148
Antinuclear antibodies (ANA). *See also* mechanisms and disease diagnosis/treatment *and* surgical principles *under specific disease/disorder*
acute pericarditis, 20
autoimmune hepatitis, 147
fibromyalgia, 285
ischemic thrombotic strokes, 319
lupus arthritis, 282
lupus erythematosus, 80
scleroderma, 80
usual interstitial pneumonitis, 509
Antioxidants, 537
Antiphospholipid antibodies, 81
Antiplatelet agents
arteriosclerotic ulcer, 78
essential thrombocythemia, 193
ischemic thrombotic strokes, 320
necrobiosis lipoidica, 83
Antipruritic agents, 209, 313, 436
Antipsychotics
affective psychoses: mania and psychotic depression, 455
Alzheimer's disease, 328
brief psychotic disorder, 457
delirium, 486
delusional disorder, 456
depression, major (unipolar), 460
history and physical keys, 324
personality disorders, 469
schizoaffective disorder, 457
schizophrenia, 454
shared psychotic disorder, 457
Antipyretics
febrile seizures, 421
orocavity, herpes simplex of the, 658
strep throat, 661
Antireflex surgery, 111
Antiretroviral therapy, 251–252

Antisocial personality disorders, 468, 473
Antistreptolysin O (ASO) titer, 62
Antithrombin III, 37
deficiency
mechanisms and disease diagnosis/treatment, 190–191
Antithymocyte globulin (ATG), 174
Anti-topoisomerase, 80
Antitoxins, 422
Antivenin, 238, 239
Anuria
ill-defined symptoms, 627–628
Anxiety
acute pancreatitis, 159
adjustment disorders, 467
amenorrhea, 352
cocaine, 230
disorders, anxiety
acute stress disorder, 466
generalized anxiety disorder, 464
obsessive-compulsive disorder, 464–465
panic disorder, 462–464
phobias, 466–467
posttraumatic stress disorder, 465–466
domestic violence, 487
epiglottitis, 435
hydrocephalus, 423
hypochondriasis, 471
hypoglycemia, 105
personality disorders, 468
premenstrual syndrome, 351
rabies, 306
sexual dysfunctions, 484
somatization disorder, 469
stimulants, 229
Aorta
aneurysms of the thoracic, 588–590, 589f
chronic valvular diseases, 24
coarctation of the, 27–28
diseases of the
aneurysms, 39–40
aortitis, 42–43
dissection, aortic, 40–41
occlusion, aortic, 41–42
essential hypertension, 30
secondary hypertension, 30
tetralogy of fallot, 27

Aortic dissection
    mechanisms and disease diagnosis/treatment, 40–41
Aortic occlusion
    mechanisms and disease diagnosis/treatment, 41–42
Aortic stenosis, 6
Aortitis
    giant cell, 43
    mechanisms and disease diagnosis/treatment, 42–43
    rheumatic, 42
    syphilitic, 42
    Takayasu's, 42
Aortography. See also mechanisms and disease diagnosis/treatment and surgical principles under specific disease/disorder
    abdominal aortic aneurysms, 164, 590
    aortic occlusion, 41, 42
    pulmonary sequestration, 447
Aphasia, 303, 320
Aplasia, 445
Aplastic anemia
    mechanisms and disease diagnosis/treatment, 173–174
Apolipoproteins, 100, 327
Appendectomy, 133, 141
Appendicitis
    mechanisms and disease diagnosis/treatment, 132–133
    peritonitis, 140
    surgical principles, 599
Appetite disturbance
    depression, major (unipolar), 459
    dysthymia, 460
    hypoglycemia, 105
    neutropenia, 194
    olfaction and taste, disorders of, 667
Applanation tonometry, 415
Apraclonidine, 416
Arachidonic acid, 239
Arachnoid cells, 326
Arcuate nucleus, 489
Argyll-Robertson pupils, 310

Arrhythmias
    atrial septal defect, 26
    basic cardiac life support, 29
    bulimia, 475
    cocaine, 230
    electrical burns, 228
    hypothermia, 240
    ischemic bowel disease, 137
    Lyme disease, 272
    psychosomatic disorders, 472
    sarcoidosis, 508
    supraventricular
        bradyarrhythmias, 16–17
        tachyarrhythmias, 17–18
    tricyclic antidepressants, 228
    ventricular
        bradyarrhythmias, 18–19
        tachyarrhythmias, 19
Arsenic, 70
    mechanisms and disease diagnosis/treatment for poisoning from, 231
    toxic disorders, 323
Arterial blood gas (ABG). See also mechanisms and disease diagnosis/treatment and surgical principles under specific disease/disorder
    acute respiratory distress syndrome, 514
    asthma and pregnancy, 389
    bronchial asthma, 198
    bronchiolitis, 434
    distributive shock, 13
    electrical burns, 228
    hypothermia, 240
    infantile botulism, 421
    pneumococcal pneumonia, 495
    Pneumocystis carinii pneumonia, 252
    pulmonary embolism, 515
    respiratory distress syndrome, 430
    right-sided heart failure, 9
    secondary erythrocytosis, 186
    tetralogy of fallot, 27
    transient tachypnea of the newborn, 429
Arterial disease
    peripheral arterial vascular disease
        acute arterial occlusion, 35–36
        chronic atherosclerotic occlusion, 34–35
        vasculitis syndromes, 36–37

Arterial ectasia, 317
Arterial embolism, 137
    surgical principles, 593–594
Arterial ulcer
    surgical principles, 569–570
Arteriography. See also mechanisms and disease diagnosis/treatment and surgical principles under specific disease/disorder
    acute arterial occlusion, 36
    aneurysms of thoracic aorta, 588
    carotid artery disease, 584
    congestive heart failure, 514
    ischemic bowel disease, 137
    stable angina pectoris, 6
Arteriosclerosis, 81, 322
Arteriosclerotic ulcer, 78
Arteriovenous fistula, 9
Arthralgias
    anemia of chronic disease, 176
    blastomycosis, 501
    coccidioidomycosis, 501
    erythema nodosum, 62
    gonococcal tenosynovitis, 272
    histoplasmosis, 500
    humoral immunodeficiency, 204
    lupus arthritis, 282
    Lyme disease, 272
    mechanisms and disease diagnosis/treatment, 273–274
    psoriasis, 53
    rubella (German measles), 267
    secondary syphilis, 52
Arthritis
    Behcet's disease, 82
    familial Mediterranean fever, 141
    glenohumeral, 298
    gouty, 280
    hoarseness, 660
    humoral immunodeficiency, 204
    lupus, 281–282
    Lyme disease, 267, 268
    mumps, 266
    psoriasis, 54
    pyoderma gangrenosum, 79
    rheumatoid, 283, 291
    rotator cuff syndrome, 298
    rubella (German measles), 267
    septic, 271–272
    vasculitis syndromes, 36
Arthrography, 298

Arthroplasty, 290
5-ASA, 134
Asacol, 134
ASA therapy, 4, 5
Asbestosis
  bronchogenic carcinoma, 518
  mechanisms and disease diagnosis/treatment, 510
  squamous cell carcinoma, 110
*Ascaris*, 160
Ascites
  cirrhosis, 155, 157
  cor pulmonale, 518
  dilated cardiomyopathy, 13
  hepatitis, 146
  hepatocellular carcinoma, 153
  ill-defined presentations, 641–642
  ovarian cancer, 344
  restrictive cardiomyopathy, 15
  Rh incompatibility, 431
  right-sided heart failure, 9
Aseptic meningitis
  mechanisms and disease diagnosis/treatment, 306
Aseptic necrosis, 176
Asherman's syndrome, 352
Ash-leaf macule, 82
Asparaginase, 179
Aspartate aminotransferase (AST)
  alcohol, 478
  cirrhosis, 155
  hepatitis, 150, 377
  intestinal obstruction, 138
  preeclampsia, 375
  pregnancy, 377
Aspergillosis, invasive
  cryptococcal infection, 502–503
*Aspergillus*, 210, 663
*Aspergillus fumigatus*, 209, 210, 503
Asphyxia, water-induced, 238
Aspiration
  acute respiratory distress syndrome, 515
  bursitis, 284
  effusion of joint, 290, 291
  gout, 280
  gram-negative bacillary pneumonias, 497
  hearing loss, 655
  mechanisms and disease diagnosis/treatment, 226
  meconium, 431
  myasthenia gravis, 312

osteomyelitis, 271
tracheoesophageal fistula, 441
Aspirin
  acute upper respiratory infection, 668
  atherosclerosis, 34
  iron-deficiency anemia, 169
  Kawasaki disease, 426
  myocardial infarction, 5
  osteoarthritis, 274
  poisoning and mechanisms and disease diagnosis/treatment, 232
  stable angina, 7
  unstable angina, 4
Assisted reproductive technology (ART), 358, 536
Asteatotic dermatitis, 56
Astelin, 201
Asthma
  acute, 504
  allergic bronchopulmonary aspergillosis, 209, 210
  bronchial, 198–200
  chronic, 504, 505f
  gastroesophageal reflux disease, 110
  mechanisms and disease diagnosis/treatment, 503–504
  pregnancy, 389
  psychosomatic disorders, 472
  substance-related disorders, 478
Astigmatism, 397
Astrocytes, 325
Ataxia
  Creutzfeldt-Jakob disease, 305
  hypothyroidism, 89
  lead toxicity, 323
  mercury toxicity, 323
  multiple sclerosis, 331
  neurosyphilis, 310
  toxoplasma encephalitis, 256
  vitamin $B_{12}$ deficiency, 172, 313
Ataxia-telangiectasia, 85
Atazanavir, 250
Atelectasis
  acute bronchiolitis, 494
  croup, 436
  postpartum sepsis, 387
  respiratory distress syndrome, 430
  surgical principles, 583–584
Atenolol, 89

Atherosclerosis
  aneurysms, 40
  cardiac transplantation, 25
  chronic atherosclerotic occlusion, 34–35
  hyperlipoproteinemia, 32
  ischemic thrombotic strokes, 319
  mechanisms and disease diagnosis/treatment, 33–34, 34f
Atherosclerotic heart disease, 137
Atherosclerotic vascular disease, 551, 553
Athletic accidents, 242
Ativan, 421
Atlantoaxial instability, 444
Atopic dermatitis
  mechanisms and disease diagnosis/treatment, 56, 206–208
Atovaquone, 252
Atresia, 654
Atrial fibrillation (AF)
  acute arterial occlusion, 36
  cardioembolic strokes, 321
  description, 17
  hyperthyroidism, 88
  sick sinus syndrome, 16
  tachyarrhythmias, 18
Atrial flutter
  description, 17
Atrial septal defect (ASD)
  acute arterial occlusion, 36
  mechanisms and disease diagnosis/treatment, 26–27
Atrial tachycardia, 17
Atropine, 413
Atrovent, 199
Attention-deficit hyperactivity disorder (ADHD)
  conduct disorder, 474
  mechanisms and disease diagnosis/treatment, 472–473
Atypical nevus
  mechanisms and disease diagnosis/treatment, 73
Auditory injury
  mechanisms and disease diagnosis/treatment, 220–221
Auer rods, 177

Auscultation and tinnitus, 657. *See also* Bruit
Autistic disease
  mechanisms and disease diagnosis/treatment, 458
Autoimmune diseases. *See also specific disease/disorder*
  hepatitis, 147–148, 150, 151, 155
  lupus arthritis, 282
  lupus inhibitor, 189
  neutropenia, 194
  sudden hearing loss, 656
  vitamin $B_{12}$ deficiency, 172
Autosomal dominant/recessive disease, 552
Avascular necrosis
  developmental dysplasia of the hip, 433
  femur, fracture of neck of, 296
  slipped capital femoral epiphysis, 278
AV block
  mechanisms and disease diagnosis/treatment, 16–17
Avitaminosis A, 413
Avoidant personality disorders, 468
AV reentry (AVRT), 17
Azathioprine
  acute pancreatitis, 160
  Behcet's disease, 82
  cardiac transplantation, 25
  Crohn's disease, 137
  lupus arthritis, 282
  lupus nephritis, 553
  pemphigus, 60
  polymyositis-dermatomyositis, 283
  pulmonary vasculitis, 517
  rheumatoid arthritis, 283
  sarcoidosis, 508
  usual interstitial pneumonitis, 509
  vasculitis, 518
Azidothymidine (AZT), 250, 251, 438, 533
Azithromycin
  cervicitis and sexually transmitted diseases, 347
  chancroid, 262
  chlamydia, 260, 533
  disseminated *Mycobacterium avium-intracellulare* complex, 256
  gonorrhea, 532
Azoospermia, 507, 535

Azotemia
  acute pancreatitis, 159
  chronic renal failure, 174, 547
  glomerulonephritis, 549
  hyperosmolar hyperglycemic nonketotic coma, 104
  metabolic encephalopathy, 315
  polycystic kidney disease, 552
  renal transplant rejection, 548

# B
Bacillus Calmette-Guèrin (BCG) vaccine, 543
*Bacillus cereus*, 122
Back pain, low. *See also* back *under* Pain
  mechanisms and disease diagnosis/treatment, 274–275
Baclofen, 317, 332
Bacteremia, 259
Bacteria. *See also individual disease/disorder/organism*
  acute enteric infections, 122
  bronchopneumonia
    gram-negative bacillary, 496–497
    *Haemophilus influenzae*, 496
    pneumococcal, 495
    staphylococcal, 496
  conjunctivitis, 393, 395, 396t
  meningitis
    mechanisms and disease diagnosis/treatment, 437
  skin infections
    cellulitis: abscess or other local infections, 49–50
    impetigo, 50
    paronychia, 49
*Bacteroides*, 358
Balneol, 63
Barbiturates
  history and physical keys, 324
  poisoning and mechanisms and disease diagnosis/treatment, 232
  seizures, 316
Barium studies. *See also* mechanisms and disease diagnosis/treatment *and* surgical principles *under specific disease/disorder*
  constipation, 139

Crohn's disease, 135
  diarrhea, 126
  gastric motility, disorders of, 118
  hereditary nonpolyposis colorectal cancer, 130
  Hirschsprung disease, 443, 444f
  intestinal obstruction, 138
  intussusception, 442, 443
Barlow sign, 433
Barometric pressure and barotrauma, 656
Barotrauma
  mechanisms and disease diagnosis/treatment, 656–657
Barrett's esophagus, 110, 113
Basal cell carcinoma
  mechanisms and disease diagnosis/treatment, 70–71, 71f
  surgical principles, 566
Basic cardiac life support, 29
Basilar fracture, 218
Basophils
  allergic rhinitis, 665
  anaphylactic shock, 239
  chronic myelogenous leukemia, 179
Battle's sign, 218
B cells
  humoral immunodeficiency, 204
  intermediate/high-grade lymphoma, 184
  low-grade lymphoma, 182
Beau's lines, 85, 85f
Beck Depression Inventory, 383
Beck's triad, 223
Bee stings, 12
Behavioral approaches/therapy
  bulimia, 477
  constipation, 140
  irritable bowel syndrome, 127, 128
  phobia, 467
  sexual dysfunctions, 484
Behavior problems/bizarre behavior
  alcohol, 479
  bulimia, 475
  child physical/sexual abuse, 486, 487
  conduct disorder, 473–474
  Huntington's disease, 329
  hypochondriasis, 471

panic disorder, 462
posttraumatic stress disorder, 465
schizophrenia, 453
substance-related disorders, 477
Behcet's disease
mechanisms and disease diagnosis/treatment, 82
Bell's palsy, 268, 272, 309
Benadryl, 187, 201–202, 238, 239, 652
Bence Jones proteins, 184
benign prostatic hyperplasia, 542
Benign prostatic hypertrophy
mechanisms and disease diagnosis/treatment, 542
surgical principles, 578
Benign urethral stricture
mechanisms and disease diagnosis/treatment, 536–537
Bentiromide, 161
Benzene, 173
Benzodiazepines
affective psychoses: mania and psychotic depression, 455
alcohol, 480
generalized anxiety disorder, 464
history and physical keys, 324
posttraumatic stress disorder, 466
schizophrenia, 454
seizures, 316
social phobia, 466
vertigo, 652
Benzoyl peroxide, 67, 448
Bereavement
depression, major (unipolar), 459
sudden infant death syndrome, 489
uncomplicated, 488–489
Berger's disease, 549
Beta-adrenergic receptors, 463
Beta blockers
aortic dissection, 41
benign prostatic hyperplasia, 542
cirrhosis, 157
dilated cardiomyopathy, 14
essential hypertension, 30
glaucoma, 416
headaches, 318
hyperthyroidism, 89

hypertrophic cardiomyopathy, 15
left-sided low output heart failure, 8, 9
malignant hypertension, 31
myocardial infarction, 5
obstructive shock, 12
pheochromocytoma, 98
psoriasis, 53
social phobia, 466
stable angina pectoris, 7
tachyarrhythmias, 18
variant angina, 6
Beta-cells, 103
Beta-hemolytic streptococci, 437
Betamethasone, 376
Bicarbonate, 104
Bichloroacetic acid, 347
Bilateral salpingo-oophorectomy (BSO), 341, 344
Biliary atresia
surgical principles, 610
Biliary tract stone disease, 160
Bilirubin
acute cholecystitis, 144
gallstones, 171
hemolytic anemia, 175
hepatitis B infection complicating pregnancy, 377
neonatal hyperbilirubinemia, 432
Rh incompatibility, 431
Rh incompatibility or isoimmunization, 381
sickle cell anemia, 176
thrombotic thrombocytopenic purpura, 193
Biofeedback, 128, 140, 351
Biopsy. *See* mechanisms and disease diagnosis/treatment *and* surgical principles *under specific disease/disorder*
Bipolar disorders
mechanisms and disease diagnosis/treatment, 461–462
schizoaffective disorder, 456
Bird breeder's lung, 210
Bird exposure and meningitis, 307
Bisphosphonates
hypercalcemia, 92
menopausal symptoms, 353
osteoporosis, 279

Bitemporal defects
mechanisms and disease diagnosis/treatment, 405
Black widow spider, 239
Bladder. *See also* Genitourinary system; Renal and urinary system
carcinoma, 575–576
cervical spine and spinal stenosis, 333
mechanisms and disease diagnosis/treatment
carcinoma, 543–544
extrophy, 429
neurogenic, 539
painful, 529–530
multiple sclerosis, 331, 332
pelvic relaxation/urinary incontinence, 350–351
posterior urethral valves, 426–427
surgical principles, 575–576
urologic trauma, 541
vesicoureteral reflux, 427, 538
*Blastomyces dermatitidis*, 501
Blastomycosis
mechanisms and disease diagnosis/treatment, 501
Bleomycin
Hodgkin's disease, 182
penile/urethral/scrotal carcinoma, 546
testicular carcinoma, 545
Blepharitis
herpes simplex keratitis, 412
mechanisms and disease diagnosis/treatment, 396
Blepharoptosis
mechanisms and disease diagnosis/treatment, 399
Blepharospasm, 410, 423
Blindness
acute sinusitis, 662
congenital cataracts, 424
herpes simplex, 52
Tay-Sachs disease, 335
Blistering diseases of the skin
bullous pemphigoid, 58–59
dermatitis herpetiformis, 60–61
herpes gestationis, 59
pemphigus, 59–60

Blood. *See also Hemo and Hema listings;* Platelets; Red blood cells; White blood cells
　abruptio placentae, 374
　chronic atherosclerotic occlusion, 35
　contusions, 292
　disseminated intravascular coagulation, 190
　disseminated *Mycobacterium avium-intracellulare* complex, 256
　epistaxis, 217
　fractures/dislocations, vascular compromise following, 299
　gastroesophageal reflux disease, 110
　ischemic heart disease, 23
　ovarian cysts, 344
　placenta previa, 374
　stable angina pectoris, 6
　sugar, 104, 105
　ventricular septic defect, 26
　von Willebrand disease, 188
Blood-loss anemia
　mechanisms and disease diagnosis/treatment, 169–170
Blood pressure
　aortic dissection, 40
　atherosclerosis, 33
　cardiogenic shock, 10
　chronic atherosclerotic occlusion, 35
　coarctation of the aorta, 28
　contusions, 331
　eclampsia, 552
　hypovolemic shock, 11
　intracerebral hemorrhage, 321
　malignant hypertension, 31
　penile, 484
　pheochromocytoma, 98
　preeclampsia, 375, 551
　secondary hypertension, 30
　vasculitis syndromes, 36
Blood urea nitrogen (BUN). *See also* mechanisms and disease diagnosis/ treatment *and* surgical principles *under specific disease/disorder*
　acute pancreatitis, 159–160

acute renal failure, 546
blood-loss anemia, 170
delirium, 486
essential hypertension, 29, 30
hypovolemic shock, 11
malignant hypertension, 31
thrombotic thrombocytopenic purpura, 192
urethral stricture, benign, 536
Blue nevus
　mechanisms and disease diagnosis/treatment, 75
Body dysmorphic disorder
　mechanisms and disease diagnosis/treatment, 472
Bone marrow
　acute lymphocytic leukemia, 178, 179
　acute myelogenous leukemia, 177, 178
　agnogenic myeloid metaplasia, 193, 194
　anemia of chronic disease, 176
　aplastic anemia, 173, 174
　cellular (T-cell) immunodeficiency, 205
　chronic lymphocytic leukemia, 180
　chronic myelogenous leukemia, 179
　disseminated *Mycobacterium avium-intracellulare* complex, 255
　essential thrombocythemia, 193
　folic acid deficiency, 170
　histoplasmosis, 500
　Hodgkin's disease, 182
　intermediate/high-grade lymphoma, 183
　iron-deficiency anemia, 169
　low-grade lymphoma, 182
　monoclonal gammopathy of undetermined significance, 185
　multiple myeloma, 184, 185
　neutropenia, 195
　osteomyelitis, 271
　polycythemia rubra vera, 185
　thalassemia-beta, 172
　trigeminal neuralgia, 317
　tuberculosis, 254
　vitamin $B_{12}$ deficiency, 173

Bone metastases. *See also* Musculoskeletal/ connective tissue disease
　mechanisms and disease diagnosis/treatment, 286–287
Bone scans
　leg/foot fractures, 296–297
　metastases to bone, 287
　osteosarcoma, 286
Borborygmi, 138
Borderline personality disorders, 468
*Bordetella pertussis,* 494, 495
*Borrelia burgdorferi,* 268, 272, 309
Botulinum, 113
Botulism, infantile
　mechanisms and disease diagnosis/treatment, 421–422
Bowel function
　benign neoplasm of the small surgical principles, 606
　bloody stool, 126, 141
　cervical spine and spinal stenosis, 333
　constipation, 139–140
　Hirschsprung disease, 443
　intestinal obstruction, 138
　intussusception, 442
　irritable bowel syndrome, 126–127
　ischemic bowel disease, 137
　large-bowel obstruction, 603
　ovarian cancer, 344
　seizures, 315
　small-bowel obstruction, 162, 601–602, 602*f*
　sounds
　　acute pancreatitis, 159
　　intestinal obstruction, 138
　　necrotizing enterocolitis, 443
　　viscus, perforation of, 223
Bowen's disease, 69
Brachytherapy, 543
Bradyarrhythmias
　mechanisms and disease diagnosis/treatment
　　supraventricular, 16–17
　　ventricular, 18–19
Bradycardia
　anorexia, 474
　hydrocephalus, 423
　hypothermia, 240

Legionnaire's disease, 497
opioids, 324
Bradykinesia, 328
Brain
　abscesses, 309
　acute sinusitis, 662
　delirium, 485
　drowning and damage to, 238
　fungal meningitis, 307
　gestational trophoblastic disease, 382
　neural tube defects, 423
　papilledema, 402
　sleep apnea, 334
　substance-related disorders, 478
　toxoplasma encephalitis, 256
　tuberculosis, 308
Brain stem auditory evoked response potentials (BAER), 424
*Branhamella catarrhalis,* 649
Breast
　cancer, 84
　　mechanisms and disease diagnosis/treatment, 353–355, 354*t*
　　metastases, 326
　　surgical principles, 570–571
　fibroadenoma, 355
　fibrocystic disease, 356
　inflammatory disease of the, 355
　menopausal symptoms, 353
　prenatal care, 365
　surgical principles
　　benign breast mass, 570
　　cancer, 570–571
Breath sounds. *See also* Crackles
　bronchogenic carcinoma, 518
　emphysema, 506
　pleural effusions, 512
　pneumothorax, 222, 513
　pulmonary tuberculosis, 499
Breech presentation, 277, 433
Breslow's level, 72
Bretylium, 19
Brief psychotic disorder
　mechanisms and disease diagnosis/treatment, 457
Brinzolamide, 416
Bromocriptine
　fibrocystic disease, 356
　overproduction syndromes (pituitary gland), 93
　Parkinson's disease, 329

Bromonidine, 416
Bronchiectasis
　allergic bronchopulmonary aspergillosis, 209
　cystic fibrosis, 507
　mechanisms and disease diagnosis/treatment, 507–508
Bronchiolitis
　acute, 494
　mechanisms and disease diagnosis/treatment, 434
Bronchitis
　acute, 494
　chronic, 505–506
　cystic fibrosis, 507
　substance-related disorders, 478
Bronchoalveolar lavage (BAL), 252, 324
Bronchodilators
　acute asthma, 504
　asthma, 504
　bronchial asthma, 199–200
　chronic asthma, 504
　emphysema, 506
　hypereosinophilic syndrome, 212
Bronchogenic carcinoma
　mechanisms and disease diagnosis/treatment, 518–519
Bronchopneumonia
　gram-negative bacillary, 496–497
　*Haemophilus influenzae,* 496
　pneumococcal, 495
　staphylococcal, 496
Bronchopulmonary dysplasia (BPD), 430
Bronchoscopy, 447, 499
Bronchospasm
　asthma, 389, 504
　atopic dermatitis, 56
　pregnancy, 389
　urticaria, 57
Brown recluse spider, 239
Brudzinski's sign, 437
Bruising. *See* Tenderness and easy bruising
Bruit
　abdominal aortic aneurysms, 39
　carotid artery disease, 584
　chronic atherosclerotic occlusion, 35
　hyperthyroidism, 88

　renovascular hypertension, 551
　thoracic outlet syndrome, 592
　tinnitus, 657
　vasculitis syndromes, 36
Buccolingual involuntary movements, 324
Bulbar muscle, 305, 312
Bulbar urethra, 537
Bulbocavernous reflex, 294
Bulimia
　mechanisms and disease diagnosis/treatment, 475–477
Bullous impetigo, 50*f*
Bullous myringitis, 498
Bullous pemphigoid
　mechanisms and disease diagnosis/treatment, 58–59
Bupropion
　anorexia, 475
　attention-deficit hyperactivity disorder, 473
　depression, major (unipolar), 460
Burger's disease, 41
Burkitt's lymphoma, 183
Burns
　electrical, 227–228
　phycomycosis, 503
　thermal, 227
Burr cells, 174
Burrow's solution, 49, 209
Bursitis
　mechanisms and disease diagnosis/treatment, 284–285
Burst fractures, thoracic spine and, 294
Buspirone
　generalized anxiety disorder, 464
Butyrophenones, 324

## C

C acetate breath tests, 118
Cachexia, 135, 441
Caffeine
　dependence, drug, 483
　fibrocystic disease, 356
　panic disorder, 464
Café-au-lait macules, 85
CAGE screen, 478
Calamine, 209

Calcification
- congenital cytomegalovirus, 439
- congenital glaucoma, 424
- congenital toxoplasmosis, 438
- contusions, 292
- histoplasmosis, 500
- silicosis, 509
- syphilitic aortitis, 42

Calcinosis, 81
Calcipotriene, 54
Calcitonin
- hypercalcemia, 92, 557
- osteoporosis, 279
- Paget's disease of bone, 290
- thyroid gland, neoplasms of the, 91

Calcium
- amyotrophic lateral sclerosis, 328
- celiac sprue, 125
- essential hypertension, 30
- febrile seizures, 421
- hypercalcemia, 91
- menopausal symptoms, 353
- osteoporosis, 279
- renal osteodystrophy, 550
- rickets, 280
- sarcoidosis, 508

Calcium channel blockers
- achalasia, 113
- diffuse esophageal spasm, 113
- hypertrophic cardiomyopathy, 15
- irritable bowel syndrome, 128
- stable angina pectoris, 7
- tachyarrhythmias, 18
- unstable angina, 4
- variant angina, 6

Calf swelling, 37
*Calilaria philippinesis*, 122
*Campylobacter*, 122
*Campylobacter jejuni*, 126, 311
*Candida*, 49, 205
*Candida albicans*
- acute enteric infections, 123
- candidiasis, oral, 48
- thrush, oral, 658

Candidiasis
- mechanisms and disease diagnosis/treatment
  - dermatology, 48–49
  - otolaryngology, 658

Cannabinoids, 482
Capsaicin cream, 47

Carbamazepine
- bipolar disorders, 462
- schizoaffective disorder, 457
- seizures, 316
- trigeminal neuralgia, 317

Carbidopa, 329
Carbohydrates and hyperosmolar hyperglycemic nonketotic coma, 104
Carbon dioxide and panic disorder, 463
Carbonic anhydrase inhibitors, 416
Carbon monoxide, mechanisms and disease
- diagnosis/treatment for poisoning from, 231

Carboxyhemoglobin, 231
Carboxyhemoglobinemia, 186
Carcinoembryonic antigen (CEA), 132, 157
Carcinoid tumors
- mechanisms and disease diagnosis/treatment, 519

Cardiac tamponade
- aortic dissection, 40
- mechanisms and disease diagnosis/treatment, 21
- obstructive shock, 12

Cardioembolic strokes
- mechanisms and disease diagnosis/treatment, 320–321

Cardiogenic pulmonary edema
- mechanisms and disease diagnosis/treatment, 514

Cardiogenic shock
- mechanisms and disease diagnosis/treatment, 10–11

Cardiomegaly, 431
Cardiomyopathy
- alcohol, 478
- hypothyroidism, 89
- ventricular tachycardia, 19

Cardiopulmonary arrest, 28–29
Cardiopulmonary resuscitation (CPR)
- anaphylactic shock, 239
- drowning, 238
- electrical burns, 228
- hypothermia, 240
- shock, 239
- skull trauma/fracture, 218
- thermal burns, 227
- traumatic injury, 239

Cardiovascular medicine
- alcohol, 478
- aorta, diseases of the
  - aneurysms, 39–40
  - aortitis, 42–43
  - dissection, aortic, 40–41
  - occlusion, aortic, 41–42
- arrhythmias
  - supraventricular, 16–18
  - ventricular, 18–19
- congenital heart disease
  - abscesses, 308
  - atrial septal defect, 26–27
  - coarctation of the aorta, 27–28
  - tetralogy of Fallot, 27
  - trisomy 18, 445
  - ventricular septal defect, 25–26
- Down syndrome, 444
- heart failure
  - left-sided, 8–9
  - right-sided, 9–10
- hypertension
  - essential, 29–30
  - malignant, 31
  - secondary, 30–31
- hypotension and acute circulatory collapse (shock)
  - cardiogenic shock, 10–11
  - distributive shock, 12–13
  - hypovolemic shock, 11–12
  - obstructive shock, 12
- ischemic heart disease
  - acute, 3–6
  - chronic, 6–7
- life support, cardiac, 28–29
- lipoproteins and atherosclerosis
  - atherosclerosis, 33–34
  - hyperlipoproteinemia, 32–33
- myocardial diseases
  - dilated cardiomyopathy, 13–14
  - hypertrophic cardiomyopathy, 14–15
  - restrictive cardiomyopathy, 15–16
- pericardial diseases
  - acute pericarditis, 20
  - cardiac tamponade, 21
  - constrictive pericarditis, 22
  - pericardial effusion, 20–21
- peripheral arterial vascular disease
  - acute arterial occlusion, 35–36

chronic atherosclerotic
occlusion, 34–35
vasculitis syndromes, 36–37
peripheral venous vascular
diseases and pulmonary
embolism
pulmonary embolism, 38
venous thrombosis, 37–38
transplantation, 25
valvular diseases
acute, 22–23
chronic, 24–25
cardioverter-defibrillator, 14
Carotenemia, 89
Carotid artery disease
surgical principles, 584–585, 585f
Carotids, bleeding from
internal/external, 217
Carpal tunnel syndrome
mechanisms and disease
diagnosis/treatment,
288–289, 310–311
Caseation necrosis, 308
Caspofungin, 503
Cataracts
amblyopia, 406
mechanisms and disease
diagnosis/treatment,
417–418, 418t
congenital, 424
Catecholamines
atherosclerosis, 34
attention-deficit hyperactivity
disorder, 473
pheochromocytoma, 98
secondary hypertension, 30
Catechol-o-methyltransferase
(COMT), 329
Catheterization. *See also*
mechanisms and disease
diagnosis/treatment *and*
surgical principles *under*
*specific disease/disorder*
acute respiratory distress
syndrome, 514
cardiac tamponade, 21
cardiogenic shock, 10, 11
choledocholithiasis, 146
chronic valvular diseases, 24, 25
congestive heart failure, 514
constrictive pericarditis, 22
cor pulmonale, 518
dilated cardiomyopathy, 13
ischemic heart disease, 23

left-sided low output heart
failure, 8
neurogenic bladder, 539, 540
peritonitis, 140
restrictive cardiomyopathy, 15
right-sided heart failure, 9
tracheoesophageal fistula, 441
urethral stricture, benign, 537
urinary tract infections, 529
urologic trauma, 541
ventricular septic defect, 26
ventricular tachycardia, 19
Cat litter, 438
Cauda equina syndrome
description, 299
spinal stenosis, 291
Cauliflower ear, 221
Cauterization, arterial, 12
Cavernous sinus thrombosis, 322,
662
CD4
atopic dermatitis, 207
cytomegalovirus, 253
disseminated *Mycobacterium*
*avium-intracellulare*
complex, 256
HIV (human immunodeficiency
virus), 248–251, 303
*Pneumocystis carinii* pneumonia,
252, 253, 498
toxoplasma encephalitis, 257
tuberculosis, 254
CD5, 180
CD8, 207
CD19, 180
Cecal diverticulitis, 133
Cefixime, 259
Cefotaxime, 260, 307
Cefotetan, 263
Cefoxitin, 263, 347
Ceftizoxime, 260
Ceftriaxone
cervicitis and sexually
transmitted diseases, 347
chancroid, 262
epididymoorchitis, 263
gonococcal tenosynovitis, 273
gonorrhea, 259, 260, 532
Lyme disease, 268, 272
pelvic inflammatory disease, 358
Cefuroxime, 493, 496
Celiac disease, 60
Celiac nerve block, 157
Celiac plexus block, 161

Celiac sprue
mechanisms and disease
diagnosis/treatment,
124–125, 124f
CellCept, 283
Cellular (T-cell) immunodeficiency
mechanisms and disease
diagnosis/treatment, 205
Cellulitis
epiglottitis, 435
ingrowing nails, 66
mechanisms and disease
diagnosis/treatment, 49–50
pharyngitis, 437
stasis ulceration, 77
substance-related disorders,
477–478
surgical principles, 564
venous thrombosis, 37
Centers for Disease Control and
Prevention (CDC), 252
Central nervous system (CNS)
amenorrhea, 352
diethyl-m-toluamide, 232
HIV (human immunodeficiency
virus), 303
hypomagnesemia, 557
infectious diseases of the
abscesses, 308–309
meningitis, 306–308
spirochetes, 309–310
viruses, 303–306
intermediate/high-grade
lymphoma, 183
lupus erythematosus, 80
Lyme disease, 268, 272
mumps, 266
neural tube defects and
malformation in the
fetus, 378–380, 379f
skull trauma/fracture, 218
toxoplasma encephalitis, 256
Central scotomas
mechanisms and disease
diagnosis/treatment,
404–405, 405f
Central sleep apnea, 524
Cephalosporin
abscesses, 309
acute otitis media, 649
gonorrhea, 259, 260
gram-negative bacillary
pneumonias, 497
pelvic inflammatory disease, 263

Cerclage, 378
Cerebral vascular diseases, 406
Cerebrospinal fluid (CSF). *See also*
	mechanisms and disease
	diagnosis/treatment *and*
	surgical principles *under*
	*specific disease/disorder*
  aseptic meningitis, 306
  bacterial meningitis, 437
  Creutzfeldt-Jakob disease, 305
  cryptococcal infection, 257, 258, 502
  facial fracture, 217
  fungal meningitis, 307
  Guillain-Barré syndrome, 311
  herpes simplex virus, 304
  HIV (human immunodeficiency virus), 303
  hydrocephalus, 423
  Lyme disease, 267, 309
  neurosyphilis, 310
  poliomyelitis, 305
  septic meningitis, 307
  skull trauma/fracture, 218
  syphilis, 261
  toxoplasma encephalitis, 256
  tuberculosis, 254, 308
Cerebrovascular accident (CVA)
  abdominal aortic aneurysm, 164
  cocaine, 324
  disorders, cerebrovascular
    cardioembolic strokes, 320–321
    intracerebral hemorrhage, 321
    ischemic thrombotic strokes, 318–320
    subarachnoid hemorrhage, 321–322
    venous thrombosis, 322–323
  elevated Lp (a) lipoprotein, 102
  essential hypertension, 30
  essential thrombocythemia, 193
  hemolytic uremic syndrome, 440
  hyperosmolar hyperglycemic nonketotic coma, 104
  lupus inhibitor, 189
  malignant hypertension, 31
  sickle cell anemia, 176, 177
  sleep apnea, 334
  sudden hearing loss, 656
  syndrome of inappropriate antidiuretic hormone secretion, 95
  vasculitis syndromes, 36

Ceruloplasmin, 458
Cerumen impaction
  mechanisms and disease diagnosis/treatment, 651
Cervical spine
  mechanisms and disease diagnosis/treatment
    fractures, 292–293
    spinal stenosis, 333
Cervicitis
  chlamydia, 260
  gonorrhea, 259
Cervix
  mechanisms and disease diagnosis/treatment
    cervical dysplasia and management of abnormal Pap smear, 347–348, 348f
    cervicitis and sexually transmitted diseases, 345–347
    incompetent, 378
    malignant neoplasm, 345
    pelvic inflammatory disease, 262, 358
    premature labor, 376
    premature rupture of membranes, 384
    spontaneous abortion, 371
Cesarean section
  labor and delivery, abnormal, 385
  neural tube defects and central nervous system malformation in the fetus, 380
  placenta previa, 374
  postpartum sepsis, 386
$C_1$-esterase inhibitor levels, 205, 206
Chalazion
  mechanisms and disease diagnosis/treatment, 397
Chancroid
  cervicitis, 346, 347
  mechanisms and disease diagnosis/treatment, 262
Charcoal, activated
  acetaminophen, 228
  poisoning and management overview, 232
  stimulants, 229
Charcot-Bouchard aneurysms, 321
Charcot's arthropathy, 276
Charcot's triad, 145

Chelation therapy
  heavy metals/arsenic, 231
  manganese toxicity, 324
  restrictive cardiomyopathy, 15
Chemical worker's lung, 210
Chemotherapy. *See also*
	mechanisms and disease
	diagnosis/treatment *and*
	surgical principles *under*
	*specific disease/disorder*
  acute lymphocytic leukemia, 179
  adenocarcinoma, 110
  bronchogenic carcinoma, 519
  carcinoid tumors, 519
  colorectal carcinoma, 132
  endometrial cancer, 341
  gastric cancer, 115
  gestational trophoblastic disease, 382
  glioblastoma, 326
  Hodgkin's disease, 182
  intermediate/high-grade lymphoma, 184
  larynx, cancer of the, 661
  metastases, 327
  multiple myeloma, 185
  oropharynx, malignant neoplasms of the, 660
  osteosarcoma, 286
  ovarian cancer, 344
  pancreatic carcinoma, 157
  penile/urethral/scrotal carcinoma, 546
  teratology, 367
  testicular carcinoma, 545
  vaginal cancer, 349
  Wilms' tumor, 545
Chest and abdominal injury
  additional information, 223
  epidemiology and prevention of chest/abdominal injury, 224
  flail chest, 223
  hemothorax, 222
  pelvic fractures, 224
  perforation of viscus, 223–224
  pneumothorax, 222
  rib cage, 221
Chest x-rays (CXRs)
  bronchiolitis, 434
  croup, 436
  low-grade lymphoma, 182
  *Pneumocystis carinii* pneumonia, 252

pulmonary sequestration, 447
respiratory distress syndrome, 430
transient tachypnea of the newborn, 429
Chickenpox. *See* Varicella
Child-Turcotte-Pugh scale, 156, 156*t*
Chills
acute enteric infections, 120
acute sinusitis, 662
blastomycosis, 501
choledocholithiasis, 145
distributive shock, 12
erythema nodosum, 62
gram-negative bacillary pneumonias, 496
histoplasmosis, 500
hypersensitivity pneumonitis, 210, 511
influenza pneumonia, 498
*Mycoplasma pneumoniae*, 497
urinary tract infections, 529
varicella (chickenpox), 46
Chlamydia
cervicitis, 346, 347
epididymoorchitis, 263
gonorrhea, 259, 532
mechanisms and disease diagnosis/treatment, 260, 532–533
*Chlamydia*, 384
*Chlamydia trachomatis*, 260
adolescent pregnancy, 370
epididymoorchitis, 263
pelvic inflammatory disease, 262, 263, 358
urethritis, 531
Chlorambucil, 82, 181
Chloramphenicol, 173, 496
Chlordiazepoxide, 480
Chloropromazine, 149
Chloroquine, 83
Chlorpropamide, 94, 95
Choanal atresia, 434
Cholangitis, 145–146
Cholecystectomy, 128, 145
Cholecystitis, 144–145
Cholecystokinin (CCK), 161
Choledochal cyst
surgical principles, 611
Choledocholithiasis
mechanisms and disease diagnosis/treatment, 145–146
surgical principles, 612

Cholelithiasis
mechanisms and disease diagnosis/treatment, 145
Cholera, 123
Cholescintigraphy, 144
Cholesteatoma, 650
Cholesterol
atherosclerosis, 34
congenital adrenal hyperplasia, 99
dysbetalipoproteinemia, type III, 100
gallstones, 145
hyperlipoproteinemia, type II, 100
hyperlipoproteinemia, type IV, 101
Cholestyramine
diarrhea, 635
hyperlipoproteinemia, 33
hyperlipoproteinemia, type II, 100
Chondroitin, 274
Chondrolysis, 296
Chondromalacia patellae
mechanisms and disease diagnosis/treatment, 450
Chorda tympani, 667
Chorea, 323, 329
Chorioamnionitis, 384, 386
Choriocarcinoma, 327
Chorionic villus sampling (CVS)
Down syndrome, 444
prenatal diagnosis, 366
trisomy, 380
Chorioretinitis
congenital cytomegalovirus, 439
congenital toxoplasmosis, 438
herpes simplex virus, 439
interstitial keratitis, 413
Chromosomal disorders, 424. *See also* Down syndrome; Trisomy
Chromosome 21, 327
Chromotography, 477
Chronic anovulation, 341
Chronic asthma, 504
Chronic atherosclerotic occlusion
mechanisms and disease diagnosis/treatment, 34–35
Chronic bronchitis
mechanisms and disease diagnosis/treatment, 505–506
Chronic cellulitis, 37

Chronic cutaneous candidiasis, 48–49
Chronic disease, anemia of
mechanisms and disease diagnosis/treatment, 176
Chronic granulocyte-colony stimulating factor (G-CSF), 195
Chronic hemolysis, 175
Chronic hemolytic anemias, 170
Chronic hepatitis, 147, 153
Chronic hypersensitivity pneumonitis, 511
Chronic lupus erythematosus, 80
Chronic lymphocytic leukemia (CLL)
idiopathic thrombocytopenic purpura, 192
mechanisms and disease diagnosis/treatment, 180–181, 180*f*
Chronic meconium ileus, 162
Chronic myelogenous leukemia (CML)
mechanisms and disease diagnosis/treatment, 179–180
Chronic obstructive pulmonary disease (COPD)
bronchiectasis, 507–508
chronic bronchitis, 505–506
coal workers' pneumoconiosis, 510, 511
cor pulmonale, 518
cystic fibrosis, 507
emphysema, 506
respiratory acidosis, 556
secondary erythrocytosis, 186
staphylococcal pneumonia, 496
Chronic pancreatitis
mechanisms and disease diagnosis/treatment, 161
pancreatic carcinoma, 157
Chronic pyelonephritis, 546
Chronic renal failure
half-and-half nails, 85
mechanisms and disease diagnosis/treatment, 174, 547
Chronic sinusitis, 663
Chronic valvular diseases
mechanisms and disease diagnosis/treatment, 24–25
Chronic venous thrombosis, 37

Chvostek's sign, 558
Chylomicronemia, type 1 familial
    mechanisms and disease
        diagnosis/treatment, 99
Chylomicrons, 32, 101
Cidofovir, 254
Cimetidine, 111, 413
Ciprofloxacin
    chancroid, 262
    diarrhea, 126
    disseminated *Mycobacterium
        avium-intracellulare*
        complex, 256
    diverticulitis, 139
    epididymitis, 531
    gonorrhea, 259, 532
    orchitis, 531
    prostatitis, 530
    tuberculosis, 255
Circulatory system. *See* Blood;
    Hematology
Cirrhosis
    alcohol, 478
    hepatitis, 146
    hepatocellular carcinoma, 153
    mechanisms and disease
        diagnosis/treatment,
        155–157
    syndrome of inappropriate
        antidiuretic hormone
        secretion, 95
    Terry's nails, 84
Cisapride, 118
Cisplatin, 544, 545
Clarithromycin, 256
Claritin, 201
Clark's level, 72
Claudication
    aneurysms, 40
    aortic occlusion, 41
    arterial ulcer, 569
    atherosclerosis, 33
    chronic atherosclerotic
        occlusion, 35
    coarctation of the aorta, 28
    peripheral arterial occlusive
        disease, 586
    spinal stenosis, 291
Clavulanate, 262, 649
Clavulinic acid
    acute epiglottitis, 493
    diverticulitis, 139
    *Haemophilus influenzae*
        pneumonia, 496

Cleft lip or palate
    mechanisms and disease
        diagnosis/treatment, 440
    otitis media, 434, 435
    trisomy 13, 445
Clindamycin
    pelvic inflammatory disease,
        263, 358
    *Pneumocystis carinii* pneumonia,
        252
    toxoplasma encephalitis, 257
Clitoromegaly, 97
Clofibrate, 33, 145
Clomiphene citrate, 536
Clomipramine, 465
Clonazepam, 332
Clonidine
    attention-deficit hyperactivity
        disorder, 473
    essential hypertension, 30
    glaucoma, 416
Closed-angle glaucoma, 416
*Clostridium*, 126
*Clostridium botulinum*, 421
*Clostridium difficile*
    acute enteric infections, 120
    Crohn's disease, 135
    diarrhea, 126
    ulcerative colitis, 134
*Clostridium perfringens*, 122
*Clostridium trachomatis*, 259
Clothing and atopic dermatitis,
    207
Clotrimazole
    candidiasis, cutaneous, 49
    candidiasis, oral, 48
    vulva/vagina, candidiasis of the,
        349
Clubbing
    allergic bronchopulmonary
        aspergillosis, 209, 210
    asbestosis, 510
    cirrhosis, 155
    nail signs and disease, 85
    pulmonary osteoarthropathy,
        287
    usual interstitial pneumonitis,
        508
Cluster headaches, 318
Coagulopathy/coagulation factor
    levels
    acute cholecystitis, 145
    cirrhosis, 155
    vitamin K deficiency, 189

Coal tar, 207
Coal workers' pneumoconiosis
    mechanisms and disease
        diagnosis/treatment,
        510–511
Coarctation of the aorta
    mechanisms and disease
        diagnosis/treatment,
        27–28
    Turner's syndrome, 445
Cocaine
    history and physical keys, 324
    poisoning and mechanisms and
        disease diagnosis/
        treatment, 230
    substance-related disorders, 478
    ulcerative colitis, 134
*Coccidioides immitis*, 502
Coccidioidomycosis
    mechanisms and disease
        diagnosis/treatment,
        501–502
Cochlear implant surgery, 655
C octanoic breath tests, 118
Codeine, 213, 521
Codman's triangle, 286
Coenzyme A (CoA), 173
Cogan's syndrome, 413, 652, 656
Cognitive-behavioral therapies
    adjustment disorders, 467
    bulimia, 477
    generalized anxiety disorder,
        464
    pain disorder, 470
    panic disorder, 464
    phobia, 467
    posttraumatic stress disorder,
        466
    sexual dysfunctions, 484
    social phobia, 466
    substance-related disorders,
        478
Cohen reimplant, 538
Coin lesion
    mechanisms and disease
        diagnosis/treatment,
        523
Colchicine
    Behcet's disease, 82
    familial Mediterranean fever,
        141
    gout, 280
Colectomy, 135, 603, 604
Colic and lead toxicity, 323

Colitis
  acute enteric infections, 123
  cytomegalovirus, 253
  diarrhea, 126
  pseudomembranous, 126
Collagen
  acute pericarditis, 20
  agnogenic myeloid metaplasia, 194
  aortic dissection, 41
  Dupuytren's contracture, 288
  livedo reticularis, 81
  menopausal symptoms, 353
  neurogenic bladder, 540
  pleural effusions, 512
  scleroderma, 81
  sick sinus syndrome, 16
  syphilitic aortitis, 42
  vascular diseases, 517
Colles' fracture, 234
Colloid solutions, 11, 13
Colon
  appendicitis, 132–133
  benign neoplasm
    surgical principles, 606, 607f
  cancer
    Muir-Torre syndrome, 84
    surgical principles, 606–607
  colorectal carcinoma, 128–132, 129t–131t
  constipation, 139–140
  diarrhea, invasive, 126
  diverticulitis, 138–139
  familial Mediterranean fever, 140–141
  inflammatory bowel disease
    Crohn's disease, 135, 136f, 137
    ulcerative colitis, 133–135, 133f
  intestinal obstruction, 138
  irritable bowel syndrome, 126–128, 127t
  ischemic bowel disease, 137
  peritonitis, 140
  viscus, perforation of, 223
Colonic aganglionosis
  mechanisms and disease diagnosis/treatment, 443–444, 444f
Colonoscopy
  colorectal carcinoma, 131
  Crohn's disease, 135
  diverticulitis, 138
  hemorrhoids, 141
  ulcerative colitis, 133

Colony-forming units (CFU), 377
Colorectal carcinoma (CRC)
  environmental risk factors, 128, 129t
  familial adenomatosis polyposis, 128
  hereditary nonpolyposis colorectal cancer, 129–131, 130t
  mechanisms and disease diagnosis/treatment, 131–132, 131t
Colostomy, 603
Colporrhaphy, 351
Colposcopy, 347, 349
Colpotomy, 359
Coma
  alcohol, 479
  Creutzfeldt-Jakob disease, 305
  diabetes mellitus, 103
  diethyl-m-toluamide, 232
  electrical burns, 227
  epidural hematoma, 330
  hepatitis B infection complicating pregnancy, 377
  hypercalcemia, 92
  hyperosmolar hyperglycemic nonketotic coma, 104
  hypoglycemia, 105
  hyponatremia, 553
  hypothermia, 240
  hypothyroidism, 89
  intracerebral hemorrhage, 321
  lead toxicity, 323
  malignant hypertension, 31
  sedatives, 229
  seizures, 316
  septic meningitis, 307
  subdural hematoma, 219
  volume depletion, 555
  volume excess, 555
Combination prophylaxis and HIV, 252
Combivent, 199
Comedo-hyperkeratosis of follicular epithelium, 448
Common acute lymphoblastic leukemia antigen (CALLA), 178
Communication issues and sexual dysfunctions, 484
Compartmental syndrome, 299

Complete blood count (CBC). *See also* mechanisms and disease diagnosis/treatment *and* surgical principles *under specific disease/disorder*
  abruptio placentae, 374
  acute myelogenous leukemia, 177
  alcohol, 480
  child physical/sexual abuse, 486
  Crohn's disease, 135
  delirium, 486
  febrile seizures, 421
  fibromyalgia, 285
  hemolytic uremic syndrome, 440
  inflammatory disease of the breast, 355
  irritable bowel syndrome, 127
  leiomyomata uteri, 342
  lupus erythematosus, 80
  neutropenia, 195
  ovarian cysts, 344, 345
  postpartum hemorrhage, 386
  preeclampsia, 375
  prenatal care, 365
  schizophrenia, 454
Complex febrile seizures, 421
Compression fractures
  lumbar spine, 294
  thoracic spine, 294
Compression stockings, 77
Computed tomography (CT), 590. *See also* mechanisms and disease diagnosis/treatment *and* surgical principles *under specific disease/disorder*
  abdominal aortic aneurysm, 164
  abscesses, 309
  acute sinusitis, 662
  allergic bronchopulmonary aspergillosis, 209
  Alzheimer's disease, 327
  aneurysms, 40, 588
  appendicitis, 132
  aseptic meningitis, 306
  autistic disorder, 458
  back pain, low, 274
  bitemporal defects, 405
  cardioembolic strokes, 320
  cervical spine, fractures of the, 293
  cervical spine and spinal stenosis, 333

Computed tomography (CT) (*continued*)
  choledocholithiasis, 145
  chronic otitis media, 649
  chronic rhinitis, 664
  chronic sinusitis, 663
  colorectal carcinoma, 132
  constrictive pericarditis, 22
  contusions, 331
  Crohn's disease, 135
  cryptorchidism, 534
  Cushing's syndrome, 97
  cystic fibrosis, 669
  epidural hematoma, 330
  epistaxis, 665
  esophageal neoplasms, 109
  femur, fracture of neck of, 296
  gastric cancer, 114
  glioblastoma, 325
  headaches, 317
  hearing loss, 654
  hepatocellular carcinoma, 154
  herpes simplex virus, 304
  Hodgkin's disease, 181
  Huntington's disease, 329
  hydrocephalus, 423
  hypersensitivity pneumonitis, 211, 511
  intracerebral hemorrhage, 321
  ischemic thrombotic strokes, 319, 319*f*
  larynx, cancer of the, 661
  lumbar disk disease, 275
  malignant otitis externa, 648
  meningioma, 326
  metabolic encephalopathy, 315
  metastases, 326
  neural tube defects, 422
  oropharynx, malignant neoplasms of the, 659
  osteoporosis, 279
  otalgia, 653
  pancreatic carcinoma, 157
  papilledema, 402
  papillitis, 403
  polycystic kidney disease, 552
  pulmonary embolism, 515
  renal cell carcinoma, 544
  seizures, 316
  septic meningitis, 307
  skull trauma/fracture, 218
  solitary pulmonary nodule, 523
  spinal stenosis, 291
  subarachnoid hemorrhage, 322
  subdural hematoma, 330
  sudden hearing loss, 655
  testicular carcinoma, 545
  thoracic spine, injuries to, 293
  tinnitus, 657
  toxoplasma encephalitis, 256
  trigeminal neuralgia, 316
  Wegener's granulomatosis, 668
Concept and application. *See* mechanisms and disease diagnosis/treatment *and* surgical principles *under specific disease/disorder*
Concussion
  mechanisms and disease diagnosis/treatment, 219
Conduct disorder
  attention-deficit hyperactivity disorder, 473
  mechanisms and disease diagnosis/treatment, 473–474
Condylomata, 52
Confidentiality and domestic violence, 488
Confusion
  antipsychotics, 324
  arsenic toxicity, 323
  brief psychotic disorder, 457
  carbon monoxide, 231
  contusions, 331
  cryptococcal infection, 502
  diabetes mellitus, 103
  heatstroke, 241
  herpes simplex virus, 303
  hypercalcemia, 92
  hyperosmolar hyperglycemic nonketotic coma, 104
  hyponatremia, 553
  hypothermia, 240
  hypothyroidism, 89
  posttraumatic stress disorder, 465
  schizophreniform disorder, 457
  sedatives, 229
  seizures, 315
  subarachnoid hemorrhage, 321
  syndrome of inappropriate antidiuretic hormone secretion, 95
  tuberculosis, 308
Congenital adrenal hyperplasia (CAH), 534, 535
Congenital anomalies
  adrenal hyperplasia
    mechanisms and disease diagnosis/treatment, 98–99
  alcohol, 478
  cardiovascular medicine
    atrial septal defect, 26–27
    coarctation of the aorta, 27–28
    tachyarrhythmias, 18
    tetralogy of Fallot, 27
    ventricular septal defect, 25–26
  deafness
    mechanisms and disease diagnosis/treatment, 424–425
  hearing loss, 654
  hip disorders
    mechanisms and disease diagnosis/treatment, 276–277
  infectious disease
    cytomegalovirus, 439
    herpes simplex virus, 439
    HIV (human immunodeficiency virus), 438–439
    rubella (German measles), 439
    syphilis, 437–438
    toxoplasmosis, 438
  melanocytic nevus, 73
  myopathies/dystrophies, 313
  ophthalmology
    blepharoptosis, 399
    cataracts, 406, 424
    disc elevation, congenital anomalous, 401–402, 401*t*, 402*t*
    glaucoma, 414, 423–424
    syphilis, 413
  platelet dysfunction, 194
  pulmonology
    cystic adenomatoid malformation, 447
    emphysema, lobar, 446–447
    laryngomalacia, 446
    pulmonary sequestration, 447
  teratology, 366–367
Congestive heart failure (CHF)
  acute renal failure, 547
  aortic dissection, 40
  AV block, 17

chronic valvular diseases, 24
Cushing's syndrome, 97
essential hypertension, 29
hypereosinophilic syndrome, 212
hyperthyroidism, 88
ischemic heart disease, 23
left-sided low output heart failure, 8
malignant hypertension, 31
mechanisms and disease diagnosis/treatment, 514
pleural effusions, 512
respiratory alkalosis, 556
tachyarrhythmias, 19
Terry's nails, 84
tetralogy of fallot, 27
ventricular tachycardia, 19
volume excess, 555
Congo red stain, 81
Conjugated hyperbilirubinemia, 150
Conjunctivitis
  acute upper respiratory infection, 667
  atopic dermatitis, 207
  measles (rubeola), 265
  mechanisms and disease diagnosis/treatment, 200–202, 393–395, 393t–396t
  ophthalmic herpes zoster, 412
  rubella (German measles), 266
Conner's scale, 473
Consciousness
  anaphylaxis, 202
  bacterial meningitis, 437
  cardiopulmonary arrest, 28
  epidural hematoma, 219, 330
  herpes simplex virus, 303
  mechanisms and disease diagnosis/treatment, 315
  metabolic encephalopathy, 315
  subarachnoid hemorrhage, 321
  subdural hematoma, 330
Constipation
  anorectal abscess, 143
  hypercalcemia, 91
  hypothyroidism, 89
  infantile botulism, 421
  mechanisms and disease diagnosis/treatment, 139–140

Constrictive pericarditis
  cardiac tamponade, 22
Contact dermatitis
  mechanisms and disease diagnosis/treatment, 55–56, 208–209
Continuous distending airway pressure (CDAP), 515
Continuous positive airway pressure (CPAP), 335, 524
Contraception. *See also* Oral contraceptives
  counseling for, general, 359
  gestational trophoblastic disease, 383
Contusions
  mechanisms and disease diagnosis/treatment, 292, 331
Conversion disorder
  mechanisms and disease diagnosis/treatment, 471
Coombs' test, indirect/direct
  chronic lymphocytic leukemia, 180
  hemolytic anemia, 175
  hemolytic uremic syndrome, 440
  mononucleosis, 264
  neonatal hyperbilirubinemia, 432
  Rh incompatibility, 431
  thalassemia-alpha, 171
Copper poisoning, 232
Cornea
  abrasion/laceration, 220
  blepharitis, 396
  congenital glaucoma, 423
  conjunctivitis, 393
  corneal arcus, 100
  disorders of the
    dry eye, 413
    globe, diseases of the, 411t
    herpes simplex keratitis, 411–412
    herpes zoster, 412–413
    interstitial keratitis, 413–414
    ulcers, 410–411
  dry-eye syndrome, 400, 413
  entropion, 398
  herpes simplex keratitis, 411
  interstitial keratitis, 413, 414
  ophthalmic herpes zoster, 412

Coronary artery bypass graph (CABG)
  myocardial infarction, 5
  stable angina pectoris, 7
  unstable angina, 4
Coronary artery disease (CAD)
  cardiopulmonary arrest, 28
  chronic atherosclerotic occlusion, 34
  decreased high-density lipoprotein, 102
  dilated cardiomyopathy, 13
  dysbetalipoproteinemia, type III, 100
  elevated Lp (a) lipoprotein, 102
  hyperlipoproteinemia, type II, 100
  hyperlipoproteinemia, type IV, 100, 101
  left-sided high output heart failure, 9
  myocardial infarction, 5
  silent ischemia, 7
  stable angina pectoris, 6
  unstable angina, 3
  variant angina, 6
Cor pulmonale
  desquamative interstitial pneumonitis, 509
  emphysema, 506
  mechanisms and disease diagnosis/treatment, 518
  sleep apnea, 523
  usual interstitial pneumonitis, 508, 509
Corticosteroids
  allergic bronchopulmonary aspergillosis, 210
  allergic rhinitis, 201, 202
  anaphylaxis, 202
  atopic dermatitis, 56, 207
  bronchial asthma, 199, 200
  bullous pemphigoid, 59
  chronic asthma, 504
  chronic bronchitis, 506
  contact dermatitis, 209
  Crohn's disease, 135, 137
  croup, 493
  cryptococcal infection, 502
  desquamative interstitial pneumonitis, 509
  drug allergy, 213
  drug reactions causing skin changes, 58

Corticosteroids *(continued)*
  emphysema, 506
  follicular cyst, 76
  giant cell aortitis, 43
  glioblastoma, 326
  headaches, 318
  hemangioma, 565
  hemolytic anemia, 175
  Henoch-Schöenlein purpura, 425
  hypereosinophilic syndrome, 212
  hypersensitivity pneumonitis, 211, 511
  idiopathic thrombocytopenic purpura, 192
  low-grade lymphoma, 183
  lupus arthritis, 282
  Lyme disease, 309
  meningioma, 326
  mononucleosis, 264
  multiple sclerosis, 332
  myasthenia gravis, 312
  myopathies/dystrophies, 313
  necrobiosis lipoidica, 83
  osteoarthritis, 274
  papillitis, 404
  pleurisy, 513
  *Pneumocystis carinii* pneumonia, 252, 498
  polymyositis-dermatomyositis, 283
  pruritus, 63
  psoriasis, 54
  pulmonary vasculitis, 517
  rheumatoid arthritis, 283
  sarcoidosis, 508
  shock, 239
  subdural hematoma, 330
  thrombotic thrombocytopenic purpura, 193
  ulcerative colitis, 134
  urticaria, 58, 203, 204
  usual interstitial pneumonitis, 509
  vasculitis, 518
Cortisol
  adrenal insufficiency, 95, 96
  congenital adrenal hyperplasia, 99
  Cushing's syndrome, 96, 97
  cutaneous manifestations of systemic disease, 98
  underproduction syndromes (pituitary gland), 94
Cortrosyn, 95
*Corynebacterium diphtheriae*, 661
Coryza
  acute upper respiratory infection, 667
  measles (rubeola), 265
  rubella (German measles), 266
Costal cartilages, 280
Cosyntropin, 95, 97
Cough
  acute bronchitis, 494
  acute epiglottitis, 493
  acute respiratory distress syndrome, 514
  acute upper respiratory infection, 667
  asbestosis, 510
  aspiration, 226
  asthma, 389, 503
  blastomycosis, 501
  bronchial asthma, 198
  bronchiectasis, 507
  bronchiolitis, 434
  bronchogenic carcinoma, 518
  carcinoid tumors, 519
  chronic bronchitis, 505
  coal workers' pneumoconiosis, 511
  coccidioidomycosis, 501
  congestive heart failure, 514
  croup, 435, 493
  cryptococcal infection, 502
  cystic fibrosis, 507, 669
  emphysema, 506
  gastroesophageal reflux disease, 110
  gram-negative bacillary pneumonias, 496
  *Haemophilus influenzae* pneumonia, 496
  histoplasmosis, 500
  hypereosinophilic syndrome, 212
  hypersensitivity pneumonitis, 210, 511
  ill-defined symptoms, 624–625
  influenza pneumonia, 498
  Legionnaire's disease, 497
  measles (rubeola), 265
  mechanisms and disease diagnosis/treatment, 520–521
  metastatic malignant tumors, 520
  otitis media, 434
  pneumococcal pneumonia, 495
  *Pneumocystis carinii* pneumonia, 252
  pulmonary embolism, 515
  pulmonary tuberculosis, 499
  rubella (German measles), 266
  sarcoidosis, 508
  silicosis, 509
  solitary pulmonary nodule, 523
  staphylococcal pneumonia, 496
  stress-related urinary incontinence, 540
  tracheoesophageal fistula, 441
  usual interstitial pneumonitis, 508
  Wegener's granulomatosis, 668
Coumadin, 321
Counseling
  alopecia areata, 69
  bulimia, 477
  contraception, 359
  genetic
    Down syndrome, 445
    fragile X syndrome, 446
    history/physical keys/diagnosis, 360
    sickle cell anemia, 177
  HIV (human immunodeficiency virus), 251
  Huntington's disease, 329
  pruritus, 63
  sterilization, 360
  sudden infant death syndrome, 489
  trisomy, 380
  Turner's syndrome, 446
Courvoisier gallbladder, 157
Couvelaire uterus, 374
Cowden's syndrome, 84
Coxsackie
  acute pancreatitis, 160
  diabetes mellitus, 103
  pleurisy, 513
Crack cocaine, 134, 478
Crackles
  acute bronchiolitis, 494
  acute respiratory distress syndrome, 514
  asbestosis, 510
  chronic valvular diseases, 24
  congestive heart failure, 514
  dilated cardiomyopathy, 13
  hypersensitivity pneumonitis, 511

left-sided low output heart
    failure, 8
Legionnaire's disease, 497
*Pneumocystis carinii* pneumonia,
    498
stable angina pectoris, 6
tracheoesophageal fistula, 441
usual interstitial pneumonitis,
    508
Cradle cap, 54
Cramping
    amyotrophic lateral sclerosis, 328
    heatstroke, 241
    hypocalcemia, 558
    hypokalemia, 554
    myopathies/dystrophies, 313
    premature labor, 376
Cranial injury. *See also* Head trauma
    auditory injury, 220–221
    concussion, 219
    epidemiology and prevention of
        ocular/auditory injury,
        221
    epidural hematoma, 219–220
    facial fracture, 217–218
    ocular injury, 220
    skull trauma or fracture, 218
    subdural hematoma, 219
    surgical principles, 580
Cranial nerves
    blepharoptosis, 399
    cryptococcal infection, 502
    hydrocephalus, 423
    malignant otitis externa, 647,
        648
    nasopharynx, masses in the, 659
    sarcoidosis, 508
    subarachnoid hemorrhage, 321
    trigeminal neuralgia, 316
    tuberculosis, 308
    venous thrombosis, 322
    vertigo, 652
Craniopharingiomas, 93, 94
C-reactive protein (CRP)
    ischemic thrombotic strokes, 318
    Kawasaki disease, 426
    osteomyelitis, 271
Creatine kinase (CK)
    amyotrophic lateral sclerosis, 328
    child physical/sexual abuse, 486
    myocardial infarction, 4
    myopathies/dystrophies, 313
    polymyositis-dermatomyositis,
        282

Creatine phosphokinase, 230
Creatine phosphokinase (CPK), 80
Creatinine
    acute lymphocytic leukemia, 179
    acute pancreatitis, 160
    acute renal failure, 546
    chronic renal failure, 547
    delirium, 486
    essential hypertension, 29, 30
    hypovolemic shock, 11
    multiple myeloma, 184
    preeclampsia, 375
    thrombotic thrombocytopenic
        purpura, 192
    tubulointerstitial disease, 548
    urethral stricture, benign, 536
CREST acronym and scleroderma,
    81
Creutzfeldt-Jakob disease
    mechanisms and disease
        diagnosis/treatment, 305
Cricopharyngeus muscle, 226
Cricothyrotomy, 435
Crigler-Najjar syndrome, 432
Crixivan, 250
Crohn's disease
    anorectal fistula, 143–144
    mechanisms and disease
        diagnosis/treatment, 135,
        136*tf*, 137
    pyoderma gangrenosum, 79
    surgical principles, 600
Cromolyn sodium
    allergic rhinitis, 665
    asthma and pregnancy, 389
    bronchial asthma, 199
    chronic asthma, 504
    conjunctivitis, 201
Croup
    mechanisms and disease
        diagnosis/treatment,
        435–436, 493
Crouzon syndrome, 425
Crural monoplegia, 322
Crying and infantile botulism, 421
Cryoglobulin, 272
Cryoprecipitate, 170
Cryotherapy, 347
Cryptococcal infection
    mechanisms and disease
        diagnosis/treatment,
        257–258
    pulmonary medicine, 502
*Cryptococcus*, 257, 307

*Cryptococcus neoformans*, 257, 502
Cryptorchidism
    intersex, 535
    mechanisms and disease
        diagnosis/treatment, 534
*Cryptosporidia*, 123
Crystalloid solutions, 11, 13
Culdocentesis, 370
Cushing's disease
    surgical principles, 573–574
Cushing's syndrome
    hydrocephalus, 423
    mechanisms and disease
        diagnosis/treatment,
        96–97, 96*f*
    overproduction syndromes
        (pituitary gland), 92, 93
    secondary hypertension, 30, 31
Cutaneous necrosis, 77
Cutis congenita, 445
Cyanosis
    acute arterial occlusion, 36
    acute respiratory distress
        syndrome, 514
    anaphylaxis, 202
    bronchiectasis, 507
    carbon monoxide, 231
    cardiopulmonary arrest, 28
    chronic bronchitis, 505
    congenital lobar emphysema, 447
    congestive heart failure, 514
    cystic fibrosis, 669
    epiglottitis, 435
    heavy metals/arsenic, 231
    preeclampsia, 375
    tetralogy of fallot, 27
    transient tachypnea of the
        newborn, 429
    usual interstitial pneumonitis,
        508
    ventricular septic defect, 25, 26
Cyclobenzaprine, 286
Cyclophosphamide
    Behcet's disease, 82
    bladder carcinoma, 543
    desquamative interstitial
        pneumonitis, 509
    lupus arthritis, 282
    lupus nephritis, 553
    pulmonary vasculitis, 517
    usual interstitial pneumonitis,
        509
    vasculitis, 518
    Wegener's granulomatosis, 668

Cycloplegia, 411, 414
Cyclosporins
    atopic dermatitis, 208
    cardiac transplantation, 25
    nephrotic syndrome, 549
    psoriasis, 54
    renal transplant rejection, 548
Cyclothymia
    mechanisms and disease diagnosis/treatment, 462
Cyperoterone, 98
Cystectomy
    bladder carcinoma, 543
    ovarian cysts, 345
Cystic adenomatoid malformation
    mechanisms and disease diagnosis/treatment, 447
Cystic fibrosis
    bronchiectasis, 507
    mechanisms and disease diagnosis/treatment, 161–162, 507, 669
Cystic fibrosis transmembrane regulator (CFTR) protein, 507
Cystitis, 353, 377
Cystoscopy. *See also* mechanisms and disease diagnosis/treatment *and* surgical principles *under specific disease/disorder*
    acute renal failure, 547
    bladder, painful, 529, 530
    neurogenic bladder, 539
    urethral stricture, benign, 536
    urinary tract infections, 529
Cystourethrocele, 350
Cytochrome P450, 118
Cytokines, 13
Cytology, 347
Cytolysis/cytotoxic agents
    chronic myelogenous leukemia, 180
    dermatomyositis, 80
    fibroadenoma, 355
    gastric cancer, 114
    glomerulonephritis, 549
    hemolytic anemia, 175
    hepatocellular carcinoma, 154
    hypereosinophilic syndrome, 212
    low-grade lymphoma, 183
    nephrotic syndrome, 549
    phycomycosis, 503
    vasculitis syndromes, 37

Cytomegalovirus (CMV)
    acute enteric infections, 123
    congenital anomalies
        cataracts, 424
        deafness, 425
        mechanisms and disease diagnosis/treatment, 253–254
    congenital anomalies, 439
Cytometry, 178
Cytoxan, 184

# D

Dacarbazine, 182
Dacrocystorhinostomy, 401
Dacron grafts, 588, 591
Dacryocystitis, acute
    mechanisms and disease diagnosis/treatment, 400–401
Dalfopristin, 496
Danazol
    endometriosis, 343
    fibrocystic disease, 356
    idiopathic thrombocytopenic purpura, 192
Dandy-Walker malformation, 423
Dapsone
    dermatitis herpetiformis, 61
    pemphigus, 60
    *Pneumocystis carinii* pneumonia, 252, 498
    pyoderma gangrenosum, 79
Darkfield exam, 52, 261, 438
Deafness, congenital. *See also* Hearing loss
    mechanisms and disease diagnosis/treatment, 424–425
Deamino-8-d-argine vasopressin (DDAVP)
    diabetes insipidus, 94
    hemophilia A and B, 188
    platelet dysfunction, 194
    von Willebrand disease, 189
Debulking therapies, 110
Decadron, 185
Decarboxylase, 83
Decongestants
    acute upper respiratory infection, 668
    allergic rhinitis, 201
    barotrauma, 657

    chronic rhinitis, 664
    chronic sinusitis, 663
Decubitus ulcer
    mechanisms and disease diagnosis/treatment, 77
    surgical principles, 568–569
Deep venous thrombosis (DVT)
    antithrombin III deficiency, 190
    lupus inhibitor, 189
    pulmonary embolism, 38, 515, 516
    surgical principles, 594–595
    venous thrombosis, 37
Defecography, 139
Defibrillators
    hypertrophic cardiomyopathy, 15
    ventricular tachycardia, 19
Degenerative disorders
    musculoskeletal/connective tissue disease
        back pain, low, 274–275
        joints, 273–274
        lumbar disk, 275–276
        neurologic disease, disorders secondary to, 276
    neurology
        Alzheimer's diagnosis, 327–328
        amyotrophic lateral sclerosis, 328
        Huntington's disease, 329
        Parkinson's disease, 328–329
Dehydration
    affective psychoses: mania and psychotic depression, 455
    anorexia, 475
    bulimia, 475
    congenital adrenal hyperplasia, 98
    hypernatremia, 554
    hyperosmolar hyperglycemic nonketotic coma, 104
    hypovolemic shock, 11
    intussusception, 442
    strep throat, 661
Dehydroepiandrosterone sulfate (DHEAS), 97, 352
Delaverdine, 251
Delirium
    heavy metals/arsenic, 231
    hypomagnesemia, 557
    mechanisms and disease diagnosis/treatment, 485–486

Delirium tremens, 480
Deltoid ligament, 237
Delusions
  affective psychoses: mania and psychotic depression, 455
  disorder, delusional
    affective psychoses: mania and psychotic depression, 456
    body dysmorphic disorder, 472
  schizophrenia, 453
  shared psychotic disorder, 457
Demeclocycline, 95
Dementia
  alcohol, 480
  Alzheimer's disease, 327
  delirium, 485
  depression, major (unipolar), 459
  fungal meningitis, 307
  HIV (human immunodeficiency virus), 303
  Huntington's disease, 329
  hypothyroidism, 89
  Lyme disease, 309
  neurosyphilis, 310
  Parkinson's disease, 328
  tuberculosis, 308
Demerol, 213
Demyelination, multiple sclerosis and, 331–332
Dependent personality disorders, 468
Depression
  adjustment disorders, 467
  alcohol, 478, 479
  anorexia, 474
  bereavement, 488
  body dysmorphic disorder, 472
  bulimia, 475
  child physical/sexual abuse, 486, 487
  conversion disorder, 471
  domestic violence, 487
  generalized anxiety disorder, 464
  hypercalcemia, 91
  hypothyroidism, 89
  mechanisms and disease diagnosis/treatment
    major (unipolar), 459–460
    obstetrics, 383–384
    psychotic, 454–455

  mother, postpartum care of the, 367
  obsessive-compulsive disorder, 464
  panic disorder, 463
  posttraumatic stress disorder, 465
  premenstrual syndrome, 351
  social phobia, 466
  somatization disorder, 469
Dermatitis
  asteatotic, 56
  atopic, 56, 206–208
  celiac sprue, 124
  contact, 55–56, 208–209
  eczematous, 50, 56–57, 57f
  herpetiformis, 124
  seborrheic, 54–55
  stasis, 57, 77, 78f
Dermatitis herpetiformis
  mechanisms and disease diagnosis/treatment, 60–61
Dermatofibroma
  mechanisms and disease diagnosis/treatment, 73
Dermatology. *See also* Skin changes
  acute exanthems
    varicella, 46
    varicella zoster, 46–47
  aortic occlusion, 41
  eruptions, skin
    blistering diseases, 58–61
    inflammatory conditions, 53–58
    insect bites and ectoparasites, 63–66
    other diseases of skin/subcutaneous tissues, 61–62
    symptoms involving the skin, 62–63
  hair and the hair follicle, diseases of
    acne vulgaris, 67
    alopecia areata, 68–69
    rosacea, 67–68
  Hodgkin's disease, 182
  infections, other
    bacterial, 49–50
    mycoses, 47–49
    secondary syphilis, 52–53
    viral, 51–52

  malignant neoplasms, cutaneous signs of internal, 83–84
  nails
    ingrowing, 66–67
    signs and disease, 84–85
  newborns, diseases/disorders of, 85
  other conditions
    acquired keratoderma, 76–77
    arteriosclerotic ulcer, 78
    decubitus ulcer, 77
    pyoderma gangrenosum, 79
    ulcer of lower limbs, 77
  surgical principles for skin disorders
    arterial ulcer, 569–570
    basal cell carcinoma, 566
    cellulitis, 564
    decubitus ulcer, 568–569
    hemangioma, 564–565
    lipoma, 564
    melanoma, 567
    neurofibroma, 565
    sarcoma, 568
    sebaceous cyst, 565–566
    squamous cell carcinoma, 566–567
    venous ulceration, 569
  systemic disease, cutaneous manifestations of
    amyloidosis, 81
    Behcet's disease, 82
    dermatomyositis, 80
    lupus erythematosus, 79–80
    necrobiosis lipoidica, 83
    porphyria cutanea tarda, 83
    scleroderma, 80–81
    tuberous sclerosis, 82–83
  tumors of the skin
    benign neoplasms, 72–75
    follicular cyst, 75–76
    premalignant and malignant neoplasms of skin, 69–72
Dermatomyositis
  mechanisms and disease diagnosis/treatment, 80
Dermatophytosis
  mechanisms and disease diagnosis/treatment, 47–48
Desensitization
  allergic rhinitis, 202, 665
  sexual dysfunctions, 484
Desferoxamine, 172

Desquamative interstitial
pneumonitis (DIP)
mechanisms and disease
diagnosis/treatment, 509
Developmental disorders
autistic disorder, 458
child physical/sexual abuse, 486,
487
congenital toxoplasmosis, 438
glaucoma, congenital, 414
HIV (human immunodeficiency
virus), 438
laryngomalacia, 446
serous otitis media, 650
Tay-Sachs disease, 335–336
Developmental dysplasia of the hip
mechanisms and disease
diagnosis/treatment, 433,
433f
Dexamethasone
adrenal insufficiency, 96
bacterial meningitis, 437
croup, 436
Cushing's syndrome, 96–97
depression, major (unipolar),
459
overproduction syndromes
(pituitary gland), 93
underproduction syndromes
(pituitary gland), 94
Dextroamphetamine, 473
Dextromethorphan, 521
Dextrose, 105
Diabetes insipidus (DI)
mechanisms and disease
diagnosis/treatment, 94
Diabetes mellitus (DM)
anorectal abscess, 143
atherosclerosis, 34
autoimmune hepatitis, 147
candidiasis, cutaneous, 48
candidiasis, oral, 48
cardiac transplantation, 25
carpal tunnel syndrome, 311
celiac sprue, 124
chronic renal failure, 547
chylomicronemia, type 1
familial, 99
cystic fibrosis, 507
Dupuytren's contracture, 288
endometrial cancer, 341
erectile impotence, 537
essential hypertension, 30
frozen shoulder syndrome, 288

fungal meningitis, 307
gastric motility, disorders of, 118
glaucoma, 414
hyperlipoproteinemia, 33
hyperosmolar hyperglycemic
nonketotic coma, 104
hypoglycemia, 105
ischemic thrombotic strokes, 318
mechanisms and disease
diagnosis/treatment
ophthalmology, 409–410
type 1, 102–103
type 2, 103–104
neurogenic bladder, 540
obstetrics
gestational, 388
overt, 389
papillary necrosis, 551
porphyria cutanea tarda, 83
sudden hearing loss, 656
vulva/vagina, candidiasis of the,
349
Diabetic ketoacidosis (DKA)
diabetes mellitus, 102, 103
hypernatremia, 554
phycomycosis, 503
Diabetic nephropathy
mechanisms and disease
diagnosis/treatment, 550
Diabetic retinopathy, 407t
mechanisms and disease
diagnosis/treatment,
409–410
Diagnosis. See mechanisms and
disease diagnosis/
treatment *and* surgical
principles *under specific
disease/disorder*
*Diagnostic and Statistical Manual of
Mental Disorders* (DSM),
468
Dialysis
chronic renal failure, 547
diabetic nephropathy, 550
folic acid deficiency, 170
hemolytic uremic syndrome, 440
hyperosmolar hyperglycemic
nonketotic coma, 104
Legionnaire's disease, 497
polycystic kidney disease, 552
renal osteodystrophy, 550
Diaphoresis
acetaminophen, 228
anaphylaxis, 202

aortic dissection, 40
cardiogenic shock, 10
congestive heart failure, 514
hypoglycemia, 105
myocardial infarction, 4
unstable angina, 3
Diaphragmatic hernia, 447, 619
Diarrhea
alcohol, 478
anorectal abscess, 143
bipolar disorders, 462
celiac sprue, 124
cellular (T-cell)
immunodeficiency, 205
Crohn's disease, 135
cytomegalovirus, 253
disseminated *Mycobacterium
avium-intracellulare*
complex, 255
dysmenorrhea, 351
hemolytic uremic syndrome,
440
HIV (human immunodeficiency
virus), 249
humoral immunodeficiency, 204
hyperkalemia, 554
hypovolemic shock, 11
ill-defined presentations,
634–635
ischemic bowel disease, 137
Legionnaire's disease, 497
mechanisms and disease
diagnosis/treatment, 120,
121t, 122–123, 124t, 126
ulcerative colitis, 133
Diazepam, 421, 652
Diazoxide, 105
Dicloxacillin, 355
Didanosine, 250
Diethylstilbestrol (DES), 349
Diethyltoluamide (DEET), 66
mechanisms and disease
diagnosis/treatment for
poisoning from, 232
Diet/nutrition
adolescent pregnancy, 369
alcohol, 478, 480
allergic rhinitis, 665
anal fissure, 142
breast cancer, 353
celiac sprue, 125
childhood schizophrenia, 458
chronic pancreatitis, 161
chronic renal failure, 547

chylomicronemia, type 1 familial, 99
colorectal carcinoma, 128
constipation, 140
cystic fibrosis, 162
decubitus ulcer, 77
diabetes, gestational, 388
diabetes mellitus, 104
diverticulitis, 139
fibrocystic disease, 356
folic acid deficiency, 170–171
gastric cancer, 114, 115*t*
hepatitis, 150
hereditary nonpolyposis colorectal cancer, 129
hyperemesis gravidarum, 385
hyperlipoproteinemia, type II, 100
hyperlipoproteinemia, type V, 101
irritable bowel syndrome, 127, 128
lactation, 368
malnutrition
  amyotrophic lateral sclerosis, 328
  hypomagnesemia, 557
  prenatal care, 365
menopausal symptoms, 353
multiple gestation, 382
necrotizing enterocolitis, 443
osteoporosis, 279
pancreatic carcinoma, 157
pruritus ani, 63
renal osteodystrophy, 550
vitamin K deficiency, 189
Diffuse esophageal spasm (DES)
  mechanisms and disease diagnosis/treatment, 113
Digestive system. *See also* Gastroenterology
  aneurysm, abdominal aortic, 164
  bulimia, 475
  celiac sprue, 124
  colon
    appendicitis, 132–133
    colorectal carcinoma, 128–132, 129*t*–131*t*
    constipation, 139–140
    diarrhea, invasive, 126
    diverticulitis, 138–139
    familial Mediterranean fever, 140–141

inflammatory bowel disease, 133–137
  intestinal obstruction, 138
  irritable bowel syndrome, 126–128, 127*t*
  ischemic bowel disease, 137
  peritonitis, 140
esophagus
  gastroesophageal reflux disease, 110–111
  malignant neoplasms, 109–110
  motor disorders, 111–114
gallbladder
  acute cholecystitis, 144–145
  choledocholithiasis and acute suppurative cholangitis, 145–146
  cholelithiasis, 145
gastrointestinal hemorrhage
  ill-defined presentations, 633–634
Henoch-Schöenlein purpura, 425
hernia
  external, 162–163
  traumatic hernias of the diaphragm, 163
hypokalemia, 554
liver
  carcinoma, hepatocellular, 153–155
  cirrhosis, hepatic fibrosis and, 155–157, 156*t*
  hepatitis, 146–150, 147*t*–149*t*, 151*t*–152*t*, 153
pancreas
  acute pancreatitis, 159–161
  carcinoma, pancreatic, 157–159
  chronic pancreatitis, 161
  cystic fibrosis, 161–162
prune-belly syndrome, 427
rectum
  abscess, anorectal, 142
  fissure, anal, 142
  fistula, anorectal, 143–144
  hemorrhoids, 141–142
  malignant neoplasm rectum. *See* Colorectal carcinoma
  pilonidal disease, 144
small intestine
  acute enteric infections, 120–124
  celiac sprue, 124–125

stomach
  acid-related disorders, 115–117
  cancer, gastric, 114–115
  motility, gastric, 118–120
surgical principles for diseases of
  achalasia, 597
  acute mesenteric ischemia, 600–601
  anorectal fistula, 605
  appendicitis, 599
  benign neoplasm of the colon, 606, 607*f*
  benign neoplasm of the small bowel, 606
  cancer of the stomach, 598
  colon cancer, 606–607
  Crohn's disease, 600
  diverticulitis, 603–604
  duodenal atresia, 608
  esophageal varices, 597–598
  gastric volvulus, 598–599
  hemorrhoids, 604
  Hirschsprung's disease, 609
  imperforate anus, 609
  large-bowel obstruction, 603
  malrotation, 608
  midesophageal traction diverticulum, 596–597
  perirectal abscess, 605
  pilonidal cyst, 605–606
  rectal tumor, 604
  small-bowel obstruction, 601–602, 602*f*
  ulcerative colitis, 599–600
  Zenker's diverticulum, 596
tuberculosis, 254
vitamin K deficiency, 189
Digitalis, 8
Digoxin
  dilated cardiomyopathy, 14
  left-sided low output heart failure, 8
  tachyarrhythmias, 18
Dilantin, 213
Dilated cardiomyopathy
  mechanisms and disease diagnosis/treatment, 13–14
Dilation and curettage (D&C), 341
Dimenhydrinate, 652
Dimercaprol, 231
Dipentum, 134

Diphenhydramine hydrochloride
    allergic rhinitis, 201
    anaphylaxis, 202, 239
    conjunctivitis, 201
    insect bites, 238
    transfusion reactions, 187
    vertigo, 652
Diphenoxylate, 128, 635
Diplopia
    alcohol, 230
    facial fracture, 217
    myasthenia gravis, 312
Direct fluorescent antibody/
        immunofluorescence
        tests, 51, 58, 59, 261. See
        also mechanisms and
        disease diagnosis/
        treatment and surgical
        principles under specific
        disease/disorder
Direct observed therapy (DOT), 255
Dislocations and separations. See
        also Fractures and
        dislocations
    mechanisms and disease
        diagnosis/treatment,
        297–298
Disseminated intravascular
        coagulation (DIC)
    abruptio placentae, 374
    diarrhea, 126
    heatstroke, 241
    hypothermia, 241
    insect and snake bites, 238
    mechanisms and disease
        diagnosis/treatment, 190
    necrotizing enterocolitis, 443
    protein C deficiency, 191
Disseminated *Mycobacterium avium-
        intracellulare* complex
    mechanisms and disease
        diagnosis/treatment,
        255–256
Dissociation, 466, 471
Distal interphalangeal (DIP) joint
    hand phalanges, closed fracture
        of, 295
    sprain
        mechanisms and disease
            diagnosis/treatment, 236
Distributive shock
    mechanisms and disease
        diagnosis/treatment,
        12–13

Disulfiram, 230, 478, 479
Diuresis
    dilated cardiomyopathy, 14
    glomerulonephritis, 549
    heart failure, left-sided high-
        output, 9
    hypercalcemia, 557
    hyperosmolar hyperglycemic
        nonketotic coma, 104
    malignant hypertension, 31
    stasis ulceration, 77
Diuretics
    acute pancreatitis, 160
    bulimia, 475
    chronic valvular diseases, 24
    constrictive pericarditis, 22
    cor pulmonale, 518
    desquamative interstitial
        pneumonitis, 509
    essential hypertension, 30
    fibrocystic disease, 356
    hypomagnesemia, 557
    left-sided low output heart
        failure, 8
    premenstrual syndrome, 352
    restrictive cardiomyopathy, 16
    right-sided heart failure, 10
    shock, 239
    usual interstitial pneumonitis,
        509
Diverticulitis
    mechanisms and disease
        diagnosis/treatment,
        138–139
    peritonitis, 140
    surgical principles, 603–604
Dizziness/light-headedness
    acute otitis media, 648
    atrial septal defect, 26
    AV block, 17
    bradyarrhythmias, 18
    cardiopulmonary arrest, 28
    hypertrophic cardiomyopathy,
        14
    hypovolemic shock, 11
    ill-defined presentations,
        629–630
    panic disorder, 463
    sick sinus syndrome, 16
    tachyarrhythmias, 18
    ventricular tachycardia, 19
    vertigo, 652
DNA analysis and prenatal
        diagnosis, 366

DNA replication, 170
DNase, 507
DNA synthesis and vitamin $B_{12}$
        deficiency, 173
Dobutamine, 9, 11
Domperidone, 118
Donepezil, 327
Dopamine
    anaphylaxis, 202
    attention-deficit hyperactivity
        disorder, 473
    basic cardiac life support, 29
    cardiogenic shock, 11
    congestive heart failure, 514
    distributive shock, 13
    Parkinson's disease, 329
    schizophrenia, 453
    shock, 239
Doppler echocardiography. See also
        mechanisms and disease
        diagnosis/treatment and
        surgical principles under
        specific disease/disorder
    antithrombin III deficiency, 191
    chronic atherosclerotic
        occlusion, 35
    deep venous thrombosis, 594
    epididymitis, 530
    erectile impotence, 537
    hypertrophic cardiomyopathy,
        14
    obstructive shock, 12
    testicular torsion, 534
Dorsal kyphosis, 280
Dorzolamide, 416
Douching and candidiasis of the
        vulva/vagina, 349
Down syndrome
    atrial septal defect, 26
    celiac sprue, 124
    mechanisms and disease
        diagnosis/treatment,
        444–445, 445f
    otitis media, 434, 435
Doxepin, 58, 62
Doxorubicin, 182, 184
Doxycycline
    cervicitis and sexually
        transmitted diseases, 347
    chlamydia, 260, 533
    epididymoorchitis, 263
    gonorrhea, 532
    Lyme disease, 268, 272, 309
    orchitis, 531

pelvic inflammatory disease, 263, 358
pleural effusions, 512
secondary syphilis, 53
urethritis, 531
Dramamine, 652
Dramatic personality disorders, 468
Dressler's syndrome, 20
Drooling
acute epiglottitis, 493
epiglottitis, 435
manganese toxicity, 323
Drowning
epidemiology and prevention, 242
mechanisms and disease diagnosis/treatment, 237–238
Drowsiness and heavy metal toxicity, 323. *See also Dizziness/light-headedness*
Drugs/medications. *See also specific drug/class of drugs*
allergy, drug
mechanisms and disease diagnosis/treatment, 212–213
amenorrhea, 352
anaphylaxis, 202
gout, 280
hepatitis, 149, 151
platelet dysfunction, 194
poisoning
acetaminophen, 228
alcohol, 230
cocaine, 230
PCP (phencyclidine), 230
sedatives, 229
stimulants, 229
tricyclic antidepressants, 228–229
skin reacting to, 58
substance-related disorders
bulimia, 475, 476
caffeine, 483
cannabinoids, 482
child physical/sexual abuse, 487
conduct disorder, 474
domestic violence, 487
factitious disorders, 472
hallucinogens, 482

inhalants, 483
malingering, 472
mechanisms and disease diagnosis/treatment, 477–478
nicotine, 483
opioids, 481
PCP (phencyclidine), 482–483
sedatives-hypnotics, 481–482
social phobia, 466
somatization disorder, 470
steroids, 483
stimulants, 480–481
sudden hearing loss, 656
toxic disorders
antipsychotics, 324
barbiturates, 324
benzodiazepines, 324
cocaine, 324
opioids, 324
urticaria, 203
Drunk driving, 242
Dry-eye syndrome
mechanisms and disease diagnosis/treatment
cornea, 413
undersecretion, 400
Dual-energy x-ray absorptiometry (DEXA)
menopausal symptoms, 353
osteoporosis, 279
Duchenne's dystrophy, 313
Dumping syndrome, 118
Duodenal atresia
Down syndrome, 444
surgical principles, 608
Dupuytren's contracture
cirrhosis, 155
hepatitis, 146
mechanisms and disease diagnosis/treatment, 288
Peyronie's disease, 537
Dusts and hypersensitivity pneumonitis, 210
Dwarfism, renal, 550
Dysarthria
amyotrophic lateral sclerosis, 328
Creutzfeldt-Jakob disease, 305
multiple sclerosis, 331
neurosyphilis, 310
Dysbetalipoproteinemia, type III
mechanisms and disease diagnosis/treatment, 100

Dysmenorrhea
endometriosis, 343
mechanisms and disease diagnosis/treatment, 351
Dyspareunia, 343, 484
Dyspepsia
gastric cancer, 114
ill-defined presentations, 636–637
Dysphagia
acute epiglottitis, 493
acute upper respiratory infection, 668
adenocarcinoma, 110
amyotrophic lateral sclerosis, 328
aortic dissection, 40
diffuse esophageal spasm, 113
epiglottitis, 435
esophageal neoplasms, 109
gastroesophageal reflux disease, 110
herpes simplex virus, 258
hoarseness, 660
ill-defined presentations, 639–640
larynx, cancer of the, 661
motor disorders of the esophagus, 111–112
oropharynx, malignant neoplasms of the, 659
Parkinson's disease, 329
rabies, 306
scleroderma, 80
strep throat, 661
thrush, oral, 658
Dysphonia, 110
Dysplastic nevus
mechanisms and disease diagnosis/treatment, 73
Dyspnea
abdominal aortic aneurysm, 164
acute bronchitis, 494
acute epiglottitis, 493
acute pericarditis, 20
acute respiratory distress syndrome, 514
anaphylaxis, 202, 239
aortic dissection, 40
asbestosis, 510
aspiration, 226
asthma, 389, 503
atrial septal defect, 26
blood-loss anemia, 169

Dyspnea (continued)
　bronchial asthma, 198
　bronchogenic carcinoma, 518
　carbon monoxide, 231
　cardiac tamponade, 21
　cardiogenic shock, 10
　cardiopulmonary arrest, 28
　chronic bronchitis, 505
　congestive heart failure, 514
　croup, 493
　cystic fibrosis, 669
　dilated cardiomyopathy, 13
　emphysema, 506
　gram-negative bacillary pneumonias, 496
　hoarseness, 660
　hyaline membrane disease, 515
　hypereosinophilic syndrome, 212
　hypersensitivity pneumonitis, 210, 511
　hyperthyroidism, 88
　hypertrophic cardiomyopathy, 14
　ill-defined symptoms, 623–624
　influenza pneumonia, 498
　iron-deficiency anemia, 169
　larynx, cancer of the, 661
　left-sided high output heart failure, 9
　left-sided low output heart failure, 8
　malignant hypertension, 31
　mechanisms and disease diagnosis/treatment, 521
　metastatic malignant tumors, 520
　obstructive shock, 12
　panic disorder, 463
　pleural effusions, 512
　pleurisy, 513
　*Pneumocystis carinii* pneumonia, 498
　pneumothorax, 222, 513
　pregnancy, 389
　pulmonary embolism, 38
　pulmonary tuberculosis, 499
　pulmonary vasculitis, 517
　restrictive cardiomyopathy, 15
　rib fracture, 221
　sarcoidosis, 508
　silicosis, 509
　staphylococcal pneumonia, 496
　transfusion reactions, 187
　unstable angina, 3
　usual interstitial pneumonitis, 508
　vitamin $B_{12}$ deficiency, 172
Dysrhythmias
　cardioembolic strokes, 320
　hypokalemia, 554
　myocardial infarction, 5
Dysthymia
　mechanisms and disease diagnosis/treatment, 460–461
Dystocia
　mechanisms and disease diagnosis/treatment, 385–386, 385t
Dystrophies
　mechanisms and disease diagnosis/treatment, 313
Dystrophin, 313
Dysuria
　chlamydia, 260
　genitourinary tract infections, 377
　gonorrhea, 259
　ill-defined symptoms, 626–627
　pelvic inflammatory disease, 358
　urethral stricture, benign, 536
　urethritis, 531
　urinary tract infections, 529
　vulva/vagina, candidiasis of the, 349

**E**

Eagle-Barrett syndrome
　mechanisms and disease diagnosis/treatment, 427
Ears
　diseases of the
　　acute otitis media, 648–649
　　barotrauma, 656–657
　　cerumen (earwax) impaction, 651
　　chronic otitis media, 649–650
　　hearing loss, 653–655
　　infectious otitis externa, 647
　　malignant otitis externa, 647–648
　　otalgia, 652
　　serous otitis media, 650–651
　　sudden hearing loss, 655–656
　　tinnitus, 657
　　vertigo, 651–652
　　foreign bodies, 225–226
　　fragile X syndrome, 446
　　injury, auditory, 220–221
　　venous thrombosis, 322
Earwax impaction
　mechanisms and disease diagnosis/treatment, 651
Eating disorders
　anorexia nervosa, 474–475
　bulimia nervosa, 475–477
Eccentric personality disorders, 468
Ecchymosis
　abruptio placentae, 374
　dislocations and separations, 297
　skull trauma/fracture, 218
　urologic trauma, 541
　venous thrombosis, 322
　vitamin K deficiency, 189
Echocardiography
　acute arterial occlusion, 35
　acute pericarditis, 20
　aneurysms of thoracic aorta, 588
　cardiac tamponade, 21
　congestive heart failure, 514
　cor pulmonale, 518
　dilated cardiomyopathy, 13
　hypertrophic cardiomyopathy, 14
　ischemic heart disease, 23
　Kawasaki disease, 426
　myocardial infarction, 4
　obstructive shock, 12
　pericardial effusion, 21
　restrictive cardiomyopathy, 15
　ventricular septic defect, 26
ECHO virus, 513
Eclampsia
　mechanisms and disease diagnosis/treatment, 375–376
　pulmonary medicine, 552
Econazole, 49
Ectopic pregnancy
　appendicitis, 133
　chlamydia, 260
　mechanisms and disease diagnosis/treatment, 370–371
Eczema, 50
　atopic dermatitis, 206, 207
　mechanisms and disease diagnosis/treatment, 56–57, 57f

Edema
  acute renal failure, 546
  acute sinusitis, 662
  anaphylaxis, 203
  anorexia, 474
  blepharoptosis, 399
  bronchiectasis, 507
  bronchiolitis, 434
  cardioembolic strokes, 320
  cardiogenic pulmonary, 514
  chronic bronchitis, 505
  chronic renal failure, 547
  corneal, 414
  cor pulmonale, 518
  croup, 436
  cystic fibrosis, 161
  diabetes mellitus with ophthalmologic manifestations, 410
  diabetic nephropathy, 550
  dilated cardiomyopathy, 13
  epiglottitis, 435
  gestational trophoblastic disease, 383
  glioblastoma, 326
  glomerulonephritis, 549
  hemolytic uremic syndrome, 440
  herpes simplex virus, 304
  hyperthyroidism, 88
  interstitial keratitis, 414
  ischemic bowel disease, 137
  Kawasaki disease, 425
  macular, 410
  malignant hypertension, 31
  manganese toxicity, 324
  meningioma, 326
  myxedema, 88
  necrotizing enterocolitis, 443
  nephrotic syndrome, 549
  papilledema, 402
  papillitis, 402
  pedal
    atrial septal defect, 26
    chronic valvular diseases, 24
    tetralogy of fallot, 27
    ventricular septal defect, 25
  preeclampsia, 551
  premenstrual syndrome, 351
  pulmonary embolism, 515
  refractory, 37
  restrictive cardiomyopathy, 15
  Rh incompatibility, 431
  right-sided heart failure, 9
  stye, 397
  Turner's syndrome, 445
  urticaria, 57
  vasogenic, 326
  villous, 383
Edrophonium chloride, 312
Education, family
  pain disorder, 471
  posttraumatic stress disorder, 466
Education, patient
  alcohol, 479
  athletic accidents, 242
  auditory injury, 221
  back pain, low, 275
  bipolar disorders, 462
  bronchial asthma, 199
  celiac sprue, 125
  drunk driving, 242
  fibromyalgia, 286
  gunshot wounds, 243
  head and spinal cord injury, 242
  injuries/wounds/accidents, 224
  irritable bowel syndrome, 127
  motor vehicle accidents, 242
  panic disorder, 464
  schizophrenia, 454
  sudden infant death syndrome, 489
  workplace accidents, 242
Efavirenz, 251
Eisenmenger's syndrome, 25, 26
Elbow dislocation, 237
Elderly patients
  abuse, 243, 488
  acute enteric infections, 122
  acute myelogenous leukemia, 178
  agnogenic myeloid metaplasia, 193
  arthralgia, 273
  bullous pemphigoid, 58
  chronic lymphocytic leukemia, 180
  delirium, 485
  depression, major (unipolar), 459
  essential thrombocythemia, 193
  femur, fracture of neck of, 295–296
  hearing loss, 654
  hemangioma, 74
  hyperosmolar hyperglycemic nonketotic coma, 104
  hypothyroidism, 90
  ischemic bowel disease, 137
  pelvic fractures, 224
  pneumococcal pneumonia, 495
  polycythemia rubra vera, 186
  polymyalgia rheumatica, 281
  posttraumatic stress disorder, 465
  rotator cuff syndrome, 298
  squamous cell carcinoma, 69
  unstable angina, 3
  vulvar carcinoma, 348
Electrical burns
  mechanisms and disease diagnosis/treatment, 227–228
Electrocardiogram (ECG). *See also* mechanisms and disease diagnosis/treatment *and* surgical principles *under specific disease/disorder*
  acute pericarditis, 20
  alcohol, 480
  AV block, 17
  bulimia, 476
  cardioembolic strokes, 320
  cardiogenic shock, 10
  congestive heart failure, 514
  constrictive pericarditis, 22
  cor pulmonale, 518
  delirium, 486
  dilated cardiomyopathy, 13
  essential hypertension, 29
  hyperkalemia, 554
  hypertrophic cardiomyopathy, 14
  hypokalemia, 554
  hypomagnesemia, 557
  hypothermia, 240
  Kawasaki disease, 426
  left-sided low output heart failure, 8
  myocardial infarction, 4
  myopathies/dystrophies, 313
  obstructive shock, 12
  pericardial effusion, 21
  pericardial tamponade syndrome, 223
  pulmonary embolism, 38, 515
  restrictive cardiomyopathy, 15
  right-sided heart failure, 9
  stable angina pectoris, 6
  unstable angina, 3
  variant angina, 5

Electroconvulsive therapy (ECT)
  affective psychoses: mania and psychotic depression, 455
  bipolar disorders, 462
  depression, major (unipolar), 460
  schizoaffective disorder, 457
Electroencephalograph (EEG)
  alcohol, 480
  Alzheimer's disease, 327
  attention-deficit hyperactivity disorder, 473
  autistic disorder, 458
  delirium, 485, 486
  depression, major (unipolar), 459
  herpes simplex virus, 304, 304f
  metabolic encephalopathy, 315
  schizophrenia, 453
Electrolytes
  acute enteric infections, 123
  acute renal failure, 546
  adrenal insufficiency, 95, 96
  anorexia, 475
  bulimia, 476
  chronic renal failure, 547
  cystic fibrosis, 161
  cytomegalovirus, 254
  delirium, 485
  diabetes insipidus, 94
  disorders, acid-base and electrolyte
    hypercalcemia, 557
    hyperkalemia, 554–555
    hypernatremia, 554
    hypocalcemia, 558
    hypokalemia, 554
    hypomagnesemia, 557
    hyponatremia, 553
    metabolic acidosis, 556
    metabolic alkalosis, 555–556
    respiratory acidosis, 556–557
    respiratory alkalosis, 556
    volume depletion, 555
    volume excess, 555
  febrile seizures, 421
  glomerulonephritis, 549
  hemolytic uremic syndrome, 440
  hepatitis, 150
  hyperemesis gravidarum, 384
  hypocalcemia, 558
  hypothermia, 240
  intestinal obstruction, 138
  metabolic acidosis, 556

panic disorder, 463
peritonitis, 140
pyloric stenosis, 441
schizophrenia, 453
tachyarrhythmias, 19
tubulointerstitial disease, 548
volume excess, 555
Electromyogram (EMG)
  amyotrophic lateral sclerosis, 328
  carpal tunnel syndrome, 311
  cervical spine and spinal stenosis, 333
  dermatomyositis, 80
  Guillain-Barré syndrome, 311
  HIV (human immunodeficiency virus), 303
  lumbar disk disease, 275
  myopathies/dystrophies, 313
  poliomyelitis, 305
  polymyositis-dermatomyositis, 282
Electronystagmography (ENG), 652, 655, 656
Electrophoresis
  decreased high-density lipoprotein, 102
  elevated Lp (a) lipoprotein, 102
  emphysema, 506
  hypercalcemia, 92
  hyperlipoproteinemia, 32
  monoclonal gammopathy of undetermined significance, 185
  multiple myeloma, 184
  sickle cell anemia, 176
  thalassemia-beta, 172
Elidel, 207
Embolectomy, 12, 36, 516
Emollients, 54, 58, 62
Emotional personality disorders, 468
Emphysema
  mechanisms and disease diagnosis/treatment, 506
  congenital lobar, 446–447
Empyema
  pleural effusions, 512
  pneumococcal pneumonia, 495
Encephalitis
  aseptic meningitis, 306
  measles (rubeola), 266
  rubella (German measles), 267

sudden hearing loss, 656
toxoplasma, 256–257
varicella (chickenpox), 265
Encephalocele, 423
Encephalopathy
  cirrhosis, 155, 157
  delirium, 485
  hepatitis, 146
  lead-poisoning anemia, 174
  Lyme disease, 309
  malignant hypertension, 31
  metabolic, 315
  thiamine deficiency, 314
  Wernicke's, 314
Endarteritis, 42
Endocarditis
  abscesses, 308
  acute arterial occlusion, 36
  cardioembolic strokes, 320, 321
  cardiogenic shock, 10
  description, 23
  history and physical keys, 23
  staphylococcal pneumonia, 496
  subacute bacterial, 85
  tetralogy of fallot, 27
  ventricular septic defect, 26
Endocervical curettage, 347
Endocrinologic shock, 12
Endocrinology
  acanthosis nigricans, 84
  adrenal gland
    congenital adrenal hyperplasia, 98–99
    Cushing's syndrome, 96–97
    hirsutism, 97–98
    insufficiency, adrenal, 95–96
    pheochromocytoma, 98
  diabetes mellitus
    hyperosmolar hyperglycemic nonketotic coma, 104
    hypoglycemia, 105
    type 1, 102–103
    type 2, 103–104
  lipoprotein disorders, clinical
    chylomicronemia, type I familial, 99
    decreased high-density lipoprotein, 102
    dysbetalipoproteinemia, type III, 100
    elevated Lp (a) lipoprotein, 102
    hyperlipoproteinemia, type II, 100

hyperlipoproteinemia, type IV, 100–101
hyperlipoproteinemia, type V, 101
livedo reticularis, 81
parathyroid gland disorders
  hypercalcemia, 91–92
pituitary gland disorders
  anterior pituitary, 92–94
  posterior pituitary, 94–95
surgical principles for diseases of
  Cushing's disease/syndrome, 573–574
  hyperparathyroidism, 572–573
  pheochromocytoma, 574
  thyroid neoplasm, 572
thyroid gland disorders
  hyperthyroidism, 88–89
  hypothyroidism, 89–90
  neoplasms of the thyroid gland, 91
undescended testis, 429
Endolymphatic sac decompression, 652
Endometrial cancer
  mechanisms and disease diagnosis/treatment, 341
Endometriosis
  infertility, 358
  mechanisms and disease diagnosis/treatment, 343, 343f
Endometritis, 262
Endomyometritis, 367, 387
Endomysial antibodies, 125
Endorectal coil magnetic resonance imaging, 542
Endoscopic retrograde cholangiopancreatography (ERCP). See also mechanisms and disease diagnosis/treatment and surgical principles under specific disease/disorder
  acute pancreatitis, 160, 161
  choledochal cyst, 611
  choledocholithiasis, 145, 146
  cholelithiasis, 145
  chronic pancreatitis, 161
  cirrhosis, 156
  pancreatic carcinoma, 157
Endoscopic ultrasonography (EUS), 109, 157

Endoscopy
  achalasia, 113
  acid-related disorders of the stomach, 116
  acute sinusitis, 662
  gastric cancer, 114
  gastric motility, disorders of, 118
  gastroesophageal reflux disease, 111
  herpes simplex virus, 258
  hypovolemic shock, 12
  intestinal obstruction, 138
  motor disorders of the esophagus, 112
  nasopharynx, masses in the, 658
  swallowing (injury/accidents), 227
  ureteropelvic junction obstruction, 541
Endothelial cells, 33
Endothelin receptor antagonist, 518
Endotoxemia, 146
Endotoxins, 13, 140
*Entamoeba histolytica*, 126
Enterochromaffin cells, 98
Enterocolitis, 376
Entropion
  mechanisms and disease diagnosis/treatment, 398
Enuresis
  mechanisms and disease diagnosis/treatment, 540
Enzyme-linked immunosorbent assay (ELISA)
  celiac sprue, 125
  HIV (human immunodeficiency virus), 248, 303
  hypersensitivity pneumonitis, 211
  Lyme disease, 272, 309
Enzymes, acute pancreatitis and digestive, 160
Eosinophil granuloma
  mechanisms and disease diagnosis/treatment, 290
Eosinophils/eosinophilia
  allergic bronchopulmonary aspergillosis, 209
  allergic rhinitis, 201, 665
  atopic dermatitis, 56, 206
  bronchial asthma, 198, 199
  chronic myelogenous leukemia, 179
  conjunctivitis, 393
  drug allergy, 213

  hereditary angioedema, 205, 206
  hypereosinophilic syndrome, 211–212
  rabies, 306
  tubulointerstitial disease, 548
Epicanthus
  mechanisms and disease diagnosis/treatment, 398–399
Epidermal growth factor, 326
*Epidermophyton*, 448
Epididymis, 532
Epididymitis
  mechanisms and disease diagnosis/treatment, 530–531
Epididymoorchitis
  mechanisms and disease diagnosis/treatment, 263
Epidural hematoma
  mechanisms and disease diagnosis/treatment
  injuries/wounds/accidents, 219–220
  neurology, 330–331
Epiglottitis
  acute, 493
  mechanisms and disease diagnosis/treatment, 435
Epilepsy, 124
Epinephrine
  anaphylactic shock, 239
  basic cardiac life support, 29
  croup, 436, 493
  drug allergy, 213
  glaucoma, 416
  hereditary angioedema, 206
  insect and snake bites, 238
  lacerations, 225
  transfusion reactions, 187
  urticaria, 204
Episiotomy, 367
Epistaxis
  idiopathic thrombocytopenic purpura, 192
  mechanisms and disease diagnosis/treatment
  overview, 217
  pulmonary medicine, 665–666, 666t
  nasopharynx, masses in the, 659
  platelet dysfunction, 194
  von Willebrand disease, 188
Epivir, 250

Epstein-Barr virus (EBV), 264, 437
Erectile impotence
  mechanisms and disease diagnosis/treatment, 537–538
Ergonovine, 5
Ergotamine, 318
Erotomanic delusions, 456
Erythema
  actinic keratosis, 69
  alcoholic liver disease, 146
  atopic dermatitis, 56
  Behcet's disease, 82
  chronic rhinitis, 664
  chronic sinusitis, 662
  chronicum migrans, 272, 309
  contact dermatitis, 55
  contusions, 292
  dermatomyositis, 80
  drug reactions causing skin changes, 58
  eyelid, 80
  glucagonoma syndrome, 84
  gonococcal tenosynovitis, 272
  gonorrhea, 259
  herpes simplex, 51
  infectious otitis externa, 647
  insect and snake bites, 238
  Kawasaki disease, 425
  lactation, 368
  livedo reticularis, 81
  lupus erythematosus, 79
  pharyngitis, 436
  postpartum sepsis, 387
  septic arthritis, 271
  thermal burns, 227
  urticaria, 203
  varicella (chickenpox), 265
Erythema migrans, 267
Erythema multiforme
  coccidioidomycosis, 501
  drug reactions causing skin changes, 58
  mechanisms and disease diagnosis/treatment, 61–62, 61f
  *Mycoplasma pneumoniae*, 498
  pemphigus, 60
Erythema nodosum
  blastomycosis, 501
  coccidioidomycosis, 501
  mechanisms and disease diagnosis/treatment, 62
  sarcoidosis, 508

Erythema toxicum neonatorum, 85
Erythrocyte sedimentation rate (ESR). *See also* mechanisms and disease diagnosis/treatment *and* surgical principles *under specific disease/disorder*
  ankylosing spondylitis, 283
  delirium, 486
  fibromyalgia, 285
  giant cell aortitis, 43
  Henoch-Schöenlein purpura, 425
  interstitial keratitis, 414
  ischemic heart disease, 23
  Kawasaki disease, 426
  osteomyelitis, 271
  pelvic inflammatory disease, 358
  polymyalgia rheumatica, 281
  rheumatoid arthritis, 283
  septic arthritis, 271
  vasculitis syndromes, 36
Erythrocytosis
  mechanisms and disease diagnosis/treatment
    primary, 185–186
    secondary, 186
Erythromycin
  acute otitis media, 649
  chancroid, 262
  chlamydia, 260
  gastric motility, disorders of, 118
  pharyngitis, 437
  pneumococcal pneumonia, 495
  syphilis, 532
Erythropoiesis, 173
Erythropoietin
  anemia of chronic disease, 176
  chronic renal failure, 174
  polycythemia rubra vera, 185
  secondary erythrocytosis, 186
*Escherichia coli*
  acute enteric infections, 122
  acute otitis media, 649
  bacterial meningitis, 437
  choledocholithiasis, 146
  chronic otitis media, 649, 650
  genitourinary tract infections, 377
  pelvic inflammatory disease, 358
  urinary tract infections, 529

Esophagitis
  cytomegalovirus, 253
  gastroesophageal reflux disease, 111
  herpes simplex virus, 258
Esophagoscopy, 653, 659
Esophagus
  gastroesophageal reflux disease, 110–111
  malignant neoplasms
    adenocarcinoma, 110
    mechanisms and disease diagnosis, 109, 109t
    squamous cell carcinoma, 109–110
  motor disorders of the
    achalasia, 113
    diffuse esophageal spasm, 113
    mechanisms and disease diagnosis/treatment, 111–113
    scleroderma, 113–114
Esotropia, 399
Essential hypertension
  mechanisms and disease diagnosis/treatment, 29–30
Essential thrombocythemia
  mechanisms and disease diagnosis/treatment, 193
Estradiol, 352, 353
Estrogen
  breast cancer, 354
  endometrial cancer, 341
  endometriosis, 343
  hyperlipoproteinemia, type IV, 101
  hyperthyroidism, 88
  meningioma, 326
  menopausal symptoms, 353
  pelvic relaxation/urinary incontinence, 351
  porphyria cutanea tarda, 83
  Turner's syndrome, 446
  ulcerative colitis, 133
  underproduction syndromes (pituitary gland), 94
Etanercept, 54
Ethambutol, 255
Ethmoid fracture, 217
Ethylenediaminetetraacetic acid (EDTA), 174, 231
Etidronate, 92, 290
Etoposide, 212, 545

Eustachian tube
nasopharynx, masses in the, 659
otitis media, 435
acute, 649
chronic, 650
serous, 650
Excess extracellular matrix (ECM), 157
Exercise echo, 6
Exercise(s). *See also* Physical therapy
adjustment disorders, 467
ankylosing spondylitis, 284
back pain, low, 275
chronic atherosclerotic occlusion, 35
diabetes mellitus, 104
emphysema, 506
fibromyalgia, 286
hypertrophic cardiomyopathy, 15
kyphosis, 449
menopausal symptoms, 353
pelvic relaxation/urinary incontinence, 351
premenstrual syndrome, 352
tendinitis, 285
Exercise stress testing
silent ischemia, 7
stable angina pectoris, 6
unstable angina, 3
Exocrine secretions, 162
Exostosis, 326
Exotoxins, 13
Extension injuries, cervical spine and, 293
Extensor plantar reflexes, 331
Extracolonic manifestations, ulcerative colitis and, 133
Eyelids, disorders of the
blepharitis, 396
blepharoptosis, 399
chalazion, 397
ectropion, 398
entropion, 398
epicanthus, 398–399
stye, 397
Eyes. *See also* Ophthalmology; Vision
barbiturates, 324
chorioretinitis
congenital cytomegalovirus, 439
congenital toxoplasmosis, 438
herpes simplex virus, 439
interstitial keratitis, 413
cytomegalovirus, 253
essential hypertension, 29
foreign bodies, 225–226
HIV (human immunodeficiency virus), 303
hyperthyroidism, 88
hypothermia, 240
injury, ocular, 220
meningioma, 326
metabolic encephalopathy, 315
multiple sclerosis, 331
neurosyphilis, 310
panic disorder, 463
sarcoidosis, 508
sedatives, 229
stimulants, 229
subdural hematoma, 330
volume depletion, 555

# F

Face chorea, 329
Facial fracture
mechanisms and disease diagnosis/treatment, 217–218
Facial plethora, 185
Factitious disorders, 472
Failure to thrive (FTT)
cellular (T-cell) immunodeficiency, 205
cystic fibrosis, 507
posterior urethral valves, 426
Falls and epidemiology/prevention, 244
Famciclovir, 264
Familial adenomatosis polyposis (FAP), 128
Familial combined hyperlipidemia, 100
Familial Mediterranean fever
mechanisms and disease diagnosis/treatment, 140–141
Family deviance/large size and conduct disorder, 474
Family history. *See also* Genetics
activated protein C resistance, 191
affective psychoses: mania and psychotic depression, 454
antithrombin III deficiency, 190
atherosclerosis, 34
attention-deficit hyperactivity disorder, 473
breast cancer, 353
child physical/sexual abuse, 486
cleft lip or palate, 440
congenital adrenal hyperplasia, 98
congenital hip disorders, 277
cyclothymia, 462
cystic fibrosis, 507
depression, major (unipolar), 459
diabetes mellitus, 103
dysplastic nevus, 73
familial Mediterranean fever, 141
hirsutism, 97
hypercalcemia, 91
hyperthyroidism, 88
hypertrophic cardiomyopathy, 14
hypothyroidism, 89
Legg-Calvé-Perthes disease, 277
melanoma, malignant, 71
panic disorder, 462
pheochromocytoma, 98
polycystic kidney disease, 552
protein C deficiency, 191
schizophrenia, 453
sickle cell anemia, 176
stable angina pectoris, 6
strabismus, 407
thyroid gland, neoplasms of the, 91
tubulointerstitial disease, 548
vesicoureteral reflux, 538
Famotidine, 111
Fanconi's syndrome, 173
Faoratriptan, 318
Fasciotomy, 36, 594
Fatigue, 13
acute lymphocytic leukemia, 178
acute myelogenous leukemia, 177
adrenal insufficiency, 95
agnogenic myeloid metaplasia, 193
alcohol, 479
anorectal abscess, 143
aplastic anemia, 173
atrial septal defect, 26
autoimmune hepatitis, 147
AV block, 17
bacterial meningitis, 437

Fatigue *(continued)*
  bereavement, 488
  blood-loss anemia, 169
  bradyarrhythmias, 18
  bulimia, 475
  cardiac tamponade, 21
  chronic myelogenous leukemia, 179
  chronic renal failure, 174
  chronic rhinitis, 664
  chronic valvular diseases, 24
  depression, major (unipolar), 459
  diabetes mellitus, 103
  dysthymia, 460
  epidural hematoma, 219
  erythema nodosum, 62
  fibromyalgia, 286
  giant cell aortitis, 43
  hepatitis B infection complicating pregnancy, 377
  herpes simplex, 52
  hypercalcemia, 91, 92
  hyperosmolar hyperglycemic nonketotic coma, 104
  hypersensitivity pneumonitis, 511
  hypoglycemia, 105
  hypomagnesemia, 557
  hypothermia, 240
  hypothyroidism, 89
  ill-defined presentations, 630–631
  influenza pneumonia, 498
  intermediate/high-grade lymphoma, 183
  iron-deficiency anemia, 169
  left-sided low output heart failure, 8
  Legionnaire's disease, 497
  lupus arthritis, 282
  Lyme disease, 272
  measles (rubeola), 265
  multiple myeloma, 184
  mumps, 266
  neutropenia, 194
  orchitis, 531
  orocavity, herpes simplex of the, 657
  overproduction syndromes (pituitary gland), 92
  PCP (phencyclidine), 230
  poliomyelitis, 305
  premenstrual syndrome, 351
  pyelonephritis, 546
  renal cell carcinoma, 544
  restrictive cardiomyopathy, 15
  rubella (German measles), 266
  sedatives, 229
  sick sinus syndrome, 16
  sleep apnea, 334
  strep throat, 660
  subarachnoid hemorrhage, 322
  tachyarrhythmias, 18
  underproduction syndromes (pituitary gland), 94
  varicella (chickenpox), 46
  vitamin $B_{12}$ deficiency, 172
Fat intake
  breast cancer, 353
  menopausal symptoms, 353
Fearful personality disorders, 468
Febrile seizures
  mechanisms and disease diagnosis/treatment, 421
Feet
  arteriosclerotic ulcer, 78
  dermatophytosis, 47–48
  fractures
    mechanisms and disease diagnosis/treatment, 296–297
  gout, 280
  Kawasaki disease, 426
  Turner's syndrome, 445
  vitamin $B_{12}$ deficiency, 313
Felty's syndrome, 194, 195
Female sexual arousal disorder, 484
Femoral hernia
  surgical principles, 617–618
Femoral neck, 278
Femur, fracture of
  mechanisms and disease diagnosis/treatment, 234, 295–296
Fenofibrate, 101
Ferritin, 135, 172, 176
Fetal alcohol syndrome, 473, 478
Fever
  acute enteric infections, 120, 122
  acute epiglottitis, 493
  acute myelogenous leukemia, 177
  acute otitis media, 648
  acute sinusitis, 662
  agnogenic myeloid metaplasia, 193
  anorectal abscess, 143
  antipsychotics, 324
  aplastic anemia, 173
  aseptic meningitis, 306
  blastomycosis, 501
  bronchiectasis, 507
  coccidioidomycosis, 501
  Crohn's disease, 135
  cryptococcal infection, 257, 502
  cytomegalovirus, 253
  diabetes mellitus, 103
  diarrhea, 126
  disseminated *Mycobacterium avium-intracellulare* complex, 255, 256
  distributive shock, 12
  drug allergy, 213
  epididymitis, 530
  erythema nodosum, 62
  familial Mediterranean fever, 141
  genital herpes, 263
  giant cell aortitis, 43
  gonococcal tenosynovitis, 272
  gram-negative bacillary pneumonias, 496
  *Haemophilus influenzae* pneumonia, 496
  hepatocellular carcinoma, 153
  hernias, external, 163
  herpes, genital, 533
  herpes simplex virus, 52, 303
  histoplasmosis, 500
  HIV (human immunodeficiency virus), 249
  hypersensitivity pneumonitis, 210, 511
  hyperthyroidism, 89
  influenza pneumonia, 498
  Kawasaki disease, 425
  Legionnaire's disease, 497
  lupus arthritis, 282
  measles (rubeola), 265
  metabolic encephalopathy, 315
  mononucleosis, 264
  mumps, 266
  *Mycoplasma pneumoniae*, 497
  ophthalmic herpes zoster, 412
  orchitis, 531
  orocavity, herpes simplex of the, 657
  osteomyelitis, 271
  otitis media, 434
  pelvic inflammatory disease, 262, 358

peritonitis, 140
pertussis, 494
pharyngitis, 436
pleurisy, 513
pneumococcal pneumonia, 495
*Pneumocystis carinii* pneumonia, 498
poliomyelitis, 305
postpartum sepsis, 387
prostatitis, 530
pulmonary sequestration, 447
pulmonary tuberculosis, 499
pyelonephritis, 546
renal transplant rejection, 548
rubella (German measles), 266
staphylococcal pneumonia, 496
strep throat, 660
thrombotic thrombocytopenic purpura, 192
transfusion reactions, 187
tuberculosis, 308
urinary tract infections, 529
varicella (chickenpox), 46
vasculitis/vasculitis syndromes, 36, 517
Fibrin, 190, 440
Fibrinogen, 374
Fibrinoid necrosis, 553
Fibrohistiocytes, 73
Fibromuscular hyperplasia, 551
Fibromyalgia
mechanisms and disease diagnosis/treatment, 285–286
Fibrosis
frozen shoulder syndrome, 288
Fibula, fracture of
mechanisms and disease diagnosis/treatment, 234
Filgrastim, 205
Fine-needle aspiration
breast cancer, 354
fibroadenoma, 355
thyroid gland, neoplasms of the, 91
Fire prevention, 244
Fire setting and conduct disorder, 474
Flail chest
mechanisms and disease diagnosis/treatment, 223
Fleas
mechanisms and disease diagnosis/treatment, 66

Flexion injuries, cervical spine and, 292–293
Flexor-extensor tendon disruption, 236
Flies
mechanisms and disease diagnosis/treatment, 65–66
Fluconazole, 502
candidiasis, cutaneous, 49
candidiasis, oral, 48
coccidioidomycosis, 502
cryptococcal infection, 258
fungal meningitis, 307
paronychia, 49
Flucytosine, 503
Fludarabine, 181, 183
Fluorescein, 413, 436
Fluorescent treponemal antibody absorption (FTA-ABS)
congenital syphilis, 438
interstitial keratitis, 414
sudden hearing loss, 655
syphilis, 261, 532
Fluoroquinolone, 259
Fluoroscopy, 446
Fluorouracil (5-FU)
actinic keratosis, 69
cervicitis and sexually transmitted diseases, 347
pancreatic carcinoma, 157
renal cell carcinoma, 544
Focal nodular hyperplasia
surgical principles, 613
Folate
alcohol, 480
celiac sprue, 125
chronic renal failure, 174
neural tube defects, 423
schizophrenia, 453
sickle cell anemia, 177
Foley catheter, 140
Folic acid
deficiency
mechanisms and disease diagnosis/treatment, 170–171
methyl alcohol poisoning, 232
neural tube defects and central nervous system malformation in the fetus, 380
Folinic acid, 257

Follicle-stimulating hormone (FSH)
amenorrhea, 352
erectile impotence, 537
infertility, 535
menopausal symptoms, 353
sexual dysfunctions, 484
underproduction syndromes (pituitary gland), 94
Follicular cyst
mechanisms and disease diagnosis/treatment, 75–76
Food-borne bacterial pathogens, 122
Forceps, obstetric
mechanisms and disease diagnosis/treatment, 387
Foreign bodies
aspiration, 226
dry-eye syndrome, 400
eye/ear/nose, 225–226
swallowed, 226–227
Fortovase, 250
Foscarnet, 253, 258
Fossa navicularis, 537
Fractures and dislocations
dislocations and separations, 297–298
extremities
femur, 234
fibula, 234
humerus, 235
radius, 234–235
tibia, 233
ulna, 235
facial, 217–218
foot and leg fractures, 296–297
hand phalanges, closed fracture of, 295
neck fractures, femoral, 295–296
open, 299
osteoporosis, 279
pelvic, 224
rib cage, 221
rotator cuff syndrome, 298–299
skull trauma/fracture, 218
spine
cervical spine, 292–293
lumbar spine, 294
thoracic spine, 293–294
sudden hearing loss, 656
urologic trauma, 541
vertebral column, 233

Fragile X syndrome
  mechanisms and disease diagnosis/treatment, 446
Frank sepsis, 546
Free fatty acid, 103
Fremitus, 513
Friction rub, 20
Frontal fracture, 217
Frostbite
  mechanisms and disease diagnosis/treatment, 240
Frozen shoulder syndrome
  mechanisms and disease diagnosis/treatment, 288
Fructose, 125
Functional endoscopic sinus surgery (FESS), 663
Fungal infections. *See also specific disease/disorder/organism*
  mechanisms and disease diagnosis/treatment
    meningitis, 307
    pediatrics, 448
  pneumonias
    blastomycosis, 501
    coccidioidomycosis, 501–502
    cryptococcus, 502
    histoplasmosis, 500–501
    invasive aspergillosis, 502–503
    phycomycosis, 503
Furosemide
  bullous pemphigoid, 59
  congestive heart failure, 514
  syndrome of inappropriate antidiuretic hormone secretion, 95
Fusion inhibitors, 251

G
Gabapentin, 47, 317, 333
Gadolinium, 93
Gag reflex, 421
Gait problems. *See also Incoordination*
  Alzheimer's disease, 327
  cervical spine and spinal stenosis, 333
  manganese, 323
  multiple sclerosis, 332
  Parkinson's disease, 328
Galactorrhea, 92
Galactosemia, 424
Galantamine, 327
Gallbladder
  acute cholecystitis, 144–145
  choledocholithiasis and acute suppurative cholangitis, 145–146
  cholelithiasis, 145
  Kawasaki disease, 426
  surgical principles
    acute cholecystitis, 610, 611*f*
    biliary atresia, 610
    carcinoma, 612
    choledochal cyst, 611
    choledocholithiasis, 612
    focal nodular hyperplasia, 613
Gallium scans, 181
Gallop, 10, 31
Gallstones, 100, 145, 146, 171
Gamekeeper's thumb, 237
Gamete intrafallopian transfer (GIFT), 358
Gamma-aminobutyric acid (GABA), 463, 480
Gamma-glutamyl transferase (GGT), 154, 230, 478
Ganciclovir, 253, 254
Gangrene
  acute arterial occlusion, 36
  chronic atherosclerotic occlusion, 35
  hemorrhoids, 142
  vasculitis syndromes, 36
*Gardnerella vaginalis*, 350
Gardner's syndrome, 72, 84
Garlic odor, 231
Gastric cancer
  mechanisms and disease diagnosis/treatment 114-115, 114–115
  thiamine deficiency, 314
Gastric lavage
  acetaminophen, 228
  diethyl-m-toluamide, 232
  tricyclic antidepressants, 229
Gastric motility, disorders of
  mechanisms and disease diagnosis/treatment, 118, 119*t*, 120
Gastric volvulus
  surgical principles, 598–599
Gastrinoma
  surgical principles, 616–617
Gastritis, 478
Gastroenterology. *See also* Digestive system
  oncology/cancer
    acanthosis nigricans, 84
    Gardner's syndrome, 84
  pediatrics
    cleft lip or palate, 440
    Hirschsprung disease, 443, 444*f*
    intussusception, 442–443, 442*f*
    malrotation of the small intestine, 441–442
    necrotizing enterocolitis, 443
    pyloric stenosis, 441
    tracheoesophageal fistula, 441
Gastroesophageal reflux disease (GERD)
  mechanisms and disease diagnosis/treatment, 110–111
  scleroderma, 113, 114
Gemfibrozil
  decreased high-density lipoprotein, 102
  dysbetalipoproteinemia, type III, 100
  hyperlipoproteinemia, 33
  hyperlipoproteinemia, type II, 100
  hyperlipoproteinemia, type IV, 101
  hyperlipoproteinemia, type V, 101
Gender. *See also* Reproduction, male/female
  anorexia, 474
  autoimmune hepatitis, 147
  Behcet's disease, 82
  bipolar disorders, 461
  congenital hip disorders, 276
  conversion disorder, 471
  dermatophytosis, 48
  epididymoorchitis, 263
  fibromyalgia, 285
  frozen shoulder syndrome, 288
  gonorrhea, 259, 532
  Henoch-Schöenlein purpura, 425
  hypereosinophilic syndrome, 212
  livedo reticularis, 81
  lupus arthritis, 281

oropharynx, malignant
neoplasms of the, 659
polymyalgia rheumatica, 281
posterior urethral valves, 426
rosacea, 67
slipped capital femoral
epiphysis, 278, 449
urinary tract infections, 529
Generalized anxiety disorder
mechanisms and disease
diagnosis/treatment, 464
Gene therapy, 205
Genetics. *See also* Family history;
Race/region
alcohol, 479
amyotrophic lateral sclerosis, 328
anorexia, 475
autistic disorder, 458
bipolar disorders, 461
bulimia, 476
cholelithiasis, 145
colorectal carcinoma, 128
conduct disorder, 474
congenital deafness, 425
counseling, 360
cystic fibrosis, 507
depression, major (unipolar),
460
glioblastoma, 326
myopathies/dystrophies, 313
obsessive-compulsive disorder,
465
otitis media, 434
panic disorder, 463
pediatrics
Down syndrome, 444–445,
445*f*
fragile X syndrome, 446
trisomy 13, 445
trisomy 18, 445
Turner's syndrome, 445–446
substance-related disorders, 478
Genital herpes, 533
mechanisms and disease
diagnosis/treatment,
263–264
Genital tract laceration, 386
Genital ulcers, 262
Genitourinary system. *See also*
Renal and urinary system
infections
mechanisms and disease
diagnosis/treatment,
376–377

pediatrics
bladder extrophy, 429
Eagle-Barrett syndrome, 427
hypospadias, 426
multicystic kidney disease,
428
polycystic disease, infantile,
428
posterior urethral valves,
426–427
prune-belly syndrome, 427
undescended testis, 428–429
vesicoureteral reflux,
427–428
Gentamicin, 263, 358
German measles. *See* Rubella
Gestational diabetes, 365
Gestational trophoblastic disease
(GTD)
mechanisms and disease
diagnosis/treatment,
382–383
Giant cell aortitis
mechanisms and disease
diagnosis/treatment, 43
Giant cell arteritis, 36
Giant cells
chalazion, 397
fungal meningitis, 307
herpes simplex keratitis, 412
varicella (chickenpox), 265
*Giardia lamblia*, 123
Giemsa stain. *See also* mechanisms
and disease diagnosis/
treatment *and* surgical
principles *under specific
disease/disorder*
herpes, 533
orocavity, herpes simplex of the,
658
*Pneumocystis carinii* pneumonia,
252
Gilbert disease, 432
Glatinamer acetate, 332
Glaucoma
cataracts, 417
herpes simplex keratitis, 412
mechanisms and disease
diagnosis/treatment,
414–416, 415*f*
congenital, 423–424
ophthalmic herpes zoster, 412
optic atrophy, 404
Glenohumeral arthritis, 298

Glioblastoma
mechanisms and disease
diagnosis/treatment,
325–326, 325*f*
Glipizide, 104
Globulin and hyperthyroidism,
88–89
Globus, 110
Glomerular filtration rate (GFR)
chronic renal failure, 547
mother, postpartum care of the,
368
tubulointerstitial disease, 548
Glomerulonephritis
mechanisms and disease
diagnosis/treatment, 549
nephrotic syndrome, 549
Glossitis, 169
Glucagon, 103
Glucagonoma syndrome, 84
Glucocorticoids
adrenal insufficiency, 96
asthma and pregnancy, 389
congenital adrenal hyperplasia,
99
phycomycosis, 503
secondary hypertension, 31
transfusion reactions, 187
vasculitis syndromes, 37
Glucosamine, 274
Glucose
alcohol, 480
chronic pancreatitis, 161
diabetes, gestational, 388
diabetes mellitus, 104
febrile seizures, 421
hyperosmolar hyperglycemic
nonketotic coma, 104
hypoglycemia, 105
metabolic encephalopathy, 315
necrobiosis lipoidica, 83
pleural effusions, 512
sexual dysfunctions, 484
syphilis, 261
thiamine deficiency, 315
Glucose-6-phosphate
dehydrogenase (G6PD)
deficiency, 175, 213
Glucosuria, 102
Glutamate excitotoxicity, 328
Glutamic acid, 176
Gluten, 60, 61, 124, 125
Glyburide, 104
Glycerin, 416

Goblet cells, 664
Gold and ulcerative colitis, 134
Gonadal dysgenesis 45, XO
  mechanisms and disease
    diagnosis/treatment,
    445–446
Gonadotropin-releasing hormone
    (GnRH)
  dysmenorrhea, 351
  endometriosis, 343
  infertility, 358
  leiomyomata uteri, 342
Gonococcal tenosynovitis
  mechanisms and disease
    diagnosis/treatment,
    272–273
Gonorrhea
  cervicitis, 345–347
  mechanisms and disease
    diagnosis/treatment,
    259–260
  renal and urinary system, 532
Goodpasture's syndrome
  mechanisms and disease
    diagnosis/treatment,
    517–518
Gottron's papules, 80
Gout
  bursitis, 284
  effusion of joint, 290
  mechanisms and disease
    diagnosis/treatment, 280
Grafts, skin, 77
Gram-negative bacillary
    pneumonias
  mechanisms and disease
    diagnosis/treatment,
    496–497
Gram-negative sepsis, 556
Gram stain. See also mechanisms
    and disease diagnosis/
    treatment and surgical
    principles under specific
    disease/disorder
  aseptic meningitis, 306
  chronic rhinitis, 664
  conjunctivitis, 393
  effusion of joint, 290–291
  fungal sinusitis, 663
  gonococcal tenosynovitis, 272
  gonorrhea, 532
  impetigo, 50
  influenza pneumonia, 498
  Mycoplasma pneumoniae, 498
  paronychia, 49
  pelvic inflammatory disease, 358
  septic meningitis, 307
  urethritis, 531
Grandiose delusions, 456
Granulocytopenia, 264
Granulomatous meningitis, 307
Granulomatous vasculitis, 517
Graves' disease, 88
Graying, premature, 172
Greenstick radial fracture, 235
Griseofulvin, 48
Groin hernias
  mechanisms and disease
    diagnosis/treatment,
    162–163
Groin pain, 295–296
Growth hormone
  underproduction syndromes
    (pituitary gland), 94
Growth hormone therapy, 446
Growth retardation, 26, 550. See
    also Intrauterine growth
    retardation
Guaifenesin, 521
Guillain-Barré syndrome (GBS)
  diarrhea, 126
  mechanisms and disease
    diagnosis/treatment,
    311–312
  mononucleosis, 264
  rubella (German measles), 267
Guilt and sexual dysfunctions, 484
Gunshot wounds, 243
Guttate psoriasis, 53, 54
Gynecologic examination and
    screening
  history/physical keys/diagnosis,
    359
Gynecomastia, 478, 545

H
Haemophilus ducreyi, 262
Haemophilus influenzae
  acute bronchitis, 494
  acute epiglottitis, 493
  acute otitis media, 649
  acute sinusitis, 662
  epiglottitis, 435
  osteomyelitis, 271
  pneumonia
    mechanisms and disease
      diagnosis/treatment, 496
  septic arthritis, 272
  septic meningitis, 307
  strep throat, 661
Haemophilus parainfluenza, 661
Hair and the hair follicle
  acne vulgaris, 67
  alopecia areata, 68–69
  arsenic toxicity, 323
  cellulitis, 49
  hirsutism, 97
  intersex, 534
  overproduction syndromes
    (pituitary gland), 92
  pilonidal disease, 144
  porphyria cutanea tarda, 83
  pubic hair, 92
  rosacea, 67–68
Half-and-half nails, 85
Halitosis, 657
Hallucinations
  alcohol, 480
  delirium, 485
  drug dependence, 482
  narcolepsy, 335
  schizophrenia, 453
Haloperidol, 458, 486
Ham test, 173
Hands. See also Clubbing
  bulimia, 475
  carpal tunnel syndrome, 310–311
  Dupuytren's contracture, 146,
    155, 288, 537
  fracture of hand phalanges,
    closed
    mechanisms and disease
      diagnosis/treatment, 295
  Huntington's disease, 329
  Kawasaki disease, 426
  panic disorder, 463
  radius fractures, 234–235
  sprains and dislocations
    distal interphalangeal sprain,
      236
    metacarpal phalangeal sprain,
      236–237
    proximal interphalangeal
      dislocation, 236
  trisomy 18, 445
  Turner's syndrome, 445
  vitamin $B_{12}$ deficiency, 313
Hartman's procedure, 604
Hashimoto's thyroiditis, 68
  diabetes mellitus, 103
  hyperthyroidism, 89

Headache
    hypothyroidism, 89
    thyroid gland, neoplasms of the, 91
Headache
    abscesses, 308
    acute lymphocytic leukemia, 178
    acute sinusitis, 662
    acute upper respiratory infection, 667
    alcohol, 478
    arsenic toxicity, 323
    aseptic meningitis, 306
    bacterial meningitis, 437
    carbon monoxide, 231
    chronic sinusitis, 662
    coarctation of the aorta, 28
    coccidioidomycosis, 501
    concussion, 219
    cryptococcal infection, 257, 502
    dysmenorrhea, 351
    epidural hematoma, 219
    essential hypertension, 29
    fungal meningitis, 307
    genital herpes, 263
    giant cell aortitis, 43
    glaucoma, 414
    glioblastoma, 325
    herpes simplex virus, 303
    histoplasmosis, 500
    HIV (human immunodeficiency virus), 303
    hydrocephalus, 423
    hypoglycemia, 105
    intracerebral hemorrhage, 321
    malignant hypertension, 31
    mechanisms and disease diagnosis/treatment, 317–318, 318f
    meningioma, 326
    metastases, 326
    mononucleosis, 264
    mumps, 266
    *Mycoplasma pneumoniae*, 497
    neurosyphilis, 310
    orocavity, herpes simplex of the, 657
    pheochromocytoma, 98
    preeclampsia, 375
    psychosomatic disorders, 472
    rubella (German measles), 266
    sleep apnea, 334, 523
    subarachnoid hemorrhage, 321
    subdural hematoma, 219, 330
    tuberculosis, 308
    underproduction syndromes (pituitary gland), 94
    varicella (chickenpox), 46
    venous thrombosis, 322
Head lice, 65
Head trauma. *See also* Cranial injury
    alcohol, 479
    conduct disorder, 474
    contusions, 331
    delirium, 485
    strabismus, 407
    subdural hematoma, 330
    surgical principles, 580
Hearing loss
    auditory injury, 220
    bacterial meningitis, 437
    barotrauma, 656
    cerumen impaction, 651
    chronic otitis media, 649, 650
    congenital cytomegalovirus, 439
    congenital deafness, 424–425
    congenital rubella infection, 439
    delusional disorder, 456
    interstitial keratitis, 413
    malignant otitis externa, 647
    mechanisms and disease diagnosis/treatment, 653–656, 654f
    nasopharynx, masses in the, 659
    noise-induced, 221, 656
    otitis media, 434, 435
    septic meningitis, 307
    sudden, 655–656
    tinnitus, 657
    vertigo, 652
Heartburn, 110, 111
Heart failure (HF)
    hemolytic uremic syndrome, 440
    left-sided
        high output, 9
        low output, 8–9
    panic disorder, 463
    pulmonary sequestration, 447
    Rh incompatibility, 431
    right-sided, 9–10
    sleep apnea, 334
Heart sounds. *See* Murmurs/heart sounds
Heatstroke
    mechanisms and disease diagnosis/treatment, 241
Heavy metals
    autistic disorder, 458
    childhood schizophrenia, 458
    mechanisms and disease diagnosis/treatment for poisoning from, 231
    teratology, 367
    toxic disorders
        arsenic, 323
        lead, 323
        manganese, 323–324
        mercury, 323
Height loss, 279
Heimlich maneuver, 226
*Helicobacter pylori*
    acid-related disorders of the stomach, 116–117, 117t
    adenocarcinoma, 110
    gastric cancer, 114
    mucosa-associated lymphoid tissue lymphomas, 115
Heller myotomy, 113
HELLP syndrome, 374
Helminths, 122
Hemangioma
    mechanisms and disease diagnosis/treatment, 74
    surgical principles, 564–565
Hemarthroses, 291
Hematochezia, 137
Hematocrit (HCT)
    acute pancreatitis, 159
    blood-loss anemia, 170
    hemolytic anemia, 175
    polycythemia rubra vera, 186
    secondary erythrocytosis, 186
    transfusion reactions, 187
Hematology. *See also* Blood; *Hema and Hemo listings*
    activated protein C resistance, 191–192
    agnogenic myeloid metaplasia, 193–194
    anemia
        aplastic, 173–174
        blood-loss, 169–170
        chronic disease, 176
        chronic renal disease, 174
        folic acid deficiency, 170–171
        hemolytic, 175
        iron-deficiency, 169
        lead-poisoning, 174
        sickle cell, 176–177
        thalassemia-alpha, 171
        thalassemia-beta, 171–172
        vitamin$_{12}$ deficiency, 172–173

Hematology (continued)
   antithrombin III deficiency, 190–191
   disseminated intravascular coagulation, 190
   essential thrombocythemia, 193
   hemophilia A and B, 187–188
   idiopathic thrombocytopenia purpura, 192
   ill-defined symptom complex and circulatory system
      murmurs, 622–623
      palpitations, 622
   lupus inhibitor, 189–190
   neutropenia, 194–195
   platelet dysfunction, 194
   polycythemia rubra vera, 185–186
   protein C deficiency, 191
   secondary erythrocytosis, 186–187
   surgical principles for circulatory diseases
      abdominal aortic aneurysmal disease, 590–591, 591f
      aneurysms of the thoracic aorta, 588
      aortic dissection, 589–590, 589f
      arterial embolism/thrombosis, 593–594
      carotid artery disease, 584–585, 585f
      deep venous thrombosis, 594–595
      infrainguinal aneurysmal disease, 592–593
      peripheral arterial occlusive disease, 586–588
      renovascular disease, 586
      superficial thrombophlebitis, 595–596
      thoracic outlet syndrome, 591–592
      varicose veins, 595
   thrombocytopenic purpura, 192–193
   transfusion reactions, 187
   Vitamin K deficiency, 189
   von Willebrand disease, 188–189
Hematopoiesis, 173
Hematuria
   bladder carcinoma, 543
   blood-loss anemia, 169
   essential hypertension, 29
   Henoch-Schöenlein purpura, 425
   papillary necrosis, 550
   urologic trauma, 541
   vitamin K deficiency, 189
   Wilms' tumor, 544
Hemiarthroplasty, 296
Hemiparesis
   contusions, 331
   glioblastoma, 325
   herpes simplex virus, 303
   intracerebral hemorrhage, 321
   ischemic thrombotic strokes, 319
   meningioma, 326
   subarachnoid hemorrhage, 321
   subdural hematoma, 330
Hemiplegia, 219
Hemithorax, 513
Hemochromatosis, 15, 150, 152
Hemoconcentration, 137
Hemodynamic monitoring
   cardiac tamponade, 21
   distributive shock, 13
   pulmonary embolism, 38
Hemoglobin
   neonatal hyperbilirubinemia, 432
   prenatal care, 365
   Rh incompatibility, 431
Hemoglobinuria, 187
Hemolysis
   acute renal failure, 546
   arsenic toxicity, 323
   hemolytic anemia, 175
   neonatal hyperbilirubinemia, 432
   Rh incompatibility, 431
   thrombotic thrombocytopenic purpura, 193
Hemolytic anemia
   disseminated intravascular coagulation, 190
   mechanisms and disease diagnosis/treatment, 175
   mononucleosis, 264
   thalassemia-alpha, 171
Hemolytic uremic syndrome, 126
   mechanisms and disease diagnosis/treatment, 440
Hemopericardium, 40
Hemophilia A and B
   mechanisms and disease diagnosis/treatment, 187–188
Hemoptysis
   blood-loss anemia, 169
   bronchiectasis, 507
   bronchogenic carcinoma, 518
   carcinoid tumors, 519
   ill-defined symptoms, 625–626
   larynx, cancer of the, 661
   mechanisms and disease diagnosis/treatment, 522
   metastatic malignant tumors, 520
   phycomycosis, 503
   pulmonary embolism, 38, 515
   pulmonary sequestration, 447
   pulmonary tuberculosis, 499
   sarcoidosis, 508
   solitary pulmonary nodule, 523
   vasculitis, 517
Hemorrhage
   auditory injury, 220
   blood-loss anemia, 169
   coarctation of the aorta, 28
   conjunctivitis, 393
   contusions, 331
   essential hypertension, 29
   essential thrombocythemia, 193
   facial fracture, 218
   glioblastoma, 325
   Henoch-Schöenlein purpura, 425
   herpes simplex virus, 304
   hypovolemic shock, 11
   ill-defined presentations gastrointestinal, 633–634
   insect and snake bites, 238
   intracerebral, 321
   ischemic bowel disease, 137
   malignant hypertension, 31
   pelvic fractures, 224
   polycythemia rubra vera, 185, 186
   postpartum, 386
   skull trauma/fracture, 218
   splinter hemorrhages, 85
   subdural hematoma, 219
   ulcerative colitis, 134
   underproduction syndromes (pituitary gland), 94
Hemorrhoidectomy, 142
Hemorrhoids
   mechanisms and disease diagnosis/treatment, 141–142
   surgical principles, 604

Henoch-Schöenlein purpura
  mechanisms and disease
      diagnosis/treatment, 425
Heparin
  acute arterial occlusion, 36
  antithrombin III deficiency, 191
  deep venous thrombosis, 594
  myocardial infarction, 5
  osteoporosis, 279
  poisoning and mechanisms and
      disease
      diagnosis/treatment, 232
  postpartum sepsis, 387
  pulmonary embolism, 38, 516,
      517
  unstable angina, 4
  venous thrombosis, 37
Hepatic adenoma
  surgical principles, 612–613
Hepatic fibrosis
  infantile polycystic disease, 428
  mechanisms and disease
      diagnosis/treatment,
      155–157
Hepatitis
  alcohol, 478
  alcoholic, 147
  autoimmune, 147–148
  B
    algorithm for therapy, 152t
    HIV (human
      immunodeficiency virus),
      251
    pregnancy complications,
      377–378
    prenatal care, 365
  C
    porphyria cutanea tarda, 83
  candidiasis, cutaneous, 49
  chronic, 147
  cirrhosis, 155, 156
  congenital syphilis, 438
  drug-induced hepatotoxicity, 147
  environmental and toxic causes,
      149t
  gonorrhea, 259
  hepatocellular carcinoma, 153,
      155
  history and physical keys, 146,
      146t
  mechanisms and disease
      diagnosis/treatment,
      146–153, 147t–149t,
      151t–152t

substance-related disorders, 477
  viral, 146–147, 147t
Hepatocellular carcinoma (HCC)
  mechanisms and disease
      diagnosis/treatment,
      153–155
Hepatomegaly
  agnogenic myeloid metaplasia,
      193
  choledocholithiasis, 145
  cirrhosis, 156
  hepatitis, 146
  hepatocellular carcinoma, 153
  right-sided heart failure, 9
Hepatorenal syndrome, 547
Hepatosplenomegaly
  chronic lymphocytic leukemia,
      180
  chylomicronemia, type 1
      familial, 99
  congenital cytomegalovirus, 439
  congenital rubella infection, 439
  congenital syphilis, 437
  hyperlipoproteinemia, type V,
      101
  infantile polycystic disease, 428
  neutropenia, 194
  secondary syphilis, 52
Hepatotoxins, 149
Hereditary angioedema
  mechanisms and disease
      diagnosis/treatment,
      205–206
Hereditary nonpolyposis colorectal
      cancer (HNPCC), 129
Hermaphrodites, 535
Hernias
  abscesses, 308
  contusions, 331
  diaphragmatic, 447
  hiatal, 111
  intestinal obstruction, 138
  mechanisms and disease
      diagnosis/treatment
      external, 162–163
      traumatic hernias of the
          diaphragm, 163
  neural tube defects, 422–423
  septic meningitis, 307
  surgical principles
    diaphragmatic, 619
    femoral, 617–618
    incisional, 618
    inguinal, 617

with obstruction, 619
    umbilical, 618
    venous thrombosis, 322
Heroin and substance-related
      disorders, 478
Herpes, genital, 263–264
  mechanisms and disease
      diagnosis/treatment, 533
Herpes gestationis
  mechanisms and disease
      diagnosis/treatment, 59
Herpes simplex keratitis
  mechanisms and disease
      diagnosis/treatment,
      411–412
Herpes simplex virus (HSV)
  atopic dermatitis, 207
  cervicitis, 345–347
  erythema multiforme, 62
  impetigo, 50
  mechanisms and disease
      diagnosis/treatment, 258
  neurology, 303–304
  pediatrics, 439
  molluscum contagiosum, 51–52,
      52f
  orocavity
    mechanisms and disease
      diagnosis/treatment,
      657–658
Herpes zoster
  ophthalmic
    mechanisms and disease
      diagnosis/treatment,
      412–413
  sudden hearing loss, 656
Herpetic keratoconjunctivitis, 52,
      412
Hexosaminidase A, 335–336
Hiatal hernia, 111
Hidradenitis suppurativa, 143
High-density lipoprotein (HDL),
      32, 101
Hip
  congenital hip disorders,
      276–277
  developmental dysplasia of the
    mechanisms and disease
      diagnosis/treatment, 433,
      433f
  Legg-Calvé-Perthes disease,
      277–278
  slipped capital femoral
      epiphysis, 449

Hirschsprung's disease, 139
   mechanisms and disease diagnosis/treatment, 443–444, 444f
   surgical principles, 609
Hirsutism
   Cushing's syndrome, 96
   mechanisms and disease diagnosis/treatment, 97–98
His-Purkinje system, 18
Histamines
   allergic rhinitis, 201
   anaphylactic shock, 239
   bronchial asthma, 199
   gastroesophageal reflux disease, 111
Histiocytoma
   mechanisms and disease diagnosis/treatment, 73
Histiocytosis, 94
*Histoplasma capsulatum*, 500
Histoplasmosis
   mechanisms and disease diagnosis/treatment, 500–501
History and physical keys. *See* mechanisms and disease diagnosis/treatment *and* surgical principles *under specific disease/disorder*
Histrionic personality disorders, 468
Hives
   mechanisms and disease diagnosis/treatment, 57–58, 203
HIV (human immunodeficiency virus)
   aseptic meningitis, 306
   candidiasis, oral, 48
   cryptococcal infection, 257–258
   cytomegalovirus, 253–254
   delirium, 486
   disseminated *Mycobacterium avium-intracellulare* complex, 255–256
   fungal sinusitis, 663
   herpes simplex virus, 258
   HIV (human immunodeficiency virus), 248–252
   intermediate/high-grade lymphoma, 183
   malignant otitis externa, 647
   mechanisms and disease diagnosis/treatment, 248–252, 249t
   neurology, 303
   pediatrics, 438–439
   renal and urinary system, 533
neurosyphilis, 310
*Pneumocystis carinii* pneumonia, 252–253, 498
scabies, 64
schizophrenia, 453
seborrheic dermatitis, 55
secondary syphilis, 53
substance-related disorders, 477
thrush, oral, 658
toxoplasma encephalitis, 256–257
tuberculosis, 254–255
varicella-zoster (shingles), 47
vulva/vagina, candidiasis of the, 349
HMG-CoA reductase inhibitors
   hyperlipoproteinemia, 33
   stable angina pectoris, 7
   unstable angina, 4
Hoarseness. *See also* Voice changes/hoarseness
   mechanisms and disease diagnosis/treatment, 660
Hodgkin's disease
   cryptococcal infection, 502
   idiopathic thrombocytopenic purpura, 192
   mechanisms and disease diagnosis/treatment, 181–182, 181f
Hollowvisceral myopathy, 118
Holter monitor, 7, 320
Home accidents, 241
Homocysteine, 318
Homocystinuria, 37, 41
Homonymous defects
   mechanisms and disease diagnosis/treatment, 405f, 406
Hormone replacement therapy (HRT), 352
Horner's syndrome, 317
Howell-Jolly bodies, 124, 176
Human chorionic gonadotropin (hCG)
   amenorrhea, 352
   ectopic pregnancy, 370
   gestational trophoblastic disease, 382, 383
   ovarian cysts, 344
   pelvic inflammatory disease, 358
   prenatal care, 365
   prenatal diagnosis, 366
   testicular carcinoma, 545
Human leukocyte antigen (HLA)
   ankylosing spondylitis, 283
   aplastic anemia, 173
   celiac sprue, 125
   chronic myelogenous leukemia, 180
   dermatitis herpetiformis, 60
   diabetes mellitus, 103
   hepatitis, 150
   multiple sclerosis, 332
Human papillomavirus (HPV)
   cervical dysplasia and management of abnormal Pap smear, 347
   cervicitis, 346, 347
   squamous cell carcinoma, 110
   verrucae, 51
Human placental lactogen (hPL), 388
Humerus, fracture of the
   mechanisms and disease diagnosis/treatment, 235
Humidification, 493
Humoral immunodeficiency
   mechanisms and disease diagnosis/treatment, 204
Hunger. *See* Appetite disturbance
Huntington's disease
   mechanisms and disease diagnosis/treatment, 329
Hutchinson's sign, 412, 413
Hutchinson teeth, 438
Hyaline membrane disease
   mechanisms and disease diagnosis/treatment, 515
Hyaline membrane formation, 430
Hydralazine, 375, 551
Hydrocele
   mechanisms and disease diagnosis/treatment, 536
Hydrocephalus
   congenital toxoplasmosis, 438
   fungal meningitis, 307
   mechanisms and disease diagnosis/treatment, 423
   neural tube defects, 380, 423
   tuberculosis, 308

Hydrochloride, 213, 652
Hydrocortisone
	adrenal insufficiency, 96
	carpal tunnel syndrome, 289
	congenital adrenal hyperplasia, 99
	hirsutism, 98
	hypothyroidism, 90
	ulcerative colitis, 134
	underproduction syndromes (pituitary gland), 94
Hydronephrosis, 427
	leiomyomata uteri, 342
	ureteropelvic junction obstruction, 541
Hydrophobia, 306
Hydrops fetalis, 431
Hydroxychloroquine, 282, 508
5-Hydroxyindoleacetic acid, 519
3-Hydroxy-3-methylglutaryl coenzyme A, 33
17-Hydroxypregnenolone, 97
17-Hydroxyprogesterone, 97
Hydroxyproline, 289
17-Hydroxysteroids, 97
Hydroxyurea
	chronic myelogenous leukemia, 180
	essential thrombocythemia, 193
	hypereosinophilic syndrome, 212
	sickle cell anemia, 177
Hydroxyzine, 62, 204, 207, 209
Hygiene
	acute enteric infections, 122
	bronchiolitis, 434
	conjunctivitis, 395
	impetigo, 50
	pruritus ani, 63
Hymenoptera, 238
Hyperactivity
	attention-deficit hyperactivity disorder, 472–474
	fragile X syndrome, 446
	stimulants, 229
Hyperaldosteronism, 30
Hyperamylasemia, 138
Hyperandrogenism, 352
Hyperbaric oxygen, 231
Hyperbilirubinemia, 145, 150, 160
Hyperbilirubinemia, neonatal
	mechanisms and disease diagnosis/treatment, 432

Hypercalcemia
	bronchogenic carcinoma, 519
	mechanisms and disease diagnosis/treatment, 91–92, 557
	multiple myeloma, 184
	renal cell carcinoma, 544
Hypercapnia
	croup, 436
	epiglottitis, 435
	respiratory distress syndrome, 431
Hyperchloremic acidosis, 554
Hypercholesterolemia, 318
Hypercoagulable states, 36, 37, 322
Hyperemesis gravidarum
	mechanisms and disease diagnosis/treatment, 384–385
Hyperemia, 434
Hypereosinophilic syndrome
	mechanisms and disease diagnosis/treatment, 211–212
Hypergastinemia, 115
Hyperglycemia
	acute pancreatitis, 159
	hyperosmolar hyperglycemic nonketotic coma, 104
	metabolic encephalopathy, 315
Hyperkalemia
	chronic renal failure, 547
	mechanisms and disease diagnosis/treatment, 554–555
Hyperkinesis, 89
Hyperlipidemia, 549
Hyperlipoproteinemia
	mechanisms and disease diagnosis/treatment, 32–33
Hyperlipoproteinemia, type II
	mechanisms and disease diagnosis/treatment, 100
Hyperlipoproteinemia, type IV
	mechanisms and disease diagnosis/treatment, 100–101
Hyperlipoproteinemia, type V
	mechanisms and disease diagnosis/treatment, 101, 101f
Hypermetabolism, 89

Hypernatremia
	diabetes insipidus, 94
	mechanisms and disease diagnosis/treatment, 554
Hypernephroma, 327
Hyperosmolar hyperglycemic nonketotic coma (HHNK)
	diabetes mellitus, 104
	mechanisms and disease diagnosis/treatment, 104
Hyperparathyroidism
	hypercalcemia, 92, 557
	pheochromocytoma, 98
	surgical principles, 572–573
Hyperperistalsis, 137
Hyperpigmentation, 77
	adrenal insufficiency, 95
	contact dermatitis, 208
	Cushing's syndrome, 96
	porphyria cutanea tarda, 83
Hyperplasia
	benign prostatic
		mechanisms and disease diagnosis/treatment, 542
	myasthenia gravis, 312
Hyperplastic arteriolitis, 553
Hyperpnea, 554
Hyperprolactinemia, 352
Hyperpyrexia, 435
Hyperreflexia, 331, 333
Hypersensitivity
	anaphylaxis, 203
	angitis, 36
	contact dermatitis, 56, 208
	hirsutism, 97
	pneumonitis, 210–211
		mechanisms and disease diagnosis/treatment, 210–211, 511
	urticaria, 57
Hypersomnia, 461
Hypertension
	abdominal aortic aneurysm, 164
	acute renal failure, 546
	alcohol, 478, 479
	anorectal abscess, 143
	atherosclerosis, 34
	atrial septal defect, 26
	cardiac transplantation, 25
	chronic renal failure, 547
	cirrhosis, 156
	coarctation of the aorta, 28
	cocaine, 230

Hypertension *(continued)*
   congenital adrenal hyperplasia, 98
   cor pulmonale, 518
   diabetic nephropathy, 550
   endometrial cancer, 341
   epistaxis, 217
   essential, 29–30
   glomerulonephritis, 549
   hemolytic uremic syndrome, 440
   hydrocephalus, 423
   hyperthyroidism, 88
   hypertrophic cardiomyopathy, 15
   infantile polycystic disease, 428
   intracerebral hemorrhage, 321
   ischemic bowel disease, 137
   ischemic thrombotic strokes, 318
   malignant, 31
   meconium aspiration, 431
   nephrosclerosis, 552, 553
   obstructive shock, 12
   panic disorder, 463
   papilledema, 402
   pheochromocytoma, 98
   polycystic kidney disease, 552
   polycythemia rubra vera, 185
   preeclampsia, 374
   pulmonary embolism, 38
   pyelonephritis, 546
   renovascular
      mechanisms and disease diagnosis/treatment, 551
   right-sided heart failure, 9
   secondary, 30–31
   sick sinus syndrome, 16
   stimulants, 229
   subarachnoid hemorrhage, 322
   tricyclic antidepressants, 228
   vesicoureteral reflux, 538
Hyperthermia
   acute pancreatitis, 159
   cocaine, 230
   glioblastoma, 326
   stimulants, 229
Hyperthyroidism
   gestational trophoblastic disease, 382
   left-sided high output heart failure, 9
   mechanisms and disease diagnosis/treatment, 88–89, 88*f*
   secondary hypertension, 30
   stable angina pectoris, 7
Hyperthyrosis, 557
Hypertriglyceridemia, 100, 101, 160
Hypertrophic cardiomyopathy
   mechanisms and disease diagnosis/treatment, 14–15
Hypertrophy
   essential hypertension, 30
   right-sided heart failure, 9
   stable angina pectoris, 6
   tetralogy of fallot, 27
Hyperuricemia, 179
Hyphema, 220
Hypnotherapy, 128, 471
Hypoactive sexual desire disorder, 484
Hypoadrenalism, 49
Hypoalbuminemia, 159, 549
Hypocalcemia
   acute pancreatitis, 159
   gastric motility, disorders of, 118
   hypomagnesemia, 557
   mechanisms and disease diagnosis/treatment, 558
Hypochloremic hypokalemic metabolic alkalosis, 441
Hypochondriasis
   mechanisms and disease diagnosis/treatment, 471–472
Hypogammaglobulinemia, 180, 204
Hypoglycemia
   delirium, 485
   mechanisms and disease diagnosis/treatment, 105
   metabolic encephalopathy, 315
   panic disorder, 463
Hypogonadism, 92
Hypokalemia
   Cushing's syndrome, 97
   gastric motility, disorders of, 118
   hypomagnesemia, 557
   mechanisms and disease diagnosis/treatment, 554
   metabolic alkalosis, 555
   secondary hypertension, 30
Hypokinesis, 9
Hypomagnesemia
   mechanisms and disease diagnosis/treatment, 557
Hyponatremia
   mechanisms and disease diagnosis/treatment, 95, 553
Hypoparathyroidism, 49, 558
Hypophosphatemia, 281
Hypoproteinemia, 161
Hypopyon, 411
Hypospadias
   cryptorchidism, 534
   intersex, 535
   mechanisms and disease diagnosis/treatment, 426, 538
Hyposthenuria, 176
Hypotension
   acute pancreatitis, 159
   adrenal insufficiency, 95
   anaphylactic shock, 239
   anorexia, 474, 475
   aortic dissection, 41
   cardiac tamponade, 21
   congenital adrenal hyperplasia, 98, 99
   constrictive pericarditis, 22
   diethyl-m-toluamide, 232
   dilated cardiomyopathy, 13
   drug allergy, 213
   hypernatremia, 554
   hypothermia, 240
   insect and snake bites, 238
   lacerations, 225
   pheochromocytoma, 98
   pneumothorax, 222
   postpartum hemorrhage, 386
   sedatives, 229
   transfusion reactions, 187
   tricyclic antidepressants, 228
   underproduction syndromes (pituitary gland), 94
Hypotension and acute circulatory collapse (shock)
   cardiogenic shock, 10–11
   distributive shock, 12–13
   hypovolemic shock, 11–12
   obstructive shock, 12
Hypothalamus and thiamine deficiency, 314
Hypothermia
   acute pancreatitis, 159
   anorexia, 474, 475

hypothyroidism, 89
    mechanisms and disease
        diagnosis/treatment,
        240–241
    opioids, 324
Hypothyroidism
    amenorrhea, 352
    candidiasis, cutaneous, 49
    carpal tunnel syndrome, 311
    dysbetalipoproteinemia, type III,
        100
    frozen shoulder syndrome, 288
    gastric motility, disorders of, 118
    mechanisms and disease
        diagnosis/treatment,
        89–90, 90f
    syndrome of inappropriate
        antidiuretic hormone
        secretion, 95
    underproduction syndromes
        (pituitary gland), 94
Hypotonia, 335
Hypovolemia
    acute renal failure, 547
    anaphylaxis, 202
    peritonitis, 140
Hypovolemic shock
    mechanisms and disease
        diagnosis/treatment,
        11–12
Hypoxemia
    acute respiratory distress
        syndrome, 514
    allergic bronchopulmonary
        aspergillosis, 209, 210
    anaphylaxis, 202
    croup, 493
    *Pneumocystis carinii* pneumonia,
        252
    pulmonary embolism, 38
    respiratory alkalosis, 556
Hypoxia
    croup, 436
    delirium, 485
    drowning, 238
    epiglottitis, 435
    metabolic encephalopathy, 315
    respiratory distress syndrome, 431
    usual interstitial pneumonitis, 509
Hysterectomy
    cervical dysplasia and
        management of abnormal
        Pap smear, 347
    endometrial cancer, 341

leiomyomata uteri, 342
ovarian cancer, 344
pelvic relaxation/urinary
    incontinence, 351
postpartum hemorrhage, 386
stress-related urinary
    incontinence, 540
Hysterosalpingogram, 356
Hysteroscopy, 341

## I

Idiopathic restrictive pulmonary
    diseases
    desquamative interstitial
        pneumonitis, 509
    usual interstitial pneumonitis,
        508–509
Idiopathic thrombocytopenic
    purpura (ITP)
    HIV (human immunodeficiency
        virus), 249
    mechanisms and disease
        diagnosis/treatment, 192
Ileal disease, 145
Ileal pouch-anal anastomosis, 135
Ileitis, 133
Ilium, fracture of, 224
Ill-defined symptom complex
    circulatory system
        murmurs, 622–623
        palpitations, 622
    presentations, ill-defined
        abdominal pain, 637–638
        ascites, 641–642
        chest pain, 632–633
        diarrhea, 634–635
        dizziness, 629–630
        dyspepsia, 636–637
        dysphagia, 639–640
        gastrointestinal hemorrhage,
            633–634
        jaundice, 640–641
        lymphadenitis, 629
        lymph nodes, enlarged,
            631–632
        malaise and fatigue, 630–631
        nausea and vomiting, 638–639
        Reye's syndrome, 635–636
        septic shock, 631
        weight loss, 642–643
    pulmonary medicine
        chest pain, 521–522
        cough, 520–521, 624–625

        dyspnea, 521, 623–624
        hemoptysis, 522, 625–626
        sleep apnea, 523–524
        solitary pulmonary nodule,
            523
        stridor, 624
        wheezing and stridor, 522–523
    renal and urinary system
        colic, renal, 626
        dysuria, 626–627
        oliguria and anuria, 627–628
        proteinuria, 628–629
Imidazole, 49
Imipenem, 139
Imipramine, 335
Immobilization
    congenital hip disorders, 277
    decubitus ulcer, 568
    leg/foot fractures, 297
    osteomyelitis, 271
    pulmonary embolism, 516
Immotile-cilia syndrome, 507
Immunemediated hemolytic
    reaction, 187
Immune modulation, 251
Immunization. *See* Vaccines
Immunofluorescence, 308. *See also*
    mechanisms and disease
    diagnosis/treatment *and*
    surgical principles *under*
    *specific disease/disorder*
Immunoglobulins (IGs)
    A
        ataxia-telangiectasia, 85
        celiac sprue, 124, 125
        dermatitis herpetiformis, 60
        Henoch-Schöenlein purpura,
            425
        humoral immunodeficiency,
            204
        hypersensitivity pneumonitis,
            211
        nephrotic syndrome, 549
        transfusion reactions, 187
    amyloidosis, 81
    bronchiectasis, 507
    E
        allergic bronchopulmonary
            aspergillosis, 209, 210
        allergic rhinitis, 201
        atopic dermatitis, 56, 206, 207
        bronchial asthma, 198
        drug allergy, 213
        urticaria, 203

Immunoglobulins (IGs) *(continued)*
G
allergic bronchopulmonary aspergillosis, 209
autoimmune hepatitis, 147
bullous pemphigoid, 59
celiac sprue, 125
hemolytic anemia, 175
HIV (human immunodeficiency virus), 303
hypersensitivity pneumonitis, 211
idiopathic thrombocytopenic purpura, 192
multiple sclerosis, 331
Rh incompatibility or isoimmunization, 381
lupus inhibitor, 190
M
Henoch-Schöenlein purpura, 425
hepatitis, 146
mononucleosis, 264
neurosyphilis, 310
Immunology and allergy
acute enteric infections, 122, 123
acute otitis media, 648
acute sinusitis, 662
allergic bronchopulmonary aspergillosis, 209–210
allergic rhinitis and conjunctivitis, 200–202
anaphylaxis/anaphylactoid reactions, 202–203
aspergillosis, invasive, 502
atopic dermatitis, 206–208
bronchial asthma, 198–200
bronchiolitis, 434
cardiac transplantation, 25
coal workers' pneumoconiosis, 511
conjunctivitis, 393, 394
contact dermatitis, 208–209
cryptococcal infection, 502
dermatophytosis, 47–48
diverticulitis, 139
drug allergy, 212–213
erythema nodosum, 62
fungal sinusitis, 663
hereditary angioedema, 205–206
herpes simplex virus, 52, 258
Hodgkin's disease, 181
hypereosinophilic syndrome, 211–212
hypersensitivity pneumonitis, 210–211
immunodeficiency
cellular (T-cell) immunodeficiency, 205
humoral immunodeficiency, 204
Legionnaire's disease, 497
ophthalmology
herpes simplex keratitis, 411
ophthalmic herpes zoster, 412
otitis media, 434
pneumococcal pneumonia, 495
*Pneumocystis carinii* pneumonia, 498
psoriasis, 54
pyoderma gangrenosum, 79
scabies, 64
squamous cell carcinoma, 70
thrush, oral, 658
tubulointerstitial disease, 548
urticaria, 203–204
varicella (chickenpox), 46, 265
vasculitis syndromes, 36
verrucae, 51
vulva/vagina, candidiasis of the, 349
Immunomodulators, 205, 208, 439
Immunotherapy, 199, 202
Imperforate anus
surgical principles, 609
Impetigo
mechanisms and disease diagnosis/treatment, 50, 50*f*
Impotence
aortic occlusion, 41
erectile, 537–538
Peyronie's disease, 537
prostate cancer, 576
sleep apnea, 334
Impulsivity and bipolar disorders, 461
Incisional hernia, 618
Incontinence
bowel
seizures, 315
mechanisms and disease diagnosis/treatment
reproduction, male/female, 350–351
stress-related, 540
urinary
neurosyphilis, 310
seizures, 315
Incoordination. *See also* Gait problems
acute otitis media, 648
alcohol, 230, 479
carbon monoxide, 231
intoeing, 278
PCP (phencyclidine), 230
India ink exam, 257, 307, 502
Indinavir, 75, 250, 252
Indirect immunofluorescence, 59
Indocin, 280
Indomethacin, 280, 376
Indonesia antibody (EMA), 125
Induced abortion
mechanisms and disease diagnosis/treatment, 372
INF-alpha2b, 72
Infancy and childhood. *See also* Newborns; Pediatrics
abuse, child, 240
acute enteric infections, 122
acute otitis media, 648
allergic rhinitis, 200
aspiration, 226
atopic dermatitis, 206
cellular (T-cell) immunodeficiency, 205
cradle cap, 54
cystic fibrosis, 161, 669
delirium, 485
*Haemophilus influenzae* pneumonia, 496
hereditary angioedema, 205
humoral immunodeficiency, 204
Huntington's disease, 329
idiopathic thrombocytopenic purpura, 192
intoeing, 278–279
Legg-Calvé-Perthes disease, 277–278
medial or lateral epicondyle fractures, 235
orocavity, herpes simplex of the, 657
osteomyelitis, 271
pneumococcal pneumonia, 495
posttraumatic stress disorder, 465
psychoses originating in childhood
autistic disorder, 458
mood disorders, 459
schizophrenia, 458

ulna, fracture of the, 235
vesicoureteral reflux, 538
Wilms' tumor, 544
Infantile botulism
  mechanisms and disease diagnosis/treatment, 421–422
Infantile polycystic disease
  mechanisms and disease diagnosis/treatment, 428
Infectious disease
  central nervous system
    abscesses, 308–309
    meningitis, 306–308
    spirochetes, 309–310
    viruses, 303–306
  dermatology
    bacterial, 49–50
    mycoses, 47–49
    secondary syphilis, 52–53
    viral, 51–52
  HIV/AIDS
    cryptococcal infection, 257–258
    cytomegalovirus, 253–254
    disseminated *Mycobacterium avium-intracellulare* complex, 255–256
    herpes simplex virus, 258
    HIV (human immunodeficiency virus), 248–252
    *Pneumocystis carinii* pneumonia, 252–253
    toxoplasma encephalitis, 256–257
    tuberculosis, 254–255
  joints, 299
  musculoskeletal/connective tissue disease
    gonococcal tenosynovitis, 272–273
    Lyme disease, 272
    osteomyelitis, 271
    septic arthritis, 271–272
  other diseases
    Lyme disease, 267–268
    measles (rubeola), 265–266
    mononucleosis, 264
    mumps, 266
    rubella (German measles), 266–267
    varicella (chickenpox), 265
  otitis externa, 647
  pediatrics
    bronchiolitis, 434
    congenital infections, 437–439
    epiglottitis, 435
    hemolytic uremic syndrome, 439
    laryngotracheitis, 435–436
    meningitis, bacterial, 437
    otitis media, 434–435
    pharyngitis, 436–437
    varicella (chickenpox), 436
  pulmonary medicine
    acute bronchiolitis, 494
    acute bronchitis, 494
    acute epiglottitis, 493
    bacterial bronchopneumonia, 495–497
    croup, 493
    fungal pneumonias, 500–503
    pertussis, 494–495
    pneumonias, atypical, 497–499
    tuberculosis, pulmonary, 499, 500$t$
  renal and urinary system
    chlamydia, 532–533
    epididymitis, 530–531
    gonorrhea, 532
    herpes, 533
    HIV (human immunodeficiency virus), 533
    orchitis, 531
    prostatitis, 530
    syphilis, 532
    urethral syndromes and painful bladder, 529–530
    urethritis, 531
    urinary tract infections, 529
  sexually transmitted diseases
    chancroid, 262
    chlamydia, 260
    epididymoorchitis, 263
    genital herpes, 263–264
    gonorrhea, 259–260
    pelvic inflammatory disease, 262–263
    syphilis, 260–262
  surgical principles for postoperative
    atelectasis and pneumonia, 583–584
    urinary tract infections, 583
    wounds, 582–583
Infertility
  chlamydia, 260
  cystic fibrosis, 507
  ectopic pregnancy, 370
  endometriosis, 343
  hypothyroidism, 89
  leiomyomata uteri, 341
  mechanisms and disease diagnosis/treatment, 356–358, 357$f$
  renal and urinary system, 535–536
  overproduction syndromes (pituitary gland), 92
  undescended testis, 428
Inflammatory bowel disease (IBD)
  anorectal abscess, 143
  Crohn's disease, 135, 136$f$, 137
  ulcerative colitis, 133–135, 133$f$
Inflammatory conditions. *See also* Infectious disease
  chalazion, 397
  musculoskeletal/connective tissue disease
    ankylosing spondylitis, 283–284, 300
    lupus arthritis, 281–282, 300
    polymyalgia rheumatica, 281, 300
    polymyositis-dermatomyositis, 282–283, 300
    rheumatoid arthritis, 283, 300
  ophthalmology
    papillitis, 402, 404
  skin
    atopic dermatitis, 56
    contact dermatitis, 55–56
    drug reactions, 58
    eczematous dermatitis, 56–57
    psoriasis, 53–54
    seborrheic dermatitis, 54–55
    urticaria, 57–58
Influenza pneumonia
  mechanisms and disease diagnosis/treatment, 498–499
Infrainguinal aneurysmal disease
  surgical principles, 592–593
Ingrowing nails
  mechanisms and disease diagnosis/treatment, 66–67
Inguinal hernia
  surgical principles, 617

Inhalants
    dependence, drug, 483
    substance-related disorders, 478
Inhibited personality disorders, 468
Injuries/wounds/accidents, 213.
        *See also* Trauma
    additional management information
        child abuse, 240
        sexual abuse/assault, 240
        shock, 239
        thermal injuries, 240–241
        traumatic injury, 239
    alcohol, 478
    anaphylactic shock, 239
    burns
        electrical, 227–228
        thermal, 227
    chest and abdominal injury
        additional information, 223
        epidemiology and prevention of chest/abdominal injury, 224
        flail chest, 223
        hemothorax, 222
        pelvic fractures, 224
        perforation of viscus, 223–224
        pneumothorax, 222
        rib cage, 221
    child physical/sexual abuse, 486
    cranial injury
        auditory injury, 220–221
        concussion, 219
        epidemiology and prevention of ocular/auditory injury, 221
        epidural hematoma, 219–220
        facial fracture, 217–218
        ocular injury, 220
        skull trauma or fracture, 218
        subdural hematoma, 219
    drowning, 237–238
    epidemiology/prevention of selected accidents
        abuse, child/spouse/elderly, 243
        athletic accidents, 242
        automobile accidents and drunk driving, 242
        drowning, 242
        falls, 244
        fire prevention, 244
        gunshot and stab wounds, 243
        head and spinal cord injury with whiplash, 242
        home accidents, 241
        ingestion of poisonous/toxic agents, 243
        sexual abuse and rape, 244
        thermal injury, 243
        workplace accidents, 242
    epistaxis, 217
    factitious disorders, 472
    foreign bodies
        aspiration, 226
        eye/ear/nose, 225–226
        swallowed, 226–227
    fractures
        extremities, 233–235
        vertebral column, 233
    insect and snake bites, 238–239
    lacerations, 225
    poisoning
        acetaminophen, 228
        additional information, 232
        alcohol, 230
        carbon monoxide, 231
        cocaine, 230
        diethyl-m-toluamide, 232
        heavy metals and arsenic, 231
        PCP (phencyclidine), 230
        sedatives, 229
        solvent sniffing, 231
        stimulants, 229
        tricyclic antidepressants, 228–229
    sprains and dislocations
        ankle, 237
        elbow, 236
        hands, 236–237
        shoulder, 236
    surgical principles
        abdominal injury, 580–582
        cranial injury, 580
        multiple injuries, 578–580
Innominate bone, 224
Insect/ectoparasite bites
    anaphylaxis, 203
    fleas, 66
    mechanisms and disease diagnosis/treatment, 238–239
    mosquitoes and flies, 65–66
    pediculosis, 65
    scabies, 63–64
Insomnia, 353
Insulin. *See also* Diabetes mellitus
    diabetes, gestational, 388
    hyperosmolar hyperglycemic nonketotic coma, 104
    hypoglycemia, 105
    underproduction syndromes (pituitary gland), 94
Intal, 199
Interferon
    atopic dermatitis, 208
    hepatitis, 150–152$t$
    hypereosinophilic syndrome, 212
    multiple sclerosis, 332
Interleukin, 544
Intermediate-density lipoproteins (IDls), 100
International Federation of Gynecology and Obstetrics (FIGO), 341
International Normalized Ratio (INR), 321
Internuclear ophthalmoplegia, 331
Intersex
    mechanisms and disease diagnosis/treatment, 534–535
Interstitial keratitis
    mechanisms and disease diagnosis/treatment, 413–414
Intestinal obstruction
    mechanisms and disease diagnosis/treatment, 138
Intoeing
    mechanisms and disease diagnosis/treatment, 278–279
Intra-aortic balloon counterpulsation (IABP), 4, 24
Intracerebral hemorrhage
    mechanisms and disease diagnosis/treatment, 321
Intracranial pressure (ICP)
    papilledema, 402
    subarachnoid hemorrhage, 322
    tuberculosis, 308
    venous thrombosis, 322
Intraocular pressure, 415–416, 424
Intrathoracic hiatal hernia, 111
Intrauterine growth retardation (IUGR)
    congenital cytomegalovirus, 439
    congenital rubella infection, 439

diabetes, overt, 389
multiple gestation, 381
trisomy 18, 445
Intravenous immunoglobulin (IVIG)
   Guillain-Barré syndrome, 312
   humoral immunodeficiency, 204
   Kawasaki disease, 426
Intravenous pyelogram (IVP), 342
Intrinsic factor, 173
Intussusception
   Henoch-Schöenlein purpura, 425
   mechanisms and disease diagnosis/treatment, 442–443, 442*f*
Invalidism, 470
Invirase, 250
In vitro fertilization (IVF), 358
Involucrum, 271
Iodine, 89
Ipecac, 228
Ipratropium bromide, 199, 506
IQ, 458, 473
Iridectomy, 416
Iridocyclitis, 393
Iritis, 52
Iron
   celiac sprue, 125
   chronic renal failure, 174
   gastroesophageal reflux disease, 110
   multiple gestation, 382
   poisoning and mechanisms and disease diagnosis/treatment, 232
   polycythemia rubra vera, 185
   porphyria cutanea tarda, 83
   squamous cell carcinoma, 109
Iron-deficiency anemia, 109
   mechanisms and disease diagnosis/treatment, 169
Irritability. *See* Anxiety
Irritable bowel syndrome (IBS)
   mechanisms and disease diagnosis/treatment, 126–128, 127*t*
   panic disorder, 463
Ischemia
   acute mesenteric, 600–601, 601*f*
   arterial ulcer, 570
   decubitus ulcer, 77, 568
   sickle cell anemia, 176
   stasis ulceration, 77
   thrombotic thrombocytopenic purpura, 192, 193
   ulcerative colitis, 134
   urethral stricture, benign, 537
Ischemic bowel disease
   mechanisms and disease diagnosis/treatment, 137
Ischemic heart disease
   acute
      myocardial infarction, 4–6
      unstable angina, 3–4
   chronic
      silent ischemia, 7
      stable angina pectoris, 6–7
   mechanisms and disease diagnosis/treatment, 23
   ventricular tachycardia, 19
Ischemic thrombotic strokes
   mechanisms and disease diagnosis/treatment, 318–319, 319*f*, 320*f*
Isoniazid (INH)
   hepatotoxins, 149
   multiple sclerosis, 332
   pulmonary tuberculosis, 499
   tuberculosis, 255, 308
Isoproterenol, 463
Isotretinoin, 68, 75
Itching. *See also* Pruritus
   allergic rhinitis, 200
   atopic dermatitis, 56
   blepharitis, 396
   conjunctivitis, 393
   dermatitis herpetiformis, 60
   drug reactions causing skin changes, 58
   dry-eye syndrome, 400
   eczema, 56
   pruritus, 63
   pruritus ani, 63
   scabies, 64
   vulva/vagina, candidiasis of the, 349
Itraconazole
   allergic bronchopulmonary aspergillosis, 210
   blastomycosis, 501
   candidiasis, cutaneous, 49
   coccidioidomycosis, 502
   cryptococcal infection, 502
   dermatophytosis, 48
   fungal meningitis, 307
   gastric motility, disorders of, 118
   histoplasmosis, 501
Ivermectin, 64

## J

Jarisch-Herxheimer reaction, 310
Jaundice. *See also* mechanisms and disease diagnosis/treatment *and* surgical principles *under specific disease/disorder*
   acetaminophen, 228
   choledocholithiasis, 145
   congenital cytomegalovirus, 439
   congenital syphilis, 438
   hepatitis, 146, 147, 377, 378
   hepatocellular carcinoma, 153
   ill-defined presentations, 640–641
   neonatal hyperbilirubinemia, 432
   pancreatic carcinoma, 157
   pregnancy, 377, 378
Jealous delusions, 456
Jerks, myoclonic, 305, 310
Jewett-Whitmore staging, 542
Joints. *See also* Arthralgias
   degenerative disease, 273–274
   dislocations and separations, 297–298
   effusion of joint
      mechanisms and disease diagnosis/treatment, 290–291
   infections, 299
Jugular venous distention (JVD)
   cardiac tamponade, 21
   constrictive pericarditis, 22
   dilated cardiomyopathy, 13
   myocardial infarction, 4
   right-sided heart failure, 9

## K

Kaletra, 250
Kaposi's sarcoma, 115
Kaposi's varicelliform eruption, 56
Kasabach-Merritt syndrome, 74
Kawasaki disease
   mechanisms and disease diagnosis/treatment, 425–426
Kegel exercises, 351
Kell-positive transfusion, 380
Keratinocytes, 75
Keratitis, 67, 413–414
Keratoconjunctivitis, 52

Keratoconjunctivitis sicca
  mechanisms and disease
      diagnosis/treatment, 413
Keratoderma, 76–77
Keratolytics, 54
Kerley's B lines, 514
Kernicterus, 431
Kernig's sign, 437
Ketoacidosis, 557
Ketoconazole
  blastomycosis, 501
  coccidioidomycosis, 502
  Cushing's syndrome, 97
  gastric motility, disorders of, 118
  histoplasmosis, 501
  seborrheic dermatitis, 55
Ketonemia, 384
Ketoneuria, 102
Ketosis, 102, 103
Kidneys. See Genitourinary system; Renal and urinary system
Kiesselbach's plexus, 217, 665, 666
Kimmelstiel-Wilson lesions, 550
*Klebsiella*, 146
*Klebsiella pneumoniae*, 497
Kleihauer-Betke test, 365
Knee
  chondromalacia patellae, 450
  osteochondritis dissecans, 449
Koebner's phenomenon, 53
Koplik's spots, 265
Korsakoff's syndrome, 314, 480
Krukenberg tumors, 114
Kussmaul's sign, 15, 22, 103
Kyphosis
  mechanisms and disease
      diagnosis/treatment, 449

## L

Labetolol, 31
Labor and delivery
  mechanisms and disease
      diagnosis/treatment
      abnormal, 385–386, 385*t*
      normal, 368–369, 369*f*
Labyrinthectomy, 652
Lacerations
  mechanisms and disease
      diagnosis/treatment, 225
Lac-Hydrin, 207
Lacrimal gland, 146
Lacrimal system, disorders of the
  acute dacryocystitis, 400–401
  undersecretion, 400

Lactate
  cardiogenic shock, 10
  distributive shock, 13
  panic disorder, 463
Lactate dehydrogenase (LDH), 138
  acute lymphocytic leukemia, 179
  folic acid deficiency, 170
  hemolytic anemia, 175
  intermediate/high-grade lymphoma, 183, 184
  low-grade lymphoma, 182
  myocardial infarction, 4
  pleural effusions, 512
  *Pneumocystis carinii* pneumonia, 498
  preeclampsia, 375
  thalassemia-alpha, 171
  thrombotic thrombocytopenic purpura, 192, 193
  vitamin $B_{12}$ deficiency, 172
Lactation
  mechanisms and disease
      diagnosis/treatment, 368
Lactic dehydrogenase, 282
Lactose and celiac sprue, 125
Lamellar mosaic bone pattern, 290
Laminectomy, 290, 292
Lamivudine, 150
Lamotrigine, 316, 317, 333
Langhans' giant cells, 397
Lanugo hair, 474
Laparoscopy
  dysmenorrhea, 351
  ectopic pregnancy, 370
  endometriosis, 343, 343*f*
  esophageal neoplasms, 109
  infertility, 358
  leiomyomata uteri, 342
  ovarian cancer, 344
  pelvic inflammatory disease, 262, 358
Laparotomy
  diverticulitis, 139
  endometriosis, 343
  familial Mediterranean fever, 141
  Hodgkin's disease, 181
  leiomyomata uteri, 342
  ovarian cancer, 344
  ovarian cysts, 345
  pelvic inflammatory disease, 359
  small-bowel obstruction, 602
  viscus, perforation of, 223

Large-bowel obstruction
  surgical principles, 603
Large cell carcinoma, 519
Laryngomalacia
  mechanisms and disease
      diagnosis/treatment, 446
Laryngoscopy. See also mechanisms and disease diagnosis/treatment *and* surgical principles *under specific disease/disorder*
  hoarseness, 660
  larynx, cancer of the, 661
  oropharynx, malignant neoplasms of the, 659
  otalgia, 653
  swallowing (injury/accidents), 226
Laryngotracheitis
  mechanisms and disease
      diagnosis/treatment, 435–436
Larynx, cancer of the
  mechanisms and disease
      diagnosis/treatment, 661
Laser photocoagulation, 410
Laser trabecular burns, 416
Latanoprost, 416
Laxatives, 140
Lead and toxic disorders, 323
Lead-poisoning anemia
  mechanisms and disease
      diagnosis/treatment, 174
Learning disabilities/disorders
  attention-deficit hyperactivity disorder, 473
  bacterial meningitis, 437
  congenital deafness, 424
Leflunomide, 283
Left-sided heart failure
  mechanisms and disease
      diagnosis/treatment
      high output, 9
      low output, 8–9
Left ventricular hypertrophy (LVH), 14
Left ventricular hypokinesis, 321
Leg fractures
  mechanisms and disease
      diagnosis/treatment, 296–297
Legg-Calvé-Perthes disease
  mechanisms and disease
      diagnosis/treatment, 277–278

*Legionella*, 497
Legionnaire's disease
　mechanisms and disease
　　　diagnosis/treatment, 497
Leiomyomata uteri
　mechanisms and disease
　　　diagnosis/treatment,
　　　341–342, 342f
Lenegre's degenerative disease, 17, 18
Lens, disorders of the
　cataract, 417–418, 418t
　glaucoma, 414–416, 415f
Leprosy, 414
Leptospirosis, 306
Leriche's syndrome, 41
Leser-Trelat, sign of, 75
Lethargy. *See* Fatigue
Leucovorin
　*Pneumocystis carinii* pneumonia, 252
Leukemia
　acute lymphocytic, 178–179
　acute myelogenous, 177–178
　chronic lymphocytic, 180–181
　chronic myelogenous, 179–180
　pyoderma gangrenosum, 79
　Sweet's syndrome, 84
Leukocyte alkaline phosphatase (LAP), 179
Leukocytes, 126, 271
Leukocytoclastic vasculitis, 517
Leukocytosis
　acute cholecystitis, 144
　anorexia, 475
　choledocholithiasis, 145
　chronic lymphocytic leukemia, 180
　diverticulitis, 138
　Henoch-Schöenlein purpura, 425
　intestinal obstruction, 138
　ischemic bowel disease, 137
　peritonitis, 140
　premature rupture of membranes, 384
　sickle cell anemia, 176
Leukopenia, 255
Leukotrienes
　allergic rhinitis, 201
　bronchial asthma, 199, 200
　psoriasis, 54
　urticaria, 204
Levafloxin, 530, 531

Levetiracetam, 316
Levodopa, 324, 329
Lev's degenerative disease, 17
Lhermitte's signs, 333
Lice, 65, 65f
Lichen simplex chronicus, 63
Lidocaine
　basic cardiac life support, 29
　epistaxis, 217
　headaches, 318
　lacerations, 225
　ventricular tachycardia, 19
Lifestyle
　back pain, low, 274
　osteoporosis, 279
Life support, basic/advanced, 29
Ligamentum arteriosum, 28
Ligase chain reaction, 260
Limb salvage surgery, 286
Lindane, 64, 65
Linezolid, 496
Lipase, 159
Lipemia retinalis, 32
Lipids and acute pancreatitis, 160
Lipoma
　mechanisms and disease diagnosis/treatment, 72
　surgical principles, 564
Lipoprotein disorders, clinical
　chylomicronemia, type I familial, 99
　decreased high-density lipoprotein, 102
　dysbetalipoproteinemia, type III, 100
　elevated Lp (a) lipoprotein, 102
　hyperlipoproteinemia, type II, 100
　hyperlipoproteinemia, type IV, 100–101
　hyperlipoproteinemia, type V, 101
Lipoproteins, 32–33
Lisfranc's joint, 296, 297
*Listeria monocytogenes*, 437
Lithium
　affective psychoses: mania and psychotic depression, 455
　bipolar disorders, 462
　cyclothymia, 462
　depression, major (unipolar), 460
　hypercalcemia, 91
　psoriasis, 53
　schizoaffective disorder, 457

Lithotripsy, 539
Little's area, 665
Livedo reticularis
　mechanisms and disease diagnosis/treatment, 81
Liver. *See also Hepat* listings
　acetaminophen, 228
　alcohol, 479
　cancer
　　carcinoma, 153–155
　　metastasis, 614, 614f
　　primary hepatobiliary cancer, 613–614
　choledocholithiasis, 146
　cirrhosis, hepatic fibrosis and, 155–157, 156t
　cor pulmonale, 518
　disseminated *Mycobacterium avium-intracellulare* complex, 255
　epistaxis, 217
　gestational trophoblastic disease, 382
　hepatitis
　　alcoholic, 147
　　autoimmune, 147–148
　　chronic, 147
　　drug-induced hepatotoxicity, 147
　　history and physical keys, 146, 146t
　　mechanisms and disease diagnosis/treatment, 146–153, 147t–149t, 151t–152t
　　pregnancy, 377, 378
　　viral, 146–147, 147t
　Hodgkin's disease, 182
　hypoglycemia, 105
　ischemic heart disease, 23
　metabolic encephalopathy, 315
　peritonitis, 140
　preeclampsia, 375
　protein C deficiency, 191
　respiratory alkalosis, 556
　restrictive cardiomyopathy, 15
　surgical principles
　　adenoma, 612–613
　　cancer, 613–614, 614f
　　focal nodular hyperplasia, 613
　　metastasis, 614, 614f
　　primary hepatobiliary cancer, 613–614
　tuberculosis, 254

Liver function tests (LFTs). *See also* mechanisms and disease diagnosis/treatment *and* surgical principles *under specific disease/disorder*
    alcohol, 480
    bulimia, 476
    delirium, 486
    renal cell carcinoma, 544
    schizophrenia, 453
    sexual dysfunctions, 484
Lobar emphysema, congenital mechanisms and disease diagnosis/treatment, 446–447
Loop electrosurgical excision procedure (LEEP), 348
Looser's lines, 280
Loperamide, 635
Loperamine, 128
Lopinavir, 250
Lorazepam, 421
Low birth weight, 365
Low-density lipoproteins (LDL)
    diabetes mellitus, 104
    hyperlipoproteinemia, 32, 33
    hyperlipoproteinemia, type II, 100
    unstable angina, 4
Lower esophageal sphincter (LES)
    achalasia, 113
    gastroesophageal reflux disease, 111
    scleroderma, 113
Lumbar puncture (LP). *See also* mechanisms and disease diagnosis/treatment *and* surgical principles *under specific disease/disorder*
    acute lymphocytic leukemia, 179
    febrile seizures, 421
    headaches, 317
    hydrocephalus, 423
    intracerebral hemorrhage, 321
    multiple sclerosis, 331
    septic meningitis, 307
    subarachnoid hemorrhage, 322
    tuberculosis, 308
    venous thrombosis, 322
Lumbar spine
    mechanisms and disease diagnosis/treatment
        disk disease, 275–276
        injuries, 294
        spinal stenosis, 333
Lumpectomy, 354, 355
Lungs and adenocarcinoma, 287. *See also* Pulmonary *and* Respiratory *listings*
Lupus arthritis
    mechanisms and disease diagnosis/treatment, 281–282
    overview, 300
Lupus erythematous
    histiocytoma, 73
    mechanisms and disease diagnosis/treatment, 79–80
Lupus inhibitor
    mechanisms and disease diagnosis/treatment, 189–190
Lupus nephritis
    mechanisms and disease diagnosis/treatment, 553
Luteal-phase deficiency, 371
Luteinizing hormone (LH)
    amenorrhea, 352
    erectile impotence, 537
    infertility, 535
    sexual dysfunctions, 484
Luteinizing hormone-releasing hormone (LHRH), 578
Lyme disease
    aseptic meningitis, 306
    carpal tunnel syndrome, 311
    mechanisms and disease diagnosis/treatment
        infectious disease, 267–268
        musculoskeletal/connective tissue disease, 272
        neurology, 309
    multiple sclerosis, 331
    papillitis, 404
Lymphadenitis
    herpes simplex keratitis, 412
    ill-defined presentations, 629
Lymphadenopathy
    acute upper respiratory infection, 668
    agnogenic myeloid metaplasia, 193
    breast cancer, 354
    chronic lymphocytic leukemia, 180
    disseminated *Mycobacterium avium-intracellulare* complex, 255
    hepatitis, 146
    herpes simplex virus, 52, 258
    HIV (human immunodeficiency virus), 248, 438
    infectious otitis externa, 647
    intermediate/high-grade lymphoma, 183
    Kawasaki disease, 425
    low-grade lymphoma, 182
    mononucleosis, 264
    nasopharynx, masses in the, 659
    pruritus, 62
    secondary syphilis, 52
Lymphangiogram, 181
Lymphedema, 445
Lymph node dissection, 72
Lymph nodes, enlarged
    ill-defined presentations, 631–632
Lymphocytes
    chronic lymphocytic leukemia, 180, 181
    contact dermatitis, 208
    HIV (human immunodeficiency virus), 533
    pertussis, 495
    tuberculosis, 308
Lymphocytosis, 264
Lymphogranuloma venereum (LGV), 346, 347
Lymphokines, 205, 283
Lymphomas
    HIV (human immunodeficiency virus), 303
    Hodgkin's disease, 181–182
    mechanisms and disease diagnosis/treatment
        intermediate/high-grade, 183–184
        low-grade, 182–183, 183*f*
Lymphoproliferative disorder, 185

# M

Macroglobulemia, 185
Macroglossia, 81
Macrolide
    acute bronchitis, 494
    Legionnaire's disease, 497
    *Mycoplasma pneumoniae*, 498
    pertussis, 495

Macrophages, 208
Macular edema, 410
Magnesium
	eclampsia, 375, 376
	headache, 318
	postpartum hemorrhage, 386
	preeclampsia, 375, 551
Magnetic resonance angiography (MRA). *See also* mechanisms and disease diagnosis/treatment *and* surgical principles *under specific disease/disorder*
	carotid artery disease, 584
	ischemic thrombotic strokes, 319
	papilledema, 402
	papillitis, 403
Magnetic resonance cholangiopancreatography (MRCP), 145
Magnetic resonance imaging (MRI). *See also* mechanisms and disease diagnosis/treatment *and* surgical principles *under specific disease/disorder*
	abdominal aortic aneurysm, 164
	Alzheimer's disease, 327
	amyotrophic lateral sclerosis, 328
	aneurysms, 40
	autistic disorder, 458
	back pain, low, 274
	cardioembolic strokes, 320
	carpal tunnel syndrome, 311
	cervical spine, fractures of the, 293
	cervical spine and spinal stenosis, 333
	cirrhosis, 156
	constrictive pericarditis, 22
	contusions, 331
	croup, 493
	Cushing's syndrome, 97
	delirium, 486
	epidural hematoma, 330
	glioblastoma, 325
	headaches, 317
	hepatocellular carcinoma, 154
	HIV (human immunodeficiency virus), 303
	Huntington's disease, 329
	intracerebral hemorrhage, 321
	ischemic thrombotic strokes, 319
	lumbar disk disease, 275
	malignant otitis externa, 648
	meningioma, 326
	metastases, 287, 326
	multiple sclerosis, 331
	myasthenia gravis, 312
	nasopharynx, masses in the, 658–659
	neural tube defects, 422
	oropharynx, malignant neoplasms of the, 659
	osteomyelitis, 271
	osteosarcoma, 286
	otalgia, 653
	overproduction syndromes (pituitary gland), 93
	pancreatic carcinoma, 157
	papilledema, 402
	papillitis, 403
	prostate cancer, 542
	radiculopathy, 334
	renovascular hypertension, 551
	rotator cuff syndrome, 298
	sclerosis, 83
	seizures, 316
	subarachnoid hemorrhage, 322
	subdural hematoma, 330
	sudden hearing loss, 655
	toxoplasma encephalitis, 256
	trigeminal neuralgia, 316
	underproduction syndromes (pituitary gland), 94
	vertigo, 652
Malabsorption
	disseminated *Mycobacterium avium-intracellulare* complex, 255
	folic acid deficiency, 170
	hypocalcemia, 558
	hypoglycemia, 105
	rickets, 281
Malaise. *See* Fatigue
Malar erythema, 79
Malathion, 65
Male erectile disorder, 484
Malformations
	pediatrics
		cataracts, congenital, 424
		deafness, congenital, 424–425
		glaucoma, congenital, 423–424
		hydrocephalus, 423
	ischemic thrombotic strokes, 319
Malingering, 470, 472
Mallet finger, 236
Malnutrition
	amyotrophic lateral sclerosis, 328
	hypomagnesemia, 557
	prenatal care, 365
Malrotation of the small intestine
	mechanisms and disease diagnosis/treatment, 441–442
	surgical principles, 608
Mammography, 354–356, 571
Mandibular fracture, 217, 218
Manganese
	toxicity and mechanisms and disease diagnosis/treatment, 323–324
Mania
	mechanisms and disease diagnosis/treatment, 454–455
	schizoaffective disorder, 456
Mannitol, 324, 416
Manometry, 111, 113, 139
Marfan's syndrome, 590
Marfan syndrome, 41, 424
Marjolin's ulcer, 566
Masked depression, 459
Masklike face, 80
Mastalgia, 356
Mast cells
	anaphylactic shock, 239
	degranulators, 213
	mediator release, 199, 202
Mastectomy, 355, 571
Mastitis, 355, 368
Mastoid fracture, 218
Maternal mortality
	mechanisms and disease diagnosis/treatment, 383
Maternal serum alpha-fetoprotein (MSAFP), 365
Maxillary fracture, 217, 218
McArdle's disease, 313
McBurney's point, 132
Mean corpuscular hemoglobin (MCH), 169
Mean corpuscular volume (MCV)
	alcohol, 478
	hemolytic anemia, 175
	iron-deficiency anemia, 169
	thalassemia-beta, 172
	vitamin $B_{12}$ deficiency, 172

Measles (rubeola)
    mechanisms and disease
        diagnosis/treatment,
            265–266
Meat, undercooked, 438
Meat tenderizer and swallowing
        (injury/accidents), 227
Mechlorethamine, 182
Meckel's diverticulitis, 133
Meclizine, 652
Meconium aspiration
    mechanisms and disease
        diagnosis/treatment, 431
Meconium ileus, 162, 507
Median distribution, paresthesias
        in the, 288–289, 311
Medications. *See*
        Drugs/medications;
        *specific drug/class of drugs*
Medroxyprogesterone, 341
Mees' lines, 231
Megacolon, toxic, 126, 134
Megakaryocytes, 192, 193
Megaureter, 541
Meibomian gland, 397
Melanocytic nevus
    mechanisms and disease
        diagnosis/treatment,
            72–73
Melanoma
    dysplastic nevus, 73
    mechanisms and disease
        diagnosis/treatment,
            71–72
    melanocytic nevus, 73
    metastases, 327
    surgical principles, 567
Melena, 441
Melphalan, 81
Menarche, 341, 353
Ménière's disease, 652
Meningeal artery, 330
Meningioma
    mechanisms and disease
        diagnosis/treatment, 326
    optic atrophy, 404
Meningitis
    aseptic, 306
    bacterial
        mechanisms and disease
            diagnosis/treatment, 437
        cryptococcal infection, 502
        fungal, 307
        gonorrhea, 259

HIV (human immunodeficiency
        virus), 303
*Mycoplasma pneumoniae*, 498
pneumococcal pneumonia, 495
septic, 306–307
skull trauma/fracture, 218
sudden hearing loss, 656
tuberculosis, 308
venous thrombosis, 322
Meningocele, 422–423
Meningoencephalitis, 266, 309,
        439
Menopause
    autoimmune hepatitis, 147
    breast cancer, 353
    endometriosis, 343
    mechanisms and disease
        diagnosis/treatment, 353
    tylosis, 76
Menorrhagia
    acute myelogenous leukemia,
        177
    idiopathic thrombocytopenic
        purpura, 192
    platelet dysfunction, 194
    von Willebrand disease, 188
Menstrual disorders
    dysmenorrhea, 351
    ovarian cysts, 344
    premenstrual syndrome, 351–352
Menstruation
    blood-loss anemia, 169
    Cushing's syndrome, 96
    disorders of, 352
    endometriosis, 343
    hirsutism, 97
    hypothyroidism, 89
    iron-deficiency anemia, 169
    ovarian cysts, 345
Mental retardation. *See also*
        Developmental disorders
    fragile X syndrome, 446
    sclerosis, 82
Mental status changes
    aseptic meningitis, 306
    bacterial meningitis, 437
    bronchiolitis, 434
    croup, 436
    cryptococcal infection, 257
    epiglottitis, 435
    hydrocephalus, 423
    hyperthyroidism, 89
    hypoglycemia, 105
    hypothyroidism, 89, 90

intussusception, 442
lead-poisoning anemia, 174
multiple myeloma, 184
necrotizing enterocolitis, 443
thrombotic thrombocytopenic
        purpura, 192
toxoplasma encephalitis, 256
tricyclic antidepressants, 229
tuberculosis, 308
vitamin $B_{12}$ deficiency, 172, 313
Mental status exam
    affective psychoses: mania and
        psychotic depression, 454
    Alzheimer's disease, 327
    panic disorder, 463
    schizophrenia, 453
Meperidine, 213
Mercaptopurine, 137
Mercury
    mechanisms and disease
        diagnosis/treatment for
            poisoning from, 231
    teratology, 367
    toxic disorders, 323
Mesalamine, 134, 137
Mesenteric lymphadenitis, 133
Mesothelioma, 510
Metabolic disease/disturbances.
        *See also* Electrolytes
    acidosis
        hemolytic uremic syndrome,
            440
        hypothermia, 240
        intussusception, 442
        ischemic bowel disease, 137
        necrotizing enterocolitis, 443
    anorexia, 475
    congenital cataracts, 424
    mechanisms and disease
        diagnosis/treatment
            acidosis, 556
            alkalosis, 555–556
            encephalopathy, 315
            pyloric stenosis, 441
            respiratory distress syndrome, 430
            sudden hearing loss, 656
Metacarpal phalangeal (MCP)
        joint, 282
    sprain
        mechanisms and disease
            diagnosis/treatment,
                236–237
Metanephric blastema tissue, 544
Metanephrines, 98

Metastases
  mechanisms and disease diagnosis/treatment
    bone, 286–287
    neurology, 326–327
    pulmonary medicine, 520
Metatarsus adductus, 278
Metformin, 104
Methadone and substance-related disorders, 478
Methanol, 230
Methergine, 386
Methicillin, 213
Methimazole, 89
Methotrexate
  bladder carcinoma, 544
  ectopic pregnancy, 370
  lupus arthritis, 282
  polymyositis-dermatomyositis, 283
  psoriasis, 54
  rheumatoid arthritis, 283
  sarcoidosis, 508
Methyl alcohol poisoning, 232
Methylcellulose, 400
Methylergonine maleate, 386
Methyliodobenzyl-guanidine imaging, 98
Methylphenidate, 335, 473
Methylprednisolone, 134, 548
Methylprostaglandin, 386
Metoclopramide, 111, 118
Metoprolol, 89
Metronidazole
  abscesses, 309
  anorectal fistula, 143
  Crohn's disease, 137
  diarrhea, 126
  diverticulitis, 139
  pelvic inflammatory disease, 263, 358
  rosacea, 68
  urethritis, 531
  vaginitis/vulvovaginitis, 350
Metyrapone, 94, 97
Metyrosine, 98
Miconazole, 118, 349
Microangiopathic hemolytic anemia
  hemolytic uremic syndrome, 440
  hypertension, 31
  thrombotic thrombocytopenic purpura, 192
Microcephaly
  congenital cytomegalovirus, 439

herpes simplex virus, 439
trisomy 13, 445
Microcytosis, 171
Microglobulin, 184
Micrognathia, 445
Microprolactinomas, 93
*Microsporum*, 448
Microtia, 654
Middle meatus, 662
Middle meningeal artery, 220
Midesophageal traction diverticulum
  surgical principles, 596–597
Migraine, 317–319
Miliaria, 85
Milk alkali syndrome, 557
Milrinone, 9
Mineralocorticoids, 98
Minimal change disease, 549
Minoxidil, 30, 69
Miosis, 324
Miotic pupils, 240
Mirtazapine, 460
Mithramycin, 557
Mitotane, 97
Mitral regurgitation, 4
Mitral stenosis, 24, 36
Mitral valve prolapse, 24, 463
Mobitz Type I/II/III block, 16–17
Modafinil, 332
Modified radical mastectomy (MRM), 571
Mohs surgery, 71, 566
Moisturizers, 56, 57, 207
Mold and allergic rhinitis, 200
Moles and gestational trophoblastic disease, 382, 383
Moll gland, 397
Molluscum contagiosum
  mechanisms and disease diagnosis/treatment, 51
Mongolian spot, 85
Monoamine oxidase inhibitors (MAOIs)
  depression, major (unipolar), 460
  Parkinson's disease, 329
  social phobia, 466
Monoclonal gammopathy of undetermined significance (MGUS)
  mechanisms and disease diagnosis/treatment, 185

Monocular defects
  mechanisms and disease diagnosis/treatment, 404–405, 405f
Mono-Diff test, 264
Monoliasis
  mechanisms and disease diagnosis/treatment, 658
Mononeuritis, 309
Mononucleosis
  mechanisms and disease diagnosis/treatment, 264
Monosodium urate crystals, 280
Monospot test, 264
Montelukast, 504
Mood disorders
  bipolar disorders, 461–462
  bulimia, 476
  childhood, psychoses originating in, 459
  cyclothymia, 462
  dysthymia, 460–461
  major (unipolar) depression, 459–460
Moon facies, 96
Morphea, 80
Morpheiform, 71
Morphine, 514
Mortality rates. *See* mechanisms and disease diagnosis/ treatment *and* surgical principles *under specific disease/disorder*
Moschowitz procedure, 351
Mosquitoes
  mechanisms and disease diagnosis/treatment, 65–66
Mother, postpartum care of the
  mechanisms and disease diagnosis/treatment, 367–368
Motor disorders
  bereavement, 489
  esophagus
    achalasia, 113
    diffuse esophageal spasm, 113
    mechanisms and disease diagnosis/treatment, 111–113
    scleroderma, 113–114
  lumbar disk disease, 275
  schizophrenia, 453
Motor vehicle accidents, 224, 242

Mouth. *See also* Otolaryngology
　allergic rhinitis, 200
　candidiasis, oral, 48
　dry-eye syndrome, 400
　neutropenia, 194
MPTP, 329
Mucin, 400, 413
Mucocutaneous junction, 142
Mucomyst, 228
*Mucor*, 503
Mucormycosis, 307
Mucosa-associated lymphoid tissue (MALT) lymphomas, 115
Muehrcke's lines, 146
Muehrcke's nails, 85
Müellerian agenesis, 352
Muir-Torre syndrome, 84
Multicystic kidney disease
　mechanisms and disease diagnosis/treatment, 428
Multiple endocrine neoplasia (MEN)
　gastric cancer, 115
　hypercalcemia, 91, 92
　multiple mucosal neuroma syndrome, 84
Multiple-gated arteriography (MUGA), 514
Multiple gestation
　incompetent cervix, 378
　mechanisms and disease diagnosis/treatment, 381–382, 382f
Multiple mucosal neuroma syndrome, 84
Multiple myeloma
　hypercalcemia, 92
　mechanisms and disease diagnosis/treatment, 184–185
　monoclonal gammopathy of undetermined significance, 185
Multiple sclerosis
　mechanisms and disease diagnosis/treatment, 331–332, 332f
　monocular defects, 405
　papillitis, 404
　sudden hearing loss, 656
　trigeminal neuralgia, 316
Mumps
　acute pancreatitis, 160
　diabetes mellitus, 103

　mechanisms and disease diagnosis/treatment, 266
　sudden hearing loss, 656
Mupirocin, 50
Murmurs/heart sounds
　cardiac tamponade, 21
　cardiogenic shock, 10
　chronic valvular diseases, 24
　dilated cardiomyopathy, 13
　ill-defined symptoms, 622–623
　left-sided low output heart failure, 8
　myocardial infarction, 4
　obstructive shock, 12
　pulmonary embolism, 38
　pulmonary sequestration, 447
　restrictive cardiomyopathy, 15
　stable angina pectoris, 6
　unstable angina, 3
　ventricular septic defect, 25
Murphy's sign, 144
Muscles
　ischemic heart disease, 23
　weakness
　　carpal tunnel syndrome, 311
　　Cushing's syndrome, 96
　　dermatomyositis, 80
　　hyperthyroidism, 88
　　hypokalemia, 554
　　myasthenia gravis, 312
　　polymyositis-dermatomyositis, 282
　　renal osteodystrophy, 550
　　secondary hypertension, 30
Musculoskeletal/connective tissue disease
　acute or emergency problems
　　cauda equina syndrome, 299
　　compartmental syndrome, 299
　　contusions, 292
　　effusion of joint, 290–291
　　fractures and dislocations, 292–299
　　joint infections, 299
　　open fractures, 299
　　spinal stenosis, 291–292
　　vascular compromise following fracture and dislocation, 299
　degenerative disorders
　　back pain, low, 274–275
　　joints, 273–274

　　lumbar disk, 275–276
　　neurologic disease, disorders secondary to, 276
　infections
　　gonococcal tenosynovitis, 272–273
　　Lyme disease, 272
　　osteomyelitis, 271
　　septic arthritis, 271–272
　inflammatory or immunologic disorders
　　ankylosing spondylitis, 283–284
　　bursitis, 284–285
　　fibromyalgia, 285–286
　　lupus arthritis, 281–282
　　polymyalgia rheumatica, 281
　　polymyositis-dermatomyositis, 282–283
　　rheumatoid arthritis, 283
　　tendinitis, 285
　inherited/congenital/developmental disorders
　　hip disorders, congenital, 276–277
　　intoeing, 278–279
　　Legg-Calvé-Perthes disease, 277–278
　　slipped capital femoral epiphysis, 278
　metabolic and nutritional disorders
　　gout, 280
　　osteoporosis, 279
　　rickets, 280–281
　neoplasms
　　bone, metastases to, 286–287
　　osteosarcoma, 286
　　pulmonary osteoarthropathy, 287
　neurology
　　carpal tunnel syndrome, 310–311
　　Guillain-Barré syndrome, 311–312
　　mechanisms and disease diagnosis/treatment, 276
　　myasthenia gravis, 312
　　myopathies and dystrophies, 313
　other disorders
　　carpal tunnel syndrome, 288–289
　　Dupuytren's contracture, 288

eosinophil granuloma, 290
Paget's disease of bone, 289–290
shoulder-hand syndrome, 288
pediatrics
chondromalacia patellae, 450
kyphosis, 449
Osgood-Schlatter disease, 449
osteochondritis dissecans, 449
scoliosis, 448–449
slipped capital femoral epiphysis, 449
stiffness, morning
ankylosing spondylitis, 283
polymyalgia rheumatica, 281
rheumatoid arthritis, 283
Mushrooms and hypersensitivity pneumonitis, 210
Mushroom worker's lung, 210
Myalgias
acute enteric infections, 120
anemia of chronic disease, 176
arsenic toxicity, 323
blastomycosis, 501
genital herpes, 263
giant cell aortitis, 43
histoplasmosis, 500
hypersensitivity pneumonitis, 210
influenza pneumonia, 498
Legionnaire's disease, 497
lupus arthritis, 282
Lyme disease, 272
mononucleosis, 264
mumps, 266
Myasthenia gravis
blepharoptosis, 399
mechanisms and disease diagnosis/treatment, 312
Mycelex troches, 658
*Mycobacterium tuberculosis*, 254, 499
*Mycoplasma*, 61
*Mycoplasma hominis*, 358
*Mycoplasma pneumoniae*
acute bronchitis, 494
acute pancreatitis, 160
mechanisms and disease diagnosis/treatment, 497–498
Mycoses
candidiasis, cutaneous, 48–49
candidiasis, oral, 48
dermatophytosis, 47–48
Mycotic aneurysms, 164
Myectomy, 15

Myelin, 173, 311, 332
Myelofibrosis, 186
Myeloma, 81
Myelomeningoceles, 423
Myocardial diseases
dilated cardiomyopathy, 13–14
hypertrophic cardiomyopathy, 14–15
restrictive cardiomyopathy, 15–16
Myocardial infarction (MI)
abdominal aortic aneurysm, 164
acute arterial occlusion, 36
acute pericarditis, 20
aortic dissection, 40
atherosclerosis, 33
bradyarrhythmias, 18
congestive heart failure, 514
essential hypertension, 30
hyperlipoproteinemia, 32
hyperosmolar hyperglycemic nonketotic coma, 104
ischemic bowel disease, 137
mechanisms and disease diagnosis/treatment, 4–5
panic disorder, 463
stable angina pectoris, 6
vasculitis syndromes, 36
Myocarditis
mononucleosis, 264
mumps, 266
rubella (German measles), 267
Myocyte injury, 14
Myofibroblast proliferation, 288
Myoglobinuria, 228, 230
Myomectomy, 342
Myopathies
mechanisms and disease diagnosis/treatment, 313
Myopia, 414
Myositis, 309
Myositis ossificans, 292
Myotomy, 113
Myotonic dystrophy, 334
Myringotomy, 651
Myringotomy tubes, 435
Myxedema, 88, 334
Myxomas, 321

N
Nadalol, 157
Nails
ingrowing, 66–67
iron-deficiency anemia, 169
signs and disease, 84–85

Naloxone, 478
Naltrexone, 479
Naphcon, 201
Naphthylamine, 157
Naratriptan, 318
Narcissistic personality disorders, 468
Narcolepsy, 335
Narcotics
familial Mediterranean fever, 141
gastric motility, disorders of, 118
osteoarthritis, 274
pancreatic carcinoma, 157
poisoning and mechanisms and disease diagnosis/treatment, 232
substance-related disorders, 477
Nasalcrom, 201
Nasal fracture, 218
Nasolacrimal duct, 400, 401
Nasonex, 201
Nasopharyngo-laryngoscopy, 659
Nasopharynx, masses in the
mechanisms and disease diagnosis/treatment, 658–659
National Cancer Institute, 129
National Surgical Adjuvant Breast and Bowel Project, 571
Nausea
abscesses, 308
acetaminophen, 228
acute cholecystitis, 144
acute enteric infections, 120
acute pancreatitis, 159
adrenal insufficiency, 95
alcohol, 479
barotrauma, 656
bipolar disorders, 462
carbon monoxide, 231
cholelithiasis, 145
concussion, 219
cryptococcal infection, 257
diabetes mellitus, 102
dysmenorrhea, 351
glaucoma, 414
headaches, 317
hyperemesis gravidarum, 384
hypoglycemia, 105
hyponatremia, 553
ill-defined presentations, 638–639
intracerebral hemorrhage, 321

Nausea (continued)
  Legionnaire's disease, 497
  neurosyphilis, 310
  orocavity, herpes simplex of the, 657
  panic disorder, 463
  pelvic inflammatory disease, 358
  prenatal care, 365
  stimulants, 229
  unstable angina, 3
  venous thrombosis, 322
  vertigo, 651
  volume excess, 555
Nearsightedness, 417
Nebulizer, home, 200, 202
Neck. See also Nose and throat; Otolaryngology
  acute lymphocytic leukemia, 178
  fractures, 234
  neurosyphilis, 310
  oropharynx, malignant neoplasms of the, 659
  rigidity
    aseptic meningitis, 306
    bacterial meningitis, 437
    fungal meningitis, 307
    herpes simplex virus, 303
    septic meningitis, 306–307
    subarachnoid hemorrhage, 321
    tuberculosis, 308
  sleep apnea, 334
Necrobiosis lipoidica
  mechanisms and disease diagnosis/treatment, 83
Necrotizing enterocolitis (NEC), 376
  mechanisms and disease diagnosis/treatment, 443
Necrotizing otitis media, 648
Necrotizing vasculitis, 36
Nedocromil, 504
Needle sharing and HIV (human immunodeficiency virus), 303
Negri bodies, 306
Neisseria gonorrhoeae
  adolescent pregnancy, 370
  epididymoorchitis, 263
  gonorrhea, 259
  pelvic inflammatory disease, 262, 263, 358
Neisseria meningitidis, 437

Neomycin, 55
Neoplasms. See also Oncology/cancer
  neurology
    glioblastoma, 325–326
    meningioma, 326
    metastases, 326–327
  pulmonary medicine
    bronchogenic carcinoma, 518–519
    carcinoid tumors, 519
    metastatic malignant tumors, 520
Neosporin, 55
Neostigmine, 399
Nephrectomy, 544, 545
Nephritis, 213
Nephropathy
  chronic myelogenous leukemia, 180
  diabetes mellitus, 103, 104
  gouty, 280
Nephrosclerosis
  mechanisms and disease diagnosis/treatment, 552
Nephrosis, 85
Nephrotic syndrome
  lupus nephritis, 553
  mechanisms and disease diagnosis/treatment, 549
  pleural effusions, 512
Nerve blocks, 47
Nerve conduction studies (NVC)
  carpal tunnel syndrome, 311
  cervical spine and spinal stenosis, 333
  Guillain-Barré syndrome, 311
  HIV (human immunodeficiency virus), 303
  myopathies/dystrophies, 313
  poliomyelitis, 305
  radiculopathy, 334
Neural tube defects
  mechanisms and disease diagnosis/treatment
    obstetrics, 378–380, 379f
    pediatrics, 422–423
Neuroblastoma, 287
Neurofibroma
  surgical principles, 565
Neurofibromatosis, 85, 424
Neurogenic shock, 12
Neuroleptic malignant syndrome
  antipsychotics, 324

Neuroleptics
  childhood schizophrenia, 458
  schizophrenia, 453
  schizophreniform disorder, 457
Neurology. See also Central nervous system; Cranial nerves
  cerebrovascular disorders
    cardioembolic strokes, 320–321
    intracerebral hemorrhage, 321
    ischemic thrombotic strokes, 318–320
    subarachnoid hemorrhage, 321–322
    venous thrombosis, 322–323
  definitions, 336–338
  degenerative diseases
    Alzheimer's diagnosis, 327–328
    amyotrophic lateral sclerosis, 328
    Huntington's disease, 329
    Parkinson's disease, 328–329
  demyelination
    multiple sclerosis, 331–332
  developmental disorders
    Tay-Sachs disease, 335–336
  Lyme disease, 267
  neoplasms
    glioblastoma, 325–326
    meningioma, 326
    metastases, 326–327
  neuromuscular disorders
    carpal tunnel syndrome, 310–311
    Guillain-Barré syndrome, 311–312
    mechanisms and disease diagnosis/treatment, 276
    myasthenia gravis, 312
    myopathies and dystrophies, 313
  nutritional and metabolic disorders
    metabolic encephalopathy, 315
    thiamine deficiency, 314–315
    vitamin $B_{12}$ deficiency, 313–314
  paroxysmal disorders
    headaches, 317–318
    seizures, 315–316
    trigeminal neuralgia, 316–317

seborrheic dermatitis, 55
sleep disorders
    apnea, sleep, 334–335
    narcolepsy, 335
spine disease
    radiculopathy, 333–334
    spinal stenosis, 333
thrombotic thrombocytopenic purpura, 192
toxic disorders
    heavy metals, 323–324
    medications, 324
trauma
    contusion, 331
    epidural hematoma, 330–331
    subdural hematoma, 330
Neuropathy
    diabetes mellitus, 103, 104
    HIV (human immunodeficiency virus), 303
    Lyme disease, 309
Neurosyphilis
    cerebrospinal fluid, 261
    mechanisms and disease diagnosis/treatment, 310
    papillitis, 404
Neutropenia
    cytomegalovirus, 254
    mechanisms and disease diagnosis/treatment, 194–195
Neutrophils
    aplastic anemia, 173
    bronchial asthma, 199
    neutropenia, 195
    pertussis, 495
    vitamin $B_{12}$ deficiency, 172
Nevirapine, 251
Newborns. *See also* Infancy and childhood; Pediatrics
    alpha-antitrypsin deficiency, 150
    chlamydia, 533
    dermatology, 85
    hepatitis B infection complicating pregnancy, 378
    hip, developmental dysplasia of the, 433, 433f
    hyperbilirubinemia, neonatal, 432
    infantile polycystic disease, 428
    mechanisms and disease diagnosis/treatment hyperbilirubinemia, 432
    immediate care of, 367
    respiratory distress syndrome, 515
    meconium aspiration, 431
    protein C deficiency, 191
    purpura fulminans, 191
    respiratory distress syndrome, 430–431, 430f
    Rh incompatibility, 431–432
    transient tachypnea of the newborn, 429
Niacin
    decreased high-density lipoprotein, 102
    dysbetalipoproteinemia, type III, 100
    elevated Lp (a) lipoprotein, 102
    hyperlipoproteinemia, type II, 100
    hyperlipoproteinemia, type IV, 101
    hyperlipoproteinemia, type V, 101
Nickel jewelry and contact dermatitis, 55
Nicotine and drug dependence, 483. *See also* Smoking
Nicotinic acid, 33
Night sweats
    disseminated *Mycobacterium avium-intracellulare* complex, 256
    mechanisms and disease diagnosis/treatment, 533
    pulmonary tuberculosis, 499
Nikolsky's sign, 58, 59
Nimodipine, 322
Nitrates
    diffuse esophageal spasm, 113
    unstable angina, 4
    variant angina, 6
Nitric oxide (NO), 113
Nitrofurantoin, 213, 377
Nitrofurantoin monohydrate macrocrystals, 529
Nitrogen, 51, 69
Nitroglycerin (NTG)
    congestive heart failure, 514
    stable angina pectoris, 7
    unstable angina, 3, 4
Nitroprusside, 31, 41, 98
Nizatidine, 111
Nocturia, 91, 529
Nocturnal penile tumescence, 484
Nodular sclerosing subtype, 181
Noise-induced hearing loss, 221, 656
Nonnucleoside reverse transcriptase inhibitors, 250–251
Norepinephrine
    anorexia, 475
    attention-deficit hyperactivity disorder, 473
    basic cardiac life support, 29
    bulimia, 476
    panic disorder, 463
Normochromic anemia, 547
Normocytic anemia, 547
Norvir, 250
Norwalk virus, 122
Norwegian scabies, 64
Nose and throat. *See also* Otolaryngology
    acute bronchiolitis, 494
    acute epiglottitis, 493
    congenital syphilis, 437, 438
    epistaxis
        idiopathic thrombocytopenic purpura, 192
        mechanisms and disease diagnosis/treatment, 217
        platelet dysfunction, 194
        von Willebrand disease, 188
    facial fracture, 217–218
    foreign bodies, 225–226
    influenza pneumonia, 498
    mononucleosis, 264
    *Mycoplasma pneumoniae,* 497
    ophthalmic herpes zoster, 412
    pharyngitis, 436
    venous thrombosis, 322
NSAIDs (nonsteroidal anti-inflammatory drugs)
    acid-related disorders of the stomach, 116
    acute upper respiratory infection, 668
    ankle injury, 237
    arthralgias, 274
    back pain, low, 275
    cervical spine and spinal stenosis, 333
    contusions, 292
    Crohn's disease, 135
    dysmenorrhea, 351
    endometriosis, 343
    epididymitis, 531

NSAIDs (nonsteroidal anti-inflammatory drugs) *(continued)*
  erythema nodosum, 62
  fibromyalgia, 286
  frozen shoulder syndrome, 288
  headaches, 318
  hereditary nonpolyposis colorectal cancer, 130
  iron-deficiency anemia, 169
  lumbar spine and spinal stenosis, 333
  lupus arthritis, 282
  orchitis, 531
  Paget's disease of bone, 290
  pain disorder, 471
  pleurisy, 513
  prostatitis, 530
  pulmonary osteoarthropathy, 287
  rheumatoid arthritis, 283
  tendinitis, 285
  ulcerative colitis, 133
Nucleoside reverse transcriptase inhibitors, 250
Nucleotides, 54
Nutriceuticals, 274
Nutrition. *See* Diet/nutrition
Nystagmus
  barotrauma, 656
  PCP (phencyclidine), 230
  vertigo, 652
Nystatin, 48, 49, 658

# O

Oat cell carcinoma, 519
Obesity
  abdominal aortic aneurysms, 590
  acanthosis nigricans, 84
  bulimia, 476
  candidiasis, cutaneous, 48
  cholelithiasis, 145
  colorectal carcinoma, 128
  Cushing's syndrome, 96
  diabetes mellitus, 104
  dysbetalipoproteinemia, type III, 100
  endometrial cancer, 341
  essential hypertension, 30
  hyperlipoproteinemia, type IV, 100
  osteoarthritis, 273
  postpartum sepsis, 387
  psychosomatic disorders, 472
  pulmonary embolism, 516
  sleep apnea, 334, 335, 524
  slipped capital femoral epiphysis, 449
  vulva/vagina, candidiasis of the, 349
Obsessive-compulsive disorder (OCD)
  anorexia, 474
  body dysmorphic disorder, 472
  mechanisms and disease diagnosis/treatment, 464–465
  overview, 468
  panic disorder, 463
Obstetrics. *See also* Pregnancy; Reproduction, male/female
  complicated pregnancy
    abruptio placentae, 374
    adolescent pregnancy, 369–370
    asthma, 389
    central nervous system malformation in fetus and neural tube defect, 378–380
    cervix, incompetent, 378
    depression, 383–384
    diabetes, gestational, 388
    diabetes, overt, 389
    eclampsia, 375–376
    ectopic pregnancy, 370–371
    forceps and vacuum extractor, 387
    genitourinary tract, infections of the, 376–377
    gestational trophoblastic disease, 382–383
    hepatitis B, 377–378
    hyperemesis gravidarum, 384–385
    induced abortion, 372
    labor, abnormalities of, 385–386
    maternal mortality, 383
    multiple gestation, 381–382
    overview, 390
    placenta previa, 373–374
    postpartum hemorrhage, 386
    postpartum sepsis, 386–387
    preeclampsia, 374–375
    premature labor, 376
    preterm premature rupture of membranes, 384
    Rh incompatibility or isoimmunization, 380–381
    septic abortion, 372
    spontaneous abortion, 371
    trisomy, 380
  uncomplicated pregnancy
    health and health maintenance, 365
    labor and delivery, normal, 368–369
    lactation, 368
    mother, postpartum care of the, 367–368
    newborn, immediate care of the, 367
    prenatal diagnosis, 366
    Rh immunoglobulin prophylaxis, 365–366
    teratology, 366–367
Obstruction stasis, 143
Obstructive chronic bronchitis, 506
Obstructive shock
  mechanisms and disease diagnosis/treatment, 12
Obstructive sleep apnea, 524
Obtundation
  epidural hematoma, 330
  glioblastoma, 325
  intracerebral hemorrhage, 321
  meningitis, 307
  opioids, 324
  subarachnoid hemorrhage, 321
  tuberculosis, 308
Octreotide, 93, 635
Ocular injury
  mechanisms and disease diagnosis/treatment, 220
Odd personality disorders, 468
Odors, foul-smelling
  anorectal abscess, 143
  chronic sinusitis, 662
  fungal sinusitis, 663
  heavy metals/arsenic, 231
  orocavity, herpes simplex of the, 657
  vaginitis/vulvovaginitis, 350
Odynophagia
  cytomegalovirus, 253
  motor disorders of the esophagus, 112
  strep throat, 660, 661
  thrush, oral, 658

Ofloxacin
    cervicitis and sexually
            transmitted diseases, 347
    chlamydia, 260
    epididymoorchitis, 263
    gonorrhea, 259
    pelvic inflammatory disease, 263
    tuberculosis, 255
Olfaction and taste, disorders of
    mechanisms and disease
            diagnosis/treatment, 667
Oligemia, 322
Oligoclonal bands, 310
Oligohydramnios, 375, 433
Oliguria
    acute renal failure, 546, 547
    aortic dissection, 41
    glomerulonephritis, 549
    hypernatremia, 554
    ill-defined symptoms, 627–628
    infantile polycystic disease, 428
    malignant hypertension, 31
    renal transplant rejection, 548
Oncology/cancer. See also
            Leukemia; Lymphomas;
            Neoplasms
    breast
        Cowden's syndrome, 84
        mechanisms and disease
                diagnosis/treatment,
                353–355, 354t
        metastases, 326
        surgical principles, 570–571
    colon
        Muir-Torre syndrome, 84
        surgical principles, 606–607
    colorectal carcinoma, 128–132,
            129t–131t
    dermatology
        actinic keratosis, 69
        benign neoplasms, 72–75
        follicular cyst, 75–76
        malignant neoplasms,
                cutaneous signs of
                internal, 83–84
        premalignant and malignant
                neoplasms of skin, 69–72
    digestive system
        acanthosis nigricans, 84
        achalasia, 113
        gastric cancer, 114–115
        stomach cancer, 598
    gallbladder
        surgical principles, 612

larynx, 661
liver, 613–614, 614f
metastases and mechanisms and
        disease diagnosis/
        treatment
    bone, 286–287
    neurology, 326–327
    pulmonary medicine, 520
multiple myeloma, 184–185
musculoskeletal/connective
        tissue disease
    bone, metastases to, 286–287
    osteosarcoma, 286
nails
    clubbed nails, 85
oropharynx, malignant
        neoplasms of the,
        659–660
pulmonary medicine
    asbestosis, 510
renal and urinary system
    benign prostatic hyperplasia,
            542
    bladder carcinoma, 543–544,
            575–576
    penile/urethral/scrotal
            carcinoma, 545–546
    prostate cancer, 542–543
    renal cell carcinoma, 544
    testicular carcinoma, 545
    Wilms' tumor, 544–545
reproduction, male/female
    ovary, 344
    uterus, 341
restrictive cardiomyopathy, 15
thyroid gland
    mechanisms and disease
            diagnosis/treatment, 91
    multiple mucosal neuroma
            syndrome, 84
Oncovin, 182
Onycholysis, 88
Onychomycosis, 47, 48
Onychosis, 84
Oophorectomy, 345
Oophoritis, 266
Open-angle glaucoma, 416
Open reduction and internal
        fixation (ORIF)
    femur, fracture of, 234
    humerus, fracture of the, 235
    medial or lateral epicondyle
            fractures, 235
    radius fractures, 235

tibia, fracture of, 233
ulna, fracture of the, 235
Ophthalmic herpes zoster
    mechanisms and disease
            diagnosis/treatment,
            412–413
Ophthalmology. See also Eyes;
        Vision
    amblyopia, 406–407
    conjunctivitis, 393–395,
            393t–396t
    cornea, disorders of the
        dry eye, 413
        globe, diseases of the, 411t
        herpes simplex keratitis,
                411–412
        herpes zoster, 412–413
        interstitial keratitis, 413–414
        ulcers, 410–411
    diabetes, 409–410
    eyelids, disorders of the
        blepharitis, 396
        blepharoptosis, 399
        chalazion, 397
        ectropion, 398
        entropion, 398
        epicanthus, 398–399
        stye, 397
    lacrimal system, disorders of the
        acute dacryocystitis, 400–401
        undersecretion, 400
    lens, disorders of the
        cataract, 417–418, 418t
        glaucoma, 414–416, 415f
    optic nerve, disorders of the
        elevation of the disc, 401–404
        pallor of the disc/optic
                atrophy, 404
    strabismus, 407–409, 408t, 409t
    visual pathways, disorders of the
        bitemporal defects, 405
        homonymous defects, 405
        monocular defects (central
                scotomas), 404–405, 405f
Ophthalmopathy, 88, 88f
Ophthalmoplegia, 330
Ophthalmoscopy
    amblyopia, 406
    cataracts, 417
    congenital anomalous disc
            elevation, 401
    congenital cataracts, 424
    monocular defects, 404, 405
    papillitis, 403
    strabismus, 407

Opioids
  dependence, drug, 481
  history and physical keys, 324
*Opisthorchis*, 160
Optic atrophy
  interstitial keratitis, 413
  mechanisms and disease diagnosis/treatment, 404
Optic nerve, disorders of the
  elevation of the disc
    congenital anomalous disc elevation, 401–402, 401*t*, 402*t*
    papilledema, 402
    papillitis, 402–404, 403*f*
    pallor of the disc/optic atrophy, 404
Optic neuritis, 404
  ophthalmic herpes zoster, 412
  rubella (German measles), 267
Oral contraceptives (OCPs)
  acne vulgaris, 67
  cholelithiasis, 145
  endometriosis, 343
  hirsutism, 98
  ischemic bowel disease, 137
  premenstrual syndrome, 352
  pulmonary embolism, 516
Orbital fracture, 217, 218
Orchiectomy, 545
Orchiopexy, 429, 534
Orchitis
  gonorrhea, 532
  mechanisms and disease diagnosis/treatment, 531
  mumps, 266
Organomegaly, 431
Orgasmic disorders, male/female, 484
Orocavity, herpes simplex of the
  mechanisms and disease diagnosis/treatment, 657–658
Oropharyngeal dysphagia, 111
Oropharynx, malignant neoplasms of the
  mechanisms and disease diagnosis/treatment, 659–660
Orthopnea
  dilated cardiomyopathy, 13
  left-sided high output heart failure, 9
  left-sided low output heart failure, 8
  obstructive shock, 12
Orthostasis, 555
Ortolani sign, 433
Oseltamivir, 494, 499
Osgood-Schlatter disease
  mechanisms and disease diagnosis/treatment, 449
Osteitis fibrosa, 547
Osteitis fibrosa cystica, 550
Osteoarthritis
  mechanisms and disease diagnosis/treatment, 273–274
  slipped capital femoral epiphysis, 278
Osteochondritis dissecans
  mechanisms and disease diagnosis/treatment, 449
Osteodystrophy
  renal
    chronic renal failure, 547
    mechanisms and disease diagnosis/treatment, 550
  rickets, 281
Osteomeatal complex, 662–663
Osteomyelitis
  mechanisms and disease diagnosis/treatment, 271
  sickle cell anemia, 176
Osteopenia, 353
Osteoporosis
  anorexia, 475
  femur, fracture of neck of, 295
  hypercalcemia, 92
  mechanisms and disease diagnosis/treatment, 279
  menopausal symptoms, 353
  Paget's disease of bone, 289
Osteosarcoma
  mechanisms and disease diagnosis/treatment, 286
Osteosclerosis, 550
Osteotomy, 278
Otalgia
  acute sinusitis, 662
  hoarseness, 660
  mechanisms and disease diagnosis/treatment, 653
  strep throat, 661
Otitis externa
  mechanisms and disease diagnosis/treatment
    infectious, 647
    malignant, 647
Otitis media
  allergic rhinitis, 200
  attention-deficit hyperactivity disorder, 473
  humoral immunodeficiency, 204
  mechanisms and disease diagnosis/treatment, 434–435
  acute, 648–649
  chronic, 648–650
  serous, 650–651
  necrotizing, 648
  sudden hearing loss, 656
Otolaryngology. *See also* Ears; Nose and throat
  mouth and throat, diseases of the
    cancer of the larynx, 661
    herpes simplex of the orocavity, 657–658
    hoarseness, 660
    malignant neoplasms of the oropharynx/hypopharynx, 659–660
    masses in the nasopharynx, 658–659
    strep throat, 660–661
    thrush, 658
Otorrhea, 648, 650
Otosclerosis, 654
Otoscopy
  acute otitis media, 648
  barotrauma, 656
  cerumen impaction, 651
  chronic otitis media, 649
  hearing loss, 654
  otalgia, 653
  otitis media, 434
  serous otitis media, 650
Ototoxic drugs, 425
Ovary
  infertility, 357–358
  mechanisms and disease diagnosis/treatment
    cysts, 344–345
    malignant neoplasm, 344
Overproduction syndromes (pituitary gland)
  mechanisms and disease diagnosis/treatment, 92–93, 93*f*

Oxazepam, 480
Oximetry, 198
Oxygen. *See also* Shock
   acute bronchiolitis, 494
   acute myelogenous leukemia, 178
   anaphylaxis, 202
   bronchial asthma, 199, 200
   bronchiolitis, 434
   carbon monoxide, 231
   cardiogenic shock, 11
   chronic bronchitis, 506
   chronic valvular diseases, 24
   congestive heart failure, 514
   cor pulmonale, 518
   cough, 521
   croup, 436
   desquamative interstitial pneumonitis, 509
   emphysema, 506
   gram-negative bacillary pneumonias, 497
   hypertrophic cardiomyopathy, 15
   Legionnaire's disease, 497
   meconium aspiration, 431
   myocardial infarction, 5
   peritonitis, 140
   pneumococcal pneumonia, 495
   *Pneumocystis carinii* pneumonia, 498
   right-sided heart failure, 10
   secondary erythrocytosis, 186
   sickle cell anemia, 177
   sleep apnea, 334, 524
   stable angina pectoris, 6, 7
   staphylococcal pneumonia, 496
   traumatic injury, 239
   unstable angina, 3
   usual interstitial pneumonitis, 509
   ventricular septic defect, 26
Oxytocin, 369, 386

## P

Pacemakers
   AV block, 17
   bradyarrhythmias, 19
   sick sinus syndrome, 16
Paclitax, 157, 544
Paget's disease of bone
   left-sided high output heart failure, 9
   mechanisms and disease diagnosis/treatment, 289–290
   osteosarcoma, 286
Pagophagia, 169
Pain
   abdominal
      acid-related disorders of the stomach, 115–116
      acute enteric infections, 120
      acute pancreatitis, 159
      adrenal insufficiency, 95
      chronic pancreatitis, 161
      chylomicronemia, type 1 familial, 99
      constipation, 139
      cystic fibrosis, 507
      diabetes mellitus, 102
      diarrhea, 126
      disseminated *Mycobacterium avium-intracellulare* complex, 255
      diverticulitis, 138
      ectopic pregnancy, 370
      gastric cancer, 114
      gastroesophageal reflux disease, 110
      hernias, external, 163
      hypereosinophilic syndrome, 212
      ill-defined presentations, 637–638
      intestinal obstruction, 138
      irritable bowel syndrome, 126
      ischemic bowel disease, 137
      mononucleosis, 264
      ovarian cysts, 344
      pancreatic carcinoma, 157
      peritonitis, 140
      pharyngitis, 436
      testicular torsion, 534
      ureteropelvic junction obstruction, 540
   back
      eosinophil granuloma, 290
      lumbar disk disease, 275–276
      mechanisms and disease diagnosis/treatment, 274–275
      psychosomatic disorders, 472
      spinal stenosis, 291
      transfusion reactions, 187
      urinary tract infections, 529
   biliary
      choledocholithiasis, 145
      cholelithiasis, 145
   bone
      multiple myeloma, 184
      osteoporosis, 279
      pulmonary osteoarthropathy, 287
      renal osteodystrophy, 550
   chest
      acute pericarditis, 20
      aortic dissection, 40
      aspergillosis, invasive, 502
      atherosclerosis, 33
      blood-loss anemia, 169
      bradyarrhythmias, 18
      bronchogenic carcinoma, 518
      cardiogenic shock, 10
      cardiopulmonary arrest, 28
      coccidioidomycosis, 501
      cryptococcal infection, 502
      diffuse esophageal spasm, 113
      esophageal neoplasms, 109
      gastroesophageal reflux disease, 110
      histoplasmosis, 500
      hypertrophic cardiomyopathy, 14
      ill-defined presentations, 632–633
      mechanisms and disease diagnosis/treatment, 521–522
      motor disorders of the esophagus, 111
      myocardial infarction, 4
      obstructive shock, 12
      panic disorder, 463
      phycomycosis, 503
      pleural effusions, 512
      pleurisy, 513
      pneumococcal pneumonia, 495
      pneumothorax, 222, 513
      pulmonary embolism, 38, 515
      stable angina pectoris, 6
      tachyarrhythmias, 18
      unstable angina, 3
      variant angina, 5
   crisis
      sickle cell anemia, 176
   disorder
      mechanisms and disease diagnosis/treatment, 470–471

Pain (continued)
  eyes
    sarcoidosis, 508
  flank
    genitourinary tract infections, 377
    papillary necrosis, 550
    pyelonephritis, 546
  groin
    femur, fracture of neck of, 295–296
  jaw
    facial fracture, 217
    giant cell aortitis, 43
  knee
    chondromalacia patellae, 450
    osteochondritis dissecans, 449
  neck
    cervical spine and spinal stenosis, 333
    larynx, cancer of the, 661
  orbital
    acute sinusitis, 662
  pelvic
    dysmenorrhea, 351
    endometriosis, 343
  perimbilical
    appendicitis, 132
  right upper quadrant
    acetaminophen, 228
    acute cholecystitis, 144
    autoimmune hepatitis, 147
    preeclampsia, 375
  shoulder
    viscus, perforation of, 223
  varicella-zoster (shingles), 46
Pallor
  anaphylaxis, 202
  aplastic anemia, 173
  arterial ulcer, 569
  blood-loss anemia, 169
  chronic renal failure, 174
  Crohn's disease, 135
  glaucoma, 414
  hemolytic uremic syndrome, 440
  hypoglycemia, 105
  iron-deficiency anemia, 169
  pheochromocytoma, 98
  Rh incompatibility, 431
  sickle cell anemia, 176
  vitamin $B_{12}$ deficiency, 172
Palmar erythema, 478
Palpitations
  arteriosclerotic ulcer, 78
  atrial septal defect, 26
  cardiopulmonary arrest, 28
  hyperthyroidism, 88
  hypoglycemia, 105
  ill-defined symptoms, 622
  panic disorder, 463
  pheochromocytoma, 98
  tachyarrhythmias, 18
  ventricular tachycardia, 19
Pamidronate, 92
Pancreas
  acute pancreatitis, 159–161, 615
  carcinoma, pancreatic
    mechanisms and disease diagnosis/treatment, 157–159
    surgical principles, 616
  chronic pancreatitis, 161
  cystic fibrosis, 161–162
  diabetes mellitus, 103
  glucagonoma syndrome, 84
  surgical principles
    acute pancreatitis, 615
    carcinoma, 616
    gastrinoma, 616–617
Pancreatitis
  acute, 159–161, 615
  alcohol, 478
  chylomicronemia, type 1 familial, 99
  cystic fibrosis, 162
  hypercalcemia, 92
  hyperlipoproteinemia, 32
  hyperlipoproteinemia, type V, 101
  mumps, 266
Pancytopenia, 170
Panic disorder
  mechanisms and disease diagnosis/treatment, 462–463
Pannus, 411
Papaverine, 538
Papillary necrosis
  mechanisms and disease diagnosis/treatment, 550–551
Papilledema, 31
  hydrocephalus, 423
  mechanisms and disease diagnosis/treatment, 402, 403f
  nephrosclerosis, 552
  optic atrophy, 404
  venous thrombosis, 322
Papillitis
  mechanisms and disease diagnosis/treatment, 402–403
Papillotomy, 146
Pap smear
  management of abnormal
    mechanisms and disease diagnosis/treatment, 347–348, 348f
  mother, postpartum care of the, 367
  vaginal cancer, 349
Paracentesis, 157
Parainfluenza virus, 436
Paranoid personality disorders, 456, 468
Paraproteinemia, 79
Parasitic pathogens and acute enteric infections, 122–123
Parathyroid gland
  disorders
    hypercalcemia, 91–92
Parathyroid hormone (PTH). See also mechanisms and disease diagnosis/treatment and surgical principles under specific disease/disorder
  hypercalcemia, 92
  hyperparathyroidism, 572
Parent's Anonymous groups, 487
Paresis/paraplegia/paralysis
  acute arterial occlusion, 35, 36
  Alzheimer's disease, 327
  carotid artery disease, 584
  infantile botulism, 421, 422
  Lyme disease, 309
  osteoporosis, 279
  poliomyelitis, 305
  spinal stenosis, 291
  thoracic spine, injuries to, 294
Paresthesia
  carpal tunnel syndrome, 288–289
  hypocalcemia, 558
  panic disorder, 463
  spinal stenosis, 291
  varicella-zoster (shingles), 46
  vitamin $B_{12}$ deficiency, 172
Parkinson's disease
  antipsychotics, 324
  mechanisms and disease diagnosis/treatment, 328–329

Paronychia
    mechanisms and disease
        diagnosis/treatment, 49
Parotid gland, 146, 266
Paroxysmal disorders
    headaches, 317–318
    seizures, 315–316
    trigeminal neuralgia, 316–317
Paroxysmal nocturnal dyspnea
    (PND), 8, 13
Parrot's pseudoparalysis, 437–438
Pars flaccida, 649
Parvovirus B19, 173, 176
Patanol, 202
Patella, 450
Patent ductus arteriosus (PDA),
    445
Pavlik's harness, 277
PCP (phencyclidine)
    dependence, drug, 482–483
    poisoning and mechanisms and
        disease diagnosis/
        treatment, 230
    substance-related disorders, 477
Peanuts and aspiration, 226
Pediatrics. *See also* Infancy and
        childhood; Newborns
    gastroenterology
        cleft lip or palate, 440
        Hirschsprung disease, 443,
            444f
        intussusception, 442–443,
            442f
        malrotation of the small
            intestine, 441–442
        necrotizing enterocolitis, 443
        pyloric stenosis, 441
        tracheoesophageal fistula, 441
    genetics
        Down syndrome, 444–445,
            445f
        fragile X syndrome, 446
        trisomy 13, 445
        trisomy 18, 445
        Turner's syndrome, 445–446
    genitourinary system
        bladder extrophy, 429
        Eagle-Barrett syndrome, 427
        hypospadias, 426
        multicystic kidney disease, 428
        polycystic disease, infantile,
            428
        posterior urethral valves,
            426–427
        prune-belly syndrome, 427
        undescended testis, 428–429
        vesicoureteral reflux, 427–428
    infectious diseases
        bronchiolitis, 434
        congenital infections, 437–439
        epiglottitis, 435
        hemolytic uremic syndrome,
            439
        laryngotracheitis, 435–436
        meningitis, bacterial, 437
        otitis media, 434–435
        pharyngitis, 436–437
        varicella (chickenpox), 436
    musculoskeletal/connective
            tissue disease
        chondromalacia patellae, 450
        kyphosis, 449
        Osgood-Schlatter disease, 449
        osteochondritis dissecans, 449
        scoliosis, 448–449
        slipped capital femoral
            epiphysis, 449
    neonatology
        hip, developmental dysplasia
            of the, 433, 433f
        hyperbilirubinemia, neonatal,
            432
        meconium aspiration, 431
        respiratory distress syndrome,
            430–431, 430f
        Rh incompatibility, 431–432
        transient tachypnea of the
            newborn, 429
    neurology
        botulism, infantile, 421–422
        febrile seizures, 421
        malformations, 423–425
        neural tube defects, 422–423,
            422f
    pulmonology
        cystic adenomatoid
            malformation, 447
        laryngomalacia, 446
        lobar emphysema, congenital,
            446–447
        pulmonary sequestration, 447
    rheumatology
        Henoch-Schöenlein purpura,
            425
        Kawasaki disease, 425–426
    skin conditions
        acne, 448
        fungal infections, 448
Pediculosis
    mechanisms and disease
        diagnosis/treatment, 65,
            65f
*Pediculosis capitis*, 65
Peer group and adjustment
        disorders, 466, 467
Pelvic fractures
    mechanisms and disease
        diagnosis/treatment, 224
Pelvic inflammatory disease (PID)
    gonorrhea, 259
    HIV (human immunodeficiency
        virus), 249
    mechanisms and disease
        diagnosis/treatment,
        262–263
    reproduction, male/female,
        358–359
Pelvic relaxation
    mechanisms and disease
        diagnosis/treatment,
        350–351
Pemoline, 332
Pemphigoid, 413
Pemphigus
    mechanisms and disease
        diagnosis/treatment,
        59–60, 60f
Pengolide, 329
Penicillamine
    copper poisoning, 232
    manganese toxicity, 324
    scleroderma, 81
Penicillin
    abscesses, 309
    cellulitis, 50
    cervicitis and sexually
        transmitted diseases, 347
    congenital syphilis, 438
    drug allergy, 213
    drug reactions causing skin
        changes, 58
    gonococcal tenosynovitis, 273
    gonorrhea, 259, 532
    gram-negative bacillary
        pneumonias, 497
    ischemic heart disease, 23
    Lyme disease, 268
    neurosyphilis, 310
    paronychia, 49
    pelvic inflammatory disease, 358
    pharyngitis, 437
    pneumococcal pneumonia, 495

Penicillin *(continued)*
  premature labor, 376
  secondary syphilis, 53
  staphylococcal pneumonia, 496
  syphilis, 261
  syphilitic aortitis, 42
Penis
  carcinoma
    mechanisms and disease diagnosis/treatment, 545–546
  erectile impotence, 537–538
  hypospadias, 426, 534, 535, 538
  Peyronie's disease, 537
  squamous cell carcinoma, 69
  urologic trauma, 541
Pentamidine
  hypoglycemia, 105
  *Pneumocystis carinii* pneumonia, 252, 498
Pentasa, 134
Pentosan polysulfate, 530
Pentoxifylline, 35, 78
Peptic ulcer disease (PUD)
  panic disorder, 463
  psychosomatic disorders, 472
*Peptostreptococcus*, 358
Percutaneous endoscopic gastrojejunostomy (PEJ), 120
Percutaneous endoscopic gastrostomy (PEG), 120
Percutaneous transhepatic cholangiography (PTC), 611
Percutaneous transluminal coronary angioplasty (PTCA)
  myocardial infarction, 5
  stable angina pectoris, 7
  unstable angina, 4
Percutaneous umbilical blood sample (PUBS), 380, 381
Perfumes and contact dermatitis, 55
Periaqueductal region and thiamine deficiency, 314
Pericardial diseases
  acute pericarditis, 20
  cardiac tamponade, 21
  constrictive pericarditis, 22
  pericardial effusion, 20–21

Pericardial effusion
  mechanisms and disease diagnosis/treatment, 20–21
  myocardial infarction, 4
  obstructive shock, 12
  Rh incompatibility, 431
Pericardial tamponade syndrome, 223
Pericardiectomy, 12, 21
Pericardiocentesis, 12, 21
Pericarditis, 264, 547
Periosteum, 286
Periostitis
  mechanisms and disease diagnosis/treatment, 437–438
  pulmonary osteoarthropathy, 287
  secondary syphilis, 52
Peripheral arterial occlusive disease
  surgical principles, 586–588
Peripheral arterial vascular disease
  acute arterial occlusion, 35–36
  chronic atherosclerotic occlusion, 34–35
  vasculitis syndromes, 36–37
Peripheral venous vascular diseases, 37–38
Perirectal abscess
  surgical principles, 605
Peritoneovenous shunting, 157
Peritonitis
  cirrhosis, 155
  diverticulitis, 139
  malrotation of the small intestine, 441
  mechanisms and disease diagnosis/treatment, 140
  pelvic inflammatory disease, 262
Peritonsillar abscess, 661
Periungual fibrous tumors, 82
Permethrin, 64
Peroxidase, 177
Persecutory delusions, 456
Personality disorders
  anorexia, 474
  anxious/fearful/inhibited, 468
  brief psychotic disorder, 457
  bulimia, 475
  conversion disorder, 471
  dramatic/emotional, 468
  factitious disorders, 472

  malingering, 472
  mechanisms and disease diagnosis/treatment, 468–469
  odd/eccentric, 468
  somatization disorder, 469
Pertussis
  mechanisms and disease diagnosis/treatment, 494–495
Pervasive developmental disorder (PDD), 458
Petechiae
  acute lymphocytic leukemia, 178
  acute myelogenous leukemia, 177
  aplastic anemia, 173
  gonorrhea, 259
  pharyngitis, 436
  septic meningitis, 307
Petrosal sinus sampling, 97
Peutz-Jeghers syndrome, 84
Peyronie's disease
  erectile impotence, 537
  mechanisms and disease diagnosis/treatment, 537
Phalen's test, 289
Pharyngitis
  acute upper respiratory infection, 667
  gonorrhea, 259
  mechanisms and disease diagnosis/treatment, 436–437
  *Mycoplasma pneumoniae*, 498
  psoriasis, 53
  rubella (German measles), 266
  secondary syphilis, 52
Pharyngitis, acute, 660–661
Ph chromosome, 179
Phenothiazines, 95, 324
Phenoxybenzamine, 98
Phentolamine, 98
Phenylketonuria (PKU), 367, 458
Phenylpropanolamine, 540
Phenytoin
  alcohol, 480
  drug reactions causing skin changes, 58
  seizures, 316
Pheochromocytoma
  hypercalcemia, 92
  mechanisms and disease diagnosis/treatment, 98

multiple mucosal neuroma
 syndrome, 84
secondary hypertension, 30, 31
surgical principles, 574
Phlebotomy, 186
pH monitoring
 distributive shock, 13
 gastroesophageal reflux disease, 111
 metabolic acidosis, 556
 metabolic alkalosis, 555
 respiratory acidosis, 557
 respiratory alkalosis, 556
 sickle cell anemia, 176
 vaginitis/vulvovaginitis, 350
Phobias
 social, 466
 specific
  mechanisms and disease diagnosis/treatment, 467
Phosphate, 497
Phosphodiesterase inhibitors, 9
Phosphorus, 550
Photon emission computed tomography (SPECT), 316, 327
Photophobia
 aseptic meningitis, 306
 congenital cataracts, 424
 congenital glaucoma, 423
 corneal ulcers, 410
 glaucoma, 414
 herpes simplex keratitis, 411
 interstitial keratitis, 413
 neonatal hyperbilirubinemia, 432
 porphyria cutanea tarda, 83
 septic meningitis, 306
Phototherapy, 54, 460
Phycomycosis
 mechanisms and disease diagnosis/treatment, 503
Physical exam. *See* mechanisms and disease diagnosis/treatment *and* surgical principles *under specific disease/disorder*
Physical therapy. *See also* Exercise(s)
 ankylosing spondylitis, 284
 back pain, low, 275
 contusions, 292
 ischemic thrombotic strokes, 320
 lumbar disk disease, 275

osteoarthritis, 274
osteoporosis, 279
radiculopathy, 334
rotator cuff syndrome, 299
tendinitis, 285
Pial vessels, 308
Pierre Robin syndrome, 425
Pigeon breeder's disease, 511
Pilocarpine, 416
Piloerection, 463
Pilonidal cyst
 surgical principles, 605–606
Pilonidal disease
 mechanisms and disease diagnosis/treatment, 144
Pimecrolimus, 56
Pinealomas, 94
Pinna, 220, 654
Pioglitazone, 104
Pipercillin, 139
Pitocin, 386
*Pitryrosporon*, 448
Pituitary gland
 disorders
  anterior pituitary, 92–93
  posterior, 94–95
 hypoglycemia, 105
*Pityrosporum ovale*, 55
Placenta and postpartum hemorrhage, 386
Placenta previa
 mechanisms and disease diagnosis/treatment, 373–374, 373f
Plaquenil, 508
Plasmapheresis
 Guillain-Barré syndrome, 312
 myasthenia gravis, 312
 thrombotic thrombocytopenic purpura, 193
 vasculitis, 518
Platelet activating factor (PAF), 199, 239
Platelets
 aplastic anemia, 173
 disseminated intravascular coagulation, 190
 essential thrombocythemia, 193
 idiopathic thrombocytopenic purpura, 192
 lupus inhibitor, 189
 mechanisms and disease diagnosis/treatment, 194
 polycythemia rubra vera, 185

preeclampsia, 375
thrombotic thrombocytopenic purpura, 193
unstable angina, 3
von Willebrand disease, 189
Platinum, 341
Pleocytosis
 abscesses, 308
 aseptic meningitis, 306
 Lyme disease, 309
 neurosyphilis, 310
 septic meningitis, 307
 tuberculosis, 308
Pleomorphism, 325
Plethysmography, 37
Pleural effusions
 mechanisms and disease diagnosis/treatment, 512, 512t
 pneumococcal pneumonia, 495
 Rh incompatibility, 431
Pleural friction rub, 502, 515
Pleural plaques/thickening, 510
Pleurisy
 mechanisms and disease diagnosis/treatment, 513
Pleuritis
 mechanisms and disease diagnosis/treatment, 513
Plummer-Vinson syndrome, 110
Pneumococcal pneumonia
 mechanisms and disease diagnosis/treatment, 495
Pneumoconiosis
 asbestosis, 510
 coal worker's pneumoconiosis, 510–511
 hypersensitivity pneumonitis, 511
 silicosis, 509–510
*Pneumocystis carinii* pneumonia (PCP)
 mechanisms and disease diagnosis/treatment
  infectious disease, 252–253
  pulmonary medicine, 498
  toxoplasma encephalitis, 257
Pneumonia
 atypical
  influenza, 498–499
  Legionnaire's disease, 497
  mycoplasma, 497–498
  *Pneumocystis carinii*, 252–253, 498

Pneumonia *(continued)*
  cystic fibrosis, 507
  fungal
    blastomycosis, 501
    coccidioidomycosis, 501–502
    cryptococcus, 502
    histoplasmosis, 500–501
    invasive aspergillosis, 502–503
    phycomycosis, 503
  humoral immunodeficiency, 204
  metastatic malignant tumors, 520
  postpartum sepsis, 387
  septic meningitis, 306
  sickle cell anemia, 176
  substance-related disorders, 477
  surgical principles, 583–584
  tracheoesophageal fistula, 441
  varicella (chickenpox), 265
Pneumothorax
  congenital lobar emphysema, 447
  mechanisms and disease diagnosis/treatment, 222, 513
  meconium aspiration, 431
Pneumovax, 177
Podophyllin, 347
Point of maximal impulse (PMI), 514
Poisoning
  accidents, 243
  drugs/medications
    acetaminophen, 228
    alcohol, 230
    cocaine, 230
    PCP (phencyclidine), 230
    sedatives, 229
    stimulants, 229
    tricyclic antidepressants, 228–229
  ingestion of toxic agents, 243
Poison ivy, 208
Polarized light microscopy, 280
Poliomyelitis
  mechanisms and disease diagnosis/treatment, 305
  sleep apnea, 334
Pollen and allergic rhinitis, 200
Polyamines, 54
Polyarteritis nodosa, 36, 413
Polyarthritis, 272
Polycystic kidney disease
  mechanisms and disease diagnosis/treatment, 552
  subarachnoid hemorrhage, 322

Polycystic ovarian disease, 352
Polycythemia rubra vera
  mechanisms and disease diagnosis/treatment, 185–186
Polydactyly, 445
Polydipsia
  diabetes insipidus, 94
  diabetes mellitus, 102, 103
  secondary hypertension, 30
Polygenic hypercholesterolemia, 100
Polyhydramnios, 381
Polymerase chain reaction (PCR)
  hemophilia A and B, 188
  herpes simplex virus, 51, 304
  HIV (human immunodeficiency virus), 438
  Lyme disease, 309
  toxoplasma encephalitis, 256
Polymerization, 176
Polymorphonuclear leukocytes, 271
Polymorphonuclear neutrophils (PMNs), 495
Polymyalgia rheumatica
  mechanisms and disease diagnosis/treatment, 281
  overview, 300
Polymyositis-dermatomyositis
  mechanisms and disease diagnosis/treatment, 282–283
  overview, 300
Polyphagia, 102, 103
Polysomnography, 334, 335, 524
Polytetrafluoroethylene (PTFE), 588, 591
Polyuria
  diabetes insipidus, 94
  diabetes mellitus, 102, 103
  secondary hypertension, 30
Popliteal artery aneurysm, 593
Porphyria cutanea tarda
  mechanisms and disease diagnosis/treatment, 83
Porphyrins, 83, 169, 323
Port-wine stain, 85
Positive end-expiratory pressure (PEEP)
  acute respiratory distress syndrome, 515
  flail chest, 223

Positron-emission tomography (PET)
  attention-deficit hyperactivity disorder, 473
  glioblastoma, 325
  Hodgkin's disease, 181
  intermediate/high-grade lymphoma, 183
  obsessive-compulsive disorder, 465
  Parkinson's disease, 328
  seizures, 316
  solitary pulmonary nodule, 523
Posterior pituitary
  disorders
    diabetes insipidus, 94
    syndrome of inappropriate antidiuretic hormone secretion, 94
Posterior urethral valves
  mechanisms and disease diagnosis/treatment, 426–427
Postexposure prophylaxis and HIV, 252
Postmenopausal women and osteoporosis, 279
Postpartum issues
  mechanisms and disease diagnosis/treatment
    hemorrhage, 386
    mother, care of the, 367–368
    sepsis, 386–387
Postpolio syndrome, 305
Posttraumatic stress disorder (PTSD)
  acute stress disorder, 466
  adjustment disorders, 467
  brief psychotic disorder, 457
  child physical/sexual abuse, 487
  domestic violence, 487
  mechanisms and disease diagnosis/treatment, 465–466
  panic disorder, 463
Potassium
  essential hypertension, 29
  hyperkalemia, 554, 555
  hypokalemia, 554
Potassium hydroxide (KOH) preparation
  blastomycosis, 501
  candidiasis, cutaneous, 48
  candidiasis, oral, 48

coccidioidomycosis, 501
dermatophytosis, 47
vaginitis/vulvovaginitis, 350
vulva/vagina, candidiasis of the, 349
Potassium iodide, 62
Potential acuity meter (PAM), 417
Pramipexole, 329
Prazosin, 6
Precipitins, 511
Prednisone
    acute lymphocytic leukemia, 179
    adrenal insufficiency, 96
    allergic bronchopulmonary aspergillosis, 210
    allergic rhinitis, 202
    amyloidosis, 81
    cardiac transplantation, 25
    chronic lymphocytic leukemia, 181
    contact dermatitis, 209
    Crohn's disease, 137
    Hodgkin's disease, 182
    insect and snake bites, 238
    intermediate/high-grade lymphoma, 184
    papillitis, 404
    polymyalgia rheumatica, 281
    sudden hearing loss, 656
    ulcerative colitis, 134
    underproduction syndromes (pituitary gland), 94
    urticaria, 204
Preeclampsia
    mechanisms and disease diagnosis/treatment, 374–375
    pulmonary medicine, 551
    multiple gestation, 381
    prenatal care, 365
Pregnancy. *See also* Obstetrics; Reproduction, male/female
    acute cholecystitis, 145
    carpal tunnel syndrome, 311
    domestic violence, 487
    folic acid deficiency, 170
    hereditary angioedema, 206
    herpes gestationis, 59
    HIV (human immunodeficiency virus), 251–252, 438
    idiopathic thrombocytopenic purpura, 192
    iron-deficiency anemia, 169

lupus inhibitor, 190
pelvic inflammatory disease, 262
pulmonary embolism, 516
Rh incompatibility, 432
stress-related urinary incontinence, 540
Turner's syndrome, 446
urinary tract infections, 529
Prehn's sign, 530
Premature junctional complex (PJC), 17
Premature labor
    mechanisms and disease diagnosis/treatment, 376
Premature rupture of membranes (PROM)
    mechanisms and disease diagnosis/treatment, 384
    premature labor, 376
Premature ventricular complexes (PVCs), 13, 17, 19
Prematurity
    deafness, congenital, 425
    hyaline membrane disease, 515
    necrotizing enterocolitis, 443
    sudden infant death syndrome, 489
Premenstrual syndrome (PMS)
    mechanisms and disease diagnosis/treatment, 351–352
Prenatal care
    mechanisms and disease diagnosis/treatment, 365
Prenatal diagnosis
    mechanisms and disease diagnosis/treatment, 366
Priapism, 176
Primaquine, 252
Primary dysmenorrhea, 351
Primary infertility, 356
Primary open-angle glaucoma, 414, 416
Primidone, 332
Prinzmetal's angina
    mechanisms and disease diagnosis/treatment, 5–6
Prions, 305
Priscilla White classification, 388*t*
Probenecid, 263, 358
Procainamide, 19, 29
Procarbazine, 182
Proctitis, 134
Proctoctomy, 135

Proctoscopy, 348
Proctosigmoiditis, 134
Proctosigmoidoscopy, 126
Progesterone
    amenorrhea, 352
    breast cancer, 354
    infertility, 356
    meningioma, 326
    premenstrual syndrome, 352
    renal cell carcinoma, 544
    spontaneous abortion, 371
Progestins
    breast cancer, 355
    endometrial cancer, 341
    fibrocystic disease, 356
    menopausal symptoms, 353
Progressive massive fibrosis (PMF), 510
Progressive multifocal leukoencephalitis (PML), 303
Progressive systemic scleroderma, 80
Prolactin, 92, 93, 484
Proliferative fibrodysplasia of the palmar subcutaneous tissue, 288
*Propionibacterium acnes*, 448
Propranolol
    aneurysms of thoracic aorta, 590
    cirrhosis, 157
    hyperthyroidism, 89
    multiple sclerosis, 332
Proptosis, 662
Propylthiouracil (PTU), 89
Prostaglandins
    allergic rhinitis, 201, 665
    bronchial asthma, 199
    dysmenorrhea, 351
    erectile impotence, 538
    glaucoma, 416
    labor and delivery, normal, 369
    premature labor, 376
Prostate cancer
    mechanisms and disease diagnosis/treatment, 542–543
    surgical principles, 576
Prostatectomy, 543
Prostate-specific antigen (PSA), 542
Prostatism, 541
Prostatitis
    mechanisms and disease diagnosis/treatment, 530

Prostatodynia, 530
Prosthesis, penile, 538
Prosthetic valves and cardioembolic strokes, 321
Protamine sulfate, 232
Protease inhibitors, 250, 506
Protein
    chronic renal failure, 547
    Creutzfeldt-Jakob disease, 305
    cystic fibrosis, 507
    disseminated intravascular coagulation, 190
    essential hypertension, 29
    Guillain-Barré syndrome, 311
    hepatitis, 150
    hypercalcemia, 92
    hyperemesis gravidarum, 384
    ischemic thrombotic strokes, 318
    Lyme disease, 309
    myopathies/dystrophies, 313
    pleural effusions, 512
    septic meningitis, 307
    syphilis, 261
    tuberculosis, 308
    venous thrombosis, 37
Protein C
    mechanisms and disease diagnosis/treatment
        activated resistance, 191–192
        deficiency, 191–192
Protein C deficiency
    mechanisms and disease diagnosis/treatment, 191
Proteinuria
    eclampsia, 552
    glomerulonephritis, 549
    ill-defined symptoms, 628–629
    lupus nephritis, 553
    nephrotic syndrome, 549
    polycystic kidney disease, 552
    preeclampsia, 551
    pyelonephritis, 546
    renal transplant rejection, 548
    thrombotic thrombocytopenic purpura, 192
Proteoglycan, 273
*Proteus*, 358, 539, 650
*Proteus mirabilis*, 649
Prothrombin/partial thromboplastin time (PT/PTT)
    abruptio placentae, 374
    blood-loss anemia, 170
    cirrhosis, 155
    disseminated intravascular coagulation, 190
    epistaxis, 217
    hemophilia A and B, 187–188
    hepatitis, 150
    lupus inhibitor, 189
    necrotizing enterocolitis, 443
    pulmonary embolism, 38
    venous thrombosis, 37
Proton-pump inhibitor (PPI)
    Crohn's disease, 137
    gastroesophageal reflux disease, 111
    scleroderma, 114
Protozoa causing diarrhea, 122–123
Protriptyline, 335
Proventil, 199
Proximal interphalangeal (PIP) joint, 282
    dislocation
        mechanisms and disease diagnosis/treatment, 236
Prune-belly syndrome
    mechanisms and disease diagnosis/treatment, 427
Pruritus. *See also* Itching
    allergic rhinitis, 200
    anaphylactic shock, 239
    atopic dermatitis, 56, 206, 207
    bullous pemphigoid, 58
    celiac sprue, 124
    chronic renal failure, 547
    dermatitis herpetiformis, 60
    drug reactions causing skin changes, 58
    mechanisms and disease diagnosis/treatment
        generalized, 62
        localized, 63
    pediculosis, 65
    scabies, 63
    seborrheic keratosis, 75
    urticaria, 203
Pruritus ani
    hemorrhoids, 141
    mechanisms and disease diagnosis/treatment, 63
Psammoma bodies, 326
Pseduodementia, 459
Pseudoaneurysm, 39
Pseudocyst, 161
Pseudodendrites, 412
Pseudogout, 290
Pseudohermaphrodites, 535
Pseudomembranous colitis, 123, 126
*Pseudomonas*
    choledocholithiasis, 146
    cystic fibrosis f, 507
    gram-negative bacillary pneumonias, 497
*Pseudomonas aeruginosa* and ear disorders, 648–650
Pseudotumor cerebri, 402
Pseudo von Willebrand disease, 188
Psoralen and ultraviolet A therapy (PUVA), 54, 56
Psoriasis
    mechanisms and disease diagnosis/treatment, 53–54, 54f
Psychiatry
    abuse syndromes
        child physical and sexual abuse, 486–487
        domestic violence, adult, 487–488
        elder abuse, 488
    adjustment disorders, 467
    anxiety disorders
        acute stress disorder, 466
        generalized anxiety disorder, 464
        obsessive-compulsive disorder, 464–465
        panic disorder, 462–464
        phobias, 466–467
        posttraumatic stress disorder, 465–466
    attention deficit/hyperactivity disorder, 472–473
    bereavement
        sudden infant death syndrome, 489
        uncomplicated, 488–489
    conduct disorder, 473–474
    delirium, 485–486
    eating disorders
        anorexia nervosa, 474–475
        bulimia nervosa, 475–477
    mood disorders
        bipolar disorders, 461–462
        cyclothymia, 462
        dysthymia, 460–461
        major (unipolar) depression, 459–460

personality disorders
　anxious/fearful/inhibited, 468–469
　dramatic/emotional, 468
　odd/eccentric, 468
pruritus, 62
psychoses
　affective psychoses: mania and psychotic depression, 454–455
　childhood, originating in, 458–459
　delusional disorder, 456
　other psychoses, 456–458
　schizophrenia, 453–454
sexual dysfunctions
　mechanisms and disease diagnosis/treatment, 484–485
somatoform disorders
　body dysmorphic disorder, 472
　conversion disorder, 471
　hypochondriasis, 471–472
　mechanisms and disease diagnosis/treatment, 469–470
　pain disorder, 470–471
　related disorders, 472
substance-related disorders
　alcohol dependence, 478–479
　alcohol syndromes, other, 479–480
　drug dependence, 480–484
　overview, 477–478
Psychosis. *See* Psychiatry
Psychosomatic disorders, 472
Psychotherapy
　acute stress disorder, 466
　adjustment disorders, 467
　bipolar disorders, 462
　body dysmorphic disorder, 472
　brief psychotic disorder, 457
　child physical/sexual abuse, 487
　cyclothymia, 462
　depression, major (unipolar), 460
　depression and obstetrics, 384
　dysthymia, 461
　irritable bowel syndrome, 128
　personality disorders, 469

psychosomatic disorders, 472
schizophrenia, 454
Psyllium, 635
Ptomaine disease, 213
Ptosis, 312, 421
Puberty, 538
Pubic hair, 92
Pudendal nerve latency, 484
Pulmonary capillary wedge pressure, 11
Pulmonary edema
　acute respiratory distress syndrome, 515
　barbiturates, 324
　cocaine, 230
　hypertension, 31
　preeclampsia, 375
　premature labor, 376
　respiratory distress syndrome, 430
Pulmonary embolism
　activated protein C resistance, 192
　antithrombin III deficiency, 190, 191
　lupus inhibitor, 189
　mechanisms and disease diagnosis/treatment, 38, 515–517, 516*f*
　obstructive shock, 12
　panic disorder, 463
Pulmonary fibrosis, 209, 210
Pulmonary function tests (PFTs). *See also* mechanisms and disease diagnosis/treatment *and* surgical principles *under specific disease/disorder*
　asbestosis, 510
　asthma, 504
　coal workers' pneumoconiosis, 511
　cor pulmonale, 518
　cystic fibrosis, 507
　desquamative interstitial pneumonitis, 509
　emphysema, 506
　hypersensitivity pneumonitis, 511
　infantile botulism, 421
　overview, 503, 504*t*
　right-sided heart failure, 9
　usual interstitial pneumonitis, 509

Pulmonary medicine. *See also* Respiratory *listings*
circulation, diseases of pulmonary
　adult respiratory distress syndrome, 514–515
　congestive heart failure, 514
　cor pulmonale, 518
　Goodpasture's syndrome, 517–518
　hyaline membrane disease, 515
　pulmonary embolism, 515–517, 516*f*
　pulmonary vasculitis, 517
diseases of respiratory system
　acute sinusitis, 662
　acute upper respiratory infection, 667–668
　allergic rhinitis, 664–665
　chronic rhinitis, 664
　chronic sinusitis, 662–663
　cystic fibrosis, 669
　epistaxis, 665–666, 666*f*
　fungal sinusitis, 663–664
　olfaction and taste, 667
　Wegener's granulomatosis, 668
ill-defined symptom complex
　chest pain, 521–522
　cough, 520–521, 624–625
　dyspnea, 521, 623–624
　hemoptysis, 522, 625–626
　sleep apnea, 523–524
　solitary pulmonary nodule, 523
　stridor, 624
　wheezing and stridor, 522–523
infectious disorders
　acute bronchiolitis, 494
　acute bronchitis, 494
　acute epiglottitis, 493
　bacterial bronchopneumonia, 495–497
　croup, 493
　fungal pneumonias, 500–503
　pertussis, 494–495
　pneumonias, atypical, 497–499
　tuberculosis, pulmonary, 499, 500*t*
neoplastic diseases
　bronchogenic carcinoma, 518–519
　carcinoid tumors, 519
　metastatic malignant tumors, 520

Pulmonary medicine *(continued)*
  obstructive pulmonary diseases
    asthma, 503–504, 504t, 505f
    chronic obstructive, 505–506
    cystic fibrosis, 505–508
    pulmonary function tests, 503
  pediatrics
    cystic adenomatoid malformation, 447
    laryngomalacia, 446
    lobar emphysema, congenital, 446–447
    pulmonary sequestration, 447
  pleural diseases
    pleural effusion, 512
    pleurisy, 513
    pneumothorax, 513
  restrictive diseases
    idiopathic, 508–509
    pneumoconiosis, 509–511
Pulmonary osteoarthropathy
  mechanisms and disease diagnosis/treatment, 287
Pulmonary sequestration
  mechanisms and disease diagnosis/treatment, 447
Pulmonary tuberculosis
  mechanisms and disease diagnosis/treatment, 499, 500t
Pulmonary vasculitis
  mechanisms and disease diagnosis/treatment, 517
Pulsatile tinnitus, 657
Pulse. *See also* mechanisms and disease diagnosis/treatment *and* surgical principles *under specific disease/disorder*
  acute bronchiolitis, 494
  anaphylaxis, 202
  aortic dissection, 40
  aortic occlusion, 41
  atherosclerosis, 33
  atrial septal defect, 26
  bradyarrhythmias, 18
  cardiopulmonary arrest, 28
  chronic atherosclerotic occlusion, 35
  *Haemophilus influenzae* pneumonia, 496
  left-sided high output heart failure, 9
  pneumococcal pneumonia, 495
  respiratory distress syndrome, 430
  sick sinus syndrome, 16
  staphylococcal pneumonia, 496
  transient tachypnea of the newborn, 429
  vasculitis syndromes, 36
Pulsus paradoxus, 21
Pupils. *See also* Eyes
  dilated ipsilateral, 219
  hypothermia, 240
  panic disorder, 463
  stimulants, 229
Purified protein derivative (PPD)
  acute pericarditis, 20
  erythema nodosum, 62
  interstitial keratitis, 414
  pulmonary tuberculosis, 499
  tuberculosis, 308
Purpura fulminans, 191
Purulent drainage/discharge
  acne, 448
  acute dacryocystitis, 400, 401
  acute otitis media, 648, 649
  acute sinusitis, 662
  acute upper respiratory infection, 667
  anorectal fistula, 143
  blastomycosis, 501
  bronchiectasis, 507
  chlamydia, 260
  chronic rhinitis, 664
  chronic sinusitis, 662, 663
  conjunctivitis, 393
  corneal ulcers, 411
  cystic fibrosis, 669
  *Haemophilus influenzae* pneumonia, 496
  premature rupture of membranes, 384
  rhinorrhea, 662
  staphylococcal pneumonia, 496
  strep throat, 660
  stye, 397
  urethritis, 531
Pyelonephritis
  genitourinary tract infections, 377
  mechanisms and disease diagnosis/treatment, 546
  postpartum sepsis, 387
Pyloric stenosis
  mechanisms and disease diagnosis/treatment, 441
Pyloromyotomy, 441

Pyoderma gangrenosum
  mechanisms and disease diagnosis/treatment, 79
Pyogenic granuloma
  mechanisms and disease diagnosis/treatment, 74–75, 74f
Pyrazinamide, 255, 308
Pyridoxine, 308
Pyrimethamine, 257, 438
Pyuria
  epididymitis, 530
  Kawasaki disease, 426
  orchitis, 531
  prostatitis, 530
  urinary tract infections, 529

## Q

Quartz particles, 509
Quinolones
  acute bronchitis, 494
  acute epiglottitis, 493
  gram-negative bacillary pneumonias, 497
  *Haemophilus influenzae* pneumonia, 496
  Legionnaire's disease, 497
  *Mycoplasma pneumoniae*, 498
Quinupristin, 496
Q waves. *See* Electrocardiogram

## R

Rabies
  mechanisms and disease diagnosis/treatment, 306
Race/region
  actinic keratosis, 69
  alcohol, 479
  blastomycosis, 501
  celiac sprue, 124
  coccidioidomycosis, 501, 502
  colorectal carcinoma, 128
  Dupuytren's contracture, 288
  epicanthus, 398
  esophageal neoplasms, 109
  familial Mediterranean fever, 140, 141
  gastric cancer, 114
  glaucoma, 414
  hepatitis, 146, 152–153
  hepatocellular carcinoma, 153, 154
  histoplasmosis, 500

irritable bowel syndrome, 127
leiomyomata uteri, 341
Lyme disease, 268, 309
melanoma, malignant, 72
Mongolian spot, 85
otitis media, 434
pemphigus, 59
prostate cancer, 576
sarcoidosis, 508
sudden infant death syndrome, 489
Tay-Sachs disease, 335
thalassemia-alpha, 171
thalassemia-beta, 171
Rachitic rosary, 280
Radiation therapy. *See also* mechanisms and disease diagnosis/treatment *and* surgical principles *under specific disease/disorder*
bladder carcinoma, 543
bronchogenic carcinoma, 519
carcinoid tumors, 519
colorectal carcinoma, 128, 132
Cushing's syndrome, 97
endometrial cancer, 341
eosinophil granuloma, 290
glioblastoma, 326
hemangioma, 565
Hodgkin's disease, 182
larynx, cancer of the, 661
low-grade lymphoma, 183
meningioma, 326
metastases, 327
metastases to bone, 287
multiple myeloma, 185
oropharynx, malignant neoplasms of the, 660
ovarian cancer, 344
overproduction syndromes (pituitary gland), 93
pancreatic carcinoma, 157
prostate cancer, 543
teratology, 367
ulcerative colitis, 134
underproduction syndromes (pituitary gland), 94
vaginal cancer, 349
vulvar carcinoma, 349
Radiculoneuritis, 309
Radiculopathy
mechanisms and disease diagnosis/treatment, 333–334

Radioallergosorbent test (RAST)
allergic rhinitis, 201, 665
anaphylaxis, 202
atopic dermatitis, 206
Radiofrequency ablation, 18
Radiography. *See also* mechanisms and disease diagnosis/treatment *and* surgical principles *under specific disease/disorder*
acid-related disorders of the stomach, 116
aneurysms, 40
ankylosing spondylitis, 283
appendicitis, 132
back pain, low, 274
bursitis, 284
cervical spine, fractures of the, 293
congenital hip disorders, 277
congenital lobar emphysema, 447
contusions, 292
cystic adenomatoid malformation, 447
developmental dysplasia of the hip, 433
diffuse esophageal spasm, 113
dislocations and separations, 297
enuresis, 540
femur, fracture of neck of, 296
glioblastoma, 326
gonococcal tenosynovitis, 272
irritable bowel syndrome, 127
kyphosis, 449
leg/foot fractures, 296
lumbar disk disease, 275
metastases to bone, 287
necrotizing enterocolitis, 443
neural tube defects, 422*f*
osteoarthritis, 273
osteochondritis dissecans, 449
osteomyelitis, 271
osteoporosis, 279
osteosarcoma, 286
Paget's disease of bone, 289
rheumatoid arthritis, 283
rickets, 280
rotator cuff syndrome, 298
scoliosis, 448
slipped capital femoral epiphysis, 278, 449
spinal stenosis, 291
thoracic spine, injuries to, 293
Radionuclear angiogram (RNA), 8

Radionuclide ventriculography (RVG), 4
Radius fractures
mechanisms and disease diagnosis/treatment, 234–235
Rai staging, 180–181
Rales. *See* Crackles
Ranson's criteria, 160
Rantidine, 111, 226
Rape, 244, 287, 466, 487
Rapid eye movement (REM), 286, 335
Rapid plasma reagin (RPR). *See also* mechanisms and disease diagnosis/treatment *and* surgical principles *under specific disease/disorder*
congenital syphilis, 438
interstitial keratitis, 414
ischemic thrombotic strokes, 319
neurosyphilis, 310
syphilis, 261, 532
Rash. *See also* Dermatitis; Petechiae; Pruritus
congenital syphilis, 437
dermatomyositis, 80
herpes simplex virus, 439
Kawasaki disease, 425
lupus arthritis, 282
measles (rubeola), 265
ophthalmic herpes zoster, 412
pharyngitis, 436
rubella (German measles), 266
syphilis, 260
varicella (chickenpox), 436
varicella-zoster (shingles), 46
Rat excreta, 306
Raynaud's phenomenon
lupus erythematosus, 79
scleroderma, 80, 81
usual interstitial pneumonitis, 508
Rectal tumor
surgical principles, 604
Rectum
abscess, anorectal, 142
fissure, anal, 142
fistula, anorectal, 143–144
hemorrhoids, 141–142
malignant neoplasm rectum. *See* Colorectal carcinoma
pilonidal disease, 144
pruritus ani, 63

Red blood cells (RBCs)
  agnogenic myeloid metaplasia, 193
  anemia of chronic disease, 176
  aplastic anemia, 173
  chronic renal failure, 174
  Crohn's disease, 135
  folic acid deficiency, 170
  genitourinary tract infections, 377
  hemolytic anemia, 175
  hemolytic uremic syndrome, 440
  iron-deficiency anemia, 169
  lead-poisoning anemia, 174
  lead toxicity, 323
  neonatal hyperbilirubinemia, 432
  polycythemia rubra vera, 185
  Rh immunoglobulin prophylaxis, 366
  Rh incompatibility, 432
  secondary erythrocytosis, 186
  thalassemia-alpha, 171
  thalassemia-beta, 172
  thiamine deficiency, 314
  thrombotic thrombocytopenic purpura, 192
  transfusion reactions, 187
  viscus, perforation of, 224
Reed-Sternberg cells, 181, 181*f*
Reflexes
  amyotrophic lateral sclerosis, 328
  bulbocavernous reflex, 294
  cervical spine and spinal stenosis, 333
  contusions, 331
  hyperthyroidism, 88
  hyponatremia, 553
  hypothyroidism, 89
  infantile botulism, 421
  multiple sclerosis, 331
  preeclampsia, 375
  toxoplasma encephalitis, 256
Reflex sympathetic dystrophy (RSD), 470
Regurgitation
  esophageal neoplasms, 109
  gastroesophageal reflux disease, 110
  necrotizing enterocolitis, 443
Remicade, 144

Renal and urinary system
  anorexia, 475
  benign conditions of the genitourinary tract
    bladder, neurogenic, 539–540
    cryptorchidism, 534
    enuresis, 540
    erectile impotence, 537–538
    hydrocele and varicocele, 536
    hypospadias, 538
    incontinence, stress-related urinary, 540
    infertility, 535–536
    intersex, 534–535
    Peyronie's disease, 537
    testicular torsion, 534
    trauma, urologic, 541
    ureteropelvic junction obstruction, 540–541
    urethral stricture, 536–537
    urolithiasis, 539
    vesicoureteral reflux, 538
  calculi
    surgical principles, 577
  delirium, 485
  electrolyte and acid-base disorders
    hypercalcemia, 557
    hyperkalemia, 554–555
    hypernatremia, 554
    hypocalcemia, 558
    hypokalemia, 554
    hypomagnesemia, 557
    hyponatremia, 553
    metabolic acidosis, 556
    metabolic alkalosis, 555–556
    respiratory acidosis, 556–557
    respiratory alkalosis, 556
    volume depletion, 555
    volume excess, 555
  Henoch-Schöenlein purpura, 425
  hypercalcemia, 91
  hypoglycemia, 105
  ill-defined symptom complex
    colic, renal, 626
    dysuria, 626–627
    oliguria and anuria, 627–628
    proteinuria, 628–629
  infectious diseases and inflammatory conditions
    chlamydia, 532–533
    epididymitis, 530–531
    gonorrhea, 532
    herpes, 533
    HIV (human immunodeficiency virus), 533
    orchitis, 531
    prostatitis, 530
    syphilis, 532
    urethral syndromes and painful bladder, 529–530
    urethritis, 531
    urinary tract infections, 529
  lead-poisoning anemia, 174
  lupus erythematosus, 80
  malignant hypertension, 31
  metabolic encephalopathy, 315
  neoplasias of the genitourinary tract
    benign prostatic hyperplasia, 542
    bladder carcinoma, 543–544
    penile/urethral/scrotal carcinoma, 545–546
    prostate cancer, 542–543
    renal cell carcinoma, 544, 576–577
    testicular carcinoma, 545
    Wilms' tumor, 544–545
  pelvic relaxation/urinary incontinence, 350–351
  prune-belly syndrome, 427
  renal disorders
    acute renal failure, 546–547
    chronic renal failure, 547
    diabetic nephropathy, 550
    eclampsia, 552
    glomerulonephritis, 549
    hypertension, 551
    lupus nephritis, 553
    nephrosclerosis, 552–553
    nephrotic syndrome, 549
    osteodystrophy, 550
    papillary necrosis, 550–551
    polycystic kidney disease, 552
    preeclampsia, 551
    pyelonephritis, 546
    transplant rejection, 548
    tubulointerstitial disease, 548
  surgical principles for diseases of
    benign prostatic hypertrophy, 578
    bladder carcinoma, 575–576
    prostate cancer, 576
    renal calculi, 577
    renal cell carcinoma, 576–577

renovascular disease, 586
testicular tumors, 575
thrombotic thrombocytopenic purpura, 192
Renal artery stenosis, 31
Renal colic
ill-defined symptoms, 626
Renal failure
acute, 546–547
chronic, 85, 174, 547
gout, 280
malignant hypertension, 31
obstructive shock, 12
septic abortion, 372
Renal papillary necrosis, 176
Renin-angiotensin-aldosterone axis
dilated cardiomyopathy, 14
left-sided low output heart failure, 8
secondary hypertension, 30
Renovascular disease
surgical principles, 586
Renovascular hypertension
mechanisms and disease diagnosis/treatment, 551
Repaglinide, 104
Repetitive movements
back pain, low, 274
bursitis, 284
carpal tunnel syndrome, 311
Reproduction, male/female. *See also* Obstetrics; Pregnancy
breast
fibroadenoma, 355
fibrocystic disease, 356
inflammatory disease of the, 355
malignant neoplasm, 353–355, 354*t*
cervix
cervical dysplasia and management of abnormal Pap smear, 347–348, 348*f*
cervicitis and sexually transmitted diseases, 345–347
malignant neoplasm, 345
health maintenance
contraception, general counseling for, 359
genetic counseling, 360
gynecologic examination and screening, 359
sterilization, 360

menopause, 353
menstrual disorders
dysmenorrhea, 351
premenstrual syndrome, 351–352
menstruation, disorders of
amenorrhea, 352
other problems
infertility, male and female, 356–358, 357*f*
pelvic inflammatory disease, 358–359
ovary
cysts, 344–345
malignant neoplasm, 344
uterus
endometriosis, 343, 343*f*
leiomyomata uteri, 341–342, 342*f*
malignant neoplasm, 341
vagina and vulva
candidiasis, 349
malignant neoplasms, 348–349
pelvic relaxation/urinary incontinence, 350–351
vaginitis and vulvovaginitis, 350
Rescriptor, 251
Residronate, 279
Respiratory acidosis
mechanisms and disease diagnosis/treatment, 556–557
Respiratory alkalosis
distributive shock, 12
mechanisms and disease diagnosis/treatment, 555
Respiratory distress/syndrome (RDS)
acute respiratory distress syndrome, 514–515
acute upper respiratory infection, 667–668
croup, 436
cystic adenomatoid malformation, 447
epiglottitis, 435
hyaline membrane disease, 515
laryngomalacia, 446
mechanisms and disease diagnosis/treatment, 430–431, 430*f*
pneumococcal pneumonia, 495

Rh incompatibility, 431
tracheoesophageal fistula, 441
Respiratory syncytial virus (RSV), 494
Respiratory system. *See* Pulmonary listings
Restrictive cardiomyopathy, 15–16
Reticulocyte count
aplastic anemia, 173
blood-loss anemia, 170
chronic renal failure, 174
hemolytic anemia, 175
iron-deficiency anemia, 169
neonatal hyperbilirubinemia, 432
Rh incompatibility, 431
thrombotic thrombocytopenic purpura, 193
Retina and essential hypertension, 29. *See also* Eyes; Ophthalmology
Retinitis, 253
Retinoblastoma, 406
Retinoic acid, 448
Retinoids, 54
Retinopathy, 103, 104
Retinopathy of prematurity, 424
Retroperitoneal lymph node dissection (RPLND), 545
Retropulsive gait, 323
Retrovir, 250
Rett's childhood disintegrative disorder, 458
Reye's syndrome, 265
ill-defined presentations, 635–636
Rhabdomyolysis
acute renal failure, 546
heatstroke, 241
hypokalemia, 554
Rheumatic aortitis, 42
Rheumatic fever
cardioembolic strokes, 320
description, 22
mitral stenosis, 24
Rheumatic heart disease, 137
Rheumatoid arthritis
bursitis, 284
carpal tunnel syndrome, 311
effusion of joint, 291
mechanisms and disease diagnosis/treatment, 283
neutropenia, 194
overview, 300

Rheumatoid factor, 283
Rheumatology, pediatric
  Henoch-Schöenlein purpura, 425
  Kawasaki disease, 425–426
RhIg and abortion, 371, 372
Rh immunoglobulin prophylaxis
  mechanisms and disease
    diagnosis/treatment, 365–366
Rh incompatibility
  mechanisms and disease
    diagnosis/treatment
      obstetrics, 380–381
      pediatrics, 431–432
    neonatal hyperbilirubinemia, 432
Rhinitis
  allergic, 664–665
  chronic, 664
Rhinocerebral disease, 503
Rhinorrhea, 217
  acute sinusitis, 662
  acute upper respiratory infection, 667
  allergic rhinitis, 664
  bronchiolitis, 434
  chronic rhinitis, 664
  chronic sinusitis, 662, 663
  fungal sinusitis, 663
*Rhizopus*, 503
RhoGAM, 432
Rhus plants, 55
Ribavirin
  acute bronchiolitis, 494
  bronchiolitis, 434
  hepatitis, 150–151
Rib fracture
  alcohol, 479
  mechanisms and disease
    diagnosis/treatment, 221
Riboflavin, 109, 318
Richter's transformation, 181
Rickets
  mechanisms and disease
    diagnosis/treatment, 280–281
  renal osteodystrophy, 550
Rifabutin, 256
Rifampin
  Legionnaire's disease, 497
  pulmonary tuberculosis, 499
  tuberculosis, 255, 308

Right-sided heart failure
  mechanisms and disease
    diagnosis/treatment, 9–10
Right ventricular outflow tract (RVOT), 27
Rigidity. *See also under* Neck
  antipsychotics, 324
  Huntington's disease, 329
  Parkinson's disease, 328
Riluzole, 328
Rimantadine, 494, 499
Ringer's solution, 227
Risperidone, 458
Ritalin, 335
Ritodrine, 376
Ritonavir, 250
Rivastigmine, 327
Rizatriptan, 318
Robeson tumor stage, 544
Rocephin, 272
Rocky Mountain spotted fever, 36
Roentgenogram, 8. *See also*
    mechanisms and disease
    diagnosis/treatment *and*
    surgical principles *under*
    *specific disease/disorder*
  acute bronchiolitis, 494
  acute bronchitis, 494
  acute epiglottitis, 493
  acute respiratory distress syndrome, 514
  allergic bronchopulmonary aspergillosis, 209
  aneurysms, 40
  asbestosis, 510
  aspergillosis, invasive, 503
  aspiration, 226
  blastomycosis, 501
  bronchial asthma, 198
  bronchogenic carcinoma, 519
  carcinoid tumors, 519
  carpal tunnel syndrome, 311
  chronic pancreatitis, 161
  chronic valvular diseases, 24
  coal workers' pneumoconiosis, 511
  coarctation of the aorta, 28
  coccidioidomycosis, 501
  congestive heart failure, 514
  cor pulmonale, 518
  cryptococcal infection, 502
  cystic fibrosis, 507
  desquamative interstitial pneumonitis, 509

  dilated cardiomyopathy, 13
  epidural hematoma, 330
  erythema nodosum, 62
  gestational trophoblastic disease, 383
  gram-negative bacillary pneumonias, 497
  *Haemophilus influenzae* pneumonia, 496
  headaches, 317
  hernias of the diaphragm, traumatic, 163
  histoplasmosis, 500
  hyaline membrane disease, 515
  hypersensitivity pneumonitis, 211, 511
  influenza pneumonia, 498
  interstitial keratitis, 414
  intestinal obstruction, 138
  Legionnaire's disease, 497
  malignant hypertension, 31
  meningioma, 326
  metabolic encephalopathy, 315
  metastatic malignant tumors, 520
  *Mycoplasma pneumoniae*, 498
  osteoarthritis, 273
  pericardial effusion, 21
  phycomycosis, 503
  pleural effusions, 512
  pneumococcal pneumonia, 495
  *Pneumocystis carinii* pneumonia, 498
  pneumothorax, 513
  poisoning and management overview, 232
  pulmonary embolism, 38, 515
  pulmonary tuberculosis, 499
  radiculopathy, 334
  sarcoidosis, 508
  silicosis, 509
  skull trauma/fracture, 218
  solitary pulmonary nodule, 523
  staphylococcal pneumonia, 496
  tibia, fracture of, 233
  transient tachypnea of the newborn, 429
  traumatic injury, 239
  usual interstitial pneumonitis, 509
  ventricular septic defect, 26
Rome I criteria, 126, 127*t*

Rosacea
  mechanisms and disease diagnosis/treatment, 67–68, 68f
Rose Bengal nuclear scan, 400, 413, 610. *See also* mechanisms and disease diagnosis/treatment *and* surgical principles *under specific disease/disorder*
Rosiglitazone, 104
Rotator cuff syndrome
  mechanisms and disease diagnosis/treatment, 298–299
Rotavirus, 122
Rubella (German measles)
  congenital
    cataracts, 424
    deafness, 425
    glaucoma, 424
  diabetes mellitus, 103
  mechanisms and disease diagnosis/treatment
    congenital anomalies, 439
    infectious disease, 266–267
  teratology, 367
Rubeola
  mechanisms and disease diagnosis/treatment, 265–266
Rumack-Matthew normogram, 228

## S
Saccadic eye movements, 303
Sacroiliitis, 283
Sacrum, fracture of, 224
Sagittal sinus thrombosis, 322
Salicylic acid
  seborrheic dermatitis, 55
  tylosis, 77
  warts, 51
Saline solution
  hypercalcemia, 92
  hyperosmolar hyperglycemic nonketotic coma, 104
  syndrome of inappropriate antidiuretic hormone secretion, 95
*Salmonella*, 122, 123, 126
Salpingectomy, 370–371
Salpingitis, 262, 370

Salt restriction
  dilated cardiomyopathy, 14
  essential hypertension, 30
  left-sided low output heart failure, 8
  restrictive cardiomyopathy, 16
Salt wasting, 98, 99
Saquinavir, 250
Sarcoidosis
  carpal tunnel syndrome, 311
  diabetes insipidus, 94
  dry-eye, 413
  erythema nodosum, 62
  hypercalcemia, 557
  mechanisms and disease diagnosis/treatment, 508
  multiple sclerosis, 331
  underproduction syndromes (pituitary gland), 94
Sarcoma
  surgical principles, 568
Sarcomatous transformation, 289
Sarna, 58, 62, 207
Satiety, early
  agnogenic myeloid metaplasia, 193
  chronic myelogenous leukemia, 179
  gastric cancer, 114
  hepatocellular carcinoma, 153
  polycythemia rubra vera, 185
Scabies
  mechanisms and disease diagnosis/treatment, 63–64, 64f
Schilling test, 173
Schiotz tonometry, 415
Schirmer test, 413
Schistosomiasis, 122
Schizoaffective disorder
  mechanisms and disease diagnosis/treatment, 456–457
Schizoid personality disorders, 468
Schizophrenia
  antipsychotics, 324
  mechanisms and disease diagnosis/treatment, 453–454
  childhood, 458
  schizoaffective disorder, 456

Schizophreniform disorder
  mechanisms and disease diagnosis/treatment, 457
Schizotypal personality disorders, 468
Scintographic assessment of gastric emptying, 118
Scleroderma
  gastric motility, disorders of, 118
  mechanisms and disease diagnosis/treatment, 80–81
  digestive system, 113–114
Sclerosis, 512, 517
Sclerotherapy, 157, 536, 595
Scoliosis
  mechanisms and disease diagnosis/treatment, 448–449
Scopalamine, 411
Scotomas, central
  mechanisms and disease diagnosis/treatment, 404–405, 405f
Scrotal carcinoma
  mechanisms and disease diagnosis/treatment, 545–546
Sebaceous cyst
  mechanisms and disease diagnosis/treatment, 75–76
  surgical principles, 565–566
Seborrheic blepharitis, 396
Seborrheic dermatitis
  mechanisms and disease diagnosis/treatment, 54–55
Seborrheic keratosis
  mechanisms and disease diagnosis/treatment, 75, 76f
Secondary dysmenorrhea, 351
Secondary glaucoma, 414
Secondary hypertension
  mechanisms and disease diagnosis/treatment, 30–31
Secondary infertility, 356
Secondary syphilis
  mechanisms and disease diagnosis/treatment, 52–53, 53f
Secretin, 161

Sedatives
    dependence, drug, 481–482
    poisoning and mechanisms and disease diagnosis/treatment, 229
    sleep apnea, 524
    substance-related disorders, 477

Seizures
    Alzheimer's disease, 327
    arsenic toxicity, 323
    bacterial meningitis, 437
    cardioembolic strokes, 320
    celiac sprue, 124
    childhood schizophrenia, 458
    cocaine, 230, 324
    conduct disorder, 474
    delirium, 485
    diethyl-m-toluamide, 232
    Dupuytren's contracture, 288
    eclampsia, 375–376, 552
    epidural hematoma, 219, 330
    febrile
        mechanisms and disease diagnosis/treatment, 421
    fragile X syndrome, 446
    glioblastoma, 325
    hemolytic uremic syndrome, 440
    herpes simplex virus, 303, 305, 439
    hypoglycemia, 105
    hyponatremia, 553
    lead toxicity, 323
    malignant hypertension, 31
    manganese toxicity, 324
    mechanisms and disease diagnosis/treatment, 315–316
    meningioma, 326
    metastases, 326
    neurosyphilis, 310
    rabies, 306
    septic meningitis, 306, 307
    stimulants, 229
    subdural hematoma, 219, 330
    Tay-Sachs disease, 335
    tricyclic antidepressants, 228
    trigeminal neuralgia, 317
    tuberculosis, 308
    tuberous sclerosis, 82
    venous thrombosis, 322, 323
    volume excess, 555

Selective estrogen receptor modulators (SERMs), 353
Selenium sulfide, 55

Self-esteem, low
    attention-deficit hyperactivity disorder, 473
    bereavement, 489
    child physical/sexual abuse, 487
    depression, major (unipolar), 459
    domestic violence, 487
    dysthymia, 460

Semen analysis, 356
Semi-Fowler position, 358
Senility, 353

Sepsis
    acute respiratory distress syndrome, 514, 515
    anorectal abscess, 143
    distributive shock, 12, 13
    gram-negative, 556
    malrotation of the small intestine, 441
    necrotizing enterocolitis, 443
    neonatal hyperbilirubinemia, 432
    postpartum, 386–387
    pyelonephritis, 546
    respiratory alkalosis, 556
    thermal burns, 227

Septic abortion
    mechanisms and disease diagnosis/treatment, 372

Septic arthritis
    gonorrhea, 259
    mechanisms and disease diagnosis/treatment, 271–272

Septic meningitis
    mechanisms and disease diagnosis/treatment, 306–307

Septic shock
    antibiotics, 239
    genitourinary tract infections, 377
    ill-defined presentations, 631
    mechanisms and disease diagnosis/treatment, 145
    peritonitis, 140
    septic abortion, 372

Sequestra, 271
Serevent, 199, 200
Serositis, 141

Serotonin
    anorexia, 475
    bulimia, 476
    personality disorders, 469

Serotonin reuptake inhibitors (SSRIs)
    alcohol, 479
    autistic disorder, 458
    body dysmorphic disorder, 472
    bulimia, 477
    conduct disorder, 474
    depression, major (unipolar), 460
    irritable bowel syndrome, 128
    obsessive-compulsive disorder, 465
    personality disorders, 469
    posttraumatic stress disorder, 466
    sexual dysfunctions, 485
    social phobia, 466

Serum protein electrophoresis (SPEP), 184. *See also* mechanisms and disease diagnosis/treatment *and* surgical principles *under specific disease/disorder*

Severity, disease. *See* mechanisms and disease diagnosis/treatment *and* surgical principles *under specific disease/disorder*

Sexual abuse/assault
    adolescent pregnancy, 369
    epidemiology and prevention, 244
    management principles, 240

Sexual activity
    adolescent pregnancy, 369–370
    cervical dysplasia and management of abnormal Pap smear, 347
    dysfunction, sexual
        child physical/sexual abuse, 487
        Cushing's syndrome, 96
        mechanisms and disease diagnosis/treatment, 484–485
        obsessive-compulsive disorder, 465
        schizophrenia, 454
        underproduction syndromes (pituitary gland), 94
    hepatitis B infection complicating pregnancy, 377
    HIV (human immunodeficiency virus), 303
    neurosyphilis, 310

Sexual ambiguity, 352
Sexual aversion disorder, 484
Sexually transmitted diseases (STDs)
  acute enteric infections, 123
  adolescent pregnancy, 369
  cervicitis, 345–347
  chancroid, 262
  chlamydia, 260
  epididymoorchitis, 263
  genital herpes, 263–264
  gonorrhea, 259–260
  pelvic inflammatory disease, 262–263
  syphilis, 260–262
  ulcerative colitis, 134
  urethral stricture, benign, 536
Shared psychotic disorder
  mechanisms and disease diagnosis/treatment, 457
*Shigella*, 122, 123, 126
Shock. *See also* Hypotension and acute circulatory collapse (shock)
  aortic dissection, 41
  cardiac tamponade, 21
  choledocholithiasis, 146
  insect and snake bites, 238
  management principles, 239
  posttraumatic stress disorder, 465
  pulmonary embolism, 38
  septic, 631
  transfusion reactions, 187
Shortness of breath (SOB)
  AV block, 17
  chronic valvular diseases, 24
  *Pneumocystis carinii* pneumonia, 252
  sick sinus syndrome, 16
  tachyarrhythmias, 18
  testicular carcinoma, 545
Short stature, 444, 445
Shoulder
  dislocation or injury, 237
  rotator cuff syndrome, 298–299
Shoulder-hand syndrome
  mechanisms and disease diagnosis/treatment, 288
Sickle cell anemia
  mechanisms and disease diagnosis/treatment, 176–177, 177*f*
  papillary necrosis, 551
  venous thrombosis, 322

Sick sinus syndrome
  description, 16
  mechanisms and disease diagnosis/treatment, 16
Sigmoidoscopy, 127
  anorectal fistula, 143
  constipation, 139
  diverticulitis, 138–139
  hemorrhoids, 141
  pelvic relaxation/urinary incontinence, 350
  ulcerative colitis, 133
Sign language, 425
Sildenafil, 485, 538
Silent ischemia
  mechanisms and disease diagnosis/treatment, 7
Silicosis
  mechanisms and disease diagnosis/treatment, 509–510
Silver sulfadiazine cream, 228
Simple compression fracture, 233
Simple febrile seizures, 421
Sinemet, 329
Singulair, 200, 204
Sinus bradycardia, 475
Sinusitis
  acute, 662
  allergic rhinitis, 200
  chronic, 662–663
  cystic fibrosis, 669
  fungal, 663–664
  humoral immunodeficiency, 204
Sinus tachycardia, 17
Sister Mary Joseph's node, 114
*Sitophilus granarius*, 210
Sitz baths, 142
Sjögren's syndrome, 124, 331, 413
Skin changes. *See also* Dermatitis; Dermatology; Erythema; Petechiae; Pruritus; Rash
  aortic occlusion, 41
  carbon monoxide, 231
  congenital rubella infection, 439
  diabetes mellitus, 103
  folic acid deficiency, 170
  frostbite, 240
  heavy metals/arsenic, 231
  herpes simplex keratitis, 412
  humoral immunodeficiency, 204
  hypothyroidism, 89
  hypovolemic shock, 11
  interstitial keratitis, 413–414

  obsessive-compulsive disorder, 464
  pediatrics
    acne, 448
    fungal infections, 448
  psychosomatic disorders, 472
  sarcoidosis, 508
  volume depletion, 555
Skull trauma/fracture
  mechanisms and disease diagnosis/treatment, 218
Sleep apnea
  cor pulmonale, 518
  mechanisms and disease diagnosis/treatment
    neurology, 334–335
    pulmonary medicine, 523–524
Sleep issues/disorders
  alcohol, 478, 479
  bereavement, 488
  bipolar disorders, 461
  chronic rhinitis, 664
  delirium, 485
  depression, major (unipolar), 459
  dysthymia, 460
  fibromyalgia, 286
  generalized anxiety disorder, 464
  herpes simplex virus, 303
  hypothyroidism, 89
  menopausal symptoms, 353
  neurology
    apnea, sleep, 334–335
    narcolepsy, 335
  pain disorder, 470
  pruritus, 62
  scabies, 64
  tinnitus, 657
Slipped capital femoral epiphysis
  mechanisms and disease diagnosis/treatment, 278, 449
Slit-lamp biomicroscopy
  cataracts, 417
  corneal ulcers, 411
  diabetes with ophthalmologic manifestations, 410
  interstitial keratitis, 414
  ophthalmic herpes zoster, 412
Slit salpingostomy, 370–371
Small bowel, benign neoplasm of the
  surgical principles, 606
Small bowel lymphoma, 125

Small-bowel obstruction, 162
  surgical principles, 601–602, 602f
Small cell carcinoma, 519
Small intestine
  acute enteric infections, 120–124
  celiac sprue, 124–125
  malrotation of the
    mechanisms and disease
      diagnosis/treatment,
      441–442
Smith's fracture, 234
Smoking
  adenocarcinoma, 110
  aortic occlusion, 41, 42
  arterial ulcer, 569
  arteriosclerotic ulcer, 78
  asbestosis, 510
  atherosclerosis, 34
  bladder carcinoma, 543
  bronchogenic carcinoma, 518
  cervical dysplasia and
    management of abnormal
    Pap smear, 347
  chronic atherosclerotic
    occlusion, 35
  chronic bronchitis, 506
  coal workers' pneumoconiosis,
    511
  colorectal carcinoma, 128
  Crohn's disease, 135
  desquamative interstitial
    pneumonitis, 509
  Dupuytren's contracture, 288
  emphysema, 506
  fibrocystic disease, 356
  hoarseness, 660
  hypercalcemia, 92
  ischemic thrombotic strokes, 318
  larynx, cancer of the, 661
  metastases, 326
  oropharynx, malignant
    neoplasms of the, 659
  osteoporosis, 279
  pulmonary embolism, 516
  renal cell carcinoma, 544
  solitary pulmonary nodule, 523
  squamous cell carcinoma, 70,
    109
  sudden infant death syndrome,
    489
  ulcerative colitis, 133
  variant angina, 5, 6
  vasculitis/vasculitis syndromes,
    37, 517

Smooth muscle antibodies (SMA),
  147
Smooth muscle cells, 342
Snake bites
  mechanisms and disease
    diagnosis/treatment, 238
Snellen letter chart, 417
Snoring and sleep apnea, 334
Social phobia
  body dysmorphic disorder, 472
  mechanisms and disease
    diagnosis/treatment, 466
Socioeconomic factors
  anorexia, 474
  bulimia, 475
  child physical/sexual abuse, 486
  conduct disorder, 474
  conversion disorder, 471
  domestic violence, 488
  schizophrenia, 453
Sodium
  chronic asthma, 504
  cystic fibrosis, 161
  essential hypertension, 30
  hypercalcemia, 557
  hypernatremia, 554
  Legionnaire's disease, 497
  metabolic encephalopathy, 315
  volume depletion, 555
Sodium bicarbonate, 230
Solitary pulmonary nodule
  mechanisms and disease
    diagnosis/treatment, 523
Solvent sniffing, mechanisms and
  disease diagnosis/
  treatment for poisoning
  from, 231
Somatization disorder
  mechanisms and disease
    diagnosis/treatment,
    469–470
Somatoform disorders
  body dysmorphic disorder, 472
  conversion disorder, 471
  depression, major (unipolar), 459
  hypochondriasis, 471–472
  mechanisms and disease
    diagnosis/treatment,
    469–470
  pain disorder, 470–471
  related disorders, 472
Somatomedin, 93
Somatosensory evoked potentials,
  592

Somatostatin, 326
Sonography
  appendicitis, 132
  pulmonary sequestration, 447
  pyloric stenosis, 441
Sotalol, 18
Soya, 125
Spasticity
  amyotrophic lateral sclerosis,
    328
  cervical spine and spinal
    stenosis, 333
  meningioma, 326
  Tay-Sachs disease, 335
Spectinomycin, 259
Spectrometry, 477
Speech, disorganized
  alcohol, 479
  delirium, 485
  depression, major (unipolar),
    459
  schizophrenia, 453
Speech problems
  cleft lip or palate, 440
Sphincter dyssynergia, 539
Sphincterotomy, 539
Sphygmomanometry, 41
Spina bifida, 380, 422
Spinal stenosis, 333
Spine/spinal cord
  accidents, 242
  dysraphism, 72
  fractures and dislocations
    cervical spine, 292–293
    lumbar spine, 294
    thoracic spine, 293–294
    vertebral column, 233
  meningioma, 326
  neural tube defects, 422–423
  neurology
    radiculopathy, 333–334
    spinal stenosis, 333
  Paget's disease of bone, 289
  poliomyelitis, 305
  scoliosis, 448–449
  spinal stenosis
    mechanisms and disease
      diagnosis/treatment,
      291–292
  vitamin $B_{12}$ deficiency, 314
Spirochetes, 42, 309, 310. See also
  specific organism
Spironolactone, 98, 99
Spleen, 223, 254

Splenectomy, 192, 194
Splenomegaly
　agnogenic myeloid metaplasia, 193
　chronic myelogenous leukemia, 179
　hemolytic anemia, 175
　hepatitis, 146
　hepatocellular carcinoma, 153
　intermediate/high-grade lymphoma, 183
　low-grade lymphoma, 182
　mononucleosis, 264
　polycythemia rubra vera, 185
Splinter hemorrhages, 85
Spongiform encephalopathy
　mechanisms and disease diagnosis/treatment, 305
Spontaneous abortion
　mechanisms and disease diagnosis/treatment, 371
Spontaneous bacterial peritonitis (SBP), 157
Spontaneous pneumothorax, 513
Spouse abuse, 243
Sprains and dislocations
　ankle
　　lateral ankle pain, 237
　　medial pain, 237
　elbow, 237
　hands
　　distal interphalangeal sprain, 236
　　metacarpal phalangeal sprain, 236–237
　　proximal interphalangeal dislocation, 236
　shoulder, 237
Spurious erythrocytosis, 186
Sputum examination. *See also* mechanisms and disease diagnosis/treatment *under specific disease/disorder*
　acute bronchitis, 494
　allergic bronchopulmonary aspergillosis, 209
　asbestosis, 510
　aspergillosis, invasive, 502
　blastomycosis, 501
　coccidioidomycosis, 501
　gram-negative bacillary pneumonias, 496–497
　influenza pneumonia, 498
　Legionnaire's disease, 497
　pneumococcal pneumonia, 495
　*Pneumocystis carinii* pneumonia, 252, 498
　pulmonary tuberculosis, 499
Squamous cell carcinoma
　bronchogenic carcinoma, 519
　cervical dysplasia and management of abnormal Pap smear, 347
　esophageal neoplasms, 109–110
　larynx, cancer of the, 661
　mechanisms and disease diagnosis/treatment, 69–70, 70*f*
　oropharynx, malignant neoplasms of the, 660
　penile/urethral/scrotal carcinoma, 546
　surgical principles, 566–567
　vaginal cancer, 349
Stable angina pectoris
　mechanisms and disease diagnosis/treatment, 6–7
Stab wounds, 243
Staphylococcal pneumonia
　mechanisms and disease diagnosis/treatment, 496
*Staphylococcus*, 49, 50
*Staphylococcus aureus*
　acute enteric infections, 122
　acute sinusitis, 662
　atopic dermatitis, 56, 207
　blepharitis, 396
　chronic otitis media, 650
　contact dermatitis, 209
　endocarditis, 23
　lactation, 368
　mother, postpartum care of the, 367
　osteomyelitis, 271
　septic arthritis, 272
　staphylococcal pneumonia, 496
*Staphylococcus epidermidis*, 396
Stapled anastomosis, 135
Startle myoclonic jerks, 305
Stasis dermatitis, 57, 77
Stasis ulceration
　mechanisms and disease diagnosis/treatment, 77, 78*f*
Status epilepticus, 316
Stauffers' syndrome, 544
Steal syndrome, 35
Steatorrhea, 161, 507
Steeple sign, 436
Stem cells, 195
Sterility, 444. *See also* Infertility
Sterilization, 360
Steroids
　abscesses, 309
　acute pericarditis, 20
　allergic rhinitis, 665
　alopecia areata, 69
　atopic dermatitis, 56
　Behcet's disease, 82
　bronchiectasis, 507
　bronchiolitis, 434
　bullous pemphigoid, 59
　carpal tunnel syndrome, 311
　chronic rhinitis, 664
　chronic sinusitis, 663
　congenital adrenal hyperplasia, 99
　conjunctivitis, 395
　contact dermatitis, 56
　corneal ulcers, 411
　Crohn's disease, 137
　Cushing's syndrome, 97
　dependence, drug, 483
　drug reactions causing skin changes, 58
　eczema, 57
　effusion of joint, 291
　erythema multiforme, 62
　erythema nodosum, 62
　fleas, 66
　glaucoma, 414, 416
　hemangioma, 74
　herpes gestationis, 59
　herpes simplex keratitis, 411, 412
　hyaline membrane disease, 515
　interstitial keratitis, 414
　iron-deficiency anemia, 169
　lupus erythematosus, 80
　lupus nephritis, 553
　miliaria, 85
　mosquitoes and flies, 66
　nephrotic syndrome, 549
　olfaction and taste, disorders of, 667
　ophthalmic herpes zoster, 413
　osteoporosis, 279
　pemphigus, 60
　premature labor, 376
　psoriasis, 53
　pyoderma gangrenosum, 79

Steroids (continued)
  respiratory distress syndrome, 431
  restrictive cardiomyopathy, 15
  sarcoidosis, 508
  scabies, 64
  seborrheic dermatitis, 55
  septic meningitis, 307
  sudden hearing loss, 656
  tuberculosis, 308
  ulcerative colitis, 600
  Wegener's granulomatosis, 668
Stevens-Johnson syndrome
  drug reactions and skin eruptions, 58, 213
  dry-eye, 413
  erythema multiforme, 61
  *Mycoplasma pneumoniae*, 498
Stimulants
  dependence, drug, 480–481
  mechanisms and disease diagnosis/treatment for poisoning from, 229
Stomach. *See also* Digestive system
  acid-related disorders, 115–117
  cancer, gastric, 114–115
  motility, gastric, 118–120
Stones
  biliary tract stone disease, 160
  bilirubin gallstones, 171
  gallstones, 100, 145, 146
  kidney, 91, 92
  urolithiasis, 539
Strabismus
  mechanisms and disease diagnosis/treatment, 407–408, 408*f*, 408*t*, 409*t*
Strep throat
  mechanisms and disease diagnosis/treatment, 660–661
*Streptococcus*
  cellulitis, 49
  erythema nodosum, 62
  impetigo, 50
  psoriasis, 53
*Streptococcus pneumoniae*
  acute bronchitis, 494
  bacterial meningitis, 437
  otitis media, 435
  pneumococcal pneumonia, 495
  strep throat, 661
*Streptococcus pyogenes*, 661

Streptokinase
  obstructive shock, 12
  pulmonary embolism, 38
  thrombosis, 594
Streptomycin, 255, 499
Stress
  acute stress disorder, 466
  adjustment disorders, 467
  bipolar disorders, 462
  brief psychotic disorder, 457
  delusional disorder, 456
  glaucoma, 414
  incontinence, urinary mechanisms and disease diagnosis/treatment, 540
  infertility, 535
  irritable bowel syndrome, 127
  panic disorder, 463
  posttraumatic stress disorder, 465
  psychosomatic disorders and managing, 472
  schizophrenia, 453
  sexual dysfunctions, 484
Stress testing, 6. *See also* mechanisms and disease diagnosis/treatment *and* surgical principles *under specific disease/disorder*
Striae, 92, 96, 96*f*
Stridor
  acute epiglottitis, 493
  anaphylaxis, 202
  croup, 435, 493
  epiglottitis, 435
  ill-defined symptoms, 624
  laryngomalacia, 446
  mechanisms and disease diagnosis/treatment, 522–523
  oropharynx, malignant neoplasms of the, 659
*Strongyloides stercoralis*, 122
Struvite stones, 539
ST segment depression/elevation. *See also* Electrocardiogram
  myocardial infarction, 4
  silent ischemia, 7
  stable angina pectoris, 6
  unstable angina, 3
  variant angina, 5
Sturge-Weber syndrome, 424
Stye
  mechanisms and disease diagnosis/treatment, 397

Subacute bacterial endocarditis (SBE), 85, 477
Subacute hypersensitivity pneumonitis, 511
Subacute lupus erythematosus, 80
Subarachnoid hemorrhage (SAH)
  cocaine, 324
  mechanisms and disease diagnosis/treatment, 321–322
Subclavian steal syndrome, 35
Subcortical cerebrovascular disease, 460
Subdural hematoma
  mechanisms and disease diagnosis/treatment, 219, 330
Substance-related disorders
  mechanisms and disease diagnosis/treatment, 477–478
Substantia nigra, 329
Succimer, 174
Sucrose, 128, 173
Sudafed, 201
Sudan black staining, 177, 178
Sudden death, 14, 15
Sudden hearing loss
  mechanisms and disease diagnosis/treatment, 655–656
Sudden infant death syndrome (SIDS), 28, 489
Suicide
  adjustment disorders, 467
  affective psychoses: mania and psychotic depression, 455
  alcohol, 479
  anorexia, 475
  arsenic, 323
  barbiturates, 324
  bereavement, 489
  bipolar disorders, 461, 462
  child physical/sexual abuse, 487
  depression, major (unipolar), 460
  domestic violence, 487
  Huntington's disease, 329
  ingestion of toxic agents, 243
  pain disorder, 470
  panic disorder, 463
  personality disorders, 469
  posttraumatic stress disorder, 465

schizophrenia, 453
shared psychotic disorder, 457
somatization disorder, 470
substance-related disorders, 477
trigeminal neuralgia, 317
Sulfadiazine, 257, 438
Sulfasalazine, 134, 135, 600
Sulfonamides, 160, 347
Sulfonylureas, 105
Sulfur compounds, 55
Sumatriptan, 318
Sunlight/sun exposure
  lupus arthritis, 282
  skin tumors and sunscreens, 69–72
Superficial keratitis, 413
Superficial thrombophlebitis, 355
  surgical principles, 595–596
Superficial venous thrombosis, 37
Superior vena cava syndrome, 40, 519
Support groups
  alcohol, 230, 479
  child physical/sexual abuse, 487
  substance-related disorders, 478
Supraglottitis
  mechanisms and disease diagnosis/treatment, 435
Supraventricular arrhythmias
  bradyarrhythmias, 16–17
  tachyarrhythmias, 17–18
Supraventricular dysrhythmias, 38
Surfactant, 430, 515
Surgical principles. *See also*
  mechanisms and disease
  diagnosis/treatment
  *under specific disease/ disorder*
  breast disorders
    benign breast mass, 569
    cancer, 570–571
  circulatory system, diseases of the
    abdominal aortic aneurysmal disease, 590–591, 591*f*
    aneurysms of the thoracic aorta, 588
    aortic dissection, 589–590, 589*f*
    arterial embolism/thrombosis, 593–594
    carotid artery disease, 584–585, 585*f*
    deep venous thrombosis, 594–595
    infrainguinal aneurysmal disease, 592–593
    peripheral arterial occlusive disease, 586–588
    renovascular disease, 586
    superficial thrombophlebitis, 595–596
    thoracic outlet syndrome, 591–592
    varicose veins, 595
  endocrine system, diseases of the
    Cushing's disease/syndrome, 573–574
    hyperparathyroidism, 572–573
    pheochromocytoma, 574
    thyroid neoplasm, 572
  gallbladder
    acute cholecystitis, 610, 611*f*
    biliary atresia, 610
    carcinoma, 612
    choledochal cyst, 611
    choledocholithiasis, 612
    focal nodular hyperplasia, 613
  gastrointestinal tract
    achalasia, 597
    acute mesenteric ischemia, 600–601
    anorectal fistula, 605
    appendicitis, 599
    benign neoplasm of the colon, 606, 607*f*
    benign neoplasm of the small bowel, 606
    cancer of the stomach, 598
    colon cancer, 606–607
    Crohn's disease, 600
    diverticulitis, 603–604
    duodenal atresia, 608
    esophageal varices, 597–598
    gastric volvulus, 598–599
    hemorrhoids, 604
    Hirschsprung's disease, 609
    imperforate anus, 609
    large-bowel obstruction, 603
    malrotation, 608
    midesophageal traction diverticulum, 596–597
    perirectal abscess, 605
    pilonidal cyst, 605–606
    rectal tumor, 604
    small-bowel obstruction, 601–602, 602*f*
    ulcerative colitis, 599–600
    Zenker's diverticulum, 596
  hernia
    diaphragmatic, 619
    femoral, 617–618
    incisional, 618
    inguinal, 617
    with obstruction, 619
    umbilical, 618
  kidney and urinary tract
    benign prostatic hypertrophy, 578
    bladder carcinoma, 575–576
    prostate cancer, 576
    renal calculi, 577
    renal cell carcinoma, 576–577
    testicular tumors, 575
  liver
    adenoma, 612–613
    focal nodular hyperplasia, 613
    metastasis, 614, 614*f*
    primary hepatobiliary cancer, 613–614
  pancreas, diseases of the
    acute pancreatitis, 615
    carcinoma, 616
    gastrinoma, 616–617
  postoperative infections
    atelectasis and pneumonia, 583–584
    urinary tract infections, 583
    wounds, 582–583
  skin and subcutaneous tissue
    arterial ulcer, 569–570
    basal cell carcinoma, 566
    cellulitis, 564
    decubitus ulcer, 568–569
    hemangioma, 564–565
    lipoma, 564
    melanoma, 567
    neurofibroma, 565
    sarcoma, 568
    sebaceous cyst, 565–566
    squamous cell carcinoma, 566–567
    venous ulceration, 569
  trauma
    abdominal injury, 580–582
    cranial injury, 580
    multiple injuries, 578–580
Sustiva, 251
Swallowing (injury/accidents)
  mechanisms and disease diagnosis/treatment, 226–227
Swan-Ganz catheter, 10, 140

Sweat chloride test, 507
Sweet's syndrome, 84
Swinging light test, 404
Sympathectomy, 35, 37
Syncope
  aortic dissection, 40
  AV block, 17
  blood-loss anemia, 169
  bradyarrhythmias, 18
  ectopic pregnancy, 370
  hypertrophic cardiomyopathy, 14
  hypoglycemia, 105
  pulmonary embolism, 38
  sick sinus syndrome, 16
  tachyarrhythmias, 18
  tetralogy of fallot, 27
  ventricular septic defect, 25
  ventricular tachycardia, 19
Syndrome of inappropriate antidiuretic hormone secretion (SIADH)
  bacterial meningitis, 437
  hyponatremia, 553
  mechanisms and disease diagnosis/treatment, 95
  volume excess, 555
Synovitis, 273
Syphilis
  aseptic meningitis, 306
  cervicitis, 346, 347
  hearing loss, 654, 656
  mechanisms and disease diagnosis/treatment
    congenital, 437–438
    infectious disease, 260–261
    renal and urinary system, 532
  multiple sclerosis, 331
  neurosyphilis, 309–310
  secondary, 52–53
  teratology, 367
Syphilitic aortitis
  mechanisms and disease diagnosis/treatment, 42
Syringobulbia, 334
Systemic disease. *See also individual disease/disorder*
  conjunctivitis, 395*t*
  cutaneous manifestations of
    amyloidosis, 81
    Behcet's disease, 82
    dermatomyositis, 80
    lupus erythematosus, 79–80
    necrobiosis lipoidica, 83
    porphyria cutanea tarda, 83
    scleroderma, 80–81
    tuberous sclerosis, 82–83
  dry-eye, 413
  herpes, genital, 533
  pruritus, 62
Systemic lupus erythematosus (SLE)
  hemolytic anemia, 175
  idiopathic thrombocytopenic purpura, 192
  lupus inhibitor, 190
  lupus nephritis, 553
  multiple sclerosis, 331
Systolic dysfunction and left-sided low output heart failure, 8

# T

Tachyarrhythmias
  hyperthyroidism, 89
  mechanisms and disease diagnosis/treatment, 17–19
Tachycardia
  acute pancreatitis, 159
  anaphylactic shock, 239
  anaphylaxis, 202
  blood-loss anemia, 169
  cardiac tamponade, 21
  cocaine, 230
  congestive heart failure, 514
  diabetes mellitus, 103
  diarrhea, 126
  dilated cardiomyopathy, 13
  hyperthyroidism, 88
  hypovolemic shock, 11
  panic disorder, 463
  peritonitis, 140
  *Pneumocystis carinii* pneumonia, 498
  pneumothorax, 222
  postpartum hemorrhage, 386
  premature rupture of membranes, 384
  pulmonary embolism, 38, 515
  sickle cell anemia, 176
  sick sinus syndrome, 16
  stimulants, 229
  tricyclic antidepressants, 228
Tachypnea
  acute pancreatitis, 159
  acute respiratory distress syndrome, 514
  anaphylaxis, 202
  bronchiolitis, 434
  epiglottitis, 435
  hyaline membrane disease, 515
  influenza pneumonia, 498
  laryngomalacia, 446
  pneumococcal pneumonia, 495
  *Pneumocystis carinii* pneumonia, 252, 498
  pulmonary embolism, 515
  tracheoesophageal fistula, 441
  transient tachypnea of the newborn, 429
Tachyzoites, 257
Tacrine, 327
Tacrolimus, 56
Takayasu's arteritis, 36, 37, 42
Talofibular ligament, 237
Tamoxifen, 341, 356
Tardive dyskinesia, 324, 454
Tar preparations, 55–57
Tarsal bone, 280
Tarsorrhaphy, 413
Taste and olfaction, disorders of
  mechanisms and disease diagnosis/treatment, 667
Tay-Sachs disease
  mechanisms and disease diagnosis/treatment, 335–336
T cells
  atopic dermatitis, 207
  histoplasmosis, 500
  HIV (human immunodeficiency virus), 438
  Hodgkin's disease, 182
  hypereosinophilic syndrome, 212
  immunodeficiency, cellular, 205
  rheumatoid arthritis, 283
Teeth
  bulimia, 475
  congenital syphilis, 438
  von Willebrand disease, 188
Telangiectasia
  ataxia-telangiectasia, 85
  rosacea, 67
  scleroderma, 81
Temperature
  acute arterial occlusion, 35
  anaphylaxis, 202
  aortic occlusion, 41
  arterial ulcer, 569
  dilated cardiomyopathy, 13

erythema nodosum, 62
hyperthyroidism, 88
hypothyroidism, 89
injuries, thermal, 240–241
livedo reticularis, 81
multiple sclerosis, 332
postpartum sepsis, 387
premenstrual syndrome, 351
rosacea, 67
venous thrombosis, 37
Temporal arteritis, 36, 37
Temporal lobe herniation, 331
Temporomandibular joint, 653, 657
Tenderness and easy bruising
abdominal aortic aneurysm, 164
acute lymphocytic leukemia, 178
acute myelogenous leukemia, 177
aplastic anemia, 173
chronic pancreatitis, 161
cirrhosis, 155
contusions, 292
epididymitis, 530
facial fracture, 217
fibromyalgia, 285
genitourinary tract infections, 377
headaches, 317
hemophilia A and B, 187
hernias, external, 163
idiopathic thrombocytopenic purpura, 192
orocavity, herpes simplex of the, 657
pelvic inflammatory disease, 262, 358
platelet dysfunction, 194
polymyalgia rheumatica, 281
postpartum sepsis, 387
prostatitis, 530
pulmonary embolism, 515
renal transplant rejection, 548
strep throat, 660
stye, 397
urolithiasis, 539
Tendinitis
mechanisms and disease diagnosis/treatment, 285
Tenesmus
diarrhea, 126
ulcerative colitis, 133
urinary tract infections, 529

Tenofovir, 251
Tenosynovitis, 259
Tensilon, 312
Tension pneumothorax, 513
Teratology
mechanisms and disease diagnosis/treatment, 366–367
Terbinafine, 48
Terbutaline, 376
Terconazole, 349
Terminal deoxynucleotidyltransferase (TdT), 178
Terry's nails, 84
Testes
acute lymphocytic leukemia, 178
alcohol, 478
cryptorchidism, 534
epididymitis, 530
intersex, 534–535
mechanisms and disease diagnosis/treatment
carcinoma, 545
undescended testis, 428–429
surgical principles, 575
testicular torsion, 534
underproduction syndromes (pituitary gland), 94
Testicular torsion
mechanisms and disease diagnosis/treatment, 534
Testosterone
amenorrhea, 352
benign prostatic hyperplasia, 542
erectile impotence, 537
infertility, 535
underproduction syndromes (pituitary gland), 94
Tetanus
black widow spider, 239
brown recluse spider, 239
frostbite, 240
lacerations, 225
Tetracycline
acute bronchitis, 494
cervicitis and sexually transmitted diseases, 347
chlamydia, 533
epididymitis, 531
gonorrhea, 259
Legionnaire's disease, 497
*Mycoplasma pneumoniae*, 498
prostatitis, 530

rosacea, 68
secondary syphilis, 53
syphilis, 261
teratology, 367
urethritis, 531
Tetralogy of Fallot
mechanisms and disease diagnosis/treatment, 27
Tetraparesis, 311
Thalamus and thiamine deficiency, 314
Thalassemia
mechanisms and disease diagnosis/treatment
alpha, 171
beta, 171–172
sickle cell anemia, 177
Thalidomide, 185
Thayer-Martin media, 531, 532
Thenar muscles, 311
Theophylline, 199
poisoning and mechanisms and disease diagnosis/treatment, 232
Thermal injuries
burns
mechanisms and disease diagnosis/treatment, 227
epidemiology and prevention, 243
frostbite, 240
heatstroke, 241
hypothermia, 240–241
Thermography, 354
Thiamine
alcohol, 480
deficiency
mechanisms and disease diagnosis/treatment, 314–315
delirium, 485
Thiazides, 58, 91
Thienopyridines, 4
Thoracentesis, 512
Thoracic aortic aneurysms, 39–40
Thoracic outlet syndrome (TOS)
surgical principles, 591–592
Thoracic spine, injuries to
mechanisms and disease diagnosis/treatment, 293–294
Thoracoscopy, 109
Thoracotomy, 222

Throat. *See* Nose and throat; Otolaryngology
Thromboangiitis, 37, 41
Thrombocythemia, essential, 193
Thrombocytopenia
  acute lymphocytic leukemia, 179
  acute myelogenous leukemia, 177
  chronic lymphocytic leukemia, 180
  congenital rubella infection, 439
  cytomegalovirus, 254
  disseminated intravascular coagulation, 190
  hemangioma, 74
  hemolytic uremic syndrome, 440
  idiopathic thrombocytopenic purpura, 192
  mononucleosis, 264
  necrotizing enterocolitis, 443
  preeclampsia, 375
  Rh incompatibility, 431
  rubella (German measles), 267
  thrombotic thrombocytopenic purpura, 192
  transfusion reactions, 187
Thrombocytosis, 169, 426
Thromboembolism, 186
Thrombolysis
  cardiogenic shock, 11
  myocardial infarction, 5
  obstructive shock, 12
  venous thrombosis, 323
Thrombophlebitis
  inflammatory disease of the breast, 355
  postpartum sepsis, 387
  substance-related disorders, 477
  superficial, 595–596
Thrombosis
  acute arterial occlusion, 36
  atherosclerosis, 34
  cavernous sinus, 662
  familial Mediterranean fever, 141
  fungal meningitis, 307
  hemorrhoids, 142
  lupus arthritis, 282
  protein C deficiency, 191
  surgical principles, 593–594
  venous thrombosis, 37, 322

Thrombotic thrombocytopenic purpura (TTP)
  hemolytic anemia, 175
  mechanisms and disease diagnosis/treatment, 192–193
Thrush
  HIV (human immunodeficiency virus), 438
  mechanisms and disease diagnosis/treatment, 658
Thymectomy, 312
Thymidylate synthesis, 170
Thymoma, 49, 312
Thymopentin, 208
Thyroglobulin, 91
Thyroid function tests
  anorexia, 475
  attention-deficit hyperactivity disorder, 473
  fibromyalgia, 285
  schizophrenia, 453
  sexual dysfunctions, 484
Thyroid gland
  bipolar disorders, 461, 462
  delirium, 485
  disorders
    hyperthyroidism, 88–89
    hypothyroidism, 89–90
    neoplasms of the thyroid gland, 91, 327, 572
  oncology/cancer
    multiple mucosal neuroma syndrome, 84
    neoplasms, 91
Thyroiditis, 266
Thyroid-stimulating hormone (TSH). *See also* mechanisms and disease diagnosis/treatment *and* surgical principles *under specific disease/disorder*
  hyperthyroidism, 88
  hypothyroidism, 89, 90
  overproduction syndromes (pituitary gland), 92, 93
  thyroid gland, neoplasms of the, 91
  underproduction syndromes (pituitary gland), 94
Thyrotoxicosis, 6
Thyrotropin-releasing hormone (TRH), 459

Thyroxine
  hyperthyroidism, 88
  hypothyroidism, 90
  neoplasms of thyroid gland, 91
  underproduction syndromes, 94
Tiagabine, 316
Tibia, fracture of
  mechanisms and disease diagnosis/treatment, 233
Tibial torsion, 278
Ticarcillin, 139
Ticks, 268, 309
Timazolamide, 326
Timolol, 416
Tinea capitis, 47
Tinea corporis, 48, 448
Tinea cruris, 448
Tinea pedis, 47, 48, 448
Tinel's sign, 289, 311
Tinnitus
  acute otitis media, 648
  barotrauma, 656
  chronic otitis media, 649
  mechanisms and disease diagnosis/treatment, 657
  sudden hearing loss, 655
Tissue necrosis
  acute arterial occlusion, 36
  electrical burns, 228
  multiple myeloma, 184
Tissue plasminogen activator (tPA), 5
Titanium dioxide, 83
Tobacco and hypersensitivity pneumonitis, 210. *See also* Smoking
Tobramycin, 507
Toluidine blue stain, 348
Tongue, 110, 334. *See also;* Mouth; Nose and throat; Otolaryngology
Tonometry, 415
Tonsillar erythema, 436
Tonsillitis, 264, 660–661
Tonsils and sleep apnea, large, 334
Topiramate, 316, 318
Total abdominal hysterectomy and bilateral salpingo-oophorectomy (TAH-BSO), 359
Total iron-binding capacity (TIBC), 169, 176
Total lung capacity (TLC), 506

Total parenteral nutrition (TPN), 134
Tourette's syndrome, 464, 465, 473
Tourniquet, 202, 238
Toxemia, 126
Toxic disorders/exposure. See also Poisoning
  acute renal failure, 546, 547
  heavy metals
    arsenic, 323
    lead, 323
    manganese, 323–324
    mercury, 323
  olfaction and taste, disorders of, 667
  tubulointerstitial disease, 548
Toxoplasma encephalitis
  mechanisms and disease diagnosis/treatment, 256–257
*Toxoplasma gondii*, 438
Toxoplasmosis
  congenital
    mechanisms and disease diagnosis/treatment, 438
  HIV (human immunodeficiency virus), 303
  teratology, 367
Tracheal-to-distal esophageal fistula, 441
Tracheoesophageal fistula (TEF)
  mechanisms and disease diagnosis/treatment, 441
Tracheostomy
  hereditary angioedema, 206
Transaminase, 282
Transfusions
  acute myelogenous leukemia, 178
  aplastic anemia, 174
  epistaxis, 665
  hemolytic uremic syndrome, 440
  HIV (human immunodeficiency virus), 303
  Kell-positive/negative, 380
  neonatal hyperbilirubinemia, 432
  reactions to
    mechanisms and disease diagnosis/treatment, 187
  Rh incompatibility, 432
Transient ischemic attack (TIA), 193, 584

Transient tachypnea of the newborn (TTN)
  mechanisms and disease diagnosis/treatment, 429
Transjugular intrahepatic portovenous shunt (TIPS), 157
Transplantation
  bone marrow
    acute lymphocytic leukemia, 179
    acute myelogenous leukemia, 178
    agnogenic myeloid metaplasia, 194
    cellular (T-cell) immunodeficiency, 205
    multiple myeloma, 185
    thalassemia, 172
  cardiac
    dilated cardiomyopathy, 14
    overview, 25
  corneal
    interstitial keratitis, 414
  kidney
    chronic renal failure, 547
    diabetic nephropathy, 550
    polycystic kidney disease, 552
    rejection, 548
  liver
    biliary atresia, 610
    carcinoma, 155
    fibrosis and cirrhosis, 157
  lung
    cystic fibrosis, 507
    silicosis, 510
    usual interstitial pneumonitis, 509
Transsphenoidal hypophysectomy, 97
Transurethral resection of the prostate (TURP)
  benign prostatic hyperplasia, 542
  benign prostatic hypertrophy, 578
  hyponatremia, 553
Transvaginal ultrasonography
  ectopic pregnancy, 370
  endometrial cancer, 341
  placenta previa, 373, 373f
  spontaneous abortion, 371
Transverse sinus thrombosis, 322

Trauma. See also Cranial injury; Fractures; Head trauma; Injuries/wounds/accidents
  acute pancreatitis, 160
  acute respiratory distress syndrome, 514, 515
  cervical spine and spinal stenosis, 333
  contusions, 292
  effusion of joint, 291
  gout, 280
  hereditary angioedema, 205
  hernias of the diaphragm, traumatic, 163
  histiocytoma, 73
  hoarseness, 660
  hypovolemic shock, 11
  impetigo, 50
  management principles, 239
  neurology
    contusion, 331
    epidural hematoma, 330–331
    subdural hematoma, 330
  olfaction and taste, disorders of, 667
  osteomyelitis, 271
  peritonitis, 140
  pneumothorax, 513
  pyogenic granuloma, 74
  splinter hemorrhages, 85
  surgical principles
    abdominal injury, 580–582
    cranial injury, 580
    multiple injuries, 578–580
  urologic
    mechanisms and disease diagnosis/treatment, 541
  venous thrombosis, 37–38
  verrucae, 51
Travaprost, 416
Treacher-Collins syndrome, 425
Treatment. See mechanisms and disease diagnosis/treatment *under specific disease/disorder;* Surgical principles
Trematodes, 122
Tremor
  alcohol, 479
  bipolar disorders, 462
  cocaine, 324
  hyperthyroidism, 88
  manganese toxicity, 323

Tremor (continued)
    mercury toxicity, 323
    multiple sclerosis, 332
    Parkinson's disease, 328
    stimulants, 229
Trendelenburg position, 202
*Treponema pallidum* and syphilis, 52, 261, 438, 532
Triamcinolone, 69
Triamcinolone acetonide, 63
*Trichinella spiralis*, 122
*Trichomonas*, 350, 531
Tricyclic antidepressants (TCAs)
    attention-deficit hyperactivity disorder, 473
    depression, major (unipolar), 460
    gastric motility, disorders of, 118
    headache, 318
    irritable bowel syndrome, 128
    poisoning and mechanisms and disease diagnosis/treatment, 228–229
    urticaria, 204
    varicella-zoster (shingles), 47
Trifascicular block, 18
Trifluorothymidine, 412
Trigeminal ganglion, 412
Trigeminal neuralgia
    mechanisms and disease diagnosis/treatment, 316–317
Triglycerides (TG)
    alcohol, 230
    chylomicronemia, type 1 familial, 99
    decreased high-density lipoprotein, 102
    dysbetalipoproteinemia, type III, 100
    hyperlipoproteinemia, 32, 33
    hyperlipoproteinemia, type IV, 101
    hyperlipoproteinemia, type V, 101
Triiodothyronine, 88, 460
Trimethoprim, 252
Trimethoprim sulfamethoxazole (TMP-SMX)
    acute otitis media, 649
    diarrhea, 126
    diverticulitis, 139
    drug reactions causing skin changes, 58

*Pneumocystis carinii* pneumonia, 252, 498
    toxoplasma encephalitis, 257
    urinary tract infections, 529
    vesicoureteral reflux, 538
Trimetrexate, 252
Trisomy. *See also* Down syndrome
    12, 180
    mechanisms and disease diagnosis/treatment, 380
    13, 445 18, 445
Trousseau's sign, 558
Trovofloxicin, 139
Tuberculosis (TB)
    acute pericarditis, 20
    constrictive pericarditis, 22
    interstitial keratitis, 414
    mechanisms and disease diagnosis/treatment, 254–255, 308
    pulmonary
        mechanisms and disease diagnosis/treatment, 499, 500t
    silicosis, 509
    underproduction syndromes (pituitary gland), 94
Tuberous sclerosis
    mechanisms and disease diagnosis/treatment, 82–83, 82f
Tubo-ovarian abscess (TOA), 262, 358
Tubulointerstitial disease
    mechanisms and disease diagnosis/treatment, 548
Tumor necrosis factor, 137
Tuning-fork studies, 649, 654
Turner's syndrome, 352
    intersex, 535
    mechanisms and disease diagnosis/treatment, 445–446
T waves. *See* Electrocardiogram
Tylenol, 668
Tylosis
    mechanisms and disease diagnosis/treatment, 76–77
    squamous cell carcinoma, 110
Tympanic membrane
    barotrauma, 656
    injury, auditory, 220

otitis media, 434
    chronic, 649
    serous, 650
Tympanometry, 434
Tzanck smear/test. *See also* mechanisms and disease diagnosis/treatment *and* surgical principles *under specific disease/disorder*
    herpes, genital, 533
    herpes simplex virus, 439
    varicella, 46, 265

**U**

Uhthoff's phenomenon, 332
Ulcerative colitis
    idiopathic thrombocytopenic purpura, 192
    mechanisms and disease diagnosis/treatment, 133–135, 133f
    psychosomatic disorders, 472
    pyoderma gangrenosum, 79
    surgical principles, 599–600
Ulcerative jejunoileitis (UJI), 125
Ulcers
    acid-related disorders of the stomach, 116–117, 117t
    acute arterial occlusion, 36
    Behcet's disease, 82
    chancroid, 262
    chronic atherosclerotic occlusion, 35
    decubitus, 77, 568–569
    herpes simplex virus, 258
    of lower limbs
        arteriosclerotic ulcer, 78
        pyoderma gangrenosum, 79
        stasis ulceration, 77, 78f
    ophthalmology
        blepharitis, 396
        entropion, 398
    oral
        lupus erythematosus, 79
    peritonitis, 140
    squamous cell carcinoma, 70
    syphilis, 260
    venous, 569
    venous thrombosis, 37
Ulna, fracture of the
    mechanisms and disease diagnosis/treatment, 235

Ultrasound. *See also* mechanisms and disease diagnosis/treatment *and* surgical principles *under specific disease/disorder*
  abdominal aortic aneurysm, 164
  acute cholecystitis, 144
  aneurysms, 40
  choledocholithiasis, 145
  cholelithiasis, 145
  cirrhosis, 156
  congenital cataracts, 424
  congenital hip disorders, 277
  developmental dysplasia of the hip, 433
  diabetes mellitus with ophthalmologic manifestations, 410
  endometrial cancer, 341
  endometriosis, 343
  gestational trophoblastic disease, 382
  intersex, 535
  leiomyomata uteri, 342
  multiple gestation, 381, 382*f*
  neural tube defects, 422
  orchitis, 531
  ovarian cysts, 344
  pelvic inflammatory disease, 359
  placenta previa, 373, 373*f*, 374
  prenatal diagnosis, 366
  prune-belly syndrome, 427
  pyelonephritis, 546
  renal transplant rejection, 548
  spontaneous abortion, 371
  teratology, 366
  undescended testis, 428
  urologic trauma, 541
  varicocele and hydrocele, 536
Ultraviolet light therapy
  atopic dermatitis, 56, 208
  contact dermatitis, 209
  pruritus, 62
  psoriasis, 54
Umbilical hernia
  surgical principles, 618
Underproduction syndromes (pituitary gland), 94
Undersecretion (dry-eye syndrome)
  mechanisms and disease diagnosis/treatment, 400

Undescended testis
  mechanisms and disease diagnosis/treatment, 428–429
UniDur, 199
Unstable angina
  atherosclerosis, 33
  mechanisms and disease diagnosis/treatment, 3–4
Urea, 77
Urea breath tests (UBT), 116
*Ureaplasma urealyticum*, 531
Uremia
  acute pericarditis, 20
  gastric motility, disorders of, 118
  hemolytic uremic syndrome, 440
  platelet dysfunction, 194
  polycystic kidney disease, 552
Ureteropelvic junction obstruction
  mechanisms and disease diagnosis/treatment, 540–541
Urethral carcinoma
  mechanisms and disease diagnosis/treatment, 545–546
Urethral stricture, benign
  mechanisms and disease diagnosis/treatment, 536–537
Urethral syndromes
  mechanisms and disease diagnosis/treatment, 529–530
Urethritis
  chlamydia, 260
  gonorrhea, 259, 532
  mechanisms and disease diagnosis/treatment, 531
Uric acid, 230, 375, 478
Urinalysis. *See also* mechanisms and disease diagnosis/treatment *and* surgical principles *under specific disease/disorder*
  enuresis, 540
  febrile seizures, 421
  genitourinary tract infections, 377
  glomerulonephritis, 549
  Henoch-Schöenlein purpura, 425
  metabolic encephalopathy, 315

  nephrotic syndrome, 549
  papillary necrosis, 550
  prenatal care, 365
  pyelonephritis, 546
  urethral stricture, benign, 536
  urinary tract infections, 529
Urinary tract infections (UTIs)
  bladder, painful, 529
  epididymoorchitis, 263
  mechanisms and disease diagnosis/treatment, 529
  pyelonephritis, 546
  surgical principles, 583
  vesicoureteral reflux, 428, 538
Urine. *See also* Genitourinary system; Renal and urinary system
  cardiogenic shock, 10
  diabetes insipidus, 94
  hypovolemic shock, 11
  neonatal hyperbilirubinemia, 432
  porphyria cutanea tarda, 83
  secondary hypertension, 30
  substance-related disorders, 477
  syndrome of inappropriate antidiuretic hormone secretion, 95
Urine protein electrophoresis (UPEP), 184
Urokinase, 594
Urolithiasis
  mechanisms and disease diagnosis/treatment, 539
Uroporphyrinogen, 83
Ursodiol, 145
Urticaria
  anaphylactic shock, 239
  anaphylaxis, 202
  drug allergy, 213
  drug reactions causing skin changes, 58
  mechanisms and disease diagnosis/treatment
    dermatology, 57–58
    immunology and allergy, 203–204
Usual interstitial pneumonitis (UIP)
  mechanisms and disease diagnosis/treatment, 508–509
Uterine atony, 386

Uterus
   abruptio placentae, 374
   labor and delivery, normal, 368–369
   mother, postpartum care of the, 367
   premature labor, 376
   reproduction, male/female
      endometriosis, 343, 343f
      leiomyomata uteri, 341–342, 342f
      malignant neoplasm, 341
Uveitis
   cataracts, 417
   Kawasaki disease, 426
   ophthalmic herpes zoster, 412

## V

Vaccines
   bacterial meningitis, 437
   bladder carcinoma, 543
   chronic bronchitis, 506
   hepatitis, 150, 151t, 153
   HIV (human immunodeficiency virus), 251, 439
   influenza pneumonia, 499
   lacerations, 225
   measles (rubeola), 266
   pneumococcal pneumonia, 495
   poliomyelitis, 305
   rabies, 306
   rubella (German measles), 267
   varicella (chickenpox), 265
Vacuum extractor
   mechanisms and disease diagnosis/treatment, 387
Vagina
   mechanisms and disease diagnosis/treatment
      candidiasis, 349
      malignant neoplasms, 349
      pelvic relaxation/urinary incontinence, 350–351
      vaginitis, 350
      menopausal symptoms and dryness, 353
      pelvic inflammatory disease, 358
Vaginismus, 484
Valacyclovir, 258, 264
Valangciclovir, 254
Valine, 176

Valium, 421
Valproate, 316
Valproic acid
   bipolar disorders, 462
   headaches, 318
   schizoaffective disorder, 457
   seizures, 316
Valsalva maneuver, 14, 322, 651
Valvular diseases
   acute
      endocarditis, 23
      ischemic, 23
      rheumatic fever, 22
   chronic, 24–25
Vanceril, 199, 200
Vancomycin
   abscesses, 309
   diarrhea, 126
   staphylococcal pneumonia, 496
Vanillylmandelic acid (VMA), 98, 574
Variant angina
   mechanisms and disease diagnosis/treatment, 5–6
Varicella (chickenpox)
   mechanisms and disease diagnosis/treatment
      dermatology, 46
      infectious disease, 265
      pediatrics, 436
Varicella-zoster virus (VZV), 265
   mechanisms and disease diagnosis/treatment, 46–47, 47f
Varicocele
   infertility, 535
   mechanisms and disease diagnosis/treatment, 536
Varicose veins
   stasis ulceration, 77
   surgical principles, 595
Vasculitis
   Behcet's disease, 82
   drug allergy, 213
   drug reactions causing skin changes, 58
   Henoch-Schöenlein purpura, 425
   lupus erythematosus, 79
   mechanisms and disease diagnosis/treatment, 517–518
   necrobiosis lipoidica, 83
   pulmonary, 517

syndromes
   mechanisms and disease diagnosis/treatment, 36–37
Vasectomy, 360
Vasoactive intestinal peptide (VIP), 113
Vasoconstriction, 11, 386
Vasodilators, 30
Vasogenic edema, 326
Vasopressin
   diabetes insipidus, 94
   enuresis, 540
   syndrome of inappropriate antidiuretic hormone secretion, 95
Vasopressors, 203, 239
Vasospasm, 322
Vena cava filter placement, 594
Vena cava interruption, 517
Venereal disease, interstitial keratitis and maternal, 413
Venereal Disease Research Laboratory test (VDRL). *See also* mechanisms and disease diagnosis/treatment *and* surgical principles *under specific disease/disorder*
   HIV (human immunodeficiency virus), 248
   neurosyphilis, 310
   syphilis, 261
Venlafaxine, 460
Venogram, 322
Venous thrombosis
   activated protein C resistance, 191
   mechanisms and disease diagnosis/treatment, 37–38, 322–323
   polycythemia rubra vera, 185
   protein C deficiency, 191
   pulmonary embolism, 516
Venous ulceration
   surgical principles, 569
Ventilation, mechanical
   acute respiratory distress syndrome, 515
   hyaline membrane disease, 515
   meconium aspiration, 431
   respiratory alkalosis, 556
   seizures, 316
   sleep apnea, 524

Ventilation-perfusion lung scan, 12
Ventricular arrhythmias
    bradyarrhythmias, 18–19
    tachyarrhythmias, 19
Ventricular fibrillation
    mechanisms and disease
        diagnosis/treatment, 19
Ventricular septic defect (VSD)
    cardiogenic shock, 10
    mechanisms and disease
        diagnosis/treatment,
        25–26
    tetralogy of fallot, 27
    trisomy 18, 445
Ventricular tachycardia
    mechanisms and disease
        diagnosis/treatment, 19
Ventriculoperitoneal shunt, 308
Ventriculoperitoneal (VP) shunt, 423
Ventriculostomy, 322, 331
Verapamil, 318
Verrucae
    mechanisms and disease
        diagnosis/treatment, 51
Vertebral column, fracture of
    mechanisms and disease
        diagnosis/treatment, 233
Vertebra plana, 290
Vertical compression injuries,
    cervical spine and, 293
Vertigo
    auditory injury, 220
    barotrauma, 656
    interstitial keratitis, 413
    mechanisms and disease
        diagnosis/treatment,
        651–652
    sudden hearing loss, 655
    tinnitus, 657
Very low-density lipoproteins
    (VLDL)
    dysbetalipoproteinemia, type III,
        100
    hyperlipoproteinemia, 32, 33
    hyperlipoproteinemia, type IV,
        101
    hyperlipoproteinemia, type V,
        101
Vesicoureteral reflux
    mechanisms and disease
        diagnosis/treatment
        pediatrics, 538
    renal and urinary system,
        427–428

V gene, 191
Vibration and low back pain, 274
Vidarabine, 412
Videx, 250
Villous edema, 383
Vinblastine, 182, 544
Vincristine
    acute lymphocytic leukemia, 179
    intermediate/high-grade
        lymphoma, 184
    multiple myeloma, 185
    Wilms' tumor, 545
Violent behavior. *See also* Abuse
        syndromes; Behavior
        problems/bizarre
        behavior
    domestic violence
        mechanisms and disease
            diagnosis/treatment,
            487–488
    PCP (phencyclidine), 230
    rape, 244, 287, 466, 487
Viral acute enteric infections,
    122
Viramune, 251
Virchow's node, 114
Virchow's triad, 37
Viread, 251
Viremia, 253
Virilization
    amenorrhea, 352
    congenital adrenal hyperplasia,
        98
    intersex, 535
Viruses. *See also individual*
        *disease/disorder*
    central nervous system
        Creutzfeldt-Jakob disease,
            305
        herpes simplex virus, 303–305,
            304f
        HIV (human immunodefi-
            ciency virus), 303
        poliomyelitis, 305
        rabies, 306
    conjunctivitis, 393–395
    skin infections
        herpes simplex, 51–52
        molluscum contagiosum, 51
        verrucae, 51
Viscus, perforation of
    mechanisms and disease
        diagnosis/treatment,
        223–224

Vision
    acute sinusitis, 662
    alcohol, 230
    cataracts, 417
    congenital cataracts, 424
    corneal ulcers, 410
    cytomegalovirus, 253
    diabetes mellitus, 103
    disorders of the visual pathways
        bitemporal defects, 405
        homonymous defects, 405
        monocular defects (central
            scotomas), 404–405,
            405f
    dry-eye, 413
    essential hypertension, 29
    giant cell aortitis, 43
    glaucoma, 414
    hemangioma, 74
    herpes simplex, 52
    herpes simplex keratitis, 411
    hypoglycemia, 105
    malignant hypertension, 31
    multiple sclerosis, 331
    optic atrophy, 404
    overproduction syndromes
        (pituitary gland), 93
    papillitis, 403
    preeclampsia, 375
    Tay-Sachs disease, 335
    venous thrombosis, 322
    vitamin $B_{12}$ deficiency, 313
    Wegener's granulomatosis, 668
Vitamins
    A
        cystic fibrosis, 162
        dry-eye syndrome, 400
        hypercalcemia, 91
        squamous cell carcinoma, 109
    $B_6$
        premenstrual syndrome, 352
    $B_{12}$
        Crohn's disease, 135
        deficiency and mechanisms
            and disease diagnosis/
            treatment, 313–314
        HIV (human immunodefi-
            ciency virus), 303
        mechanisms and disease
            diagnosis/treatment,
            172–173
        schizophrenia, 453
    C
        squamous cell carcinoma, 109

Vitamins (continued)
    D
        celiac sprue, 125
        Crohn's disease, 135
        cystic fibrosis, 162
        hypercalcemia, 91, 92
        hypocalcemia, 558
        osteoporosis, 279
        prune-belly syndrome, 427
        renal osteodystrophy, 550
        rickets, 281
    E
        Alzheimer's disease, 327
        cystic fibrosis, 162
    K
        cystic fibrosis, 162
        mechanisms and disease
            diagnosis/treatment, 189
        protein C deficiency, 191
Vitiligo, 68
    autoimmune hepatitis, 147
Vitrectomy, 410
Voice changes/hoarseness
    acute epiglottitis, 493
    aortic dissection, 40
    aspiration, 226
    bronchogenic carcinoma, 518
    croup, 435, 493
    epiglottitis, 435
    gastroesophageal reflux disease, 110
    hypothyroidism, 89
    thoracic aortic aneurysms, 39
    thyroid gland, neoplasms of the, 91
Voiding cystourethroscopy
    posterior urethral valves, 426
    urinary tract infections, 529
    vesicoureteral reflux, 427
Volmax, 204
Volume depletion
    mechanisms and disease
        diagnosis/treatment, 555
Volume excess
    mechanisms and disease
        diagnosis/treatment, 555
Vomiting
    abscesses, 308
    acetaminophen, 228
    acute cholecystitis, 144
    acute enteric infections, 120
    acute pancreatitis, 159
    adrenal insufficiency, 95
    alcohol, 230, 479

    barotrauma, 656
    bulimia, 475
    cholelithiasis, 145
    concussion, 219
    cryptococcal infection, 257
    diethyl-m-toluamide, 232
    glaucoma, 414
    headaches, 317
    heavy metals/arsenic, 231
    Hirschsprung disease, 443
    hydrocephalus, 423
    hyperemesis gravidarum, 384
    hypovolemic shock, 11
    ill-defined presentations, 638–639
    insect and snake bites, 238
    intestinal obstruction, 138
    intracerebral hemorrhage, 321
    intussusception, 442
    ischemic bowel disease, 137
    Legionnaire's disease, 497
    neurosyphilis, 310
    orocavity, herpes simplex of the, 657
    pelvic inflammatory disease, 358
    poliomyelitis, 305
    posterior urethral valves, 426
    psychosomatic disorders, 472
    pyloric stenosis, 441
    stimulants, 229
    subarachnoid hemorrhage, 321
    venous thrombosis, 322
    vertigo, 651
von Willebrand disease
    hemophilia A and B, 188
    mechanisms and disease
        diagnosis/treatment, 188–189
Voriconazole, 503
Vulva
    mechanisms and disease
        diagnosis/treatment
            candidiasis, 349
            malignant neoplasms, 348–349
            vulvovaginitis, 350
Vulvectomy, 349
Vulvovaginal candidiasis, 249


W
Waardenburg's syndrome, 425, 654
Warfarin
    cardioembolic strokes, 321
    protein C deficiency, 191

    pulmonary embolism, 516, 517
    teratology, 367
    venous thrombosis, 38
Warts
    mechanisms and disease
        diagnosis/treatment, 51
Wasting syndrome, 253
Water deprivation test, 94
Water drinking, compulsive, 95
Weakness. See also under Muscles
    amyotrophic lateral sclerosis, 328
    aortic dissection, 40
    aplastic anemia, 173
    arsenic toxicity, 323
    bronchiectasis, 507
    bulimia, 475
    carpal tunnel syndrome, 289
    cervical spine and spinal stenosis, 333
    diabetes mellitus, 103
    Guillain-Barré syndrome, 311
    hypercalcemia, 91
    hyperkalemia, 554
    hypothyroidism, 89
    hypovolemic shock, 11
    infantile botulism, 421
    insect and snake bites, 238
    iron-deficiency anemia, 169
    ischemic thrombotic strokes, 319
    lumbar disk disease, 275
    lumbar spine and spinal stenosis, 333
    meningioma, 326
    multiple sclerosis, 331
    myopathies/dystrophies, 313
    poliomyelitis, 305
    radiculopathy, 333–334
    restrictive cardiomyopathy, 15
    rotator cuff syndrome, 298
    sick sinus syndrome, 16
    spinal stenosis, 291
    subarachnoid hemorrhage, 321
    tendinitis, 285
    vitamin $B_{12}$ deficiency, 172, 313, 314
    volume excess, 555
Wegener's granulomatosis, 517
    mechanisms and disease
        diagnosis/treatment, 668
Weight, refusal to bear
    femur, fracture of neck of, 295
    Legg-Calvé-Perthes disease, 277
    osteoarthritis, 273

osteomyelitis, 271
septic arthritis, 271
Weight gain
  bipolar disorders, 462
  depression, major (unipolar), 459, 460
  hypothyroidism, 89
  obsessive-compulsive disorder, 465
  premenstrual syndrome, 351
  schizophrenia, 454
Weight loss
  adrenal insufficiency, 95
  agnogenic myeloid metaplasia, 193
  amenorrhea, 352
  anemia of chronic disease, 176
  bronchiectasis, 507
  bronchogenic carcinoma, 518
  chronic myelogenous leukemia, 179
  chronic pancreatitis, 161
  Crohn's disease, 135
  cystic fibrosis, 161
  cytomegalovirus, 253
  depression, major (unipolar), 459
  diabetes mellitus, 102
  disseminated *Mycobacterium avium-intracellulare* complex, 255
  dysbetalipoproteinemia, type III, 100
  esophageal neoplasms, 109
  gastric cancer, 114
  gastroesophageal reflux disease, 110
  HIV (human immunodeficiency virus), 533
  Hodgkin's disease, 182
  hyperemesis gravidarum, 384
  hyperlipoproteinemia, type IV, 101
  hyperthyroidism, 88, 89
  ill-defined presentations, 642–643
  multiple myeloma, 184
  osteoarthritis, 273
  pancreatic carcinoma, 157
  penile/urethral/scrotal carcinoma, 546
  pulmonary tuberculosis, 499
  renal cell carcinoma, 544
  vasculitis syndromes, 36
Wernicke's encephalopathy, 314, 480
Western blot test, 309
Western blot test and Lyme disease, 272, 309
West Nile virus, 66
Wet work and cutaneous candidiasis, 48
Wheat miller's lung, 210
Wheezing
  acute bronchiolitis, 494
  anaphylaxis, 202
  aspiration, 226
  asthma, 389, 503
  bronchial asthma, 198
  bronchiolitis, 434
  bronchogenic carcinoma, 518
  carcinoid tumors, 519
  congestive heart failure, 514
  emphysema, 506
  mechanisms and disease diagnosis/treatment, 522–523
  metastatic malignant tumors, 520
  sarcoidosis, 508
  tracheoesophageal fistula, 441
Whiplash, 242
White blood cells. *See also* mechanisms and disease diagnosis/treatment *and* surgical principles *under specific disease/disorder*
  acute lymphocytic leukemia, 178
  acute myelogenous leukemia, 177, 178
  bursitis, 284
  chronic lymphocytic leukemia, 180
  chronic myelogenous leukemia, 179
  distributive shock, 13
  effusion of joint, 290, 291
  essential thrombocythemia, 193
  genitourinary tract infections, 377
  gram-negative bacillary pneumonias, 497
  Guillain-Barré syndrome, 311
  Henoch-Schöenlein purpura, 425
  inflammatory disease of the breast, 355
  influenza pneumonia, 498
  ischemic heart disease, 23
  Kawasaki disease, 426
  Legionnaire's disease, 497
  *Mycoplasma pneumoniae*, 498
  neutropenia, 195
  osteomyelitis, 271
  pelvic inflammatory disease, 358
  pertussis, 495
  polycythemia rubra vera, 185
  pyelonephritis, 546
  septic arthritis, 271, 272
  transfusion reactions, 187
  urinary tract infections, 529
Wilms' tumor, 287
  mechanisms and disease diagnosis/treatment, 544–545
Wilson's disease, 150
WinRhoD, 192
Wolff-Parkinson-White syndrome, 18
Wood's light, 47, 83
Workplace accidents, 242
Wound infections, surgical principles for post-operative, 582–583. *See also* Injuries/wounds/accidents
Wright stain, 533

X

Xanthomas
  chylomicronemia, type 1 familial, 99
  dysbetalipoproteinemia, type III, 100
  hyperlipoproteinemia, 32
  hyperlipoproteinemia, type II, 100
  hyperlipoproteinemia, type V, 101, 101f
X-rays. *See also* Chest x-rays
  abdominal aortic aneurysms, 590
  croup, 493
  Legg-Calvé-Perthes disease, 277
  squamous cell carcinoma, 70

Y

Yeast infections, 349
*Yersinia*, 126

## Z

Zalcitabine, 250
Zanamivir, 494, 499
Zantac, 204, 226
Zarfirlukast, 504
Zeis gland, 397
Zenker's diverticulum
   surgical principles, 596
Zetar, 207
Ziagen, 250
Zinc oxide, 83
Zinc pyrithione, 55
Zinc superoxide dismutase gene, 328
Zolmitriptan, 318
Zonalon, 207, 209
Zonisamide, 316
Zrivada, 250
Zyflo, 199
Zyrtec, 201